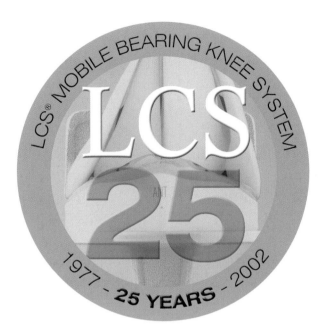

Springer

Berlin
Heidelberg
New York
Hong Kong
London
Milan
Paris
Tokyo

KAREL J. HAMELYNCK • JAMES B. STIEHL (EDS.)

LCS® Mobile Bearing Knee Arthroplasty

A 25 Years Worldwide Review

With 497 Figures and 6 Tables

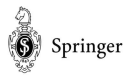
Springer

KAREL J. HAMELYNCK, MD, PhD
Hospital Slotervaart Ziekenhuis
Louwesweg 6
1066 EC Amsterdam
The Netherlands

JAMES B. STIEHL, MD
Orthopaedic Hospital of Wisconsin
575 West Riverwoods Parkway, #204
Milwaukee, Wisconsin, 53212
USA

ISBN 3-540-43284-1 Springer-Verlag Berlin Heidelberg New York

Die Deutsche Bibliothek - CIP-Einheitsaufnahme
LCS® mobile bearing knee arthroplasty : a 25 years worldwide review / Karel J. Hamelynck ;
James B. Stiehl (ed.). - Berlin ; Heidelberg ; New York ; Hong Kong ; London ; Milan ; Paris ;
Tokyo ; Springer, 2002
    ISBN 3-540-43284-1

Springer-Verlag Berlin Heidelberg New York
a member of BertelsmannSpringer Science+Business Media GmbH

http://www.springer.de

© Springer-Verlag Berlin Heidelberg 2002
Printed in Italy

DePuy®
The Components comprising the complete APC are protected by European Patent 0519 873 B1; USA Patent 5395 401, Japanese
Patent 2741 644 and Swiss Patent 689 539 which are licensed to DePuy International Limited by Mr. André R. Baechler, Kapsteig
44, CH 8032 Zurich, Switzerland.
LCS® and Porocoat® are registered trademarks and Milestone™, Completion™ and DuoFix™ are trademarks of DePuy
Orthopaedics, Inc.
The use of general descriptive names, registered names, trademarks, etc. in this publication does not imply, even in the absence
of a specific statement, that such names are exempt from the relevant protective laws and regulations and therefore free for
general use.
Product liability: The publishers cannot guarantee the accuracy of any information about the application of operative
techniques and medications contained in this book. In every individual case the user must check such information by
consulting the relevant literature.

Cover design: *design & production,* Heidelberg
Typesetting: medio Technologies AG, Berlin
SPIN: 10859079   18/3130/ag   5 4 3 2 1 0 – Printed on acid-free paper

Foreword

Twenty-five years have come and gone like the "blink of an eye"! In our world of LCS knee replacement, this quarter century marks a unique time for us to reflect upon the events and especially the people who have contributed toward the worldwide success of this controversial yet extremely versatile, mobile-bearing knee replacement system.

The events, of course, are now history but are worth sharing briefly. The initial prime moving event was the meeting and collaboration of two motorcycle riders, one an orthopaedic surgeon and the other a mechanical engineer in 1974 at Martland Hospital in Newark, New Jersey. This chance meeting of two dissimilar personalities linked by a common hobby and a common orthopaedic development goal, led to personal friendship, personal sacrifice and thousands of hours of research and development in the field of human joint replacement technology. The friendship still lasts, the personal sacrifice has been rewarded and research and development still continues to this day, a testimony to the concept of perseverance!

Other extremely notable events include: the exposure to the Oxford meniscal bearing concept, exposure to the Insall tibial-cut-first surgical technique, completion of FDA cemented and cementless clinical trials in the United States, mechanical failure of the Porous Coated Anatomic (PCA) knee replacement and development of an international LCS market.

The people involved most notably include the faithful United States and International orthopaedic surgeons, who despite extreme peer pressure, decided to use a knee replacement device based on sound mechanical engineering and biological principles rather than commercial hype. Their acceptance of advanced mobile-bearing concepts will forever give us a feeling of great affection and pride; for in a sense, they accepted our baby child, the LCS knee, before it had matured into a worthy adult!

Other extremely notable people include: the United States sales, marketing and engineering departments of DePuy in Warsaw, Indiana; the sales, marketing and engineering staffs of DePuy International in Leeds, England as well as the LCS Knee Product Managers worldwide. Without their timely resources and educational seminars, dissemination of our mobile-bearing concepts around the world would not have happened. We sincerely appreciate all of their efforts.

Thus, it is with a sense of nostalgia and pride that we remember the development of the New Jersey Low-Contact-Stress Knee Replacement System together with the association of the many fine surgeons, engineers and salesmen around the world that contributed to its success. We hope that the mobile-bearing principles that we have established will continue to be embraced encouraged and improved upon for the future good of our patients.

We would like to thank all of you for the opportunity to be of service to mankind!

Sincerely,
FREDERICK F. BUECHEL, SR., MD FACS
MICHAEL J. PAPPAS, PHD, PE

Preface

Worldwide experience with the LCS® mobile bearing total knee prosthesis has been unparalleled both in terms of enduring popularity and outstanding long-term clinical results. Buechel and Pappas's design was based on the principles of; restoring anatomical joint function to as near normal as possible, minimising contact stresses to avoid wear and damage to the bearing surfaces. and finally the idea that constraint should reflect the need for mobility, to avoid shear stresses and loosening of the implant. In 1977, the LCS® knee was implanted by Dr. Frederick Buechel. This was the first mobile bearing, tri-compartmental knee implant. This was also the first to successfully address the key issues of loosening, wear and patello-femoral problems associated with earlier designs. The unique design solution was the creation of a common articulating geometry for the tibia and patella on the distal femoral surface. This resulted in a tibial and patellar articulation that was mobile in nature, but with an identical radius of curvature and conformity.

The mobile bearing concept was considered sufficiently novel and unproven that the US FDA (Food & Drug Administration) required that it be validated in an Investigational Device Evaluation (IDE). An FDA IDE study involving 25 US surgeons was initiated in 1981. Validation of the clinical success of the device in this study resulted in FDA approval of the LCS, Knee (for cemented, tri-compartmental use) in 1985. The IDE study was extended to validate the cementless and fixed stem revision designs which were approved for sale in the US in 1990.

European use of LCS, began in 1984. During this period, surgeons around the world became intrigued with the prosthesis and its potential for long term clinical performance due to the problems experienced with existing knee designs. The fact that the LCS design has remained almost entirely unchanged is a tribute to the design excellence of the LCS® Knee system. Any future refinements will not violate the LCS proven design principles.

During the past 25 years, a large body of literature has accumulated regarding total knee arthroplasty. Some of the theories of total knee performance have been proved as scientific fact whilst others have fallen out of favour. The LCS implant remains "futuristic" to the extent that recent kinematic inquiries have confirmed the ingenious elements of the design. Such research has spurred interest in the mobile bearing concept from other total knee designers.

This book will carefully document the history, development, and clinical outcome to date of this unique device. The vista for the future is evolutionary advances in knowledge of knee function, which will guide surgeons to better surgical technique and instrumentation.

Finally we wish to thank our publishing editor Thomas Guenther of Springer Verlag for his competent support and organization without which this project would not have been completed.

K. J. HAMELYNCK AND J.B. STIEHL (EDS.)

Table of Contents

The Editors

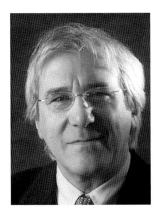

Karel J. Hamelynck, MD, PhD

Dr. Hamelynck is specialised in General Surgery at the Wilhelmina Hospital of the University of Amsterdam, the Netherlands, and later in orthopaedic surgery at the Dijkzigt Hospital of the University of Rotterdam. In 1979 he returned to Amsterdam to become head of the department of Orthopaedic and Rheumatoid Surgery of the Slotervaart Hospital and the Jan van Breemen Institute, Centre for Rheumatogy, in 1981. He developed a special interest in the surgery of rheumatoid arthritis and joint replacement and in particular the biomechanics and design of prostheses.

He was the first surgeon in Europe to use the LCS® total knee prosthesis. After the introduction of the prosthesis in the Slotervaart Ziekenhuis in 1984, this Amsterdam centre became the learning centre for total knee replacement for many surgeons from all over the world. More than 2000 surgeons have visited Amsterdam to improve their knowledge and skills.

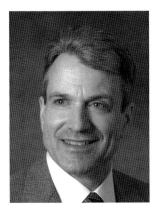

James B. Stiehl, MD

Dr. Stiehl is Director of the Midwest Orthopaedic Biomechanical Laboratory, an organisation that collaborates with the Rocky Mountain Musculoskeletal Research Laboratory in Denver where he has pioneered several new methodologies investigating the kinematics of total knee arthroplasty. He is a member of the US Knee Society and has served on the program committee of American Academy of Orthopaedic Surgeons on the reconstructive knee section. He reviews for JBJS, CORR, and the Journal of Arthroplasty in Reconstructive Surgery, and has authored over 100 publications. He is in private practice at Columbia Hospital in Milwaukee, Wisconsin.

Members of the Review-Board

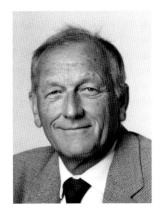

Professor Werner Mueller

Professor Mueller is specialised in Orthopaedic Surgery at the University Hospital of Basle, Switzerland, from 1960 to 1967. After a specialisation in traumatology he became head of the Orthopedic Traumatologic Department in 1970. In 1978 he became head of the Department of Orthopaedic Surgery and Traumatology of the Kantonspital Bruderholz. In 1982 he published his book "The Knee" in three languages, which brought him fame all over the world. In 1990 he was appointed as a full professor at the University of Basle. His profound knowledge of the anatomy and function of the knee made him an eminent teacher for many knee surgeons. He gives numerous lectures at International and National orthopaedic meetings. Among many other activities he is a former president of ESSKA, the European Society for Surgery of the Knee and Arthroscopy.

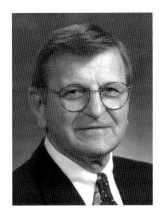

Peter A. Keblish, MD

Dr. Keblish is a former Chief and Director of Total Joint Learning Center at Lehigh Valley Hospital, Allentown, Pennsylvania, USA. Clinical Assistant Professor Orthopaedic Surgery, Hershey, Pennsylvania State University, Pennsylvania, USA.

Dr. Keblish is an "orthopaedic veteran" of the Vietnam War, with extensive interest and experience in trauma / rehabilitation and reconstructive surgery. Over the past 35 years he has had experience with total joint surgery, paralleling the development of THA and TKA. His knee experience included early use of hinge knees, hemiarthroplasty, and fixed-bearing design knees in the 1970s. He has been involved with the LCS project since its inception with the FDA trial in 1980 and has been utilizing and reporting the LCS mobile bearing primary, uni-, and revision total knee system. His primary interests have been development of surgical approaches and he has assisted in the development of UKA and TKA with the LCS group.

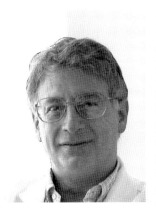

Jean-Louis Briard, MD

Dr. Jean Louis Briard received his orthopaedic training in the Assistance Publique de Paris Programme. He also spent one year as an orthopaedic resident at the Children's Hospital in Boston, USA. In 1981, Dr Briard moved to Rouen where he has a private practice. His major interest is surgery of the knee joint, in particular sports medicine and total knee replacement. His passion for knee biomechanics led him to use unicompartmental prostheses. After 10 years it became evident that the polyethylene issue was the most important aspect of survivorship. In 1987 he implanted his first LCS®. He is very involved in teaching and has run a total knee course every 2 years for the last 15 years. This has been an exciting experience, which forces surgeons to better understand knee replacement and also share their knowledge with other surgeons.

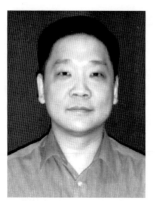
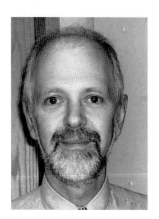

Authors

AIGNER, CHRISTIAN
Universitaet Graz
Klinische Abteilung fuer Orthopaedie
Auenbruggerplatz 9
8036 Graz
Austria

AUGER, DANIEL D.
DePuy Orthopaedics Inc
700 Orthopedics Drive
Warsaw, IN 46581-0988

BEVERLAND, DAVID E.
Musgrave Park Hospital
Stockman's Lane
Belfast, BT9 7JB
Ireland, UK

BOLDT, JENS G.
St. Vincent-Krankenhaus
Schlossstrasse 85
40477 Düsseldorf
Germany

BRIARD, JEAN-LOUIS
Clinique du Cèdre
Bois Guilleaume
F-76235 Rouen-Cedex
France

BUECHEL, FREDERICK F.
Biomedical Engineering Trust
South Mountain Orthopaedic Associates
61 First Street
South Orange
New Jersey 07079
USA

CHIU, PETER K. Y.
Queen Mary Hospital, Univ. of Hongkong
Department of Orthopaedic Surgery
Division of Joint Replacement Surgery
5th Floor, Professorial Block, Room 509
Hong Kong

COLLIER, JOHN P.
Dartmouth Biomedical Engineering Center
8000 Cummings Hall
Dartmouth College
Hanover, NH 03755
USA

DROBNY, THOMAS K.
Schulthess-Klinik
Lengghalde 2
CH-8008 Zürich
Switzerland

FARRAR, RICHARD
DePuy International Ltd.
St Anthony's Road
Leeds LS11 8DT
England

FISHER, DAVID A.
Methodist Hospital, Clavian Health Care
Indiana University
1801 N. Senate, Suite 200,
Indianapolis, IN 46202
USA

FISHER, JOHN
Medical and Biological Engineering
School of Mechanical Engineering
University of Leeds
Leeds, LS2 9JT
UK

FITZEK, JOSEF G.
Kreiskrankenhaus Mechernich, Orthopädie
St. Elisabeth-Str. 2-8
53894 Mechernich
Germany

FRIEDERICH, NIKLAUS F.
Klinik für Orthopädische Chirurgie und
Traumatologie des Bewegungsapparates
Kantonsspital
CH - 4101 Bruderholz
Switzerland

GOODFELLOW, JOHN W.
4 Uplands Park Road
Summertown, Oxford OX2 7RU
UK

GREENWALD, SETH A.
Ortho Research Lab/Lutheran Hospital
Cleveland Clinic Health System
The Mt Sinai Medical Center
1730 W 25th Street
Cleveland, OH 44106
USA

HAAS, BRIAN
Colorado Joint Replacement Center
2425 South Colorado Blvd., Suite 270
Denver, CO 80222
USA

HAMELYNCK, KAREL J.
Slotervaart Ziekenhuis
Louwesweg 6
1066 EC Amsterdam
The Netherlands

HOOPER, GARY
Leinster Orthopaedic Center
51 Leinster Road
Christchurch
New Zealand

JONES, RICHARD "DICKEY" E.
Southwest Orthopaedic Institute
5920 Forest Park Road
Suite 600,
Dallas, TX 75235
USA

JONES, V. C.
Medical and Biological Engineering
School of Medical Engineering
University of Leeds
Leeds, Ls29JT
UK

JORDAN, LOUIS R.
Jordan-Young Institute, P.C.
5501 Greenwich Road, Suite 200
Virginia Beach, VA 23462
USA

KASHIWAGI, TERU YUKI
Orthopedic Associates of Allentown
Suite 2500
1243 South Cedar Crest Boulevard
Allentown, PA 18103
USA

KEBLISH, PETER A
Orthopedic Associates of Allentown
Suite 2500
1243 South Cedar Crest Boulevard
Allentown, PA 18103
USA

KEENE, GREGORY C.
Sports Med SA
32 Payneham Road
SA 5069 Adelaide
Australia

KILGUS, DOUGLAS J.
Bowman Gray School of Medicine
Medical Center Boulevard (WFUSSM)
Department of Orthopaedic Surgery
Winston-Salem North Carolina, NC 27157
USA

KOMISTEK, RICHARD D.
Rose Musculoskeletal Research Lab.
2425 S Colorado Blvd., Suite 280
Denver, CO, 80222
USA

LIAO, YEN-SHUO
DePuy Orthopaedics Inc.
700 Orthopaedics Way
Warsaw
IN 46851-0988
USA

MAYOR, MICHAEL B.
147 Three Mile Road
Hanover
NH 03755-3908
USA

McEVEN, HANNAH M.
Medical and Biological Engineering
School of Mechanical Engineering
University of Leeds
Leeds, LS2 9JT
UK

McNULTY, DONALD E.
DePuy Orthopaedics Inc.
700 Orthopaedics Way
Warsaw
IN 46851-0988
USA

MERCHANT, ALAN C.
2500 Hospital Drive
Building 7
Mountain View, CA 94040
USA

MUELLER, WERNER
Spechtweg 10
CH - 4125 Riehen
Switzerland

MUNZINGER, URS K.
Schulthess-Klinik
Lengghalde 2
CH-8008 Zürich
Switzerland

O'CONNOR, JOHN J.
Quarry Manor
Beaumont Road,
Headington, Oxford, OX3 8JN
UK

OAKESHOTT, ROGER D.
Sports Med SA
32 Payneham Road, Stepney
SA 5069 Adelaide
Australia

OLIVIO, JANE L.
Jordan-Young Institute, P.C.
5501 Greenwich Road, Suite 200
Virginia Beach, VA 23462
USA

PAPPAS, MICHAEL, J. PH.D., P.E.
Biomedical Engineering Trust
South Mountain Orthopaedic Associates
61 First Street, South Orange, New Jersey 07079
USA

RUETHER, WOLFGANG
Universitaetsklinikum Hamburg-Eppendorf
Klinik und Poliklinik fuer Orthopaedie
Martinistr. 52
20251 Hamburg
Germany

SORRELLS, R. BARRY
US Orthopaedics Center
8907 Kanis Road, Suite 300
Little Rock, Arkansas 72205
USA

STIEHL, JAMES B.
Orthopaedic Hospital of Wisconsin
575 West Riverwoods Parkway, #204
Milwaukee, WI 53212
USA

STONE, MARTIN H.
Medical and Biological Engineering
School of Mechanical Engineering
University of Leeds
Leeds, LS2 9JT
UK

STRAUSS, MATTHIAS J.
Rheumaklinik Bad Branstedt
Oskar-Alexander-Strasse 26
24576 Bad Bramstedt
Germany

THOMAS, BERT J.
UCLA Medical Center
10833 LeConte Ave # 76-134
Los Angeles, CA 99095
USA

THUEMLER, PETER
St. Vincent-Krankenhaus
Schlossstrasse 85
40477 Düsseldorf
Germany

VOORHORST, PAUL E.
DePuy Orthopaedics Inc
700 Orthopedics Drive
Warsaw, IN 46581-0988

WALTER, WILLIAM K.
Sidney Northside Hip & Knee Surgeons
Level 3, 100 Bay Road, Waverton, NSW 2060
Australia

WILLIAMS, I.R.
Medical and Biological Engineering
School of Mechanical Engineering
University of Leeds, Leeds, LS2 9JT
UK

WINDHAGER, REINHARD
Universitaet Graz
Klinische Abteilung fuer Orthopaedie
Auenbruggerplatz 9
8036 Graz
Austria

ZICAT, BERNIE
Sidney Northside Hip & Knee Surgeons
Level 3, 100 Bay Road
Waverton, NSW 2060
Australia

History

I

Introduction:
Evolution of Meniscal Bearings

Karel J. Hamelynck

Today mobile bearing knee arthroplasty is known throughout the world of orthopaedics and probably has become the new "state of the art" of knee replacement. Two of the most important challenges of total knee arthroplasty, wear of polyethylene and mechanical loosening of components, were resolved by the introduction of mobile bearings, which had congruity to overcome the problem of high contact stresses causing wear, and which were mobile to eliminate constraint forces and so to reduce mechanical loosening.

In the seventies this knowledge was not at all common and wear was not considered a serious problem. With the growing of knowledge of the biomechanics of knee replacement and the reasons for success and failure, new design criteria were formed including the demand for free unconstraint anatomical motion. In knee replacement systems with fixed bearings this free anatomical movement could only be realised by incongruity between the articulating surfaces of the components. This resulted in even higher wear rates in these knees. The solution was found in compromise or in ignoring that there was a problem.

Some engineers and surgeons had better ideas, Dr John O' Conner, engineer, and Dr John Goodfellow, orthopaedic surgeon, were the first to present the concept of meniscal bearings in knees to replace the damaged cartilage. The polyethylene "menisci" were to be used in one or both compartments of the knee, preferably in the presence of intact cruciate ligaments. This concept has tremendously influenced the development of the New Jersey Knee Replacement System, later named the Low Contact Stress knee system.

The editors of the book are very grateful to both authors for their contribution to the book celebrating the 25th anniversary of the LCS knee system.

With their "classic" paper "The mechanics of the knee and prothesis design", originally published in the Journal of Bone and Joint Surgery, Vol. 60B, No 3: 35368, 1978, they introduced the new principle for artificial knee design clearly.

And another name should be mentioned: Doug Noiles. Doug Noiles was an engineer at U.S. Surgical Corporation. He designed a hinge knee system with a rotating platform type of mobile bearing and later he designed a posterior stabilised rotating platform. Dickey Jones will report about his activities in chapter 2.

The designers of the LCS knee were Michael J. Pappas, mechanical engineer, and Frederick F. Buechel, orthopaedic surgeon. The story of the development of the LCS knee will be told by Fred Buechel in chapter 3.

The editors of the book wanted to start the book with a little bit of history to give full credit to those engineers and surgeons, who were ahead of all others and gave a total new dimension to total knee arthroplasty.

After reading their stories and the chapters in the book you may realise it is true what has been said about the LCS: "So much behind it and so much ahead"!!!

Chapter 1
The Mechanics of the Knee and Prosthesis Design*

J. W. Goodfellow, J. O'Connor[1]

The mechanisms controlling and limiting movement and serving to transmit load between the femur and the tibia are discussed. Having accounted for the transmission of all components of force and couple across the joint and noted the load-bearing role of the menisci, some principles which might guide the design of knee prostheses are deduced. It ist shown that current designs transgress some of these principles. An experimental prosthesis is then described, which incorporates analogues of the natural menisci. The possible practical application of this novel principle has been studied in cadaveric human joints and in living patients.

They hung her from the ceiling,
Yes, they hung up Miss Gee;
And a couple of Oxford Groupers
Carefully dissected her knee

W. H. Auden

Anatomical descriptions of animal joints are customarily limited to the capsule of the joint and contents. From its functional viewpoint, this custom is unsatisfactory and it is more useful to regard the animal limb as a chain of rigid bars joined together by soft tissues, which include the muscles and their tendons no less than the ligaments. A function of all elements in a skeleton is to transmit load, an we describe the specialised structures of the human knee and its muscles in these terms.

Load transmission. All loads can be expressed in terms of forces acting in three directions at right angles to each other and couples acting about axes in those three directions. For the knee, it is convenient to choose the anteroposterior and mediolateral directions. (Fig. 1) Since it is customary to describe movements at the joint with respect to these three directions.

Thus, a force in the direction of the tibial axis resists interpenetration of the bones if compressive, distraction of the bones if tensile. Forces in the anteroposterior and mediolateral directions resist (or induce) relative translations of the bones in those directions respectively. A couple about the mediolateral axis resists (or induces) flexion or extension. A couple about the anteroposterior axis resists (or induces) flexion or extension. A couple about the anteroposterior axis resists (or induces) abduction or adduction. And lastly, a couple about the tibial axis resists (or induces) medial and lateral rotation. This convention describes not only all possible move-

* Reprint from J Bone Joint Surg 60B, 3: 358-368, 1979
[1] Based in part on lectures given to the Sixth Combined Meeting, London, 1976 an dto the Twenty-third Meeting of the Orthopaedic Research Society, Las Vegas, 1977.
John Goodfellow, F.R.C.S., Nuffield Orthopaedic Centre, Headington, Oxford OX3 7 LD, England.
John O'Connor, B.E., M.A., Ph.D., Department of Engineering Science, University of Oxford, Parks Road, Oxford OX1 3PJ, England.
Requests for reprints should be sent to Mr John Goodfellow.

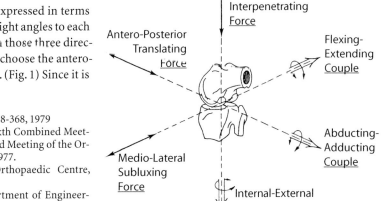

Fig. 1. Reference directions for the knee

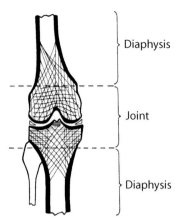

Fig. 2. Tubular and juxta-articular bone. The joint consists of all the material between the dotted lines

ments at the joint but all possible loads to which the limb is subject.

We must distinguish between the mode of transmission of loads along the shafts of the tubular bones and the mode of their transmission from one bone to another (Fig. 2). Within and along the diaphyses, all six components of load are transmitted by means of tensile, compressive and shear stresses, continuously distributed troughout the bony material. The tubulated form reflects the function of diaphysial bone. By contrast, at the joint, all these six components are transmitted from one bone to the other in some combination of pressure at the articular surfaces and tension in the soft tissues spanning the joint. The articular surfaces of synovial joints are so smooth and well lubricated as to offer minimal resistance to sliding movements and can therefore transmit no significant shear stress on to another. They do not adhere and cannot therefore transmit tensile stress. They can transmit only compressive stress (pressure) normal to their surfaces. The soft tissues can transmit only tension in the line of their fibres.

Consequently, the expanded juxtra-articular bone at the ends of the shafts and embraced by the ligaments is subjected predominantly to compression, applied to it by the articulating surfaces which it supports. We assume that the trabeculated form of the juxta-articular bone reflects its function and distinguishes it from the tubulated bone which lies beyond the ligamentous insertions. The distinction suggests that different considerations may apply to the design of prostheses which use intramedullary stems to gain attachment to the tubulated bone on the other hand, and those which are attached directly to the trabecular bone on the other.

Mobility and stability. Mobility at a joint is conferred by the provision of low-friction bearing surfaces between

the bones. Stability is a measure of the degree to which relative movement at the bearing surfaces is limited or resisted.

We should distinguish between passive stability, a measure of the limitation imposed by the length of the ligaments and the contour of the joint surfaces, and active stability when the forces of gravity, ground reaction and muscle action are added. The range of movement in activity cannot lie beyond the range allowed passively.

In most joints, and particularly those of the lower limb, stability is of greater functional importance than mobility and it is possible to describe the natural knee in terms of the mechanisms that resist movement and transmit load. Our purpose is to explain what may appear to be a paradox: that a condylar replacement prosthesis my best confer stability upon the living joint if it is itself completely unstable. We will show that, since natural articular surfaces contribute to joint stability merely by resisting interpenetration of the bones, the only function required of prosthetic surfaces is to do the same.

We shall first describe the forces and couples required to control or limit each of the six possible between active and passive stability. Since force is required either to initiate or to limit movement, the mechanisms that control movement are the same as those used for the transmission of load. The ligaments and tendons that span the joint are favourably oriented to resist distraction of the bones and to develop the tensile component of the couples needed to resist flexion or extension and abduction or adduction. They are less favourably oriented to resist those movements that involve sliding of the articular surfaces – rotation about the tibial axis and translation of the bones in the mediolateral and anteroposterior directions.

These sliding movements are not resisted until the sof tissues tighten and, as they tighten, pull the articular surfaces together (Fig. 3). A balance is reached and further movement is resisted when the component of the soft tissue tension perpendicular to the articular sur-

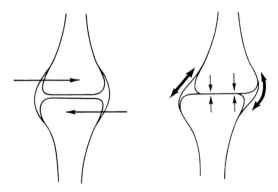

Fig. 3. General method of limiting sliding movements

faces equals the compressive force on the condyles and the component parallel to the articular surfaces equals the applied shearing force. The range of sliding movement available in any joint, therefore, depends on the rate at which the soft tissues tighten in response to a translation or rotation of the bones which, in turn, depends on al complex relationship between the geometry of the articular surfaces and the disposition oft the soft tissues.

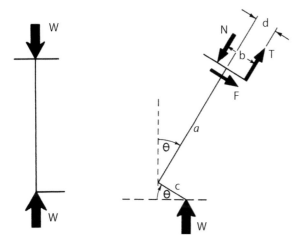

Fig. 4. Equilibrium of the tibia. When vertical, a compressive force at the knee can keep the tibia in equilibrium. When inclined to the vertical, tensile, compressive and shear forces are required. From statics:

$$N = W\left[\frac{a}{b}\sin\theta - \left(\frac{c-d}{b}\right)\cos\theta\right]; T = W\left[\frac{a}{b}\sin\theta - \left(1 + \frac{c-d}{b}\right)\cos\theta\right];$$

$$F = W\sin\theta$$

The factor $\frac{a}{b}$ in these equation has a value of at least 8

These generalisations apply to the control of all translatory movements. It is convenient to consider flexion and extension with anteroposterior translation because the former movements occur naturally with the latter. We will treat abduction and adduction with mediolateral translations for the same reason.

Flexion and extension with anteroposterior translation. Off all the ways in which the femur and the tibia might move relative to one another, only flexion from the anatomical position is free of passive limitation.

Flexion from any position is resisted actively by the couple of tension in the patellar tendon and compression at the contact areas between the two bones. This couple acts about a lever arm b (Fig. 4), the distance between the line of action of the quadriceps at the insertion of its tendon and the centre of pressure of the contact forces. The large compressive forces described in the caption arise because couples acting through generally short lever arms along the joint surfaces must resist couples acting through lever arms which can be as long as the shafts of the bones.

In all positions except full extension, the normal knee allows a limited range of anteroposterior gliding of its articular surfaces.

Kapandji (1970) and Huson (1974) have shown that, mainly because of the crossed form of the cruciate ligaments, flexion of the knee is accompanied not only by a sliding movement of the femoral condyles upon the tibia but also by an obligatory rolling movement which carries the contact areas backwards on the tibia in flexion and forwards in extension. The two-dimensional model in Figures 5, 6 and 7, in which the components are held

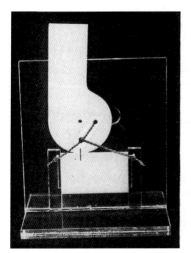

Fig. 5

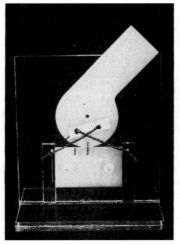

Fig. 6

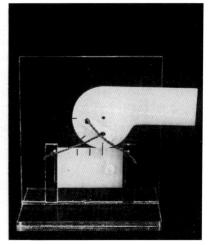

Fig. 7

Fig. 5–7. Two-dimensional model. Marks on the model bones show that the four-bar linkage commands posterior rolling of the femur on the tibia while flexing. The discrepant distances between successive points of contact indicate that posterior rolling is accompanied by anterior sliding in a ratio of about to one

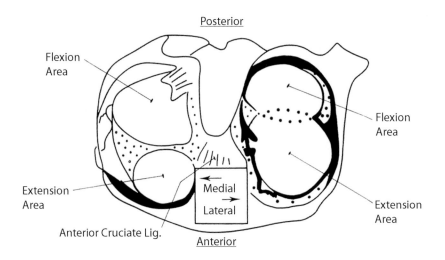

Fig. 8. Movement of the contact areas on the tibial plateau, as determined by Michael Harding using a dye-exclusion technique on a cadaveric specimen

together by crossed wires to simulate the cruciate ligaments, demonstrates that the two bones and the two ligaments constitute a four-bar linkage which commands such movement. Passive stability in the anteroposterior direction is mainly dependent upon the integrity of the direction of such movements. Kapandji (1970) has also shown that the collateral ligaments have a similar crossed form when viewed from the side, and they, too, contribute to the mechanism.

The contact areas of a cadaveric knee in extension and flexion are shown in Figure 8. Their obligatory excursion is of the order 0.8 to 1.2 centimetres. Reference to the caption of Figure 4 will show that this backward movement of the contact areas in flexion maximises the power of the quadriceps to extend the knee (or to resist flexion) and minimises the compressive force at the articular surfaces by making the lever arm b as large as possible.

Within the narrow range of uncertainty allowed by the ligaments, active control of the position of the contact areas depends, at any moment, on the balance of the relevant muscle forces. For example, when the quadriceps muscle contracts, the patellofemoral component of its action tends to push the femur backwards on the tibia while the posterior component of the hamstring action tends to pull the tibia backwards on the femur.

Passive limitation of extension depends on the action of a couple of compression at the tibiofemoral contact areas and tension in the soft tissues. It is tibiofemoral contact areas and tension in the soft tissues. It is common practice to assign specific roles to specific ligaments in producing this couple, but it is probably more accurate to say that tension in any of the longitudinally disposed ligaments lying posterior to the centre of pressure of the contact forces must contribute. The posterior capsular ligament clearly enjoys a mechanical advantage over the other ligamentous structures.

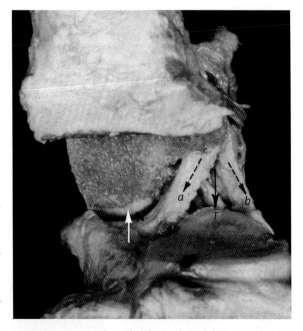

Fig. 9. Specimen with medial femoral condyle removed. Anterior cruciate ligament (*a*) and posterior capsular ligament (*b*) both tight at passive limit of null extension. Note anterior location of the contact area between the bones. The resultant T of the tensions in the ligaments and the compressive force N provide the couple which limits the extension

Active limitation of extension derives from the flexor muscles which employ a lever arm similar to that of the posterior capsular ligament. In both cases the length of the lever arm is maximised by the forward location of the contact areas ordained by the cruciate mechanism. In Figure 9, both the posterior capsular and the anterior cruciate ligaments are seen to be tight at the passive limit of extension. In the absence of external forces, the two cruciates act together to locate the contact areas, but it is the anterior ligament that mainly resists forces tending to move them backwards on the tibia.

It is commonly supposed that is the greater radius of curvature of the anterior parts of the femoral condyles which accounts for the tightening of the ligaments and the "locked" state of the fully extended knee. However, a similar state develops even when the natural condyles are replaced by perfectly spherical components, provided that the contact areas can move forward in extension. It is the combination of anterior location of the contact areas and posterior location of the tension elements which allows the development of a couple capable of resisting hyperextension.

Rotation. In all positions short of full extension, a range of rotational freedom is available. It has been measured by Markolf, Mensch and Amstutz (1976) in the minimally loaded joint and found to be about 30 degrees with the joint flexed to a right angle.

Several authors have atributed particular responsibilities in resisting medial and lateral rotation to particular ligaments. However, all the tension-bearing elements that span the joint are capable, when they are rendered tight, of contributing to the couples that resist rotation, For example, the circumferential components of the tension forces in all the capsular structures may provide such a couple.

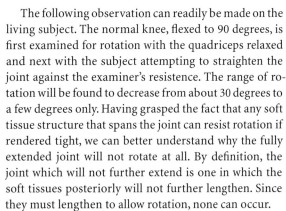

The following observation can readily be made on the living subject. The normal knee, flexed to 90 degrees, is first examined for rotation with the quadriceps relaxed and next with the subject attempting to straighten the joint against the examiner's resistence. The range of rotation will be found to decrease from about 30 degrees to a few degrees only. Having grasped the fact that any soft tissue structure that spans the joint can resist rotation if rendered tight, we can better understand why the fully extended joint will not rotate at all. By definition, the joint which will not further extend is one in which the soft tissues posteriorly will not further lengthen. Since they must lengthen to allow rotation, none can occur.

The presence of the tibial eminence may give rise to a subsidiary mechanism in limiting rotation (Fig. 10). During rotation, the contact areas move on the tibia, one anteriorly, the other posteriorly. Any tendency of the femur to mount the tibial eminence would be resisted by tension forces in the soft tissues spanning the joint, tension which would be balanced by compression on the articular surfaces. If the tibial eminence is brought into contact, the components of the compressive forces in the plane of the tibial plateau could provide a couple to balance an applied torque. The lever arm of the couple arises form the relatively anterior position of one contact area and the posterior position of the other (Fig. 10).

We believe the contribution of the tibial eminence couple to be small. Deane (1970) has noted that the tibial plateau is tracked to allow the anteroposterior movement of the contact areas with relatively little distraction. Figure 11 shows the measured[2] range of tibial rotation of a cadaveric knee. The relative unimportance of the tibial eminence in resisting rotation my be deduced from the fact that the range of rotation remained much the same when a distracting force which separated the articular surface was applied. We will show (Fig. 22) that a similar range of tibial rotation was optained when the tibial plateau was replaced by flat prosthetic surfaces which did not mimic the tibial eminence.

Abduction and adduction with mediolateral translation. A mediolateral force applied through the foot tends both to abduct and adduct the knee and to translate the bones relative to each other in the mediolateral direction. For a state of equilibrium to exist, an equal and opposite mediolateral force and a couple about the anteroposterior axis are transmitted across the joint (Fig. 12).

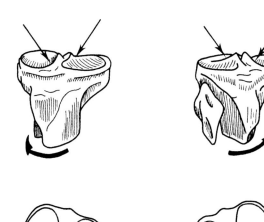

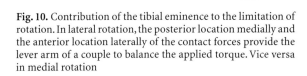

Fig. 10. Contribution of the tibial eminence to the limitation of rotation. In lateral rotation, the posterior location medially and the anterior location laterally of the contact forces provide the lever arm of a couple to balance the applied torque. Vice versa in medial rotation

---

[2] Detail of the experimental method and further results are given in the paper by Bourne, Goodfellow and O'Connor (1978).

The collateral ligaments are the most advantageously disposed to resist abduction and adduction, in couple with compression on the colateral condyles. The longest lever arms available are thereby employed. The collateral ligaments are not, however, the only structures which an passively resist such movements. The diagram suggests that tension in the cruciate ligaments can resist abduc-

tionor adduction though working through a shorter lever arm than do the collateral ligaments. We have found that each compartment of the knee has a degree of inherent stability independent of the other. If, in a cadaveric joint, one femoral condyle is excised, considerable stability is retained in both directions. The retained collateral and cruciate ligaments, acting albeit through a much shorter lever arm than in the intact joint, nevertheless effectively resist angulation.

At first sight, it might appear that ligamentous mechanisms are the only ones available to resist abduction or adduction at the knee, and that the joint's stability about ths axis must, unlike other modes of stability, be the same during function as it is under minimal load. But, although there are no muscles able to induce abduction or adduction, it by no means follows that there are none capable of resisting such movements. Reference to Figure 12a will show that if the fulcrum of an adduction movement is within the contact area of the medial femoral condyle, all tension-bearing structures that span the joint lateral to that fulcrum contribute to the couple that resists adduction. Thus tension in the patellar tendon can resist both abduction and adduction movement. In full extension, the tight posterior capsule exerts a similar effect for the same reasons. We test for the passive stabilising effect of the collateral ligaments with the knee slightly flexed. If this clinical test were done with the knee fully extended, the stability engendered by the tight posterior capsule would mask any deficiency in the collateral ligaments.

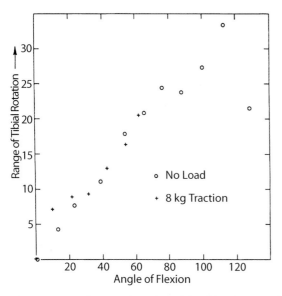

Fig. 11. Measured range of rotation of the tibia relative to the femur in a cadaveric knee under no load and under a traction force of 8 kilograms applied along the ankle-hip axis

Fig. 12. (a) Simple couple resisting abduction or adduction. Dotted tension force represents active contribution of, for instance, patellar tendon force. (b) Abduction or adduction is usually accompanied by mediolateral translation which is resisted in part by the mediolateral component of the contact force. (c) Simple analysis of the tibia gives $N = T = F\dfrac{a}{b}$ where $\dfrac{a}{b}$ is approximately equal to 6

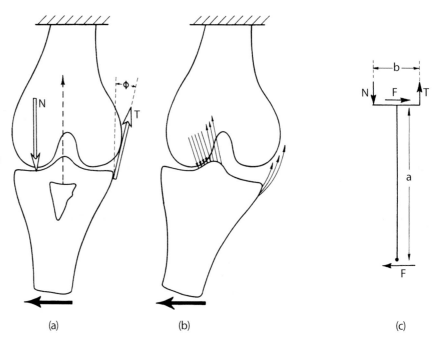

(a)   (b)   (c)

It is easy to show from statics (fig. 12c) that the tensile and compressive forces needed to resist abduction and adduction must be several times larger than the value of the mediolateral force applied. The lever arm available along the tibia to the joint forces. If the mechanism of Figure 3 were to operate alone to resist mediolateral translation, we estimate that an inclination of the soft tissues forces of about 10 degrees (the angle Ø in Figure 12a) would be needed to balance the applied force. Such an inclination would imply mediolateral translation of the bones of about 5 millimetres, rather more than is observed. The joint is much more congruous when viewed from the front; the contact force could be transmitted, in part, by the tibial eminence and the mediolateral component of that force could help to balance the applied load.

The function of the menisci. Fairbank (1948) suggested that the menisci transmit load between the femur and the tibia, and several recent investigations have confirmed the truth of his opinion (Seedholm, Dowson and Wright 1974; Shrive 1974; Walker and Erkman 1975; Krause *et al.* 1976). Estimates vary, but all are agreed that at least 50 per cent of the compressive force between the bones is carried by the menisci. They are relatively free to distort and can be displaced forwards and backwards upon the tibial condyles in order to maintain contact with the femur in all positions (Karpandji 1970). Such movements have been observed by arthroscopy to occur in the living during flexion, extension and rotation of the joint (Henry 1976).

The menisci act as conforming mobile bearing pads which spread the load transmitted between the femur and the tibia, increasing by a factor of about two the area of their contact, and thereby reducing the average pressure on the articulating surfaces.

Résumé
We have accounted for the control of all possible relative movements between the tibia and the femur, and described the transmission of all possible loads across the joint in terms of articular surface compression and soft tissue tension. The ability of the joint to transmit all possible loads and resist all possible movements derives lolely from the ability of the articular surfaces to resist interpenetration and of the soft tissues to resist distraction.

The normal joint invites analogy with a well-pitched tent, which resists all forces tending to distort it by the development of tension in its guy-ropes and compression in its pole. It is the function of the articular surfaces to keep the bones apart; it is the function of the soft tissues to keep the bones together. The compressive stress

is always at right angles to the articular surface, and the juxta-articular bone is therefore subject to this stress and designed to withstand it.

These generalisations are true of all synovial joints; they vary only in the proportion in which the soft and hard tissues contribute to stability. Instability results as readily from failure of an articulare surface as it does from lengthening or rupture of a ligament, and in both cases the load-bearing function of the joint is prejudiced.

In offering this general description of the mechanics of the knee, we have not reported estimates of the magnitude of the forces in the various structures nor even, in any detail, specified the particular tension-carrying elements involved in the transmission of any particular component of load. Such calculations may be prone to considerable error. Smith (1975) has shown that small errors in the estimates of the lengths of the lever arms can lead to large errors in the estimates of the forces. The joint, in mechanical terms, is a highly indeterminate structure. Crowningshield, Pope and Johnson (1976) had to use a model consisting of thirteen soft tissue elements to study the passive stability of the joint; were the features which contribute to active stability to be added, the calculation would be still more complex. Fortunately, to design a condylar replacement prosthesis it is not necessary to know the precise distribution of stress throughout the soft tissues so long as it is realised that the ligaments confer passive stability by setting limits to the range of possible positions which the bones may adopt and that, within that range, the forces of gravity, of ground reaction and of muscle action determine their precise disposition. For these mechanisms to work, it is necessary that the articular surfaces, of themselves, should resist any relative movement of the bones other than their interpenetration.

1 The Design of a Prosthesis

The foregoing suggests some principles to guide the design of prostheses which replace diseased or worn articular surfaces while retaining the ligaments and muscles.

The components should be shaped to allow distracting, sliding and rolling movements between the bones; the components should apply only compressive stress to the juxta-articular bone; all surviving soft tissues should be kept and restored to their natural tensions; and the areas of contact between the prosthetic surfaces should be large enough to maintain the pressure under load at a level which the prosthetic materials can withstand.

It is not possible to attempt the design of prosthetic articular surfaces without immediately encountering

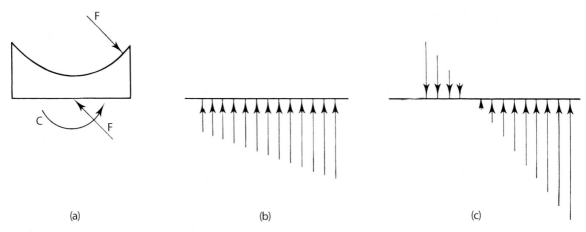

Fig. 13. (a) Contact force on a socket-like tibial component is balanced by an equal and opposite force and a couple. (b) The normal stress applied to the juxta-articular bone is entirely compressive if the couple is small but (c) can be tensile over part of the interface if the couple is large

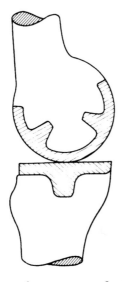

Fig. 14. Convex femoral components on flat tibial components

a dilemma. If the components are to bear their loads through large areas of contact, they must fit one another in all postures of the joint – and the only shapes which will do so are spheres in spherical sockets. If two such devices are employed, one on each side of the joint, there can be but one axis of movement, a circumstance allow, and one which may rob the joint of certain valuable mechanical advantages. Such a joint is kinematically indistinguishable from a simple hinge with a transverse axle and rotation can only occur by dislocation of its surfaces By their shapes the tibial elements in this design *resist* rotation, anteroposterior and mediolateral translation and must therefore *transmit* the assciated forces and couples. Rocking moments are thus engendered, and it would not be surprising if the elements in such a

design were to come loose. All prostheses employing interlocked surfaces transmit shear and tension stresses to the bones, as demonstrated, for example, in Figure 13.

However, if we reject the ball-and-socket principle in favour of two articular surfaces which do not match, we necessarily transgress the fourth principle above. Figure 14 is the archetype of such designs. It may be ideal kinematically, allowing the convex femoral components to roll, slide and spin upon the tibia as the ligaments ordain, and its components (if friction between tehm is ignored) transmit largely compressive stress to the bones beneath them. But the contact areas are small, and the pressures to be sustained by the materials are therefore high, with the likelihood of excessive creep and wear.

Many current designs seek compromise solutions to the dilemma; their components are made so that the opposed contours almost match, but not quite. Such compromises represent an acceptance of some of the disadvantages of incongruity of the components to gain some of the advantages of unconstrained movement. The large variety of such designs differ from each other mainly in the fine detail of the surface geometry considered necessary to complement the function of the soft tissues. Accuracy of implanation then becomes critical to the stability of the resulting arthroplasty.

There is one way of avoiding the need to compromise at all which is similar to the natural solution. Figures 15, 16 and 17 show the same model as in Figures 5 to 7 but with the addition of a closely fitting but unconstrained washer trapped, only by its shape, between the two articular surfaces. A perfect fit with good load-bearing can be achieved without altering the kinematics of the model at all. The function of the natural menisci is similar to that served by the washer in the model, though the

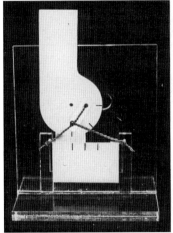
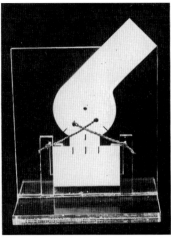
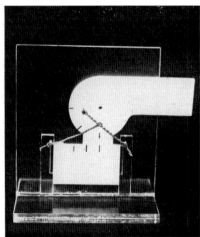

Fig. 15   Fig. 16   Fig. 17

Fig. 15–17. Two dimensional model with a meniscal "washer". Movement of femur relative to tibia is the same as in Figures 5 to 7 but the contact areas are larger

mechanism of load-transmission *within* the menisci is quite different. In the model, a rigid and undeformable washer transmits load in compression, while the natural meniscus transmits compressive force by the development of tension in its collagen fibres which are mainly aligned with its circumference (Bullough et al. 1970).

Figures 18 and 19 show a cadaveric knee into which a prosthesis has been implanted. The femoral components are spherical; the tibial components are flat. These elements were cemented to the bone ends. Between them lie plastic washers, each spherically concave above and flat below, exactly fitting the shapes of the metal components. The washers were made in several thicknesses (in 1 millimetre steps) and, from this range, two were chosen which "snapped" into place, rendering the ligaments tight. This prosthesis has been implanted into twenty-five cadaveric joints. Femoral components of the same size (radius 24 millimetres) were used in all. The femoral elements were so adjusted on the bone, by appropriate cuts, that the gaps existing between their surfaces and those of the tibial elements were the same at full extension as they were at 90 degrees of flexion. The washers filled those gaps and were trapped in position because of their shape.

Flexion and extension. Comparison of Figures 18 and 19 shows that, as the joint flexes and extends, the washers move backwards and forwards upon the tibial flats, as did the washer in the two-dimensional model. This movement of the washers was found to be obligatory, for if it was artificially blocked, the joint "locked" and would neither flex nor extend. The excursion of the washers was between 0.6 and 1.2 centimetres during flexion to 90 degrees.

In those cadaveric joints that initially enjoyed a full range of movement this was reproduced after implanta-

tion of the device. Beyond about 120 degrees of flexion, the backwards excursion of the washers brought their posterior edges to the posterior limit of the tibial plateaux and sometimes beyond, but posterior dislocation never occurred.

Rotation. Comparison of Figures 20 and 21 shows that medial and lateral rotations were allowed by reciprocal backward and forward movements of the femoral condyles upon the tibia, a movement accomodated by the washers sliding backwards and forwards upon the tibial flats.

In Figure 22, the range of rotation available at various positions of flexion an an intact cadaveric knee is compared with the same joint after implantation of the prosthesis. The range of rotation was determined with the joint unloaded, an in both cases the measured range ws similar to that of Markolf, Mensch and Amstutz (1976).

Stability. The most striking feature of the function of the implant was the degree of passive stability which it could confer and the fine control which choice of washer thickness exercised. An appropriate choice gave complete lateral stability throughout the range of flexion; extension was accurately limited and the joint locked in full extension as in the normal knee, allowing no rotation in that position (Fig. 22). The drawer test, performed with the knee flexed, demonstrated a normal range of anteroposterior glide of the femoral condyles and their washers upon the tibial flats.

All these features of passive stability, depending as they do on the development of tension in the ligaments, could be diminished or enhanced by reducing or increasing the thickness of the washers. Reproduction of

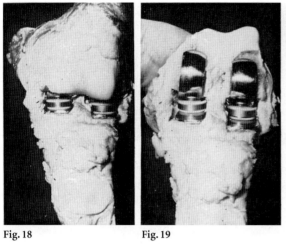

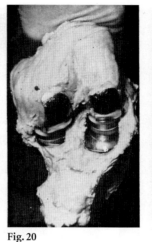

Fig. 18   Fig. 19

Fig. 20   Fig. 21

Fig. 18,19. The "meniscal" prosthesis demontrating the obligatory anteroposterior movement of the washers. **Fig. 18** in extension; **Fig. 19** in flexion

Fig. 20,21. Rotation of the tibia, demonstrating the reciprocal movement of the washers. **Fig. 20** lateral rotation; **Fig. 21** medial rotation

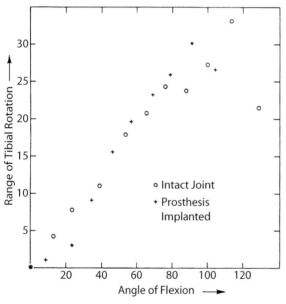

Fig. 22. Measured range of tibial rotation of a cadaveric knee under no load before and after implantation of the "meniscal" prosthesis

tive, the range of rotation increased, and stability in abduction and adduction diminished. These changes occurred because the washers, which had hitherto been of adequate thickness to tension the ligaments, were now obviously too thin.

As thicker washers, in millimetre steps, were inserted, the lateral stability of the joint was gradually regained and its rotary freedom diminished to near normal again. The control of the anteroposterior location of the washers on the tibial flats also improved, but never achieved the precision of a joint with intact cruciate ligaments.

Clinical application

Having shown that the prosthesis was capable of restoring passive stability and natural mobility in the cadaveric knee, and that the uncontrained washers did not displace, some implants have been undertaken in patients suffering from advanced rheumatoid arthritis or osteoarthritis. In due course the results of the clinical trial will be reported in full. It is already possible to state that, in joints rendered grossly unstable by disease, stability can be re-established by the use of this prosthesis almost as readily at operation as in the laboratory.

In the two disease processes mentioned, instability was found to result mainly from erosion of the articular surfaces. Once the surfaces had been replaced, the remaining ligaments proved capable of resuming their former function. In some cases, the anterior cruciate ligament was absent, but we have not yet encountered a joint which lacked both cruciates.

In the living, we have been able to observe the additional effects of muscle force, ground reaction and gravity upon the passive stability provided by the tightened

normal stability required an accuracy to within 1. to 2 millimetres.

Effects of division of the cruciate ligaments. In some cadaveric joints, one and then both the cruciate ligaments were divided after implantation of the prosthesis. The effect was always to render the joint less stable. Backward and forward movements of the washers still occurred with rotation and flexion or extension, but with much less precision. The drawer test became posi-

ligaments. The recovery of active stability has been the most remarkable feature in the small series of patients operated upon.

2 Discussion

In our mechanical analysis of the human knee, we concluded that it was the function of the articular surfaces to hold the bones apart. The prosthesis just described does that – and nothing else. Its components can offer no significant resistance to shear or tension stresses, and all loads must be transmitted through the reconstructed knee, as they are through the natural joint, by a combination of pressure normal to its articulating surfaces and tension in the soft tissues. The results of the experiments just described confirm that, if the prosthesis fulfils this one function, the retained soft tissues can faithfully reproduce the freedoms and limitations of movement seen in the natural joint. But the soft tissues can only do so if the "spacer effect" of the prosthesis accurately adjusts their tension and maintains it troughout the range of movement. This it can do only if its design imposes nor arbitrary axes upon such movements.

In addition to the clear advantage of spreading the load, the use of interposed washers confers upon the design an important advantage, that the tension in the ligaments can be adjusted *after* the metal components have been fixed to the bones.

Since it may be significant in its practical application, we draw attention to the behaviour of the prosthesis in those cadaveric joints in which the cruciate ligaments were divided. The experiment confirms the commanding role the cruciates play in the control of the intact joint, but it also demonstrates that the other soft tissues, designed as they are to *accommodate* the natural combination of rolling and sliding movements, can themselves *command* such movements if the cruciates are not functioning. They command such movements only if they are rendered tight enough to do so by implanting thicker washers than the intact cruciates will allow.

The experiments also confirm that the polyaxial movements of the human knee are the result of the crossed form of its ligaments and not a direct consequence of the polycentric curvatures of the femoral condyles. It is at first difficult to understand how a circular surface on a flat one can keep the ligamentous structures at a lifelike tension throughout the range of movements. That they can do so is shown by the fact that all aspects of passive stability were reproduced, as evidenced, for example, by the similarity of the two graphs in Figure 22. It appears that the significance of the generally helical shape of the femoral condyles has been wrongly over-

emphasised. The explanation of the fact that a crossed system of ligaments can accommodate an infinite number of pairs of surfaces provided that they are free to roll and slide upon one another is given in some detail in the Appendix to this paper.

The question whether the inclusion of unconstrained washers within a prosthesis will prove a practical as well as a theoretical solution to the design dilemma referred to cannot yet be answered. In twenty-five cadaveric joints, tested in a rig which allowed normal knee movements, the washers did not dislocate.

If a washer of the right size is inserted in the first instance, it could dislocate only if the gap between the fixed components subsequently were to open. This could happen if the ligaments were to stretch or if one or other fixed component were to sink into the bone.

No form of attachment has been used to hold the washers in place other than the entrapment provided by their geometry. The retained soft tissues, by resisting distraction of the joint, resist dislocation of the prosthesis just as they resist dislocation of the normal joint. Indeed, were there to be any other restraint in the form of tracks or stops to limit the freedom of the washers to translate within the range defined by the ligaments, such restraints would inevitably cause the fixed components to transmit shear and tension stresses to the bone. Experiments with "semi-constrained" washers showed that constraints which operated within the range of the ligaments did indeed result in rocking of the tibial components. If such tracks or stops only came into operation outside the range normally allowed ty the ligaments, they could give an extra security against dislocation when the joint is unloaded and its surfaces liable to distract.

Will the soft tissues of diseased joints maintain for as long as the function demanded of them in this design? We have shown that they can reassume initial control and we rely on the general observation that biological materials thrive when functioning within their design range. If, however, this hope is not realised, then the prospects for all condylar replacement prostheses must be poor. For, if the tensile components of load are not wholly borne by the soft tissues, then the prosthetic surfaces cannot escape transmitting shear and tension stress to the bones to which they are attached. Any form of interlocking of the prosthetic surfaces must have this effect. Our mechanical analysis suggests that juxta-articular bone may fail when stressed in this way, and it explains why constrained designs of prostheses may require intramedullary stems to carry the forces across the intracapsular bone to the shaft, the tubulated form of which is designed to resist all components of load.

The problems of wear and creep common to all joint prostheses are limited in this design to the washers. Laboratory tests show that creep in the plastic washer can be much reduced by placing a metal ring around its circumference (Figs. 18 to 21). By preventing radial expansion, in the manner of a tyre on a farmyard cartwheel, the ring reduces the maximum shear stress in the washer and, therefore, its propensity to flow. Wear rates, deduced from the data of Dowson, Atkinson and Brown (1975), can be expected to be small.

At the inception of these studies, Dr. N. g. Shrive demonstrated the weight-bearing role of the menisci (Shrive, N. G. (1974) D. Phil. Thesis, University of Oxford) and was involved int the preliminary discussions which led to the design of the "meniscal" prosthesis (Goodfellow, J. W., O'Connor, J. J., and Shrive, N. G. (1974). British Patent Application No. 49794/74).

Appendix: Geometry of Condylar Surfaces

The kinematics of the two-dimensional model (Figs. 5 to 7) can be analysed to demonstrate the characteristics of crossed ligament designs and the surface shapes they can accommodate.

The instant centre of the femur relative to the tibia, the point about which either bone may be considered to be spinning relative to the other, is always located at the point at which the two ligaments cross. As the joint flexes and extends, the point of cross-over moves relative to both bones. The paths of the instant centre, on both bones, may be determined by finding the location of the cross-over point relative to each bone for several positions of the joint. These paths consist of pairs of points, one attached to each bone, each pair coinciding for one position of the joint and, when coincident, moving with exactly the same velocity. The two paths therefore represent the shapes of those surfaces, one attached to each bone, which would complement the ligament design and roll without slip on each other. The curves are called the centrodes of the mechanism. For a given mechanism the centrodes alt unique.

Three sets of centrodes are shown in Figure 23 for three different designs. The femoral centrode in each case is closely circular but the tibial centrode is concave upward, concave downward or flat, depending on whether the femoral attachment distance is less than, greater than or equal to half the tibial attachment distance. In the latter case, the design is called the Chebychev straight-line mechanism (Hall 1961), used to roll a circular surface upon a flat surface without slip.

The measured dimensions[3] of the cruciate ligaments in the human knee (AB = 22 millimetres, CD = 12 milli-

metres) approximate to those of the mechanism 2 in the figure, and so the centrodes of the human cruciates are approximately a circle on a flat.

A circle of relatively smaller or relatively larger radius than that of the centrode can be used, but in both instances some sliding movements between the surfaces are introduced. If a circle of radius less than that of the centrode is employed, the sliding will be in the same direction as the rolling movement. If a larger radius is used, the sliding and rolling occur in opposite directions. For the surfaces to make contact at about the level of attachment of the cruciates to the tibia, a circle of larger diameter than that of the femoral centrode is required, and such a surface will roll backwards while sliding forwards, and vice versa (Figs. 5 to 7).

The number of pairs of surfaces which a crossed four-bar linkage can accomodate is, in fact, infinite. The shape of one surface having been chosen quite arbitrarily, it is possible by simple geometry to deduce the shape of the only surface which will complement it, and each pair of surfaces will exhibit a particular combination of rolling and sliding movements. We deduce that the articular surfaces of the knee form one of many possible combi-

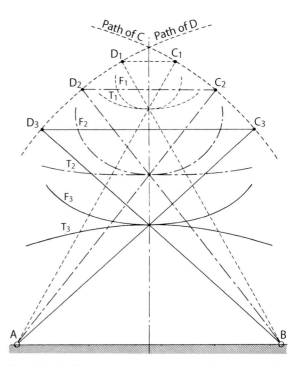

Fig. 23. Loci of instantaneous centre (centrodes) relative to the femur (F_1, F_2, F_3) and relative to the tibia (T_1, T_2, T_3) for three designs of cruciate mechanism having femoral attachment distances (C_1D_1, C_2D_2, C_3D_3) equal to 0.2, 0.5 and 0.8 of the tibial attachment distance AB. Within a certain range of flexion, the femoral centrodes are circular. Tibial centrode T_2 is flat within a flexion range of about 60°

---

[3] Although Kapandji (1970) states that posterior cruciate is three-fifths the lengh of the anterior, when viewed from the side they appear much more nearly equal in length.

nations which could complement its ligaments. The circle on the flat is a good approximation to another.

Since circles of differing radii can all be accomodated by a ligament design of fixed dimensions, it follows that a circle of fixed radius can accomodate ligaments of varied dimensions. If the ligaments of large and small human knees vary only in their absolute and not in their proportional dimensions, a circular femoral prosthetic surface of one radius can accomodate them all, and only the relationship of the level of the articulation to the cross-over point of the cruciates need vary. This is the theoretical explanation for the observations reported in this paper that, in forty-one human knees, femoral components of radius 24 millimetres accomodated the ligaments in every case, the level of the articulation varying as did the quantity of bone removed from the tibia and the thickness of the interposed washers.

References

1. Bullough, PG, Munuera, L, Murphy, J, and Weinstein, AM (1970) The strength of the menisci of the knee as it relates to their fine structure. Journal of Bone and Joint Surgery, 52-B, 564–570
2. Bourne, R, Goodfellow, JW and O'Connor, JJ (1978) A functional analysis of various knee arthroplastics. Proceedings of the 24th Meeting, Orthopaedic Research Society, Dallas
3. Crowningshield, R, Pope, MH, and Johnson, RJ (1976) A analytical model of the knee. Journal of Biomechanics, 9, 397–405
4. Deane, G (1970) Contact Print Studies in the Human Knee Joint. M.Sc. Thesis, University of Surrey.
5. Dowson, D, Atkinson, JR, and Brown, K (1975) The wear of high molecular weight polyethylene with particular reference to its use in artificial human joints. Advances in Polymer Friction and Wear, 5B, 533
6. Fairbank, TJ (1948) Knee joint changes after meniscectomy. Journal of Bone and Joint Surgery, 30-B, 664–670
7. Hall, AS (1961) Kinematics and Linkage Design. Englewood Cliffs: Prentice-Hall
8. Henry, A (1976) Personal Communication
9. Huson, A (1974) The functional anatomy of the knee joint: the closed kinematic chain as a model of the knee joint. In The Knee Joint, pp. 163–168. International Congress Series No. 324. Amsterdam: Excerpta Medica
10. Kapandji, IA (1970) The Physiology of the Joints. Volume 2. Lower Limb, p. 120. London and Edinburgh: Churchill Livingstone
11. Krause, WR Pope, MH, Johnson, RJ, and Wilder, DG (1976) Mechanical changes in the knee after meniscectomy. Journal of Bone and Joint Surgery, 58-A, 599–604
12. Markolf, KL, Mensch, JS, and Amstutz, HC (1976) Stiffness and laxity of the knee – the contributions of the supporting structure. A quantitative in vitro study. Journal of Bone and Joint Surgery, 58-A, 583
13. Seedhom, BB, Dowson, D, and Wright, V (1974) The load-bearing function of the menisci: a preliminary study. In The knee study. In The Knee Joint, pp. 37–42. International Congress Series No. 324. Amsterdam: Excerpta Medica
14. Shrive, N (1974) The weight-bearing role of the menisci of the knee. Journal of Bone and Joint Surgery, 56-B, 381
15. Smith, AJ (1975) Estimates of muscle and joint forces at the knee and ankle during a jumping activity. Journal of Human Movement Studies, 1, 78–86
16. Walker, PS, and Erkman, MJ (1975) The role of the menisci in force transmission across the knee. Clinical Orthopaedics and Related Research, 109, 184–192

Chapter 2
The Historical Perspective of Mobile-Bearing Knee Implants

R. D. Jones

1   Introduction

Conventional fixed-bearing total knees have mid to long-term follow-ups of 10–15 years demonstrating good results [6, 12, 13]. The patients in most studies of fixed-bearing implants have been older patients with low activity levels, and subsequently low demands on the implant [4]. Twenty to twenty-five year results with fixed-bearing designs are unknown at this time.

Studies have shown that the contact stresses of condylar total knees can surpass the yield strength of ultra-high molecular weight polyethylene [1]. The contact stress can be even greater when the prosthesis design has low tibiofemoral conformity and cyclic sliding occurs which produces significant polyethylene wear [2]. The non-conforming articular designs of total knees in the 1970's and 1980's have been replaced by more conforming designs in the late 1990's. Polyethylene wear can also occur on the undersurface of the tibial insert with micromotion between it and the tibial baseplate in modular, fixed-bearing designs [10, 16]. Such "backside wear" cannot be eliminated as long as we continue to use fixed-bearing, modular tibial designs. The creation of small polyethylene particles (<5 microns) from abrasive wear has led to significant osteolysis [11, 16]. The generation of polyethylene debris, wherever it occurs, is detrimental to the long-term survival of total knee arthroplasty.

With the recent trend for more conforming fixed-bearing designs, the implant constraint becomes higher and less forgiving. This increasing conformity transfers stress to the tibial insert-tibial baseplate interface, just as non-modular designs transfer stress to the bone implant interface [10]. Therefore, the challenge of total knee arthroplasty is to improve the wear potential and long-term function by resolving that kinematic conflict between a conforming, low stress articulation and rotational freedom.

Mobile-bearing implant designs diminish the surface and sub-surface polyethylene stresses by increasing the bearing contact area and the conformity. Such mobile-bearing total knees can allow femoral articular conformity with rotation, while fixed-bearing designs compromise rotation significantly when conformity is increased.

2   The Rotating Platform Mobile-Bearing Knee Implant

The original patent on a rotating platform type of mobile-bearing knee implant was given to Doug Noiles, an engineer at U.S. Surgical Corporation. This implant was used in a hinge knee system called the Noiles Hinge Knee. Noiles' patent went with him as he joined Joint Medical Products of Stamford, CT to produce the Noiles Hinge Knee. Later, the Noiles-PS knee prosthesis, a rotating platform, posterior stabilized design was introduced. Subsequently, all rotating platform knee designs had to pay licensing fees to Noiles and Joint Medical Products until the patent expired in 1997. The expiration of the patent triggered wide-spread activity among many orthopedic device manufacturing companies in further development of mobile-bearing total knee arthroplasty. This has led to the introduction of many other companies' mobile-bearing knee implants. While some have unique designs, many are directly based on the rotating platform concept.

Buechel and Pappas originally developed the New Jersey Knee (DePuy, Warsaw, IN) as a meniscal bearing mobile knee using two polyethylene bearings in curved tracks along the medial and lateral aspects of the metal tibial baseplate. The design allowed for cruciate retention. Shortly thereafter Buechel and Pappas introduced the rotating platform mobile-bearing knee and it was renamed the LCS (low contact stress – DePuy, Warsaw, IN). The LCS is the most widely used mobile-bearing knee system in the world. Sorrells has reported a 94.7% survivorship at 11 years [14] and Callaghan et al reported excellent results and no revisions in over 100 patients at 9–12 years follow-up [5].

3   Conclusions

The rotating platform mobile-bearing knee evolved from the need to create a better knee arthroplasty system. Such knees resolve the kinematic conflict between increasing conformity and rotational freedom, thusly creating high contact but low contact stress. Experimental studies have shown that highly congruent surfaces undergoing unidirectional articulation have negligible wear. Rotating platforms with flat poly bearing surfaces on a highly polished chrome cobalt tibial base plate diminish the problem of "backside wear" of polyethylene. The results of the rotating platform total knee arthroplasty compare favorably to results found with fixed-bearing total knee systems [4]. If wear is the predominant failure mode, longer term studies should confirm a superiority with the rotating platform type of total knee arthroplasty designs.

References

1. Bartel DL, Bicknell VL, Wright TM (1986) The effect of conformity, thickness, and material on stresses in ultra-high molecular weight components for total joint replacement. J Bone Joint Surg 68 A: 1041–1051
2. Blunn GW, Walker PS, Joshi A, Hardinge K (1991) The dominance of cyclic sliding in producing wear in total knee replacements. Clin Orthop 273: 253–260
3. Callaghan JJ (2000) Reduction of polyethylene wear in mobile-bearing knees. Orthopaedics Today, Thorofare, NJ
4. Callaghan JJ, Insall JN, Greenwald AS, Dennis DA, Komistek RD, Murray DW, Bourne RB, Rorabeck CH, Dorr LD (2000) Mobile-bearing knee replacement: concepts and results. J Bone Joint Surg 82 A:1020–1037
5. Callaghan JJ, Squire MW, Goetz DD, Sullivan PM, Johnston RC (2000) Cemented rotating-platform total knee replacement: a nine to twelve-year follow-up study. J Bone Joint Surg 82 A: 705–711
6. Colliza WA, Insall JN, Scuderi GR (1995) The posterior stabilized total knee prosthesis: assessment of polyethylene damage and osteolysis after a ten-year-minimum follow-up. J Bone Joint Surg 77 A: 1713–1720
7. Goodfellow JW, O'Connor JJ (1992) The anterior cruciate ligament in knee arthroplasty: a risk factor in unconstrained meniscal prostheses. Clin Orthop 276: 245–252
8. James P (2000) Making the transition from a fixed-bearing to a mobile-bearing design. Orthopedics Today, Thorofare, NJ
9. Jones VC, Barton DC, Fitzpatrick DP, Auger DD, Stone MH, Fisher J (1999) An experimental model of tibial counterface polyethylene wear in mobile bearing knees: the influence of design and kinematics. Biomed Mater Eng 9: 189–196
10. Parks NL, Engh GA, Topoleski LDT, Emperado J (1998) Modular tibial insert micromotion: a concern with contemporary knee implants. Clin Orthop 356: 10–15
11. Peters PC, Engh GA, Dwyer KA, Vinh TN (1992) Osteolysis after total knee arthroplasty without cement. J Bone Joint Surg 74 A: 864–876
12. Ranawat CS, Flynn Jr WF, Saddler S, Hansraj KK, Maynard MJ (1993) Long-term results of the total condylar knee arthroplasty: a 15-year survivorship study. Clin Orthop 286: 94–102
13. Schai PA, Thornhill TS, Scott RD (1998) Total knee arthroplasty with the PFC system: results at a minimum of ten years and survivorship analysis. J Bone Joint Surg 80B: 850–858
14. Sorrells RB (1996) Primary knee arthroplasty: long-term outcomes. the rotating platform mobile bearing TKA. Orthopedics 19: 793–796
15. Trent PS, Walker PS (1976) Ligament length patterns, strength, and rotational axes of the knee joint. Clin Orthop 117: 263–270
16. Wasielewski RC, Parks N, Williams I, Surprenant H, Collier JP, Engh G (1997) Tibial insert undersurface as a contributing source of polyethylene wear debris. Clin Orthop 345: 53–59

Chapter 3
The LCS Story

F. F. Buechel

1 The Early Beginning

As a first year orthopaedic surgery resident at New Jersey Medical School in Newark, New Jersey, I first met Michael J. Pappas, PhD, my biomechanics teacher from New Jersey Institute of Technology, (NJIT) (also in Newark, N.J.). It was early in 1974 when my orthopaedic chairman, Anthony F. DePalma, MD (a feisty, world renowned shoulder surgeon and founder of Clinical Orthopaedics and Related Research) decided that his orthopaedic residents needed to have an understanding of engineering principles as they applied to bone and joint surgery. To that end he enlisted two mechanical engineering volunteers from NJIT, Harry Herman, PhD and his junior associate Michael J. Pappas, PhD.

They gladly came to Martland Hospital in Newark once weekly to give us lectures on Forces, Kinematics and Structural design. The orthopaedic residents were overwhelmed by the mathematics involved and perceived lack of relationship to the field of orthopaedics. I was one of those intimidated residents, but I recall asking questions like: "Dr. Pappas, bridge building is all well and good, but can these principles help us to identify stronger nails and plates used to fix fractures?" Dr. Pappas responded by asking to be shown the various internal fixation appliances so he could mechanically evaluate them for strength and durability. I promptly supplied some old Jewett, Massie, and Holt nails for his review and he promptly used cantilever-bending equations, combined with strength of materials science to give us the answers. To me, it was enlightening to know that our field of orthopaedics could be more fully understood by understanding basic mechanical engineering principles. Time-based senior surgeon knowledge of bone remodeling could be compressed by understanding the nature of bone loading forces and their biomechanical consequences.

In addition, the field of joint replacement, which was quite new in 1974, could be more easily understood with mechanical engineering concepts, and in fact, was not intelligible without them. Concepts such as compressive, tensile and shear loading as well as material property strengths were for the first time integrated into our orthopaedic knowledge base. Kinematic motion studies gave us an improved understanding of normal joint function while suggesting the direction for prosthetic joint function.

2 The First Mobile-Bearing

After an unsuccessful attempt to develop a satisfactory fixed-bearing, cylindrical total ankle replacement, [5] Dr. Pappas and I developed the first mobile-bearing joint replacement in 1974, called the "Floating-Socket" total shoulder (Fig. 1) [2]. This device had two spheres with offset pivot points that extended the range of motion of simple ball-socket systems and had application in constrained knee and hip embodiments, which were never clinically tested. The floating-center prosthetic joint United States patent, [3] which was filed in 1974, issued in 1975 after a successful interference was concluded against the kinematically similar "Spherocentric" shoulder replacement. Our earlier conception, diligence and reduction to practice prevailed in the interference proceeding.

This "Floating-Socket" shoulder device seemed to solve a basic lack of motion problem seen in early ball-socket implants. Clinical and animal (chimpanzee) research with this device [1] gained national attention as the Founder's Award Paper at the Eastern Orthopaedic Annual Meeting at the Breaker's Hotel in Palm Beach, Florida in 1976.

3 Commercial Interest in Mobile-Bearings

Several implant companies, most notably DePuy, became interested in the floating-socket shoulder replacement and offered a licensing agreement for the right to

Fig. 1 a–d. Early models of
the LCS Knee Repalcement.
a Mark I fully congruent fixed
bearing tibial and patellar replacements. b Lateral Mo-
bile bearing with constrained
AP motion and fixed me-
dial bearing. c Medial straight
track mobile bearing and lateral curved track mobile
bearing. d Both mobile bearings have curved tracks

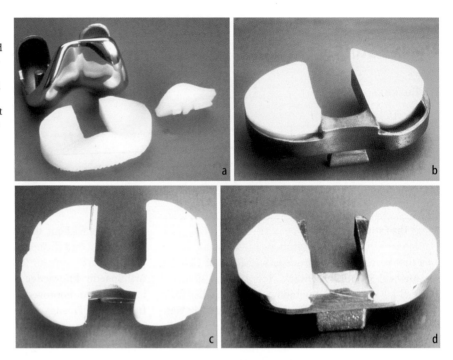

manufacture and sell it. Dr. Pappas and I were interested
in the offer, but wished to pursue development of a knee
replacement system as part of the deal, and specifically
linked our acceptance of the agreement to the acceptance of our knee system once it was developed. This
was put into writing in 1977 and marked the initiation of
formal development of the New Jersey Integrated Knee
Replacement System.

4   Knee Design Challenges of the 1970's

Dr. Pappas and I had been working on a fixed-bearing knee replacement in 1975 and 1976 to improve
upon similar implants of the time. Challenges to be addressed in TKR surgery at that time were lowering contact stresses on the poly in both the patellofemoral articulation as well as tibiofemoral articulation to reduce
wear. Additionally, overconstraint was seen to cause
loosening, so minimizing or eliminating constraint in
knee replacement was an important issue. More uniform bone loading using metal support was also an important concept to be explored to eliminate poly bending of tibial and patella bearing surfaces.

5   The Meniscal Bearing Connection

A key moment in time was February 1977 at the annual AAOS meeting in Las Vegas, when Dr. Pappas and

I attended a research society meeting in which Dr. John
O'Conner, (a mechanical engineer from Oxford, England) presented a concept of meniscal washers (bearings) to be used with intact cruciate ligaments to allow
normal knee kinematics after TKR. This presentation
stimulated me tremendously, although Dr. Pappas was
less enthused. By allowing congruity with mobility, the
artificial knee could reduce contact stress on the bearing surface and eliminate constraint forces – the two major challenges of the time. Of course, there were drawbacks to a completely free-floating meniscal bearing in
the knee joint, most notably irreducible dislocation.

We did not collaborate at all with the Oxford Group.
The reason that our knee inventions, which were licensed to DePuy in 1977, required a sublicense from the
Oxford Group was that our Floating-Center prosthetic
joint patent claims, which superceded the Oxford patent, were too narrow to govern the Oxford claims, a mistake of our patent attorney, R. Gale Rhodes, Jr., when he
filed in 1974. The additional wording of "a floating-bear-
ing with a curvature of infinite radius" would have covered meniscal bearings! Our loss was Oxford's gain. The
trade-off was acceptable.

6   Developing The LCS Knee

The early days of knee replacement development, after signing the license agreement with DePuy in 1977,
led to a methodical program of mobile-bearing design

including models and cadaver trials (Fig. 2). My own knee X-rays were used to document normal roll back of the femur on the tibia. Fresh above-knee amputation specimens were then used to assess similar meniscal bearing roll back in our radial track meniscal bearing prototype models (Fig. 3). This process was quite rapid and occurred over a six month period. My access to anatomical specimens at N.J. Medical School and N.J. Orthopaedic Hospital as well as Dr. Pappas' access to model making and machining facilities both locally and at N.J. Institute of Technology made for rapid turn around of models and prototypes. Additionally, since there were no committees involved to curtail our development activities, we became of one mind and direction. By August 1977, we had sufficient confidence in the mobile-bearing knee design that implantable prototypes were fabricated at a dental laboratory in Irvington, New Jersey, the town in which we both lived at that time.

7 Initial LCS Knee Implantation

On September 22, 1977, I implanted the first cemented, medial, unicompartmental mobile-bearing knee replacement (later to be known as the New Jersey Knee) at N.J. Orthopaedic Hospital in Orange, N.J. The patient was a 64 year old 178 lb. 5 foot 7 inch tall, osteoarthritic man who had a medical meniscectomy 5 years before. He died 10 years later of heart failure, but enjoyed a normally functioning knee replacement until the end. This first implant was a prototype design, made of induction casted Co-Cr-Mo, which was ethylene oxide sterilized. The meniscal bearing was sculpted with a scalpel at surgery to give it a better shape to prevent bony and soft tissue impingement. This sculpted bearing shape was then mechanically defined by Dr. Pappas and future meniscal bearings were fabricated to the sculpted dimensions.

In 1978 the first cemented bicruciate retaining meniscal bearing TKR with a rotating bearing patella was implanted in a 72 year old 125 lb, 5'6" tall osteoarthritic female who enjoyed her knee without complication for 16 years until her death in 1994.

The first cemented rotating platform prototype was also implanted in 1978 in a 59 year old rheumatoid man who had a failed Geomedic knee after 2 years. He enjoyed his prosthesis for 16 years until his death. His family granted us retrieval rights to his knee replacement which showed minimal signs of wear on his ethylene oxide sterilized bearings (Fig. 4). We developed the initial wooden models and molds for lost wax casting of Co-Cr-Mo rotating platforms and bicruciate retain-

ing meniscal bearing tibial components as well as the femoral component and rotating patella metallic backplate, all were of one size (standard). The wooden models were made by Nelson Model Makers in Bloomfield, N.J. and the original machining of metal and polyethylene prototype implants were done by machinists Jack Wilkins, Herb Schraft and Rudy Neuhauser at Alco Machine & Tool Co, also in Bloomfield, New Jersey. We used to eat at the King George Restaurant around the corner from their shop to discuss the complexities of machining these unique parts.

8 Depuy Decides to Manufacture the LCS Knee

In 1979, with 2 years of clinical experience, Dr. Pappas and I put together a significant slide presentation based upon our early biomechanical studies; mechan-

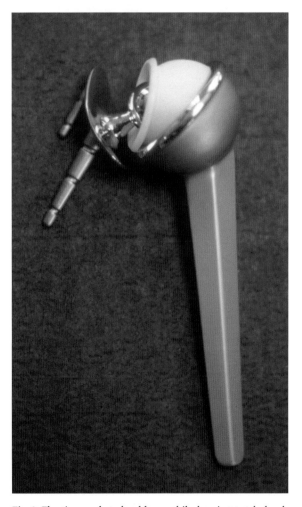

Fig. 2. Floating socket shoulder, mobile bearing total shoulder replacement

Fig. 3. Cadaveric Models used to assess rollback and component design. As the knee is flexed, the bearings are shown to move posterior

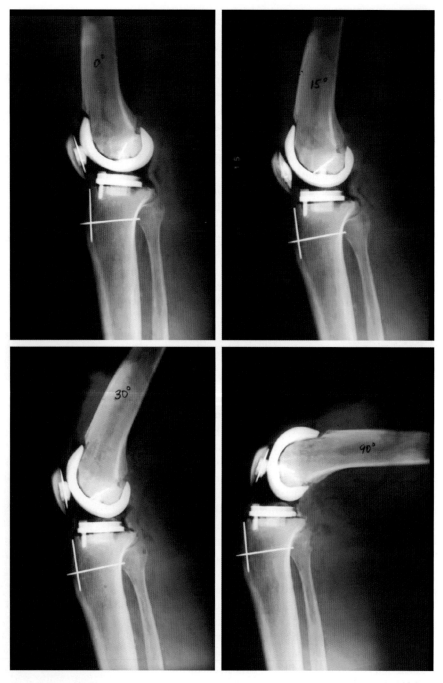

ical simulator studies comparing meniscal bearings to total condylar and Townley tibial bearings; short term clinical studies and retrieval studies. This presentation which was given at the Ocean Reef Club in Key Largo, Florida demonstrated the improved wear performance of meniscal bearings over conventional fixed-bearings and documented highly acceptable clinical performance of these cemented implants. The audience assembled for this meeting included orthopaedic professors

from around the United States, who collectively composed the implant advisory panel of DePuy. After the presentation of the New Jersey Integrated Knee Replacement System was concluded, the panel asked me questions, then voted as to whether or not DePuy should proceed with marketing this new total knee design. The vote of the approximately 10 panel members was a unanimous yes! This meeting gave DePuy confidence that this knee replacement system had viability in the market-

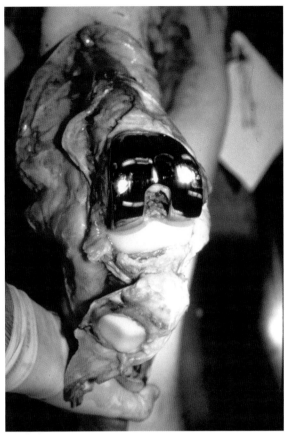

Fig. 4. Sixteen year retrieval of an active rotating platform showing minimal signs of wear

place. Richard Nikolaev, the executive vice-president of DePuy, in charge of the total knee project gave the "go ahead" to engineering and manufacturing at that meeting to go into production of the New Jersey Knee, as it was then called.

9   Other Surgeons and the FDA

Shortly thereafter in mid 1979, Dr. Barry Sorrells from Little Rock, Arkansas flew his own plane with his operating room staff to Warsaw, Indiana and then to New Jersey to learn about the New Jersey Knee System. He was having loosening problems with the overconstrained Geomedic knee replacement and was looking for a good tricompartmental substitute. After a "wee hours" hotel room presentation in Livingston, New Jersey, Dr. Sorrells fell in love with the rotating platform components of the knee system and began using them exclusively. Twenty years later he continued to successfully use the rotating platform and became a key speaker for DePuy around the world. He was both eloquent and down-to-earth in

his presentations and Learning Center Courses, which were well received and very influential, especially internationally.

In the meantime, also in 1979, the United States Food and Drug Administration (FDA) refused to allow sale of the New Jersey Knee as a 510 K device (grandfathered device similar to devices in existence prior to 1976, when FDA medical device legislation was enacted). Despite compelling arguments by Dr. Pappas and myself at FDA headquarters in Rockville, Maryland, the FDA determined that this mobile-bearing device required a Pre-Market Approval (PMA) and Investigational Device Exemption (IDE) clinical trial to prove safety and efficacy before being allowed to be sold on the United States medical market.

10   FDA Multicenter Clinical Trials

DePuy organized the multi-center FDA clinical trial for the New Jersey Knee System and began seeking clinical investigators for me to surgically train. Dr. Blackwell "Buzz" Sawyer from Point Pleasant, New Jersey was extremely interested in this knee and signed on early to do meniscal bearings. He was a kind, father-figure who was involved with Dr. Emmet Lunceford (the father of the AML hip) in an orthopaedic scuba diving society called OST (Orthopaedic Surgery and Trauma). I was invited to speak at their annual diving meeting and became an active member and later President. During my initial years with the diving group I was fortunate to meet Dr. Peter Keblish from Allentown, Pennsylvania. He was a strong-willed, veteran orthopaedic surgeon with Vietnam war experience, who became extremely interested in the meniscal bearing and rotating platform concepts, and like Dr. Sawyer and Dr. Sorrells, he signed-on early as a clinical investigator. Dr. Keblish became extremely valuable to the New Jersey Knee project as a speaker and training surgeon both at home in his Allentown Learning Center and around the world.

Many other United States orthopaedic surgeons also became involved both during and after the FDA clinical trials to advance the mobile-bearing knee concepts, for which Dr. Pappas and I remain eternally grateful.

The cemented FDA clinical trials were presented in Washington, D.C. on July 11, 1984 and involved 918 knee replacements followed for a minimum of 2 years from 23 orthopaedic surgeons. Clinically, over 90 % of patients were doing quite well, but a question from the FDA panel engineer nearly stopped the process in its tracks. The question, "What are the simulator results?" was asked. Dr. Pappas and I had only preliminary one million cycle results on one set of meniscal bearings, used as a screening test against the higher wearing total condylar and Town-ley devices. I thought our trial would be rejected, when out of the audience, as if riding a "white horse", came Dr. Seth Greenwald who cheerfully reported, "I have 10 million cycle simulation on three sets of meniscal bearings which show minimal wear and an improvement over fixed-bearings". With this mechanical data and our medium term clinical data, the panel voted unanimously to approve the New Jersey Knee System for cemented use. Formal FDA approval arrived in 1985, after which DePuy began seriously marketing the device. The FDA cementless New Jersey LCS clinical trials were then successfully completed between 1984 and 1991 with nearly identical results to the cemented trials.

11   Resistance to the Mobile-Bearing Concept

In the United States there was strong resistance to the mobile-bearing concept by the "Boston – New York – Baltimore Influenced" knee replacement surgeons. At most meetings in the mid-1980's I was the only speaker on the subject of mobile-bearing design. Quite often I was ridiculed during panel discussions and shunned at social gatherings. Although troublesome, I always enjoyed private camaraderie and was exposed to some great wines and exotic places. Today, many of these same surgeons are friendly colleagues who embrace the mobile-bearing concept.

12   International Influence

Knee replacement concepts began to change when the Porous Coated Anatomic (PCA) Knee replacement began to fail in the mid 1980's. In 1984, a wonderfully-bright Dutch orthopaedic surgeon from Amsterdam visited me at New Jersey Orthopaedic Hospital in Orange, New Jersey. Dr. Karel Hamelynck, who has become one of my best friends, was on a "Don Quixote" mission from Holland to find the biomechanical "best knee" in the world. After spending one full day in my operating room watching how meniscal bearings function in vivo, he was convinced that it was the New Jersey Knee. He went back to Amsterdam with this new knowledge and began the first European cementless New Jersey Knee implantations. His good results were similar to my results and we began to collaborate openly. His speaking knowledge of five languages and his open and friendly manner made him an invaluable resource for DePuy and the European orthopaedic community. At his learning centers in Amsterdam he would host surgeons from around the world and speak to them in their native lan-guage. I was always happy when he decided to speak English, of course!

Dr. Hamelynck and I with the help of Dr. Pappas developed biomechanical presentations that explained the PCA Knee wear problem and the general wear or loosening problems associated with fixed-bearing knee designs. Because the wear issue was so important the term low-contact-stress (LCS) began to dominate our discussions. So dominant was this LCS concept that DePuy decided to change the name of our knee to the New Jersey LCS Knee System.

The LCS Knee, as it came to be called later, had the solution to the wear problems seen with the failing PCA knee and other fixed-bearing knee systems. As such, the European orthopaedic community as well as the New Zealand and Australian communities embraced the advanced mobile-bearing concepts and without regret put them to work for their patients. This growing influence of the LCS concept has led to worldwide acceptance of mobile-bearings and in fact now dominates the international market for total knee devices. It has been wonderful to see that "the truth shall prevail".

13   John Insall Endorses the Mobile-Bearing Concept

In the United States, however, the LCS concept had been slow to flourish, until Dr. John Insall himself, "came out-of-the-closet" in favor of mobile-bearings over fixed-bearings as the best way to improve long term wear performance in total knees [4]. His untimely death in 2000 may unfortunately stall his supporters from changing to mobile-bearing from the traditional Insall-Burstein designs which he began to abandon. Additionally, the dominance of fixed-bearing knee designers in the United States has produced an economically based group which will be slow to divest their interests.

14   Reflection on the LCS Knee

It is with great affection and pride that Dr. Pappas and I recall the development of this unique New Jersey LCS Mobile-Bearing Total Knee System together with the association of the many fine surgeons, engineers and salesman around the world that contributed to its success. It remains the only knee system to have been formally approved by the FDA in both cemented and cementless embodiments through the clinical trial process before being released for sale. We are also extremely grateful to those progressive orthopaedic surgeons around the world who have had the fortitude to use a device based on sound mechanical engineering and biological prin-

ciples rather than commercial hype. We hope these principles will continue to be embraced, encouraged and improved upon for the future good of our patients.

References

1. Buechel FF (1977) Shoulder replacement in the chimpanzee:
   surgical and post-operative management. J Med Primatol-
   ogy 6: 274–283
2. Buechel FF, Pappas MJ, De Palma AF (1978) "Floating-Socket"
   total shoulder replacement: anatomical, biomechanical and
   surgical rationale. J Biomed Mater Res 1: 89–114
3. Buechel FF, Pappas, MJ (1975) U.S. Patent No. 3,916,451;
   "Floating-Socket Joint"
4. Insall JN (1998) Adventures in mobile-bearing knee design:
   A mid-life crisis. Orthop 21: 1021–1023
5. Pappas MJ, Buechel FF, De Palma A F (1976) Cylindrical total ankle joint replacement: surgical and biomechanical rationale. Clin Orthop 118: 82–92

Design of the LCS

II

Chapter 4
Biomechanics of Total Knee Arthroplasty (TKA)

K. J. Hamelynck, J.-L. Briard, M. J. Pappas

1   Introduction

When discussing the biomechanics and some tribological aspects of total knee replacement (TKR), it makes sense to look at normal knee anatomy and function in order to understand the natural motions and forces about the knee joint. However it should be realized that a replaced knee may look like a normal knee on the outside but in fact it is very different from the normal knee. Additionally, the knee being replaced is itself not normal, but a knee changed by pathology.

Components of total knee replacement systems may look like the natural surfaces of the femur and tibia but their geometry is quite different; the medial and lateral femoral condyles in knee replacement systems are usually identical which is never the case in the normal knee. These components need to be fixed to bone whilst taking into account their shape and size.

No replacement system can be designed taking into account all possible individual varieties of knee anatomy, among other problems it would simply be impossible for financial reasons.

2   The Normal Knee

The knee is an extremely complex joint comprising of three bones, femur, tibia and patella. This skeletal structure is stabilized by capsular and ligamentous structures and has the ability to move in six different directions and to sustain external loads of 6–8 times body weight without loosing stability. The knee is able to carry out well controlled movements at the same time.

Looking at the anatomy of the joint it is hard to say whether form determines function or function determines form. The interrelationship between the anatomical structures, motions and the loading forces about the knee joint is of extreme importance. Motion characteristics of the knee may be studied separately, but it remains of more interest to look at the knee as one whole

system. During activities, there is a constant need for a total balance in the joint between loading forces and resisting structures, this guarantees stability of the knee but also allows for motion.

2.1   Knee Motion

The movements of the knee are multi-directional and complex. Six movements may be distinguished, three rotations and three translations (Fig. 1). These movements may be described separately, but it must remain clear that most movements are made in combination with other movements. These movements are determined by the passive motion characteristics of the knee and external loads [3, 6].

The flexion-extension movement is the most prominent of all movements of the knee joint. The shape of the articular surfaces and menisci, and the presence of ligaments especially the cruciate ligaments define this movement induced by muscular force. The normal flexion-extension range is typically considered to be about 145° [14]. The maximum active flexion is about 135 degrees whereas maximum passive flexion is about 162° [9]. Any restriction of this motion is undesirable as it adversely affects knee function and can produce undesirable knee loading.

During normal knee flexion, the action of the posterior cruciate and the shape of the articulating surfaces produce roll back of the femur on the tibia. Roll forward during extension is produced by the action of the anterior cruciate. As a result of this rollback phenomenon, flexion of the knee is improved because no impingement of the femoral diaphysis on the tibia will occur, and the force and effectiveness of the extensor mechanism is optimized because the lever arm is of maximal length.

Roll back on the more congruent medial condyle is about 5 mm while the roll back on the relatively incongruent lateral condyle is about 15 mm [12]. The dis-

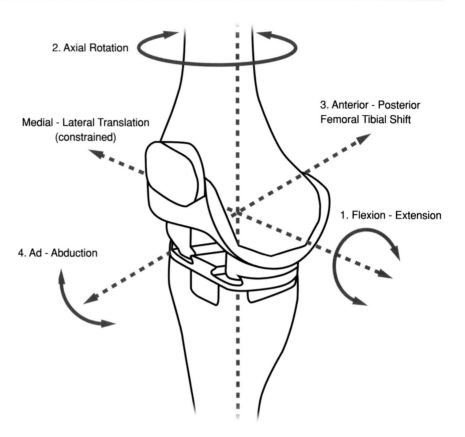

ruption of the cruciate ligaments disrupts the normal
roll back function making anterior-posterior motion
unpredictable. Typically without the anterior cruciate
function, the posterior cruciate ligament may pull the
femorotibial contact posteriorly in extension, and with
weightbearing, there is paradoxical roll forward.

The axial rotatory laxity varies from 0 degrees in full
extension to 40–60 degrees in 90 degrees of flexion [2].
This freedom of rotation is almost independent of the
amount of torque applied expressing the fact that the
limits of the envelope of passive motion are very stiff. The
structures limiting rotation are different for internal and
external rotation; resisting internal rotation is a function
of the cruciate ligaments, where external rotation is
controlled by the collateral ligaments. The cruciate
ligaments having a short moment arm are not strong
enough to control internal rotation alone. The cup shaped,
articular surface of the medial tibial condyle provides an
important contribution. In external rotation the collateral
ligaments are almost strong enough to take all loads.

Axial rotation can potentially occur during normal
human activities, such as rising from a chair or from a
seated position on the floor [9]. During walking axial rotation is about +/– 6° [5].

Additionally, ad/abduction is normal during
many human activities, for example during walking

about 8° of abduction occurs [5, 14]. Varus-valgus
rotations, when compared to flexion-extension and
axial rotations are relatively small, but the fact that
they occur is of great importance when discussing
the biomechanics of total knee replacement. If this
fact is ignored and varus-valgus movements are not
permitted by the prosthesis, the oscillating varus –
valgus movements and loads may cause mechanical
loosening of a component (Fig. 2).

What is more, as a result of the varus-valgus movements, compression of the articular surfaces will not be
evenly distributed over the medial and lateral surface.
Loading constantly changes from the medial to the lateral tibial condyle and vice versa. This has serious implications for the materials to be used in an artificial knee,
as most of the load during walking will be transmitted
to one condyle only.

Patellofemoral motion is essentially dependent on
tibiofemoral motion. The axial rotation of the tibia with
respect to the femur, produces a medial-lateral excursion of the patella tendon insertion resulting in axial rotation of the patella relative to the femur. Rotation produced during walking is about 6 degrees of internal rotation and 8 degrees of external rotation [14]. Rotation
can be more than double these amounts for other normal activities.

Fig. 2. Oscillating varus-valgus movements of the knee

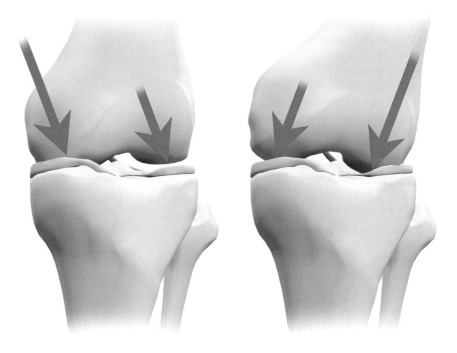

The patella does not articulate with the sulcus of the femur until about 30 of flexion due to the oblique pull of the quadriceps. The patella tends toward a lateral tilt until about 45 degrees where high compressive loads force contact with the femur on both lateral and medial middle facets of the patella [12].

Apart from the aforementioned three rotations that the knee may exert, three translations also have to be taken into account; one in the axial direction when the knee is loaded and the articular surfaces compressed, one in medial-lateral direction and one in anterior-posterior direction. In a knee with intact collateral and cruciate ligaments medial and lateral translation is small and the forces causing this translation well balanced, but this situation may change a lot in the absence of cruciate ligaments. The anterior-posterior translations in a knee well balanced by intact cruciate ligaments and articular surfaces remain well within the envelope of passive motion and anterior-posterior forces have little effect. However any change in geometry of the surfaces and absence of a cruciate ligament may result in a totally different situation. This is a situation generally seen or created during total knee replacement.

The passive motion characteristics of the knee, as described above, may demonstrate clearly that freedom of passive motion is strongly dependent on the flexion-extension position of the knee; almost complete rigidity in extension and far greater freedom in flexion.

2.2   Stability of the Knee

The knee is stabilized in three different ways, there is the intrinsic stability given by the geometry of the articular surfaces and menisci and the extrinsic stability given by the restraint of the surrounding soft tissues; ligaments and capsule.

The most powerful stabilizers are the muscles stabilizing the knee dynamically. The muscles carry out activities to make the knee move, to resist external loads and to stabilize the joint. Some of these activities are being carried out consciously by the individual, but it must be realized that most activities are done sub-consciously and guided by mechanisms like proprioceptis and reflex. The information the muscles need to function effectively is provided by the neuroreceptors, which may be found in all soft tissues around the joint; muscles, capsule and ligaments.

In the normal knee, several structures stabilize the joint and resist varus-valgus loads. The amount of restraint exerted by these structures is again dependent on the position of the knee. The medial restraining structures are the medial collateral ligament (mcl), the posteromedial capsule and the cruciate ligaments. The mcl is the most important stabilizer. In the fully extended position the mcl takes 57.4% of the load. The contribution of the cruciate ligaments is important, accounting for 14.8% of the load, but the contribution of the posteromedial capsule is remarkable taking 17.5% [5]. In flexion, the contribution of the posteromedial capsule is minimal and reduced to 3.6%.this is due to the fact that the posterior capsule is slack in the flexed position. However, the restraining activity of the posteromedial capsule is strong enough to almost completely stabilize the fully extended knee even when the mcl is cut!

Lateral restraint against varus motion is provided for by the lateral collateral ligament (lcl), the lateral and posterior capsule and the cruciate ligaments. The contribution of the lcl is important as is the contribution of the posterior arcuate complex, but like on the medial side, this is only true in the extended position. The contribution of the cruciate ligaments is also important, taking 22.2% of the loads in 5 degrees of flexion and 12.3% in 25 degrees of flexion [5].

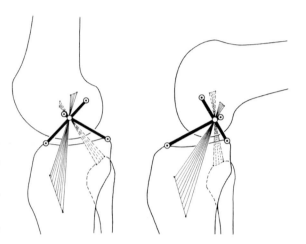

Fig. 3. Close cooperation of cruciate and collateral ligaments in extension and flexion [8]

2.3   The Role of the Cruciate and Collateral Ligaments

It has become clear that the cruciate ligaments play an important role in controlling the rollback movement of the femur during flexion movements. The amount of function of the cruciate ligaments is very much dependent on the position of the knee and the direction of the forces. Anterior translation is mostly restrained by the acl, especially in the extended position and posterior translation by the pcl, conversely, especially in the flexed knee.

The cruciate ligaments also provide a considerable contribution to medial and lateral stabilization of the knee and in restraining rotation. The stabilizing role of the cruciate ligaments is generally underestimated, particularly in total knee arthroplasty where cruciate ligaments are seldom retained. The cruciate ligaments may well be considered as the collateral ligaments of the compartments: the anterior cruciate ligament (acl) for the lateral compartment and the posterior cruciate ligament (pcl) for the medial compartment [8]. It needs to be noticed that as in flexion-extension, where the cruciate ligaments work together to control rollback, in restraining varus-valgus loads, the cruciate ligaments do not function independently of each other especially in near full extension. This is particularly important as this is the position where most loads are applied at the joint.

What is more, most activities are exerted in close cooperation with the collateral ligaments (Fig. 3).

Ligaments are strong structures and may conduct considerable loads. In physiological conditions they are loaded up to about 30% of their ultimate strength, so rupture of a ligament will not easily occur. The ligaments may stretch up to 3% and recover. With further stretching, plastic deformity will take place and at 9%

the ligament will rupture [16]. Ligaments in the knee do in fact conduct considerable loads [7] and in this respect all ligaments of the knee are important stabilizers. During total knee replacement the surgeon is often confronted with the question of whether the cruciate ligaments should be retained or sacrificed. The surgeon must realize that absence of a ligament as a result of disease or trauma, or as a result of a surgical intervention (!) will cause a redistribution of forces over the available ligaments. This may overload and stretch, or rupture the ligament, depending on mechanical factors such as activity, weight and the quality of the ligament.

2.4   The Loading Forces About the Knee Joint

During activities of daily living considerable forces are being applied at the knee. These forces are dependent considerably on the kind of activity (level walking, running, stair climbing or descending) and also by anatomical abnormalities outside the knee joint (a stiff hip, a varus deformity of the tibia), habits – perhaps change to lifestyle, posture, body weight and velocity of the action.

Compressive forces are by far the greatest. They are usually expressed in terms of body weight, as there is a strong correlation between body weight and compressive force. The kind of activity defines the magnitude of the compressive force, for instance, running or descending stairs causes much higher compressive forces than level walking.

The compressive forces active at the knee (Fig. 4) may amount to 6–7 times body weight during normal physical activities [11]. During walking there is a high load shortly after heel strike and a peak load when the

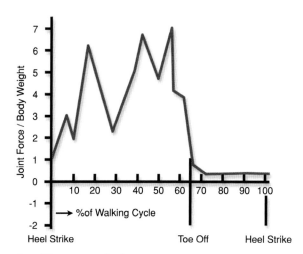

Fig. 4. The compressive forces

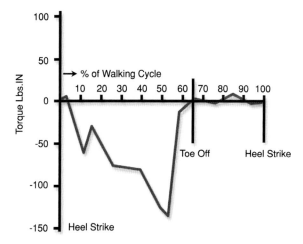

Fig. 5. Torque, highest before "toe-off"

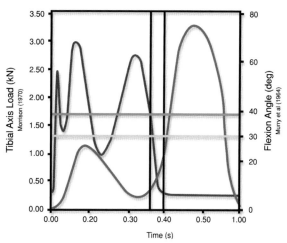

Fig. 6. Highest compressive forces are seen after heelstrike and before "toe-off", when the knee is in 10–25 degrees of flexion

This moment of push off is extremely important. At that moment, not only does most compressive loading occur, but also at the same time lateral shear forces and torque try to dislocate the knee laterally creating external rotation. It is interesting to observe that the knee, during the moments of peak loading, is in a position between 0 and 20 degrees of flexion (Fig. 6).

This may explain why in the natural knee the articular tibial surface is not perpendicular to the tibial axis but in 7–10 degrees of flexion. This must have implications for the design of tibial components of total knee replacement systems and their placement relative to the tibia. Another important detail is that at the time of maximal loading, the knee is close to full extension and all ligaments are under tension.

foot is pushing the body off, to go in a forward direction. Directly after this push-off activity the foot looses contact with the ground, "toe-off", after which moment the compressive forces are reduced to almost 0 and the swing phase of walking commences. This pushing moment just before toe-off is a very important one because not only are the compressive forces at their greatest, but so to are the shear and rotational forces.

An anterior shear force of 1 times body weight is exerted after heel strike and a posterior shear force of 2 times body weight at push off. During the whole stand phase of walking a relatively small shear force is directed medially, but at the moment of push off this force is converted into a lateral shear force of 1.5 times body weight.

During walking a rotational force is exerted at the knee, which is again highest at push off (Fig. 5).

3   The Replaced Knee

During total knee replacement, the intrinsic stability of the knee, shaped by the geometry of the articular surfaces and the menisci, is destroyed by the surgeon. This is in order to create a joint space big enough to implant a new spacer, the prosthesis. Also, part of the extrinsic stability is removed as very often during knee replacement the cruciate ligaments are sacrificed.

By removing the cruciate ligaments, often necessary in order to create room for the introduction of a central peg for fixation of the tibial component, the mechanical function of the ligaments is sacrificed. Their neurological function (propriocepsis) which provides active stabilization of the knee by muscles is sacrificed as well. The muscles themselves may also be somewhat damaged during surgery.

3.1 The Goal of Total Knee Replacement

Because the complaints of patients requiring TKA are serious pain, lack of motion and instability, the goal of TKR is to provide the patient with a knee, which is free of any pain, with a good stability and a physiological range of motion. Once these goals are achieved the result should last forever, fixation must be permanent and wear of the materials used minimal.

3.2 Stability of the Replaced Knee

Stability is the most important need in knee replacement. Without stability walking is not possible, but stability may counteract other goals of TKA. Thus, the way in which stability of the replaced knee is achieved is very important. As written before, the intrinsic stability of the knee and some of the extrinsic stabilizers are removed during knee replacement, so there is a need to restabilize the joint. The more extrinsic stability is lost by the pathology of the patient or by action of the surgeon (often dictated by the design of a prosthesis), the more intrinsic stability of the prosthesis is required to stabilize the knee.

Most of this new stability needs to come from the geometry of the prosthetic components and their positioning. One should realize that the geometry of these components providing stability to the knee does and must restrain movements. As a consequence forces causing these movements, but being restricted by the geometry of the components, will be transmitted through the prosthesis to the bone-prosthesis interface. The greater the intrinsic constraint provided by the geometry, the greater the force conducted to the interface. This results in a prosthesis that is more likely to show mechanical loosening [11]. Rotational and shear forces should be minimally conducted to the interface and movement should not be fully restricted by the geometry of components. Free anatomical motion is one of the requirements of successful TKA.

There are other reasons to restrict the movement of the knee and to force the knee into a certain motion. The roll-glide mechanism of the natural knee responsible for maximal flexion and optimal effectiveness of the extensor mechanism, does not function anymore after removal of the articular surfaces and the cruciate ligaments. It remains desirable to fulfill the demands of the patient in all sorts of daily activities. In several designs of total knee a post and cam or other form of posterior stabilization, forces rollback effectively. But one must bear in mind, that whenever a motion is forced by a component, more forces will be conducted to the inter-

face and loosening is more likely to occur. Whether loosening, in reality will occur, is a matter of how good the fixation is and how strong the forces are.

3.3 The ligaments of the replaced knee

As stability of the replaced knee is of utmost importance and stability by intrinsic constraint is detrimental for lifelong fixation, it is needed to look again at the natural extrinsic stabilizers of the knee; muscles, capsule and the collateral and cruciate ligaments in particular. The ligaments are made to passively stabilize the knee joint and play an important role in the active stabilization because of their proprioceptive properties. Their presence, under normal conditions does not cause harm to the prosthesis, so it seems wise to use these stabilizers while performing TKA.

The reasons to retain or not retain the cruciate ligaments will be discussed seperately in this book. In this chapter it should be clearly stated that retaining the cruciate ligaments may largely contribute to the extrinsic stability of the knee and to normal kinematics, especially if both cruciate ligaments are retained. When all ligaments are intact, only one articular envelope is possible. Retention of the posterior cruciate ligament only, does not create normal knee motion, as demonstrated in fluoroscopic studies [17], but retaining the posterior cruciate ligament may have a role for other reasons like stabilizing the knee in the frontal plane.

In summary, the more intrinsic stability, provided by the articular surface, and extrinsic stability, provided by the cruciate ligaments is removed the greater the need for intrinsic stability of the prosthetic component. This may be paradoxically detrimental for lifelong fixation. Again, free anatomical motion is one of the important requirements of successful TKA.

3.4 Anatomical Motion

Anatomical motion is desirable for most patients, but the needs of patients may differ a lot, in the Asian population, maximal flexion is needed for the normal sedentary position, but European patients may be happy when they are able to ride a bike for which 110 degrees of flexion is sufficient.

Biomechanically speaking, anatomical motion after TKR is important to prevent mechanical loosening of prosthetic components. When motion is not restricted by intrinsic constraint the rotational and shear forces will be conducted through the soft tissues rather than the prosthetic components and the fixation of components is not overloaded, so loosening is prevented.

In most knee replacement systems free anatomical motion between femoral and tibial components is only possible when these components have different radii of curvature, or the tibial component is relatively flat. This will provide the knee with a greater freedom of passive motion in anterior-posterior and medial-lateral direction and also in rotation. To prevent instability the freedom of motion is limited, the tibial surface is not to flat and prominences prevent dislocation. The situation may be described as a compromise between too much intrinsic stability and too much freedom of motion.

This compromise may be beneficial for many patients when the fixation of the prosthetic components is good and the activity level of the patients not too high. The fixation of components needs to be good because as a result of the given freedom in translation, loading of the knee will not always occur at the same spot. This means that the load transfer to the underlying bone may differ from situation to situation with possible negative consequences for fixation.

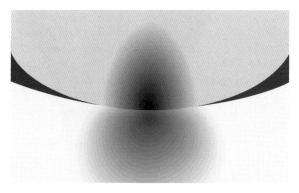

Fig. 7. Concentration of high subsurface stresses in a knee prosthesis with limited contact between the articulating surfaces

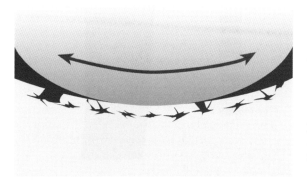

Fig. 8. Pitting, cracking and delamination as a result of multi-directional movement

Freedom of motion provided for by the incongruence of components may however have an important drawback! The contact area between the femoral and tibial component is reduced to only a point or a line in the designs where the components have different radii. All loading occurs on a very small area and the contact stresses are extremely high (Fig. 7). It has been experimentally demonstrated and calculated that these contact stresses widely exceed the maximum permitted contact stress for the commonly used material for tibial bearings: ultra-high-molecular-weight-high-density polyethylene [10]. As a result the bearings may wear, especially under the influence of multi-directional movements occurring at the surfaces (Fig. 8).

3.5 Polyethylene Wear

The polyethylene wear seen in knee prostheses, is partly different from the kind of polyethylene wear usually seen in total hip prostheses where abrasion and adhesion, occurring at the surface, are the dominant types of wear. In the knee, as a result of the high contact stresses, more often pitting, cracking and delamination is observed and the phenomena of fatigue wear originating in the subsurface area of the polyethylene (see Fig. 8).

Wear of polyethylene is not only the result of excessive contact stress. The way polyethylene is produced (moulded vs. machined) and the method of sterilization (gamma-radiation in air which may cause subsurface oxidation and weakening of polyethylene) contribute to the possibility of wear. But the type of wear seen in knee replacement systems is very typical for high contact stresses and cyclic stress variations.

Polyethylene wear may cause a painful synovitis, which is very troublesome for the patient.

But even more important: phagocytosis of the smaller wear particles by macrophages may induce the production of cytokines, which stimulate the osteocytes to produce osteolysis. This osteolysis could result in aseptic loosening of the prosthesis [17]. This is certainly not the goal of TKA so everything needs to be done to prevent excessive wear of polyethylene. This is not only true for today's practice but even more for the future as more and more prostheses are being implanted in younger and more active patients.

Contact stresses may be reduced by using thicker polyethylene components [20] but the contact stresses are still to high when a 20 mm component is used in a non conforming articulation.

Enlarging the contact area is the only way to sufficiently reduce fatigue wear of polyethylene. This implies greater congruency between the articular surfaces, the only possible situation where a contact area is created that is sufficiently large to reduce the contact stresses below the desired level of 10 MPa. By increasing the congruency between the components the contact stresses are reduced to below 5 MPa when a load of 2200 Newton is applied [10]. It should be realized that abrasive and adhesive wear occurring at the surface, are not prevented by creating congruency.

Congruency between components may be effective in minimizing polyethylene wear but looking at the complex kinematics of the knee, there is a consequence of congruency that needs to be addressed. When congruency is created in the full range of flexion-extension movement, a new problem becomes apparent. Total congruency in the full range of motion implies a single radius of curvature of the femoral condyles, which may cause a limitation of the flexion movement of the knee because the radius is too long. Or, when a shorter radius of curvature is chosen, this may create a design problem for the patellofemoral articulation. There is an overlap of the tibiofemoral and the patellofemoral articulation in a knee joint.

In most designs of knee prostheses, the radius of the posterior condyle is reduced in order to create a better degree of flexion. If the radius of curvature is reduced, a large contact area becomes impossible. The contact will be reduced to a spherical line. This may be acceptable because most flexion of the knee occurs in the unloaded swing phase of gait. A large, congruent contact area is most important in the loaded knee. Maximum loads are normally seen when the knee is almost in full extension, or between 0 and 30 degrees of flexion.

Unfortunately there is an even greater disadvantage of congruency between components. Congruency between the femoral condyles and the surface of the tibial component, results in intrinsic constraint between the components enabling flexion-extension movements. The possibility of some varus-valgus rotation also occurs but not axial rotation, medial-lateral translation or anterior-posterior translation. In the absence of important extrinsic stabilizers most rotational and shear forces will be directly conducted to the bone-prosthesis interface and mechanical loosening of the component may occur. Thus what is best for reducing wear, is worst for maintaining fixation of the components! Congruency between femoral and tibial components (and between patellar and femoral components) is therefore a mistake in design when the tibial (and patellar) components have fixed bearings, bearings that cannot move relative to the fixation plate.

3.6 Fixation of prosthetic components

Several factors define the quality of fixation of prosthetic components. The quality of bone is probably the most important one. During TKA the surgeon destabilizes the knee, as mentioned before, because the articular surfaces and part of the extrinsic stabilizers are removed.

Removing the articular surfaces has another important disadvantage. The strongest bone, the subchondral bone immediately underneath the most loaded surfaces, is removed, leaving much softer bone for fixation of the components. The effects of disease diminish the strength of this bone. The stiffness of the cancelous bone of the proximal tibia, which normally is 1287 N/mm, in osteoarthritis is reduced to 1116 N/mm on average and in rheumatoid arthritis even more: 675 N/mm [4, 20]. The central spongious bone of the proximal tibia is the weakest bone. An important question, is how the

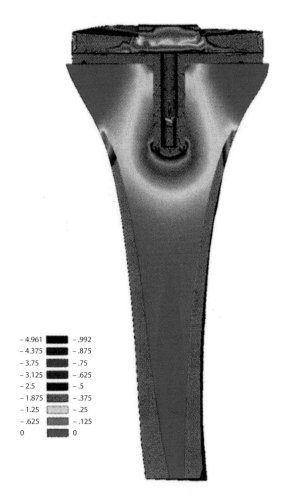

− 4.961	− .992
− 4.375	− .875
− 3.75	− .75
− 3.125	− .625
− 2.5	− .5
− 1.875	− .375
− 1.25	− .25
− .625	− .125
0	0

Fig. 9. Spread of compressive loads on the bone of the proximal tibia, when a short central stem is used (according to Witzel [18])

loading forces are transmitted to the cortex of the tibia, which distally is the strong structure.

It may be expected that forces will follow the shortest pathway to the stronger supporting structures (Fig. 9).

This may be seriously affected by the fixation principle of the prosthesis [18]. If the tibial component is provided with a long intramedullary stem, the forces will be transmitted to the distal cortex almost directly and the proximal tibia will be bypassed and not physiologically loaded (Fig. 10). According to Wolff, bone needs a certain amount of load share (bone if not loaded will atrophy [19]. In terms of knee replacement, the consequence is mechanical loosening of the component.

Tibial components may need central pegs to improve fixation in the relatively weak bone of the proximal tibia to resist the alternating loading forces. The considerable risk of stress bypass and stress shielding remains as the forces will be conducted from the point of the peg to the distal cortex and an area is created underneath the tibial component with very low tension and strain. To prevent atrophy of bone good primary and secondary stability to resist the loading forces is necessary and a physiolog-

ical spread of load to all bone must be maintained.

By removing the articular surfaces and some of the extrinsic stabilizers of the knee followed by implantation of a prosthesis the loading forces of the knee do not disappear but the direction of the forces and the spread of load may considerably be influenced by the geometry of the new articular surfaces and the absence of cruciate ligaments. Absence of the restraint provided by the cruciate ligaments may enhance varus-valgus rotations and contribute to condylar lift off. As a result, one tibial condyle will be overloaded. This may cause compression of tibial bone medially but traction on the lateral side.

In knee replacement systems in which the rollback mechanism of the knee is forced by a post on the tibial surface, abnormal forces will be conducted to the bone-prosthesis interface. The same is true for the rotational forces no longer resisted by the natural restraining structures but by geometry of prosthetic components.

Another factor contributing to the change of load transfer to the underlying bone are: elasticity and thickness of the prosthetic materials [1]. Both factors may influence the spread of load over the tibia surface. By us-

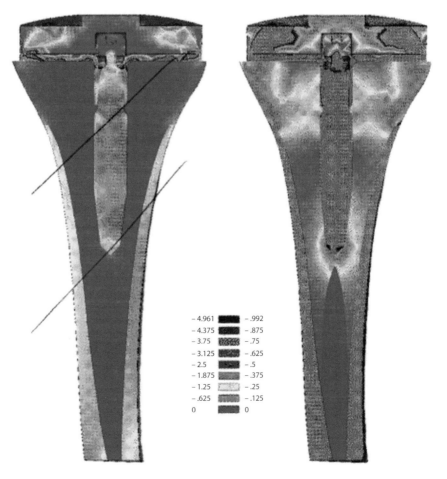

Fig. 10. Spread of compressive loads on the bone of the proximal tibia, when a long stem And two small pegs are used (according to Witzel [18])

ing a metal tibial fixation plate the forces may be more evenly distributed [1].

Fixation of prosthetic components is extremely important for the long-term success of TKA. Many factors contribute to the ultimate result. The quality of bone and the quality of the primary and secondary fixation are the primary important factors. After successful surgical fixation the biomechanical concept of the prosthesis and the activity of the patients are probably the most important factors defining the outcome.

Whether the use of bone cement for fixation plays an important role is disputable, though the literature and the results of long term follow up show more favorable results of cemented fixation [13].

4   Conclusion

The goal of total knee replacement is to solve the problem of pain caused by destruction of the articular cartilage, and to provide the patient with a knee that is stable during weight bearing activities and has anatomical motion as well. Stability, should ideally be created by extrinsic stabilizers (muscles, ligaments and capsule) thus avoiding stability by intrinsic constraint of components. This intrinsic constraint may be the cause of mechanical loosening. Anatomical motion should not be the result of incongruency between components as incongruency may cause high contact stresses on the articular surfaces and subsequent wear. Wear particles may cause a painful synovitis and/or osteolysis and subsequent aseptic loosening of components.

Fixation of components is dependent on surgical technique, the quality of bone, the fixation principle of the prosthesis, and very much on the biomechanical principle of the replacement system.

References

1. Bartel DL, Bicknell VL, Wright TM (1986) The effect of conformity, thickness, and material on stresses in UHMWPE components for total joint replacement. J Bone Joint Surg 68 A: 1041–1051
2. Blankevoort L, Huiskes R, Lange A de (1988) The envelope of passive knee joint motion. J Biomech 21: 705–721
3. Blankevoort L (1991) Passive motion characteristics of the human knee joint. Dissertation, University of Nijmegen, NL
4. Finlay JB, Bourne RB, Kraemer WJ, Moroz TK, Rorabeck CH (1989) Stiffness of bone underlying the tibial plateaus of osteoarthritic and normal knees. Clin Orthop 247: 193–201
5. Grood ES, Noyes FR, Butler DL, Suntay WJ (1981) Ligamentous and capsular restraints preventing straight medial and lateral laxity in intact human cadaver knees. J Bone Joint Surg 63 A: 1257–1269
6. Markolf KL, Bargar WL, Shoemaker SC, Amstutz HC (1981) The role of joint load in knee stability. J Bone Joint Surg 63 A: 570–585
7. Morrison JB (1970) The mechanics of the knee joint in relation to normal walking. J Biomech 3: 51–61
8. Mueller W (1981) Das Knie. Form, Funktion und ligamentäre Wiederherstellungschirurgie. Springer, Berlin Heidelberg New York
9. Nakagawa S, Kadoya Y, Todo S et al. (2000) Tibiofemoral movement 3: full flexion in the living knee studied by MRI. J Bone Joint Surg 82B: 1199–1203
10. Pappas MJ, Makris G, Buechel FF (1986) Contact stresses in metal-plastic total knee replacements. Biomedical Enginering Technical Report
11. Postac PD, Matejczyk MB, Greenwald AS (1989) Stability characteristics of total knee replacements. AAOS 56th Annual meeting (scientific exhibit) in Las Vegas, Nevada
12. Renstrom P, Johnson RL (1990) Anatomy and biomechanics of the menisci. Clin Sports Med 9:523–528
13. Robertson O, Knutson K, Lewold S, Goodman S, Lidgren L (1997) Knee arthroplasty in rheumatoid arthritis. A report from the Swedish Knee Arthroplasty Register on 4,381 primary operations 1985–1995. Acta Orthop Scand 68: 545–553
14. Smidt GL (1973) Biomechanical analysis of the Knee. J Biomech 6:79–102
15. Stiehl JB, Komistek RD, Dennis DA et al. (1995) Fluoroscopic analysis of kinematics after posterior-cruciate-retaining knee arthroplasty. J Bone Joint Surg Br 77: 884
16. Vildik A (1980) The mechanical properties of parallel fibered collagenous tissue. In: Vildik A, Vuust J (eEds) Biology of collagen. Academic Press, London, pp 237–255
17. Willert H (1996) Tissue reactions to plastic and metallic wear products of joint endoprosthesis. Clin Orthop 333: 4–14
18. Witzel U (2000) Biomechanische und tribologische Aspekte der Kniegelenkendoprothetik. In: Eulert J, Hassenpflug J (Hrsg) Praxis der Knieendoprothetik. Springer, Heidelberg, Berlin, New York Tokyo
19. Wolff J (1892) Das Gesetz der Transformation der Knochen, Hirschwald, Berlin
20. Yang JP, Woodside TD, Bogoch ER, Hearn TC (1997) Stiffness of the tibial trabecular bone in rheumatoid arthritis of the knee. J Arthroplasty 12: 798–803

Chapter 5
Engineering Design of the LCS Knee Replacement

M.J. Pappas

1   Introduction

Engineering design of orthopedic joint replacements is a complex, interdisciplinary, process that requires a substantial base of knowledge in sciences associated with both orthopedics and design of moving mechanical elements (Machine Design). It is essential therefore to understand, to some degree, certain fundamental scientific concepts in order to understand the design rationale associated with joint replacements. Further it is important to understand the design process itself if one is to understand this rationale.

This chapter will first present the most important of these scientific and design concepts in order to provide a basis for the understanding of the LCS knee design. It then will present the design rationale itself with a description of its effect.

2   Orthopedic Biomechanics

The science associated with the motion and forces in the knee as well as its functional anatomy is critical to the proper design of a knee. Ideally a replacement should simulate the biomechanics of the normal knee. Important knee structures are, however, usually absent, nonviable, or compromised, after replacement. One needs to attempt to understand and compensate for the effect of such pathology. The ability to do this is strongly dependent on an understanding of the biomechanics and functional anatomy of the knee and its structures.

2.1   Motion

A body in space has six degrees of freedom and therefore there are six possible relative motions or variables associated with a joint. There are three positional and three angular variables required to specify its position and orientation in space or relative to some other body.

If one is concerned about interconnected bodies not all of these variables are necessarily independent.

In the case of the knee joint the position and orientation of the tibia relative to the femur can be represented by the following variables:

- Flexion-Extension Rotation
- Ab-Adduction Rotation
- Axial Rotation
- Anterior-Posterior (A/P) Translation
- Medial-Lateral (M/L) Translation
- Superior-Inferior Translation.

In the normal knee the medial-lateral translation is limited by the interaction between the femoral condyles and the tibial spine coupled with the action of the collateral ligaments. Superior-inferior translation is limited in compression by the interaction of the femoral and tibial condyles and in tension by the action of the knee ligaments and tendons. Anterior-posterior translation is dependent to a large degree on the degree of flexion as the result of the action of the cruciate ligaments and the shapes of the condylar surfaces. It is, within some slack allowed by these structures, not an independent motion variable.

Only the rotational motion variables are independent to a significant degree. Even for these there is some degree of dependence on flexion. Near full extension axial rotation and ab-adduction are very limited due to the screw-home action of the cruciate ligaments. In flexion significant axial rotation can occur independently of' flexion as can some limited ab-adductional rotation.

Disruption of the structures of the knee both bony and ligamentous can dramatically effect the kinematics of knee motion. Such disruption is always associated with knee replacement. The extent that this replacement reproduces the constraining effect of these disrupted structures will affect the motion, or kinematic properties of the replaced knee.

The normal Flexion-Extension range is typically considered to be about 145° [15]. Later work indicates a maximum active flexion of about 135° and maximum passive flexion of about 162° [8]. Any restriction of this motion is undesirable as it adversely affects knee function and can produce undesirable knee loading.

Normal maximum axial rotation is about +/– 20° through the range of motion during non-weight-bearing. Such rotation can potentially occur during normal human activities, such as arising from a chair or from a seated position on the floor [8]. During walking axial rotation is about +/– 6° [17]. Ad-Abduction is normal during many human activities. The Abduction during normal walking is about 8° [15, 17].

The action of the posterior cruciate and the shape of the articulating surfaces produce roll back of the femur on the tibia during normal knee flexion. Roll forward during extension is produced by the action of the anterior cruciate. Roll back on the more congruent medial condyle is about 5 mm while the roll back on the relatively incongruent lateral condyle is about 15 mm [13]. The disruption of the cruciate ligaments disrupts the normal roll back function making anterior-posterior motion unpredictable. Typically without the anterior cruciate function, the posterior cruciate ligament may pull the femorotibial contact posteriorly in extension, and with weightbearing, there is paradoxical roll forward.

Patellofemoral motion is essentially dependent on tibiofemoral motion. The axial rotation of the tibia with respect to the femur produces a medial-lateral excursion of the patella tendon insertion resulting in axial rotation of the patella relative to the femur. Rotation during walking is about 6 degrees of internal rotation and 8 degrees of external rotation [17]. Rotation can be more than double these amounts for other normal activities.

The patella does not articulate with the sulcus of the femur until about 30 degrees of flexion due to the oblique pull of the quadriceps. The patella tends toward a lateral tilt until about 45 degrees of flexion where high compressive loads force contact with the femur on both lateral and medial middle facets of the patella [18].

Control of the positional and orientational variables is of importance not only in the design of a knee replacement, but also in the development of the surgical procedure and instrumentation for implantation of the device. Thus one must seek to control a total of 18 variables, six for each component, in establishing the proper position and orientation of the components of a typical knee replacement. This matter is discussed in detail in chapter 10.1.

2.2   Forces

The tibiofemoral forces in the knee during walking are on the order of about 1.8 to 2.5 times body weight in

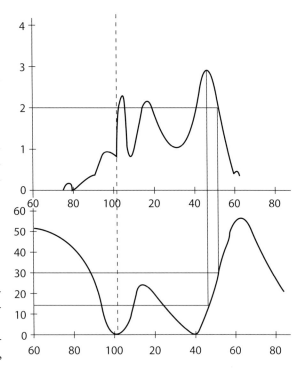

Fig. 1. Joint forces and motion for normal gait

normal gait [7]. Peak forces occur at about 15° of flexion but substantial forces are present from 0 to 35° as may be seen in Fig. 1.

The loading is not equally shared by the condyles. Rather, the bulk of the loading in the high loading phase occurs in the more congruent medial condyle. This high loading phase is accompanied by significant lateral collateral ligament loading and abduction. The less congruent lateral condyle is more highly loaded during the lightly loaded swing phase. Thus the knee experiences an oscillating varus-valgus loading, which makes tibial fixation difficult. Patellofemoral compression forces are quite low near full extension but reaches a maximum weight in deep flexion.

2.3   Functional Anatomy

The primary function of the menisci is to reduce the effective incongruity of the knee articulation. This incongruity is needed to provide mobility. The menisci act to spread the contact between condyles over an increased area. In the high load bearing phases near full extension the menisci greatly increase the area over which condylar contact occurs. During deep flexion, however, the menisci have less effect. It is for these reasons that it has been found that removal of the menisci, or frequent

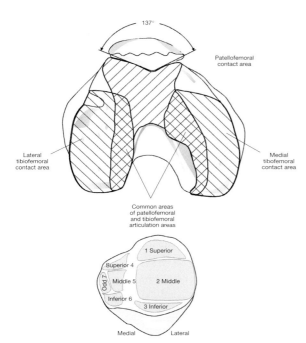

Fig. 2. Patellofemoral articulation and patellar facets

deep knee bend activity leads to damage of the articular cartilage of the knee.

The cruciate ligaments are the primary A/P stabilizers of the knee. As described above, they also generate A/P translation and inhibit axial tibial rotation relative to the femur at full extension.

The collateral ligaments are the primary valgus-varus stabilizers of the knee. They act through a lever arm of length equal to the distance from each ligament to the point of contact between the tibial and femoral condyles on the articulation opposite to the acting ligament. Replacement devices should not reduce the length of this lever arm if they are to maintain normal valgus-varus stability.

The posterior inclination of the normal tibial articulating surface has been determined to be about 10° for Caucasian based populations and about 12° for Asian peoples [6]. This slope indicates the force on the tibia is essentially perpendicular to this surface and thus is not directed along the tibial shaft. Use of a perpendicular tibial resection and replacement articular surface will produce undesirable, and unnecessary, shearing loads at the prosthetic and replacement articular interfaces. Further use of a perpendicular replacement articular tibial surface will adversely affect the action of the ligaments of the knee since the ligament lengths and attachments are adapted for an inclined surface.

The patellofemoral articulation consists of the femoral sulcus and the posterior surface of the patella. The patellar-articulating surface consists of seven facets as shown in Fig. 2. The medial facets are smaller than the lateral facets and tend to be convex rather than concave. This indicates that the lateral loading on the patella is substantially greater than the medial. The medial ridge of the patella is located either slightly laterally, or centrally, in the sulcus [1].

2.4 Fixation

The most important principle of fixation is straightforward. Avoid tension at the prosthesis bone interface. Load the interface by compression.

2.5 Wear and Bearing Fatigue

Although polyethylene wear has received much attention recently due to catastrophic problems with metal-backed patellar [16] and tibial prostheses [2] such wear has been recognized by scientific investigators and clinicians as a major problem for some time [2, 9]. Wear related problems involve wear-through, break-up, and the physiological effects of wear [19].

To better understand the wear phenomena, and what can be done to reduce wear, and its undesirable effects one needs to examine; abrasive, adhesive, three body, and fatigue related wear; contact pressures and stresses; and the relationship between design and wear.

Abrasive wear results from direct contact between the metal and plastic components. Even polished surfaces are microscopically rough. If the metal is allowed direct contact with the plastic the peaks (asperities) on the metal surface will slowly gouge (abrade) away the plastic as the metal surface moves over the plastic surface, much as very fine sandpaper abrades away a wooden surface. The rate of abrasion is a function of the smoothness of the metal surface, the rate declining as the height of the asperities decline (the metal becomes smoother) [4].

Most machinery bearings are in relatively constant, unidirectional motion. When the sliding velocity is sufficient a lubricating film separates the surfaces, avoiding direct contact, and therefore avoiding abrasion. This is a hydrodynamic effect where the load is supported by a film resulting from a relative velocity between the surfaces. The parts float on this film of lubricant much as high velocity, relative to the water, supports a water skier. Under such conditions wear is negligible.

Unfortunately, human joint motion is oscillatory and therefore has substantial periods of low and zero velocity where a hydrodynamic film cannot be sustained. In such cases one has either boundary film lubrication, where some lubrication components act to partially separate the surfaces, or dry lubrication where there is no separating effect of the lubricant. Human joint motion may be characterized by a predominance of boundary and the more destructive dry lubrication.

Adhesive wear results from localized bonding and tearing, rather than gouging, of the contacting surfaces. When opposing asperities contact each other the localized attraction of the opposing atoms of the two materials in contact creates a bond. Translation of one with respect to the other will then produce tearing or rupture of one or both of the asperities. This phenomenon is dominant after the development of a polyethylene transfer film on the Co-Cr surface of the articulating couple. Just as the Co-Cr abrades the UHMWPe, the UHMWPe will also abrade the Co-Cr (albeit much more slowly). This roughened Co-Cr provides a base for the adherence of an UHMWPe film. One then has similar materials in contact, and thus the proper conditions for adhesive wear. The wear rate under these adhesive conditions can be much higher than that associated with smooth surface abrasive wear [12].

The presence of contaminants such as cement, bone debris, and loose metallic beads, as well as the wear debris of the articulating couple, also contribute to wear. This contribution is called "three-body wear". Typically the harder bodies become embedded in the soft. These bodies then can rapidly abrade the metal surface increasing abrasive and adhesive wear.

The dominant wear (perhaps better called failure) mode in knee replacements is fatigue related. Incongruent bodies in contact under load will deform and produce an area of contact, or a contact patch. The highest Von-Mises, or crack initiating stress, will be about 1 mm below the surface of the UHMWPe near the center of the patch for typical incongruent knee replacement articulations. As the metal component slides and rolls over the surface of the weaker plastic surface the point of peak stress will move under the surfaces of the plastic. If the stress is high enough cracks will initiate below the surface. The cracks then coalesce to produce pitting, delamination, and by propagation through the part, catastrophic failure. This is a classic mode of surface failure in rolling contact [14].

Equations, sufficient for use in knee prostheses, for the computation of the contact stress of two bodies in contact were developed in the 1930's [14]. These equations are given and discussed in Pappas et al. [9]. They reduce to $s = K (P)^{1/3}$ where s is the stress, P the applied load, and K a constant that is a function of the difference in the principal radii of curvature of the bodies at the point of contact and the stiffness of the bodies. Increased stiff-

ness and difference in contact radii produce increased stress. On the other hand, contact stress is related to the inverse cube root of the applied load, thus negating the effect of high body weight as a predominant source of wear. This analytical methodology is adequate for preliminary design evaluations but final evaluations should be performed using finite element analysis, which will produce more accurate estimates of contact stress.

3 Historical Lessons

An understanding of the prior art in a field its failures and successes is important in the development or evaluation of new designs. One must learn from this earlier experience and apply its lessons.

3.1 First Generation

Early hinge designs of the 1950's, such as the "Waldius" and later the "GUEPAR" knees restricted motion to a single flexion-extension axis. Although they initially worked reasonably well when they were simply press-fit into the bone, they showed early loosening when used with cement. This loosening is attributed to over-constraint resulting from lack of axial and ad-abduction rotation producing large axial and varus-valgus torques.

3.2 Second Generation

Later resurfacing designs of the late 1960's, such as the "Geomedic" and "Geometric", also rapidly failed due to lack of axial rotation and lack of provision for roll back. Less constrained designs such as the "Marmor" and "Gunston" designs of the late 60's failed due to excessive contact stress and material overloading. The 1970's saw the introduction of improved resurfacing designs, which provided for patellar replacement. The "Total Condylar" and "Townley" designs worked reasonably well. The principal problems were; lack of adequate flexion, patellar wear and loosening problems, posterior subluxation of the Total Condylar; and tibial loosening and excessive pitting type wear with both devices. Tibial loosening problems resulted in the introduction of metal-backed bearings, which dominate today. Use of metal-backed patellar components introduced to attempt to reduce patellar loosening were a jump from the "frying pan into the fire" as the reinforcement of the relatively thin patellar components created a worse problem.

Attempts were made to develop hinge designs with axial rotation. The "Spherocentric" knee provided axial rotation and even some varus-valgus motion. Failure of this design was; however, quite rapid due to loosening which was the result of varus-valgus constraint combined with excessive bone removal and inadequate stem fixation.

3.3 Third Generation

The mid, and late, 1970's saw the introduction of mobile bearing knee designs, such as the "Oxford" and "New Jersey LCS" knees. These designs provide mobility and congruency by use of a second bearing surface articulating against a metal tibial platform. The mobile bearing concept provided a basis for the solution to the dilemma of congruency vs. constraint facing knee designers of the time.

The Oxford knee has demonstrated some success as a medial compartment unicondylar replacement. It is contraindicated for lateral or bicompartmental replacement. The Oxford design has several design deficiencies that limit its use. These are, excessive A/P displacement during flexion due to a single radius of curvature, lack of adequate axial rotation, and lack of a patellofemoral articulation. The lack of the ability to replace some or all of these articulating surfaces is a serious limiting factor in the application of the Oxford design to a large percentage of patients. Furthermore, the original designers found that normal kinematics with preservation of both the anterior and posterior cruciates were needed to prevent bearing dislocations.

3.4 Lessons from the three generations

The primary lessons of these early designs are:

- Avoid unnecessary prosthetic constraints if possible. Allow the soft tissue constraints to act. If the soft tissue constraints are not available and prosthetic constraints must be used, provide sufficient fixation to resist the expected loading resulting from these constraints.
- Accommodate typical total knee motion and loading. Failure to provide for total knee motion and loading can produce excessive stresses in the prosthesis and at the bone-prosthesis interface.
- Mobile bearings are needed to provide the necessary degree of congruity and mobility to provide a long service life using materials currently available for knee prostheses.
- The design of a successful knee replacement is complex and careful design is necessary to avoid serious design defects.

3.5 Misconceptions

There is a feeling that this excessive contact stress will disappear as a result of some combination of deformation and "bedding in" which will somehow provide the congruency needed to sustain normal loads since the original design geometry clearly cannot. This concept is nonsense since the complex motion of the knee means that the femoral condyles move over the surface of the tibial articulating surface and thus point loading occurs over a region of the tibial surface rather than at discrete points on the surface where bedding in could occur. Thus, for one loading cycle, deformation or wear will occur at one point, and at some other point for the next loading cycle. This random motion will not produce significant bedding in since the location and shape of femoral condylar contact continuously changes. For significant bedding in there must be a reasonable consistency of contact region and shape. Bedding in does occur in fixed axis of rotation mechanical simulator tests where the conditions for bedding in are present [10], but they will not occur in a knee replacement.

This may be seen from Fig. 3. Here the two-year, total condylar, shows evidence of surface fatigue due to overloading rather than some bedding in process.

Another misconception is that if a tibial bearing is 6 mm thick it is satisfactory with respect to contact stress. This misconception comes from a misinterpretation of Bartel et al. [2]. This study simply indicates that at a thickness below 6 mm stress becomes significantly larger than that of a much thicker component. It does not indicate that a 6 mm thick component is safe.

An annotated version of the data of Bartel et al. [2] is given in Fig. 4. Added here are the values of compressive yield strength [9], the manufacturers maximum recommended compressive stress for RCH-1000 UHMWPe [5],

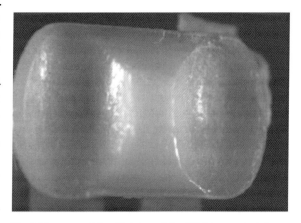

Fig. 3. Two year retrieval total condylar tibial component showing fatigue pits

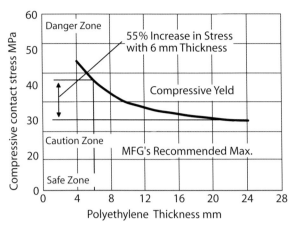

Fig. 4. Contact stress as a function of UHMWPe thickness in incongruent contact knee bearings

and the increase in stress resulting from metal backing where a 6 mm thick bearing is used. It may be seen that the 6 mm bearing studied in Bartel et al. [2] produces an increase in stress of more than 50 % a stress above the yield strength of the UHMWPe. Even at the greatest thickness, however, the contact stresses are clearly excessive.

This graph is associated with a particular articulation configuration studied in Bartel et al. [2]. More congruent articulations have lower contact stress and are less sensitive to thickness. Less congruent configurations have higher contact stress and are more sensitive to thickness. Thus each design must be judged individually and cannot be judged simply on the basis of bearing thickness. No fixed tibial bearing designs we have studied approach satisfactory values of contact stress.

4   The Design Process

Engineering design is a complex and iterative process requiring creativity, objectivity and science to produce well-designed devices. In particular the ability to understand and apply often-complex and interdisciplinary scientific principles and knowledge is of critical importance in engineering design. Further design is an art. As such it requires both talent as well as knowledge to do well. The process described below is not to be considered a recipe but rather an example of how engineering design is done by many of its practitioners. The design process typically starts with the identification of a need to modify some element of a device to prevent failure or improve performance. Or there may be a need for a new device, which can supply new effects or those, superior to other known devices. After identification of a

need a feasibility study is often performed to establish whether the need can or should be satisfied. Coupled with this study is the development of design specifications describing the characteristics and needed performance of the device is developed. Not all projects need a formal study. Often the ability or requirement to satisfy a need is obvious.

Once feasibility is established creative processes are used to synthesize solutions to the problem of satisfying the need. These designs are then carefully evaluated to determine their desirability. This is a complex process, which is well understood by experienced design practitioners and is well founded in science and often makes extensive use of advanced scientific principles. This evaluation, or analysis, determines or estimates the performance and characteristics of the device and thus whether or not it meets the defined engineering specifications.

Usually such analysis will disclose the need to modify, or even abandon, the preliminary designs, and can produce a need to again evaluate feasibility. In most cases one final design is finally developed after a number of analysis-redesign cycles until the design team is satisfied that, within the time and budget it has available, the design is the best, which can be developed.

It should be noted that the selection of design features is often a compromise. Often the design criteria are conflicting. Further there are typically several solutions to a problem. Each solution has its advantages and disadvantages. An important element of successful design is to understand and properly attribute weight to these features and choose the most effective combinations of solutions to the series of design problems associated with the design of a device.

A prototype of the resulting design is then made and evaluated, usually with some form of experimental testing. It should be noted that it is common to build models and perform test on them as part of the feasibility and synthesis process in order to obtain knowledge needed to complete these earlier steps. The purpose of this phase of the general design process is to perform a final evaluation of a model of what is expected to be the final production design. Mathematical analysis tools used earlier have limitations. Thus generally formal mechanical and even field-testing are needed to verify characteristics and performance.

After verification and establishment that the prototype meets specifications the design is released for production where a whole new series of design process are invoked to satisfy the needs established by the need to produce the device.

It should be noted that the steps in the design process are interrelated and the process is highly iterative. The feasibility study or the synthesis or evaluation phase may discover new needs that in turn produce additional synthesis and evaluation effort. Development of the manufacturing capability may require or suggest the need for redesign to make production efficient, or even practical. Experience in the field with the production device, or other field developments usually also generate a need for design modification. Thus the process is continuous and lasts until the device is abandoned.

5 Design of the NJ-LCS

5.1 The Need

Our early work in the knee is described in chapter 3. It became clear during our early effort that variation of the existing designs at the time could not produce a design with sufficient mobility coupled with sufficient load bearing capacity to produce a replacement providing long-term service and reasonably normal function. This realization initiated the need for a new device that would.

5.2 Feasibility

The mid, and late, 1970's saw the introduction of mobile bearing implant designs, such as our "Floating Socket Shoulder", our " Trunion Ankle" and the "Oxford" knee. These devices provided mobility and congruency by use of a second bearing surface articulating against a metal platform. The mobile bearing concept provided the basis for the solution of the dilemma of congruency vs. constraint facing knee and ankle replacement designers of this time. Thus mobile bearings provided a possible means to satisfy the need.

In 1977 the year the design development of the NJ-LCS was started our work was essentially research oriented. We were concerned with exploring means for significantly improving the performance of joint replacements. Thus the usual feasibility concerns relating to expected commercial success were not involved. Our only real concern was could it be done. Our analysis of the Oxford knee indicated that a mobile bearing is only part of the solution in that excess translation of the bearing also had to be avoided. Thus establishment of feasibility required a solution to that problem as well.

The solution emerged from an understanding of the behavior and anatomy of the natural knee. Although, considering the effect of the menisci, the knee was almost congruent for most of its range of motion during normal activities it was not congruent in some of the range, particularly in deep flexion. The natural knee has a decreasing radius of curvature at the contact of the femoral condyles in flexion. This shape clearly allowed the large range of motion associated with this condylar joint.

Thus it was decided to follow the example of nature and use a femoral component with a decreasing radius of curvature. This decision violated the basic tenet of mobile bearings, that such bearings allow both congruity and mobility. Such a compromise appeared to us to be needed if excess bearing translation was to be avoided and normal knee flexion allowed. The question now was the cost of this compromise.

From Fig. 1 it may be seen that peak walking loads occurred at flexion of less than about 25° during normal walking. Thus at least for this activity it may be possible to accept some incongruity at deeper flexion. Using a mobile bearing design with a femoral articular surface with decreasing posterior radius still provided line contact in flexion. Such contact typically produces lower contact stresses than the typical point contact of fixed bearing devices with similar mobility. Our calculations indicated that at the expected loads during walking in the flexion phases where line contact would occur contact stresses were acceptable. Now since walking is by far the most frequent activity with regard to its number of loading cycles, and since our analysis of stresses for much less frequent activities indicated they could be tolerated, lead us to conclude that the cost of the compromise was justified. Thus feasibility was established for our purposes.

The design criteria that emerged from this study were:

- Medical and Engineering Criteria
  - Material and wear product compatibility
  - Adequate mechanical strength
  - Minimization of the joint reaction forces
  - Minimization of fixation interface shear
  - Avoidance of fixation interface tension
  - Uniformity of interface compression
  - Duplication of anatomical function
  - Adequate fit for the patient population
  - Manufacturability
  - Inventory costs
- Medical and Surgical Criteria
  - Treatment of a broad variety of pathologies
  - Maximal preoperative options
  - Maximal intraoperative options
  - Maximal postoperative options in case of failure
  - Salvageability
  - Tolerance for misalignment
  - Ease of implantation

Some of these criteria are conflicting, but most are complimentary. A full discussion of all these criteria is, unfortunately, beyond the scope of this text.

The primary design objectives for the NJ-LCS can be summarized as:

- Restoration of Anatomical Function and Motion
- Long Term Fixation
- Excellent Wear Properties

These criteria are complimentary.

Further it was decided that a system of different designs were needed since it did not appear that a single design could achieve these objectives in the bulk of those cases requiring knee replacement.

There were additional design considerations. It is a simple matter to produce a fully congruent design. Congruency, by itself, is not sufficient. This is evidenced by the early Geomedic-Geometric designs, which fail to provide adequate provision for axial rotation or femoral rollback. Mobility is needed along with congruity. Many later, incongruent, designs also fail to provide adequate axial rotation

In fixed bearing designs axial rotation can substantially change the nature of the surface contact. In a properly designed mobile bearing device the nature of the contact does not need to change since the bearing can move with the femoral component.

There must also be provision for abduction. Abduction of the knee occurs during the loading and swing phase of the walking cycle, and during other normal activities. To minimize wear the articulating surfaces must accommodate such motion. This means the avoidance of flat on flat articulating surfaces. The PCA, the Miller-Gallante knee, and Natural knee were classic cases of failure to accommodate such motion by their use of flat on flat articulating surfaces.

5.3 Synthesis

Over several months a number of designs were created and models constructed and were evaluated visually some after insertion into cadaver. The learning process and experience gained from these early models completed our preparation for the creation of the final design.

The final system designs were created, and engineering drawings prepared in three days of effort in August of 1977. The design rationale and analysis used will be described in detail below in the description and discussion of the design.

5.4 Prototyping and Testing.

We quickly made implantable prototypes. It should be noted that DePuy, the ultimate manufacturer of the NJ-LCS system, was not involved in the design or manufacture of the system at this stage of development. Local firms working under contract to us handled all manufacturing.

The testing took two principal forms, mechanical simulation and clinical evaluation. A knee joint simulator, including a patellofemoral testing capability was designed and made to perform motion and loading testing. The device was used to test the NJ-LCS, the Total Condylar and the Townley knee. The Total Condylar and Townley developed fatigue pits similar to those of Fig. 3 within a few hundred thousand cycles. The NJ-LCS showed only minimal burnishing of the meniscal bearings after several million cycles. Thus the superiority of mobile bearings in wear seemed confirmed.

Dr. Buechel performed several implantations of the versions of the system, as it existed at the time. These were the unicompartmental, bicompartmental and rotating platform devices. The need for a design modification emerged from this study. It was found that ligament tension was very unpredictable. This triggered a reexamination of the instrumentation system and lead to its abandonment. A tibia first approach learned from Insall was adapted for the NJ-LCS system. Using this approach the posteriorly inclined tibial resection used with the NJ-LCS required the use of a distal femoral resection of matching slope if one were to create a joint space with parallel sides. Such a space was desirable to allow its reliable measurement that is not greatly dependent on the relative A/P position of the femur and tibia at measurement. Thus the distal fixation surface of the femoral component was changed from a perpendicular to a 15° inclination so that, considering the natural femoral bow and the slight hyperextension present when determining the extension gap, the surfaces of the gap were essentially parallel.

5.5 Release for Production

We had in 1977 signed an agreement with DePuy entitling them to the design of the NJ-LCS system. After our testing and initial clinical study DePuy decided to accept our system and thus the system was released for production. Unfortunately the novel design did not, at least in the opinion of the FDA, fall within the "grandfather" 510 k exemption used to allow the sale of all other knees of the time. A formal clinical trial and submission to the FDA for acceptance was needed to make these devices generally available. Fortunately the management personnel at DePuy had the foresight and understanding of the importance of this design to sponsor a decade long series of clinical trials to obtain FDA approval to market this system.

5.6   The Design and Its Rationale

As illustrated in Fig. 5 the NJ-LCS uses a common generating curve to form its articular surfaces. The sulcus region of the curve was carefully developed to provide appropriate lateral stability of the patella. It was designed to reasonably approximate the natural patellar sulcus so as to allow use of the retained, natural, patella.

This generating curve is swept around a series of parallel axes to form the femoral articular shape. The same curve is used to form the tibial and patellar articulating surfaces insuring that at least line contact will be maintained for all motion phases.

This generation is illustrated in Fig. 6 for the femoral component. Segment 2 the "Principal Load Bearing Segment" is generated by rotating the generating curve about an axis through the centers of the two "A" radii of Fig. 5. This produces two spherical regions in the Principal Load Bearing Segment. The tibial bearings have similar complimentary spherical surfaces, and thus all articulation in this region has congruent area contact. This produces congruent tibiofemoral contact during peak load phases of walking and congruent patellar articulation during all motion phases except near full extension where patellofemoral compressive loads are very small.

This spherical surface allows varus-valgus motion and patellar tilt without loss of congruent contact (Fig. 7).

Beyond around 35° of flexion the tibiofemoral articulation is typified by line contact. A reduced posterior radius of curvature for the femoral condyles is needed to provide anatomical motion without bearing extrusion. This is a compromise also occurring in the natural knee. The designers of the Oxford Knee failed to make this compromise resulting in excessive lateral meniscal bearing dislocation.

The generating curve is designed to provide substantial medial-lateral stability since the intercondylar bony structures naturally providing this stability are resected (Fig. 8).

In the case of the Cruciate Sacrificing device needed anterior-posterior stability is provided by the congruency of the articulating surfaces and the posterior inclination of the tibial component (Fig. 9).

Design Criteria A2–A4 and A7 dictate the use of a mobile bearing tibial platform. Fixed bearings are not

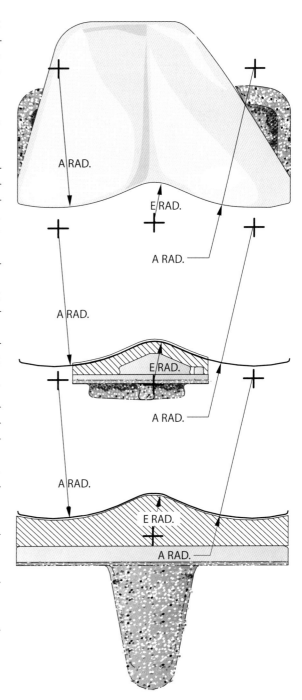

Fig. 5. Common generating curve

capable of providing needed mobility, without unnecessary constraints and associated shear and tensile forces, while keeping contact stresses within reasonable limits, for long term, high activity use.

The use of a metal platform, which is desirable in light of criteria A5 and A6, required with mobile bearings, is highly desirable in itself. Mobile bearings sim-

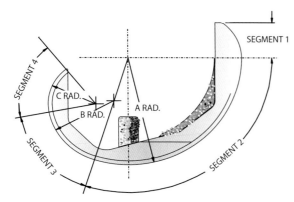

Fig. 6. Articulating surface segments

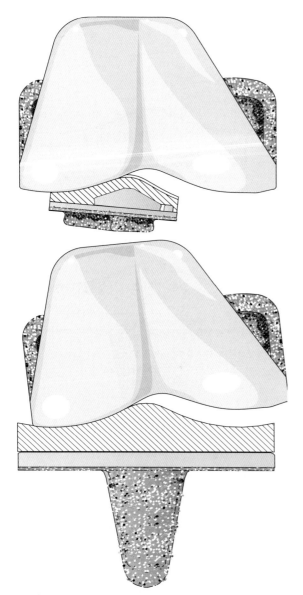

Fig. 7. Varus-valgus tilt and patellar without loss of congruent contact

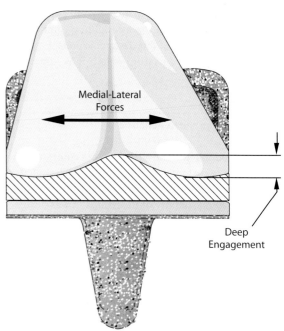

Fig. 8. Medial-lateral stability provided by the articular surfaces

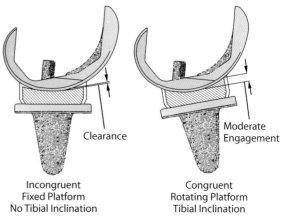

Incongruent
Fixed Platform
No Tibial Inclination

Congruent
Rotating Platform
Tibial Inclination

Fig. 9. Improved anterior-posterior stability resulting from congruity and posterior tibial component inclination

ply make optimal use of the metal platform. Those now urging a return to all poly tibial components have forgotten the lessons of the past where the flexibility of these components has been strongly implicated in loosening. Metal backing is desirable if used properly, that is when used with congruent mobile bearing elements.

Criteria A3–A7 dictate the use of the natural posterior tibial plane inclination. If the tibial component is placed perpendicular to the tibial axis, as was the norm at the time, shearing forces are introduced at the articulating surfaces and prosthetic interfaces.

Further, since with a perpendicular tibial bearing surface the normal ligament pattern is not duplicated, flexion must be accompanied by stretching of the ligaments. This may result in loss of flexion and added posterior compression force producing anterior lift (and tension). This action may increase the joint reaction force, and reduces compression uniformity. The lack of posterior tibial inclination can be responsible for flexion problems with the PCA and it is a likely the reason the designers of the PCA used an anterior screw in an attempt to avoid anterior lift. A compromise solution was used in the "Insall-Burstein" Knee that used a perpendicular resection but a wedge type tibial component producing a posteriorly inclined prosthetic plane.

This approach eliminates shear at the articular surface providing a partial solution. Unnecessary shear at the bone-prosthesis interface remains, however. It should be noted that a perpendicular cut requires additional anterior tibial resection compared to an inclined cut. Further, since the tibial plane is not parallel to the distal femoral resection, an anterior-posterior variation in the position of the femur relative to the tibia will produce a variation in prosthetic gap since the path of the femur is along the inclined plane and is not parallel to the distal femoral resection. Thus inclining the articular surface, but not the tibial resection, provides only a partial solution to the problems of a perpendicular tibial cut.

On the other hand, a posteriorly inclined tibial and femoral resection used with NJ-LCS meniscal bearing tibial components, results in the elimination of A-P interfacial shear and a consistent prosthetic gap.

The tibial spine prevents posterior bearing dislocation of the meniscal bearings. The anterior soft tissues prevent anterior dislocation. Early, infrequent, problems of meniscal bearing fracture and dislocation have been resolved by a minor design change, use of improved polyethylene, and criteria for tibial component selection.

The NJ-LCS Meniscal Bearing Cruciate Retaining Tibial Platforms differ substantially from the earlier Oxford design. The one-piece NJ-LCS platform replaces both tibial condyles avoiding the problem of platform alignment that exists with the Oxford design. Curved dovetailed tracks are used with the NJ-LCS. A dovetail track is used to greatly reduce the possibility of bearing dislocation. Through use of the dovetails the bearing must move sufficiently to fully disengage the male and female dovetails for dislocation to occur. Such motion is in excess of +/-30° motion, and thus dislocation should not occur if the ligaments are sufficiently tight to hold the femoral component against the bearing.

The NJ-LCS tibial component uses curved tracks, rather than the straight side guide of the Oxford de-sign described earlier, to provide for adequate axial rotation. The radius of curvature of the tracks is designed to provide for a variety of axial rotational and A-P translational movement.

The thickness of the thinnest section of the platform was calculated so that expected loads will produce stresses well within the fatigue limit of the material. Similarly the anterior bridge connecting the tibial plateaus was carefully designed to resist bending and torsion if four times body weight is applied to the unsupported side.

Where shear loading is substantially unidirectional, as it is in this case since there is essentially no A/P shearing force, fins are more effective in resisting loads since a fin provides the same projected area to resist such loads with much less bone loss than a round peg.

The fixation of the rotating platform tibial component, however, requires multidirectional shear load resistance since it provides both A/P and M/L stability and thus is subject to shear forces in both directions. Since the entire distal stem tip typically sees alternating tension and compression, ingrowth or long-term cement fixation is not expected at the tip. Thus stress protection of the proximal tibia does not result from the fully porous coated stem. Rather the coating allows ingrowth of fibrous tissue that is felt to provide some degrees of tension load resistance and protection against pressure necrosis. When used with cement the coating prevents cement delamination from the metal and thus reduces the possibility of associated cement wear debris and bone lysis.

A conical peg is chosen for several reasons. These are:

- Simplified preparation of the bone.
- Ability to easily adjust the axial, and transitional position of the tibial component.
- The ability to easily achieve a press fit, important in Cementless use.
- Provides a region for an effective load and wear resistant bearing connection.
- Bone loss is limited to the central tibia where there is little bone of load carrying quality, and thus bone loss is not of great importance. Loss of bone in the condylar regions of the tibia associated with the fixation stem, where bone loss is of great importance is completely avoided.
- Stress concentrations in the load bearing subchondral region associated with the sharp edges of the fins used in crossed fin stems are avoided.

The principal advantage of a crossed fin or rectangular stem to improve torsional resistance is not important in this design since the rotating platform is free of axial constraints and therefore does not exert significant torque on the interface. Thus, for this application, a conical stem is far superior to a crossed fin stem.

Where both cruciates are absent, lack of sufficient anterior-posterior soft tissue restraints, requires that A-P stability be provided by the interaction of the bearing and the femoral component. The forces associated with these constraints must be supported by the interfaces between the bearing and the tibial platform. The Rotating Platform Bearing is thus designed to provide adequate shear resistance against fracture and wear at the bearing-platform connection due to A-P shearing forces.

The NJ-LCS Patellar Component utilizes a trunion rotating connection to provide needed axial rotation of the patella relative to the femur. Although thin, and metal-backed, this patella has demonstrated exceptional long-term reliability, which is established by several long-term clinical studies involving thousands of patients (see chapter 3). This proves that claims that metal-backed patellae do not work are erroneous. Improperly designed metal-backed patellae will rapidly fail. Properly designed metal backed patellae have been proven to be reliable and durable.

As shown in Figs. 5 and 10 the generating curve of the LCS femur matches that of the patellar articulating surface producing at least line contact as opposed to the point contact of typical fixed bearing designs.

Further, during flexion phases where there is significant patellar compression loading, the patellar surface congruently matches the primary load bearing of the femur resulting in area contact of the patellofemoral articulation for almost the entire range of motion of the patella. Line contact occurs only near full extension where the patella compression load is very low (Fig. 11).

It may be seen that, except near full extension, the nature of the contact does not vary during the motion of the patellar component over the surface of the femoral component. This feature allows any minor manufacturing imperfections to bed in providing improved congruity of articulation.

A similar situation exists where the patella is retained. Since the patella contacts the same surface over its load bearing range of motion remodeling can accommodate the mismatch in shape between the natural patellar articulating surface and the femoral component. Thus the shape of the LCS femoral component allows retention of the natural patella in many cases.

It may be seen from Fig. 10 that the center of the patella is in its normal medial-lateral position after replacement. Symmetrical patellar designs lateralize the patella increasing the need for a medal release.

6   The Properties of the Resulting Design

A theoretical and experimental study of contact stress [9] demonstrates the superiority of the NJ-LCS mobile bearing tibiofemoral articulation. Using a load of 2200 N (450 lbs) and 15° of flexion the contact stress is computed using the equations given in [9, 14]. The con-

Fig. 10. Anatomic prosthetic articulation and patellar prosthesis facets

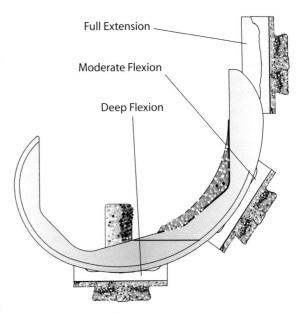

Fig. 11. Prosthetic patellofemoral contact

tact stress values were then checked using pressure sensitive film. The study tested four typical articulations.

The results are shown in Fig. 12.

It may be seen that only the contact stresses in the area (mobile bearing) type are within reasonable limits. The other types (fixed bearings) have stresses, greatly exceeding acceptable limits, even approaching, or exceeding, the compressive yield stress of UHMWPe [5, 10]. A similar situation exists in typical patellofemoral articulations [3].

Contact stress cannot be considered by itself in evaluating the articular surfaces of a knee replacement. Mobility must also be considered. Fixed bearing designs can have either mobility or congruency, but not both. Thus those designers of fixed bearing knees that consider contact stress seriously must compromise between the conflicting requirements for mobility and congruency. This dilemma is eliminated by use of mobile bearings.

The stability study of Postac et al. [11] demonstrates the mobility of the LCS proving that low constraint forces match the low contact stress of the LCS.

7   Changes and New System Elements

Other than the introduction of a posterior cruciate retaining tibial tray the system sold by DePuy in the USA until 2001 is identical to that released release for production in 1978 except for a minor change in the outside shape of the meniscal bearing used to reduce the incidence of bearing fracture.

In the late 1980's we developed and introduced into Dr. Buechel's clinical use additional modifications and new elements. These include: a deep dished rotating platform revision tibial insert, a modified femoral component increasing the range of congruent contact by

about 7°, more dislocation resistant meniscal and rotating bearings, a more anatomical, universal, tibial tray, all poly patella and tibial tray, two peg unicompartmental femoral component fixation, ceramic articulating surfaces, a new rotating hinge knee and a "FlexGlide" (AP-Glide) rotating bearing with A/P translation ability.

DePuy has adapted almost all of these changes and is now selling most of these new and modified devices.

8   Conclusion

The NJ-LCS system design has been remarkably successful. Still a more complete understanding of the needs associated with knee replacement and a more complete understanding of the science involved means that additional advances are possible. We are now involved in the design of new devices, such as an early engagement posterior stabilized knee, as well as the clinical and mechanical testing of the other more recently developed devices.

References

1. American Academy of Orthopaedic Surgeons, Committee on Biomedical Engineering (1992) The patella in TKR – biomedical considerations. Scientific Exhibit, 59th Ann Meeting of the AAOS, Washington D.C.
2. Bartel DL, Bicknell VL, Wright TM (1986) The effect of conformity, thickness and material on stresses in ultra-high molecular weight polyethylene components for total joint replacement. J Bone Joint Surg 68A: 1041–1051
3. Buechel FF, Pappas MJ, Makris G (1991) Evaluation of contact stress in metal–backed patellar replacements: A predictor of survivorship. Clin Orthop Rel Res 273: 190–197
4. Dowson et al. (1985). ACS Symp Ser 287:171–187
5. Hostalen GUR (1982) Hoechst Aktiengesellschaft, Verkauf Kunststoffe, 6230 Frankfurt am Main 80:22.
6. Ishinishi T, Ogata K, Nishino I et al. (1990) Comparison of Asian and Caucasian normal and osteoarthritic knees. Trans ORS 562–563
7. Morrison JB (1970) The mechanics of the knee joint in relation to normal walking. J Biomech 3: 51–61
8. Nakagawa S, Kadoya Y, Todo S et al. (2000) Tibiofemoral Movement 3: Full Flexion in the Living Knee Studied by MRI. J Bone Joint Surg 82B: 1199–1203
9. Pappas MJ, Makris G, Buechel FF (1986) Contact stresses in metal–plastic total knee replacements: A theoretical and experimental study. Biomed Engin Tech Report
10. Pappas MJ, Makris G, Buechel FF (1992) Wear in prosthetic knee joints. Scientific Exhibit, 59th Ann Meeting of the AAOS, Washington D.C.
11. Postac PD, Matejczyk MB, Greenwald AS (1989) Stability characteristics of total knee replacements. Scientific Exhibit, 56th Ann Meeting of the AAOS, Washington D.C.
12. Rabinowiez E (1965) Friction and wear of materials. Wiley, New York
13. Renstrom P, Johnson RL (1990) Anatomy and biomechanics of the menisci. Clin Sports Med 9: 523–528
14. Seely FB, Smith JO (1958) Advanced mechanics of materials. Wiley, New York

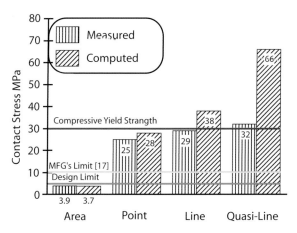

Fig. 12. Surface contact stresses for the four contact types evaluated

15. Smidt GL (1973) Biomechanical analysis of the knee. J Bio-
    mechanics 6: 79–102
16. Stulberg SD, Stulberg BN, Hamati Y et al. (1988) Failure
    mechanisms of metal-backed patellar components. Clin
    Orthop Rel Research 236: 88–105
17. Townsend MA, Izak M, Jackson RW (1977) Total knee mo-
    tion goniometry. J Biomech 10: 183–193
18. Tria AJ, Klein KS, Li RZ (1992) Biomechanics. In: Bowman-
    Schulman E (ed) An illustrate guide to the knee. Churchill
    Livingstone, New York, pp 31–39
19. Willert HG, Semlitsh M (1977) Reaction of the articular
    capsule to wear products of artificial joint prosthesis. J
    Biomed Mat Res 11: 134–164

Chapter 6
Stability Characteristics of the Tibial-Femoral and Patellar-Femoral Articulations*

A.S. Greenwald

1   Introduction

The Low Contact Stress (LCS) knee system was introduced in 1977 as an attempt to improve the survivorship and clinical function of total knee replacement. From its outset, the design goals of this mobile bearing knee system were to decrease the prospect of polyethylene material damage, minimize constraint and optimize patient implant kinematics. The gait-congruent LCS design, in its origin, was proposed as a system inclusive of both cruciate-sparing meniscal bearing and PCL-sacrificing rotating platform variants, with the latter gaining the majority of popular usage over time. Both systems employ a dynamic tracking metal-backed rotating patellar component that articulates with the femoral sulcus.

Fixed plateau knee designs have two extremes. At one end, minimal geometric constraint against displacement results in small contact areas and high contact stresses. The benefit is the transmission of minimal torques to fixation interfaces but at the increased risk of polyethylene articulation damage. Alternately, more highly conforming devices distribute peak stresses over increased contact surfaces, but with the consequence of increased constraint and interface force transmission.

Mobile bearing knees represent a design optimization of these extremes. They offer significant increases in articulation conformity, reducing contact stresses, while at the same time, through insert mobility, they minimize constraint forces transferred to fixation interfaces [1, 3, 6, 9, 13].

Dual surface articulation between a UHMWPE insert and a metallic femoral and tibial tray characterizes this unique knee design. For this reason, the Food and Drug Administration required both laboratory and prospective clinical evaluations to demonstrate its safety and efficacy [2, 4, 7, 11, 18]. This paper describes the stability characteristics of the LCS meniscal bearing and rotating platform designs.

2   Tibial-Femoral Stability

The restoration of normal knee function through surgical reconstruction is highly dependent upon load sharing between the implant, surrounding ligaments and other supporting soft tissue structures. Excision, surgical release and progressive pathological weakening of ligamentous structures results in an increased dependency upon the implant system for stability. Intrinsic stability, achieved in non-hinged, total knee replacements through geometric variation of the condylar surfaces, is influenced by the relationship to the active and passive soft tissue structures. Stability in this regard is the capacity of the implant to limit rotational, anterior-posterior, and medial-lateral displacements to within normal physiologic ranges [8, 9, 10].

The bar graphs depicted in Fig. 1 and 2 describe the stability characteristics of LCS system designs under physiological compression loading for both posterior and rotational directions. Comparative data for fixed plateau designs has also been included [16]. The horizontal lines depict the maximum posterior shear force and rotatory torque that have been reported for normal knee function [15, 17]. One may deduce that implants whose bars are below the reference line are indicative of the need for soft tissue involvement to achieve stability under the forces of gait. Parenthetically, it may be appreciated that the distance between the top of the bar graph and the reference line is a measure of the soft tissue competency demanded to achieve overall stability. This competency may be provided by active collateral, cruciate and capsular soft tissue structures as well as by particular muscle activity. It is of further interest that an early argument against meniscal bearing use was that the bearing tracks would become soft tissue ingrown, inhibiting rotatory motion. A further experiment in

* I would like to thank Maryrose Bauschka, B.A., for invaluable assistance in the preparation of this manuscript.

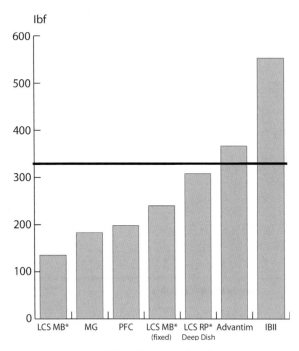

Fig. 1. Posterior stability characteristics for contemporary knee designs (0° extension, 650 lbs compression loading, at 50% of the gait cycle, n = 3). *MB Meniscal Bearing, RP Rotating Platform

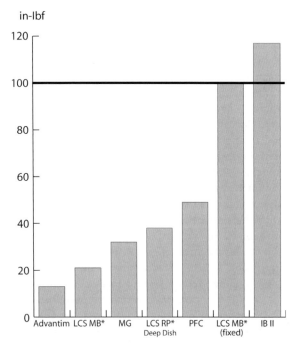

Fig. 2. Rotational stability characteristics for contemporary knee designs (15° flexion, 430 lbs compression loading, at 50% of the gait cycle, n = 3). *MB Meniscal Bearing, RP Rotating Platform

which the bearings were fixed indicates a significant increase in the intrinsic rotational stability provided by the geometry of the condyles. This points to a significantly more constrained system, less dependent on soft tissue involvement and potentially transferring higher interface stresses to the implant-bone interface. Given the low incidence of *in vivo* tibial component loosening with the LCS designs, it is an inference of bearing motion [2, 11]. Like many of their fixed plateau counterparts, the LCS is seen to be dependent on soft tissue involvement for stability during function. This load sharing enhanced by plateau motion is regarded as a positive factor in achieving *in vivo* implant durability.

3 Patellar-Femoral Stability

While the need for patellar resurfacing remains a contentious issue, the majority of American use favors replacement. Yet patellar replacement remains one of the more frequent reasons for knee failure. Clinical outcome is dependent upon patient factors, technical proficiency and implant design. The normal patella tracks in an anatomical groove on the anterior distal femur. Compressive and lateral forces acting at the patellar-femoral joint increase with knee flexion. In the normal valgus knee, a lateral resultant force is produced by the quadriceps mechanism. The magnitude of this reaction depends upon individual anatomy and soft tissue balance. Although not precisely defined, estimates suggest significant force generation. Excessive lateral forces can cause patellar subluxation or dislocation contributing to component failure.

A series of experiments to define the resistance of contemporary patellar-femoral articulations to lateral subluxation under physiological compressive loads inclusive of the LCS lend insight into anticipated design performance. The bar graphs in Fig. 3–5 depict the intrinsic lateral stability of the LCS patellar-femoral implant at varying degrees of flexion. For comparative purposes, data for all-polyethylene, cemented patellar designs are included [19]. The estimated lateral load components for the normal knee are represented by the horizontal line [5, 12, 14]. The interaction of condylar and patellar geometry defines the resistance offered to lateral subluxation. The lateral stabilities of the LCS system, as well as those of the other designs, vary with knee flexion angle. Inherent geometrical constraint should correspond with anticipated *in vivo* lateral loading. The results suggest that sufficient intrinsic stability is provided by the patellar-femoral geometry of the LCS design over the gait cycle. Overall patellar-femoral stability is defined by the interaction between these geometries and the ex-

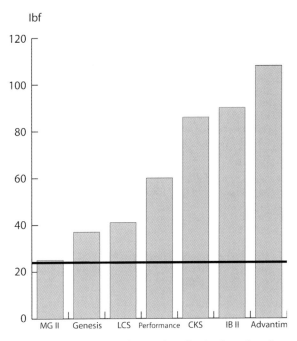

Fig. 3. Lateral subluxation forces of patellar implants (150 flexion, 95 lbs compression loading, n = 3)

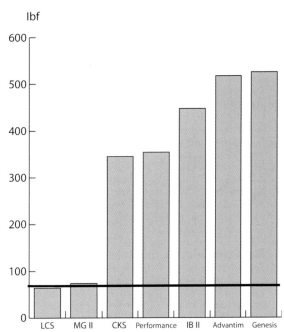

Fig. 5. Lateral subluxation forces of patellar implants (900 flexion, 478 lbs compression loading, n = 3)

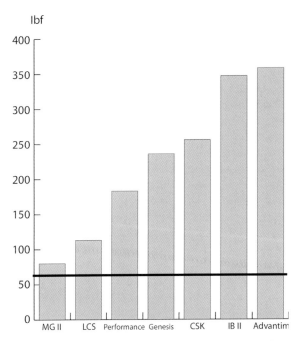

Fig. 4. Lateral subluxation forces of patellar implants (450 flexion, 395 lbs compression loading, n = 3)

tensor mechanism. Within any design, this process is assisted by component placement and correction of varus-valgus deformity through soft tissue release and bone resection. It is of note that this data supports the long-term clinical reports promoting the efficacy of the LCS rotating patellar component [2,11,18].

4 Summary

The LCS mobile bearing knee system is approaching two decades of clinical utility since its FDA approval in 1984. The dual surface nature of this design facilitates implant stability that derives from load sharing between conforming geometries and the soft tissues which surround them. Further, through the mobility of the bearing surfaces, the design decreases force transmission to fixation interfaces and accommodates the geometric constraint afforded by expansive condylar conformity. The laboratory descriptions of tibial-femoral and patellar-femoral stability through the range of functional gait support the ongoing clinical use of this design.

References

1. Argenson JN, O'Connor JJ (1992) Polyethylene wear in meniscal knee replacement. A one to nine-year retrieval analysis of the Oxford knee. J Bone Joint Surg Br 74(2): 228–32
2. Buechel FF Sr, Buechel FF Jr, Pappas MJ, D'Alessio J (2001) Twenty-year evaluation of meniscal bearing and rotating platform knee replacements. Clin Orthop 388: 41–50
3. Buechel FF, Pappas MJ, Makris G (1991) Evaluation of contact stress in metal-backed patellar replacements. A predictor of survivorship. Clin Orthop (273): 190–7

4. Callaghan JJ, Squire MW, Goetz DD, Sullivan PM, Johnston RC (2000) Cemented rotating-platform total knee replacement. A nine to twelve-year follow-up study. J Bone Joint Surg Am 82(5): 705–711
5. Cepulo AJ, Black JD, Moran JM, Matejczyk M, Stahurski TM, Greenwald AS (1982) Mechanical characteristics of patello-femoral replacements. Trans Orthop Res Soc 8: 41
6. Goodfellow JW, O'Connor J (1986) Clinical results of the Oxford knee. Surface arthroplasty of the tibiofemoral joint with a meniscal bearing prosthesis. Clin Orthop 205: 21–42
7. Greenwald AS, Bacon RK, Smith TS (1984) FDA Pre-market application LCS meniscal bearing knee simulator studies.
8. Greenwald AS, Black JD, Matejczyk MB (1981) American Academy of Orthopaedic Surgeons Instructional Course Lectures, Mosby, St. Louis, pp 301–312
9. Heim CS, Postak PD, Plaxton NA, Greenwald AS (2001) Classification of mobile bearing knee design: mobility and constraint. J Bone Joint Surg Am 83 (Suppl 2): 32–37
10. Heim CS, Postak PD, Plaxton NA, Greenwald AS (2000) Mobility characteristics of mobile bearing total knee designs – Series II. Proceedings of the American Academy of Orthopaedic Surgeons Annual Meeting 1: 618
11. Jordan, LR, Olivo JL, Voorhorst PE (1997) Survivorship analysis of cementless meniscal bearing total knee arthroplasty. Clin Orthop 338: 119–123
12. Maquet PGJ (1976) Biomechanics of the Knee, Springer, New York, pp 13–170
13. Matsuda S, White SE, Williams VG II, McCarthy DS, Whiteside LA (1998) Contact stress analysis in mensical bearing total knee arthroplasty. J Arthroplasty 13(6): 699–706
14. Matthews LS, Sonstegard DA, Henke JA (1977) Load bearing characteristics of the patello-femoral joint. Acta Orthop Scand 48: 511–516
15. Morrison JB (1970) The mechanics of the knee joint in relation to normal walking. J Biomech 3: 51–61
16. Postak PD, Matejczyk MB, Greenwald AS (1987) Stability characteristics of total knee replacements. Scientific Exhibit, AAOS Annual Meeting, San Francisco, 1987
17. Seireg A, Arvikar RJ (1975) The prediction of the muscular load sharing and joint forces in the lower extremities during walking. J Biomech 8: 89–102
18. Sorrells RB (1996) Primary knee arthroplasty: long-term outcomes of the rotating platform mobile bearing TKA. Orthopedics 19: 793–796
19. Steubben CM, Postak PD, Greenwald AS (1993/94) Mechanical characteristics of patello-femoral replacements. Orthop Trans 17(4):1126

Chapter 7
Kinematics of the LCS Mobile Bearing Total Knee Arthroplasty

J.B. Stiehl, R.D. Komistek

1 Introduction

The determination of three-dimensional femoral-tibial kinematics dramatically improved with the introduction of in vivo weight bearing fluoroscopic studies. It is now believed that these techniques are highly accurate and reproducible as compared to earlier non-fluoroscopic methods. From literature review, those older techniques included in vitro cadaver studies, in vivo non-weight bearing radiographic studies, gait analysis, goniometric studies, and photogrammetry (RSA). In vitro cadaver studies measured the passive effects of the primary and secondary ligament constraints but were unable to add the physiologic muscle forces or the dynamic loading of actual human weight bearing. The disadvantage of gait studies and goniometric fixtures was the significant error introduced by non-stationary soft tissues which has been shown to be substantial. Roentgenographic stereophotogrammetry (RSA) can be stated as highly precise with accuracy of 0.03 mm but the method must be considered non-weight bearing as subjects are not able to walk, stair climb, deep knee bend, etc.

Without exception, all published in vitro cadaveric studies have suggested that posterior cruciate retaining TKA specimens have the possibility of posterior femorotibial rollback as described by the normal knee. Schlepckow et al. measured the ligamentous versus prosthetic constraint of three different implant designs to compare unconstrained (LCS), semiconstrained (TriconM), and constrained (Mark II). Though posterior rollback and rotation of the total knees was stated, a concern about implant stability was noted with increasing flexion [25]. Menchetti and Walker utilized the radiographic cadaver technique described by Kurosawa to analyze a mobile bearing TKA (MBK). Posterior rollback from –1.4 to –7 mm (net 4.6 mm) was seen from 0° to 120° flexion. Also increased lateral condyle translation accounted for tibial internal rotation [19, 20].

Garg and Walker used a computer generated model based on 23 anatomical specimens to assess flexion and

rollback. They concluded that rollback was possible if the PCL was maintained and the posterior slope of the tibia matched that of the normal patient [14]. Using similar methods, Soudry et al. concluded that rollback was present in posterior cruciate retaining designs and was not influenced by weight bearing loads. Their study did not however examine weight-bearing loads [26].

El Nahass et al. used a electrogoniometric fixture to assess anterior-posterior translation and internal-external rotation of the tibia in weight bearing gait and stair climbing. For total knees, there was 5°–10° of internal rotation and 9–14 mm of posterior femoral rollback from 0° to 90° [11]. Andriacchi et al. reported recently that total knees had anterior-posterior translation of 2.9 cm with normal knees moving 1.9 cm. The method used was a point cluster system that possibly suffers error due to soft tissue translation [1]. Nilsson used RSA to evaluate total knee kinematics placing tantulum markers in the bone about implants and obtaining perpendicular radiographs of the knees. Spatial calculations of the markers were used to determine femorotibial movements. This method was done non-weight bearing in the prone position with simple loads applied [21]. Nilsson studied a fixed (MG I) and mobile bearing (LCS) posterior cruciate retaining design and a posterior cruciate sacrificing design finding an increased posterior position in extension though there appeared to be significant posterior translation or rollback with increasing flexion. Prosthetic knees showed 3° to 4° of internal rotation with flexion while normal knees averaged 6.5° of internal rotation [22]. Lateral radiographs of these subjects confirmed the relatively posterior femorotibial contact position. Kim et al. performed a similar non-weight bearing study utilizing lateral radiographs at 0° and 90° flexion finding essentially no change in anterior/posterior position and concluded that there was no rollback [18].

2   First Generation In vivo Video Fluroscopy

The idea of fluoroscoping a subject following total knee arthroplasty began with Banks and Hodge in 1991. They studied four LCS meniscal bearing implants and found a paradoxical anterior translation of femorotibial contact with flexion [3]. Stiehl et al. modified this technique slightly using a two dimensional computer vector analysis to study anterior/posterior translation of the lateral condyle in posterior cruciate retaining total knee arthroplasty (Fig. 1).

The lateral condyle was chosen from the belief that the greatest motion would be seen on the lateral side. That study found that the lateral condyle started on average about 10 mm posterior to the midsagittal plane of the tibia in extension and translated anteriorly 15 mm to a point 5 mm anterior to the midsagittal tibia. It was noted that the pattern of motion in total knees was highly variable and was irreproducible showing jerky discontinuous motion. In addition, the first evidence of lateral condylar lift-off using in vivo fluoroscopy was demonstrated (Fig. 2) [33].

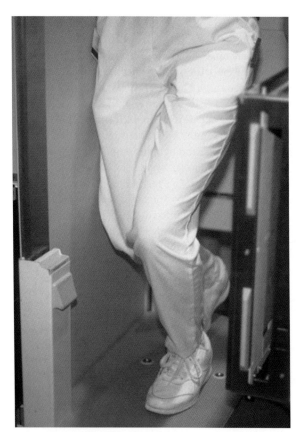

Fig. 1. Illustration of in vivo fluoroscopy technique with standard imaging table turned verticle with technician following knee on deep knee bend

It was postulated that in the normal knee, the ACL was maximally loaded in extension with a highly active quadriceps while the PCL was minimally loaded. The quadriceps without the restraint of the ACL tended to pull the femur posteriorly during full extension, hence the posterior femorotibial contact position. On weight bearing, the normally posteriorly directed shear force on the proximal tibia caused the prosthetic femur to translate anteriorly. An interesting feature of that early study was that five different posterior cruciate retaining "flat on flat" condylar total knee designs were evaluated from nine community surgeons. Despite the diversity of results, the patterns of motion were uniform reflecting the lack of the ACL and the pull of the quadriceps. This study suffered early criticism as it was felt that the surgeons were not skilled in correctly balancing the posterior cruciate ligament. Also, the analysis which was done only with a deep knee bend, was not felt to be a realistic measure of normal gait, the most common ambulatory activity. We were drawn, however to the clear cut results, and the implication of not having reproducible posterior femoral rollback with these "flat on flat" condylar implants.

The LCS mobile bearing total knee was investigated with posterior cruciate retention (meniscal bearing) or sacrifice (rotating platform) again evaluating the sagittal plane kinematics of the lateral femorotibial joint [29, 32]. The implant, which has very high conformity from 0° to 30° of flexion and diminished line contact with further flexion. The femoral implant has a total condylar shape with decreasing radii of curvature into deep flexion. The tibial implant has a highly conforming geometry to match the femoral side both in the coronal and sagittal plane and a cone or runners to allow unrestrained rotational freedom. The only significant implant difference in this study was the surgical technique with reference to the posterior cruciate ligament. The posterior cruciate retaining LCS meniscal bearing implant demonstrated consistent femorotibial contact posterior to the midsagittal tibial reference point. There was early posterior rollback up to 30° but anterior translation was noted at 60° and 90° of flexion. The posterior cruciate sacrificing LCS rotating platform design remained virtually midline on the proximal tibia throughout range of motion. There was however a minor trend for early rollback with anterior translation in deep flexion (Fig. 3).

Our interpretation of these studies was that the rotating platform knee demonstrated midline sagittal plane proximal tibia position throughout the deep knee bend and gait cycle which is optimal for congruency and weight bearing. The minor early posterior femoral rollback could be attributed to the high conformity of this

Fig. 2. Lateral condyle femoral tibial contact patterns of four different total knees compared to normal on deep bend using original vector analysis. Note irreproducible jerky discontinuous motion of total knees. (Reprinted from [33])

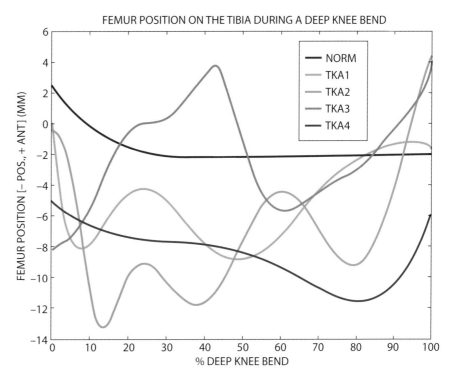

design up to 30° of flexion, while the anterior translation seen from 60° to 90° related to the freedom due to the smaller radii of curvature of the posterior femoral condyles. The most desirable features were the midline position related to the design conformity and the lack of major anterior posterior translation over the proximal tibia which could be detrimental both for tibial base plate fixation and wear. The meniscal bearing LCS implant showed femoral tibial contact posterior to the midsagittal plane of the tibia in virtually all positions. Again there was a fairly predictable posterior femoral rollback with early flexion up to 30° which could be attributed to the high conformity of the design in this position. After 60° flexion, there was anterior translation of the condyles that persisted with flexion up to 90°. Again this results from the decreased conformity of the design in higher degrees of flexion with the smaller radii of curvature of the posterior femoral condyles and from the freedom of excursion in the tracks.

3   Second Generation In vivo Video Fluoroscopy

Dennis et al. refined the computer vector analysis to utilize 3-dimensional computer assisted design models of the tibial and femoral components. A large library of 3-dimensional images (861) for the prosthesis then described spatial orientation through six degrees of freedom. The computer technician matched the appropri-

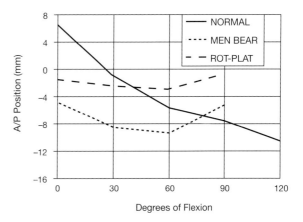

Fig. 3. In vivo kinematic comparison of LCS posterior cruciate retaining (Meniscal Bearing) versus posterior cruciate sacrificing (Rotating Platform) assessing lateral condyle motion using second generation image matching technique

ately oriented image to the two dimensional image, and then subtracted that image allowing computer analysis [7]. Though cumbersome and time consuming, it was then possible to evaluate three dimensional kinematics of both femoral condyles from each video image (Fig. 4).

This was a major technology jump with the ability to obtain unlimited imaging information to fully understand the complex motions of implants through motion.

Fig. 4. Automated image matching shows technique of placing CAD model onto the two dimensional fluoroscopic image in the appropriate spatial orientation

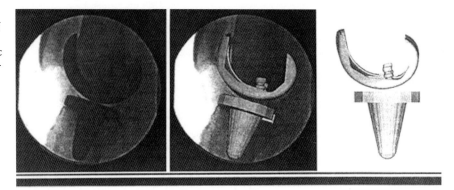

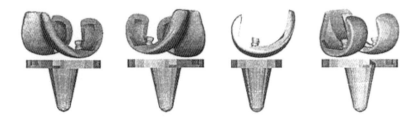

Dennis et al. evaluated and compared the kinematics of posterior cruciate retaining and posterior cruciate substituting total knee arthroplasties with normal knees and anterior cruciate deficient knee. Anterior cruciate deficient knees revealed a posterior femorotibial contact in extension followed by varying and erratic degrees of anterior translation from 30° to 90° of flexion (Fig. 5).

On average, this amounted to 0.5 mm but one case translated as far as 13.7 mm through flexion. According to Dennis, posterior cruciate retaining TKA started with an average position 5.1 mm posterior to the midsagittal tibia in extension with anterior translation from 30° to 90°. One knee moved anteriorly 7 mm. Posterior cruciate stabilized total knees started at the midline and translated posteriorly on average 7.71 mm.

Appropriate conclusions from Dennis's study were that posterior cruciate retaining total knees suffered from anterior cruciate deficient kinematics and that weight bearing kinematics in total knees were substantially effected by both implant geometry and ligamentous constraints as determined by surgical technique. Thusly, tight posterior cruciate ligament tensioning caused the implant to remain posterior when the PCL is tight while laxity caused the femorotibial contact to translate anteriorly, occasionally in exaggerated fashion. Posterior cruciate stabilized total knees had femorotibial contact controlled by the geometry of the implant with a cam/post engagement causing posterior rollback with increasing flexion.

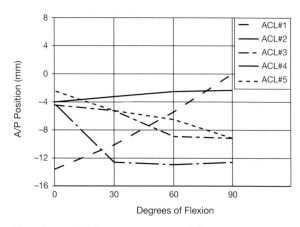

Fig. 5. Femorotibial contact patterns of five anterior cruciate deficient knees. Note variability with trend for anterior translation with flexion. (Reprinted from [7])

Dennis, et al. evaluated in vivo passive versus weight bearing range of motion in patients finding that all knees, including normal, posterior cruciate retaining TKA, and posterior cruciate substituting TKA had significantly less active weight bearing versus passive range of motion ($p < 0.02$). This could result from the increased constraint of combining ligament restraints with articular surface geometry, muscle contraction, and femorotibial kinematics. On in vivo weight bearing, posterior cruciate retaining TKA had significantly less motion that posterior cruciate substituting TKA ($p < 0.05$) with a max-

Fig. 6. Whiteside "flat on flat" posterior cruciate retaining total knee femorotibial invivo kinematics with a deep knee bend. (Reprinted from [31])

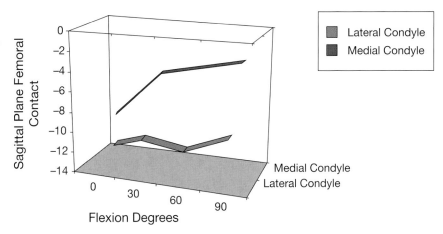

imum flexion of 103° versus 115° in PS knees. From the authors' perspective, rollback or posterior translation seemed to be preserved in the PS TKA while paradoxical anterior femorotibial translation of PCR TKA may limit the amount of flexion possible [8].

Stiehl et al. investigated medial and lateral femorotibial contact in a variety of total knees to assess in vivo kinematics. The "flat on flat" condylar Whiteside prosthesis demonstrated posterior contact of both condyles in extension, exaggerated medial condylar sliding, and relative lateral condyle pivot on deep knee bend (Fig. 6).

Though not as prominent with gait, anterior medial sliding was still greater than lateral motion and no rollback was demonstrated. Rotation was unpredictable showing up to 9° of internal rotation and 1.5° of external rotation. Our greatest concern was the detrimental medial condyle sliding of considerable distance of 6–14 mm which could result in significant in significant pattern wear [31]. Blunn et al. have implicated a sliding, ploughing motion as the most likely cause of polyethylene implant delamination and catastrophic wear. We have a retrieval specimen of a Whiteside tibial insert after eight years of use that shows a large medial delamination zone with a small lateral "pivot" zone that would be similar to the predicted kinematics for this particular prosthesis (Fig. 7).

Retrieval studies of other "flat on flat" condylar designs have shown similar pattern wear [4]. Gabriel et al. suggested an additional problem with exaggeration of tibial fixation interface stresses resulting from posterior femorotibial contact [13].

Stiehl et al. evaluated the results of a bicruciate or anterior cruciate retaining total knee arthroplasty, the Cloutier prosthesis [27]. This implant had spherical line contact but would be considered an unconstrained implant, similar to the Whiteside prosthesis. This implant overall resulted in posterior femoral rollback on early flexion with some anterior translation in deep flexion (Fig. 8, 9).

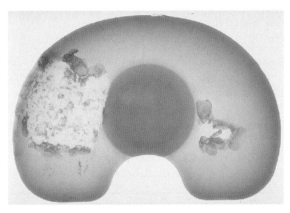

Fig 7. Eight year retrieval of Whiteside tibial insert showing broad medial condyle delamination zone and small lateral "pivot" zone reflecting abnormal kinematics

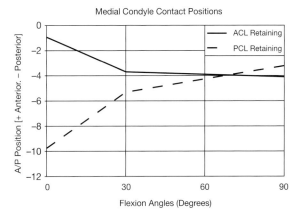

Fig. 8. In vivo kinematic analysis of average medial condyle contact positions comparing the Cloutier bicruciate (anterior cruciate retaining) and Whiteside posterior cruciate retaining total knees with deep knee bend

However, all implant positions were posterior to the midsagittal tibial line. The conclusion was that while about 50 % of cases had an improvement over posterior

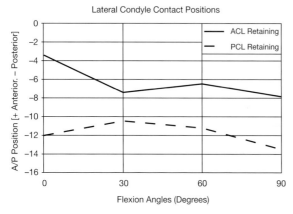

Fig. 9. In vivo kinematic analysis of average lateral condyle contact positions comparing the Cloutier bicruciate (anterior cruciate retaining) and Whiteside posterior cruciate retaining total knees with deep knee bend

cruciate retaining implants, the remainder probably had a nonfunctioning anterior cruciate ligament possibly due to inaccurate prosthetic placement or ligament balancing. A number of cases had a flexion contracture of 10°–15° which could represent a minor imbalance or tightness of the anterior cruciate ligament.

4   Third Generation In vivo Video Fluoroscopy

More recently, Komistek et al. have developed a sophisticated computer method of interactive model fitting that allows true three dimensional spatial determination. Initially, digitizing of the 3-D CAD models was done manually by the technician(second generation). The current technique has an automated system where the computer seeks the best fit scenario of the 3-D CAD model on the fluoroscopic image (see Fig. 4) This third generation method allows calculation of all six degrees of freedom such as sagittal plane anterior/posterior motion, internal/external (screw home) rotation and abduction/adduction (condylar lift-off). For purposes of this discussion, the most obvious enlightenment was simultaneous calculation of both coronal and sagittal plane medial and lateral condyle femorotibial contact while prior studies had evaluated only one plane of imaging. The other technological advance was the use of automation of 3-D CAD model matching that is done by the computer instead of the technician, thus dramatically facilitating the speed and accuracy of the method [6].

Dennis et al. recently analyzed medial and lateral femorotibial contact positions of the PFC total knee arthroplasty with options of a flat, dished, or posterior stabilized tibial polyethylene insert utilizing gait and stair

climbing modes [6]. Both flat and dished posterior cruciate retaining implants had posterior femorotibial contact in extension followed by anterior translation primarily of the medial condyle in midflexion and terminal flexion. Anterior translation was rarely observed on the lateral condyle. Nearly 50% of posterior cruciate substituting designs had some degree of medial condyle anterior translation but virtually 100% demonstrated lateral condyle posterior rollback from extension to 90° flexion compared with 51% flat and 58% dished tibial inserts. The cam post geometry of the posterior substituting implants explained posterior rollback similar to normal knees while the unconstrained posterior cruciate retaining knees had anterior translation consistent with earlier studies.

Argenson et al. investigated the results of a unicondylar total knee arthroplasty using video fluoroscopy [2]. Preoperative indications included the presence of a normal anterior cruciate ligament. During a deep knee bend, although the average motion was small, each subject having a medial or lateral unicondylar arthroplasty exhibited highly variable motions in the anteroposterior direction. The average contact position at full extension for subjects having a MUA was –0.8 mm (10.7 to –6.8), –1.4 mm (8.6 to –10.5) at 30 degrees of knee flexion, –2.4 mm (2.7 to –9.9) at 60 degrees of knee flexion, and –1.7 mm (3.3 to –5.4) at 90 degrees of knee flexion. At full extension, the average contact position for subjects having a LUA was –4.0 mm (1.2 to –9.2), –7.9 mm (–1.6 to – 15.3) at 30 degrees of knee flexion, –5.7 mm (–1.0 to –8.3) at 60 degrees of knee flexion, and –5.7 mm (–1.2 to –12.5) at 90 degrees of knee flexion. Seven subjects having a MUA and two subjects having a LUA experienced paradoxical anterior femoral translation during increased knee flexion. Only six subjects having a MUA and one subject having a LUA experienced anterior contact at full extension. The authors concluded that anteroposterior translation of unicompartmental arthroplasty (UKA) were more similar to TKA than the normal knee with posterior contact in full extension and paradoxical anterior femoral translation. The results suggest that progressive laxity of the ACL may occur over time and inconsistent ACL function following UKA could account for premature polyethylene wear occasionally seen in UKA.

Stiehl et al. investigated sagittal plane patellofemoral kinematics in subjects while performing a weight-bearing deep knee bend under fluoroscopic surveillance [30]. The knees tested included normal knees, posterior cruciate retaining fixed bearing total knees and posterior cruciate substituting fixed bearing total knees with a dome shaped all polyethylene patellae, and the LCS rotating platform posterior cruciate sacrificing total knee, with or without a mobile bearing metal backed patella. Measures analyzed included the patellofemoral contact which determines a point superior or inferior to the sagittal midpoint of the dorsal surface of the patella, patellar tilt angle which is the angle formed by the sagittal plane longitudinal axis of the patella compared to the axis of the tibial shaft, and patellar separation measured in extension followed by flexing the knee to determine the engaged position. Total knee arthroplasty patellae experienced superior patellofemoral contact and higher patellar tilt angles compared to the normal and ACL deficient knees ($p < 0.05$). Patellofemoral separation at 5° (+/– 3°) extension was seen in 86 % cruciate retaining and 44 % cruciate stabilized total knees, and 8 % anterior cruciate deficient knees, but not in the normal or mobile bearing TKA ($p < 0.05$). The authors concluded that patella kinematic patterns for subjects having a total knee arthroplasty were more variable than subjects having either a normal or ACL deficient knee. However, the LCS patellae, most significantly the patella in unresurfaced total knees had kinematic performance closest to the normal knee than any other option. This may reflect the multiple design aspects of the LCS that favor the patellofemoral joint such as the 15° sloped distal cut in femoral preparation, the deep anatomical intercondylar femoral groove and optimized geometry that favors high conformity and articulation throughout motion. Ultimately, kinematic abnormalities of the prosthetic patellofemoral joint may reduce the effective extensor moment function after total knee arthroplasty.

With the ability to determine three dimensional kinematics has also come the possibility to precisely measure actual lift-off and screwhome rotation of total knees [9, 28]. Stiehl et al. examined in vivo kinematics of 20 patients with the rotating platform LCS and noted that 90 % of patients had significant lift-off (> 0.75 mm) during the stance phase of gait. Condylar lift-off was seen in both the lateral and medial condyles with the maximal medial lift-off of 2.12 mm while the greatest lateral lift-off was 3.53 mm. Screwhome rotation was quite variable and there could be internal tibial rotation in knee flexion as high as 9.6° or external tibial rotation with a maximum observed of 6.2°. The average screwhome rotation for the group was 0.5° [28]. Most designers have considered the amount of rotation necessary for fixed bearing designs, on the order of 20°, but this lead to the need for relatively flat articulations and line to line contact. The LCS implants tested demonstrated the extremes of condylar rotation, but an optimal performance from the design point of view as the LCS is rotationally unconstrained. Recently designed fixed bearing implants with higher "dishing" would have a tendency to diminish this rotation and to aggravate wear issues such as post impingement and "sliding" translation. Condylar lift-off is a more ubiquitous problem when one understands that it is obviously present in the normal knee. The LCS may have substantial lift-off while remaining in virtual normal conformity. This is opposed to "flat on flat" designs which may be prone to edge loading or peripheral pattern wear. Condylar lift-off in the extreme setting may be problematic and be a mechanism of late failure in the chronically unstable total knee. With the LCS, implants with lift-off greater than 9 millimeters are prone to implant dislocation.

Haas et al. analyzed the femorotibial kinematics of patients with either the LCS rotating platform or a rotating platform with a posterior stabilized cam and post mechanism [15] (Fig. 10, 11).

With deep knee bend, the rotating platform cruciate sacrificing implant showed midline positioning, slightly posterior to the midline tibia in extension. There was posterior translation to 60° flexion with anterior trans-

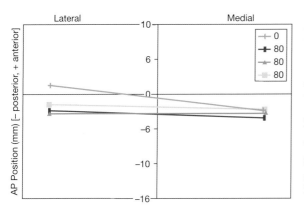

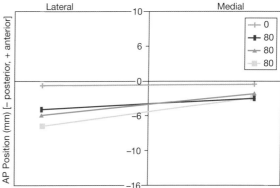

Fig. 10. In vivo kinematic analysis of the LCS Rotating Platform with deep knee bend from 0°–90° flexion showing near midline position throughout

Fig. 11. In vivo kinematic analysis of the LCS PS Rotating Platform with deep knee bend from 0°–90° flexion showing gradual posterior rollback primarily on the lateral condyle

lation to 90°. During gait, translation was minimal with near midline positioning. The posterior cruciate stabilized implant had positioning slightly anterior to the midline tibia in extension. With deep knee bend, there was progressive posterior rollback of both condyles, greater on the lateral. Gait showed less posterior translation with medial condyle showing anterior translation in three knees. Positive screw home rotation or tibial internal rotation was seen with the posterior stabilized implant during deep knee bend and gait. The rotating platform had positive screw home with deep knee bend but negative screw home with gait. All implants showed medial condylar lift-off. Lateral condyle lift-off was seen with both implants on deep knee bend but only one rotating platform with gait. The comparison of the two implants demonstrated that posterior rollback with deep knee bend requires implant constraint of the cam/post mechanism but during gait, kinematics were similar for both implants.

5   Fourth Generation In vivo Fluoroscopy

The most recent evolution of video fluoroscopy in total knee arthroplasty has been to evaluate in different planes such as the frontal or coronal plane. This approach utilizes the same auto CAD technology but now uses special C-arm fluoroscopy machines that allow gait and deep knee bends done in the frontal plane. Stiehl et al. investigated 10 patients with either the LCS rotating platform or the posterior stabilized rotating platform evaluating both condylar lift-off and medial-lateral coronal plane translation [34] (Fig. 12).

They found that the amount of medial/lateral translation and condylar lift-off was statistically different for the two groups (p < 0.05). On average, subjects having a LCS PS TKA experienced only 1.7 mm (1.1–2.6) of medial/lateral translation. Subjects having a LCS RP TKA experienced 4.3 mm (3.4–7.4) of medial/lateral translation. This difference could be explained by the conflict of the PS post. On average, subjects having a LCS PS TKA experienced 1.2 mm (0.6–2.8) of condylar lift-off during the medial/lateral shift, while subjects having a LCS RP TKA experienced 2.0 mm (1.1–3.1) of condylar lift-off. The results from this study determined that during condylar lift-off, the contact of the condyle remaining on the tibia shifts away from the medial peripheral edge toward the center of the joint. The LCS rotating platform device allows for high conformity despite the lateral femoral displacement. With the posterior stabilized rotating platform tibial insert, both condylar lift-off and medial/lateral translation were limited by the spine/box interference. This study was unique in that the amount of tibial translation of the rotating platform was unexpected but not surprising given the prior results of both skeletal pin gait lab studies and stereoroentgenographic photogrammetry which have shown five to six millimeters of translation in the normal knee [5, 10, 16, 17].

Oakshott et al. have evaluated the kinematics of the AP Glide LCS which is a posterior cruciate retaining device [23]. That device performed in many ways similar to the original meniscal bearing LCS but with higher technical resolution of the kinematic fluoroscopy some interesting features were noted. The average range of motion of 10 patients was 119° weight bearing and 129° non-weight bearing. Condylar lift-off and rotation were comparable to other studies but there was a range of nearly 20° of tibial rotation non-weight bearing while most of the rotation weight bearing was up to 10° of external rotation. Finally, contact was significantly more anterior with greater degrees of flexion in non-weight bearing. This would highlight the potential problem of anterior impingement demonstrated by some surgeons using this implant and encourage a fairly accurate flexion space.

6   Discussion

The summary of known kinematic information regarding the knee can be stated as follows. From the magnetic resonance studies of Freeman et al. the normal knee has a complex pattern of motion with tibial internal rotation on flexion related to posterior translation or rollback of the lateral condyle about a relatively fixed medial pivot point [12, 24]. Posterior cruciate retaining total knees have abnormal kinematics that most likely re-

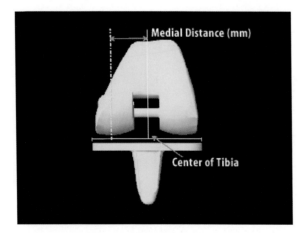

Fig. 12. Frontal plane kinematics showing reference point of medial femoral condyle and measurement of lift-off and translation

late to surgical technique, specific implant geometry, and absence of the anterior cruciate ligament. There is posterior femorotibial contact in extension followed by varying degrees of anterior translation with flexion and virtually no predictable rollback. Surgical technique determined whether or not the femorotibial contact positions would slide forward (PCL too loose) or remained in a relatively posterior position (PCL too tight). "Flat on flat" condylar designs were popularized to allow retention of the posterior cruciate ligament and a simplified surgical technique. Tibial insert design was flat to minimize constraint suggested to be the most likely cause of failure, i.e. mechanical loosening of the tibial tray. Virtually no attention was given to the impact this approach may have to implant wear.

We have shown that range of motion of all knees, i.e. normal and posterior cruciate retaining, posterior cruciate sacrificing, and posterior cruciate stabilized total knees have significantly less active weight bearing range of motion than passive non-weight bearing motion. Those total knees that have posterior rollback such as the posterior stabilized total knees have significantly more motion than those such as the posterior cruciate retaining total knees that do not. It is clear to see how the anterior femoral translation typical of posterior cruciate retaining implants could explain this problem. Therefore, we question the validity of non-weight bearing range of motion at least as it relates to predicting ambulatory function.

We have been able to demonstrate abnormal medial condylar sliding or roll forward seen with some "flat on flat" condylar designs. When combined with a young, high demand patient, this mechanism can explain the wear problems of osteolysis and catastrophic implant failure seen with these designs. An additional feature of abnormal kinematics is loss of normal "screwhome" rotation or internal rotation in certain cases. Whilst internal rotation of up to 10° has been confirmed in total knee arthroplasty, external rotation of over 6° is also seen. With abnormal tibial component placement, this irregularity can cause potential component wear in certain fixed bearing designs.

With our fourth generation modeling technique, we have been able to measure significant condylar lift-off of one condyle in relation to the other. This phenomenon is seen in normal knees and most total knees regardless of method. We believe this finding will help explain pattern and peripheral wear identified in recent publications regarding implant retrievals. Current studies are being done to correlate wear patterns with abnormal condylar lift-off and femorotibial translation.

Those implant designs with high conformity such as the mobile bearing LCS, or posterior stabilized de-

signs that have a cam/post mechanism for articulated anterior/posterior motion have obligatory posterior femoral rollback as a function of implant geometry. Stated simply, the design engineer can enforce a degree of posterior rollback by creating a unique design. In the LCS, this results from the maximal femorotibial conformity in extension which will tend to drive the contact posteriorly with flexion. The posterior stabilized designs rely on a cam post device which engages at about 50° flexion and drives the contact posteriorly.

The LCS system now offers multiple possibilities of surgical technique including the original bicruciate retaining device(ACL preserving), the original meniscal bearing implant and the anterior-posterior glide insert (PCL preserving), the rotating platform insert (PCL Sacrificing), and the LCS revision system (PCL Substituting). The kinematic performance of these devices has been well described by the numerous above quoted studies. From a scientific investigation point of view, this experience is optimal as the prosthetic femoral, tibia and patellar geometry are virtually identical in all of these studies. Ultimately, knee function relates to a complex interaction of surgical technique, weight bearing forces, muscle contractions and kinematic features which are likely to be abnormal or non-physiologic in total knee patients. With a thorough understanding of these issues, the surgeon may make the optimal choices for surgical implementation in his patients and we can hope with the help of computered assisted surgery in the future.

References

1. Andriacchi TP, Tanrowski LE, Berger RA, Galante JO (1999) New insights into femoral rollback during stair climbing and posterior cruciate ligament function. Transactions 45th Annual Meeting, Orthopaedic Research Society, Anaheim, Ca, p 20
2. Argenson JN, Komistek RD, Stiehl JB et al. (2001) In vivo 3D determination of kinematics for subjects having a normal knee, unicompartmental or total knee arthroplasty. Proceedings 68th Annual Meeting of AAOS, San Francisco, CA, p 663
3. Banks SC, Riley PO, Spector C, Hodge WA (1991) In vivo bearing motion with meniscal bearing TKR. Proceedings of the 37th Annual Orthopaedic Research Society Meeting, Annheim, Ca, p 563
4. Blunn GW, Walker PS, Joshi A, Hardinge K (1991) The dominance of cyclic sliding in producing wear in total knee replacements. Clin Orthop 273: 253–260
5. Dejour H, Bonnin M (1994) Tibial translation after anterior cruciate ligament rupture. J Bone Joint Surg 76B: 745–749
6. Dennis DA, Komistek RD, Colwell CE, Ranawat CS, Scott RD, Thornhill TS, Lapp MA (1998) In vivo anteroposterior femorotibial translation of total knee arthroplasty: a multicenter analysis. Clin Orthop 356: 47–57
7. Dennis DA, Komistek RD, Hoff WA, Gabriel SM (1996) In vivo kinematics derived using an inverse perspective technique. Clin Orthop 331: 107–117

8. Dennis DA, Komistek RD, Stiehl JB, Walker SA, Dennis KN (1998) Range of motion after total knee arthroplasty. J Arthroplasty 13: 748–752

9. Dennis DA, Komistek RD, Walker SA, Cheal EJ, Stiehl JB (2001) Femoral condylar lift-off in vivo total knee arthroplasty. J Bone Joint Surg 83B: 33–39

10. Draganich LF, Andriacchi TP, Andersson GBJ (1987) Interaction between intrinsic knee mechanics and the knee extensor mechanism. J Orthop Res 5: 539–547

11. El Nahass B, Madson NM, Walker PS (1991) Motion of the knee after condylar resurfacing – an in vivo study. J Biomech 24: 1107–1117

12. Freeman MAR, Railton GT (1988) Should the posterior cruciate ligament be retained or resected in condylar nonmeniscal knee arthroplasty? J Arthroplasty 1 (Suppl): 3–12

13. Gabriel SM, Dennis DA, Koomistek RD, Hoff WA, Stiehl JB (1996) In vivo TKA kinematics with consequences for system stresses and strains. Proceedings 42nd Annual Meeting Orthopaedic Research Society, Atlanta, Georgia, p 201

14. Garg A, Walker PS (1990) Prediction of total knee motion using a three-dimensional computer-graphics model. J Biomech 23: 45–58

15. Haas B, Stiehl JB, Komistek RD (2002) Kinematic comparison of posterior cruciate sacrifice versus substitution in a mobile bearing total knee arthroplasty. (Accepted)

16. Jonsson H, Kärrholm J (1994) Three-dimensional knee joint movements during a step-up: Evaluation after anterior cruciate ligament rupture. J Orthop Res 12: 769–779

17. Kärrholm J, Selvik G, Elmqvist LG, Hansson LI (1988) Active knee motion after cruciate ligament rupture. Acta Orthop Scand 59: 158–164

18. Kim H, Pelker RR, Gibson DH, Irving JF, Lynch JK (1997) Rollback in posterior cruciate ligament-retaining total knee arthroplasty. J Arthroplasty 12: 553–561

19. Kurosaw H, Walker PS, Abe S, Garg A, Hunter T (1985) Geometry and motion of the knee for implant and orthotic design. J Biomech 18: 487–499

20. Menchetti PP, Walker PS (1997) Mechanical evaluation of mobile bearing knees. Am J Knee Surg 10: 73–81

21. Nilsson KG, Kärrholm J, Ekelund L (1990) Knee motion in total knee arthroplasty. A roentgen stereophotogrammetric analysis of kinematics of the Tricon-M knee prosthesis. Clin Orthop 256: 147–161

22. Nilsson KG, Kärrholm J, Gadegaard P (1991) Abnormal kinematics of the artificial knee. Roentgen stereophotogrammetric analysis of 10 Miller-Galante and five New Jersey LCS Knee. Acta Orthop Scand 62: 440–446

23. Oakshott R, Stiehl JB, Komistek RD, Haas BR (2002) Kinematics of a posterior cruciate retaining mobile bearing total knee arthroplasty. J Arthroplasty (Accepted)

24. Pinskerova V, Iwaki H, Freeman MAR (1999) The movements of the knee: A cadaveric magnetic resonance imaging and dissection study. Transactions of the Annual Meeting, American Academy of Orthopaedic Surgeons, Anaheim, CA, p 82

25. Schlepckow P (1992) Three-dimensional kinematics of total knee replacement systems. Arch Orthop Trauma Surg 111: 204–209

26. Soudry M, Walker PS, Reilly DT, Kurosawa H, Sledge CB (1986) Effects of total knee replacement design on femoral-tibial contact conditions. J Arthroplasty 1: 35–45

27. Stiehl JB, Dennis DA, Komistek RD (1998) The cruciate ligaments in total knee arthroplasty: a kinematic analysis. Orthop Trans 22: 150

28. Stiehl JB, Dennis DA, Komistek RD, Crane HS (1999) In vivo Determination of condylar lift-off and screw-home in a mobile-bearing total knee arthroplasty. J Arthroplasty 14: 293–299

29. Stiehl JB, Dennis DA, Komistek RD, Keblish PA (1997) Kinematic analysis of a mobile bearing total knee arthroplasty. Clin Orthop 345: 60–65

30. Stiehl JB, Dennis DA, Komistek RD, Keblish PA (2001) In vivo kinematics of the patellofemoral joint in total knee arthroplasty. J Arthroplasty 16: 706–714

31. Stiehl JB, Komistek RD, Dennis DA (1999) Detrimental kinematics of a flat on flat total condylar knee arthroplasty. Clini Orthop 364: 46–56

32. Stiehl JB, Komistek RD, Dennis DA (2000) In vivo kinematic comparison of posterior cruciate retention or sacrifice with a mobile bearing total knee arthroplasty. Am J Knee Surg 13: 13–18

33. Stiehl JB, Komistek RD, Dennis DA, Paxson RD (1995) Fluoroscopic analysis of kinematics after posterior cruciate-retaining knee arthroplasty. J Bone Joint Surg 77B: 884–889

34. Stiehl, JB, Komistek, RD, Haas BR, Dennis DA (2001) Frontal plane kinematics after mobile bearing total knee arthroplasty. Clin Orthop 392: 56–61

Chapter 8
Wear Studies of the LCS

8.1   Wear-analysis of Mobile Bearing Knee*

H. M. J. McEwen, D. E. McNulty, D. D. Auger, R. Farrar, Y. S. Liao, M. H. Stone and J. Fisher

1   Introduction

Improvements in total knee replacement (TKR) designs, materials and sterilization techniques during the past decade have led to improved clinical performance of these joints by reducing the prevalence of delamination and structural fatigue of the ultra high molecular weight polyethylene (UHMWPE) bearings. However, in the longer term, concern remains regarding the surface wear of total knee components as the generation and accumulation of micrometre and submicrometer size wear particles has been observed in tissues surrounding knee prostheses that were revised for infection in the early years of implantation [5]. This may lead to osteolysis and long-term failure mechanisms similar to those found in total hip replacements [6]. The generation of UHMWPE wear debris from articulating surfaces in knee prostheses is controlled by a number of factors. These include damage or scratching to the femoral and tibial counterfaces, kinematic input conditions (in particular the amount of internal-external rotation) and the design of the knee components.

Current TKR devices can be subdivided into two groups based on different fundamental design principles: fixed bearing knees, where the UHMWPE insert snap or press fits into the tibial tray, and mobile bearing designs which facilitate movement of the insert relative to the tray. As the polymer insert in fixed bearing knees is constrained in the tibial tray, rotation of the knee occurs at the femoral-insert articulation. Anterior-posterior (AP) translation and internal-external (IE) rotation also occur at this interface. Therefore, a multidirectional wear path results. However, in some mobile bearing knee designs, it is possible to decouple the bearing motions, by allowing rotation at the tray-insert counterface, hence reducing the degree of rotation at the femoral-insert articulation.

We hypothesize that the rotating platform mobile bearing TKR design translates complex knee kinematics into more linear motions at the superior and inferior surfaces of the polyethylene bearing, thus reducing polyethylene wear. This chapter reviews recent studies which have compared the wear of rotating platform mobile bearing knees with that of fixed bearing components under different kinematic and counterface conditions. The influences of mobile bearing and fixed bearing knee designs on surface wear and osteolytic potential are discussed.

2   Materials

The wear of fixed bearing and rotating platform mobile bearing TKRs was compared using the Leeds ProSim six-station force/displacement controlled knee simulator and also using an AMTI six-station displacement controlled simulator [10, 12]. Size 3, Press Fit Condylar (PFC) Sigma fixed bearing TKR components were tested (DePuy). Curved tibial inserts (GUR1020 UHMWPE) of 10 mm thickness were assembled by snap fit into titanium alloy (Ti-6Al-4 V) tibial trays. The bearings articulated with posterior cruciate retaining, right, Co-Cr-Mo alloy femoral components. Low Contact Stress (LCS) Rotating Platform (RP) mobile bearing TKR were also investigated (DePuy). On the Leeds simulators, Standard size, cruciate sacrificing, right, Co-Cr-Mo alloy femoral components articulated with LCS Universal, Standard, 10 mm thick inserts which were machined from GUR1020 UHMWPE. The bearings freely rotated within size 3, LCS Universal, Co-Cr-Mo alloy tibial trays. Similar LCS systems were tested on the AMTI simulator but consisted of Std+ size components with Deep Dish Rotating Platform inserts of 10 mm thickness.

Six (n=6) TKR of a single design were tested under each set of conditions on the Leeds simulator whereas

* DePuy International, a Johnson and Johnson company, provided a studentship for H.M.J. McEwen. Funding for the Leeds ProSim knee simulators was received from EPSRC and ARC. Thank you to Steve Swope for technical expertise with performance of the AMTI knee simulator.

three (n=3) replicate mobile bearing TKR or six (n=6) replicate fixed bearing components were tested simultaneously in each AMTI simulator study. All tibial inserts were packaged in foil pouches prior to sterilisation by a nominal dose of 4.0 MRad gamma irradiation in a vacuum (1020 GVF).

3   Methods

3.1   Standard Conditions

Femoral axial loading (maximum 2600 N) and extension-flexion (0°–58°) input profiles were adopted from the ISO 14243–1 [7] draft standard for simulator studies at both test centers (Fig. 1).

For testing using the Leeds simulator, tibial rotation was displacement controlled with internal-external rotation of ±5° based on the natural knee kinematics described by Lafortune et al. [9]. AP sliding translation of the tibial trays was displacement controlled (0–10 mm) for the fixed bearing knees according to natural knee profiles [9]. However, the ISO 14243–1 [7] AP force profile (–262 N to 110 N) was input to the mobile bearing knees as the rotating platform design restricts AP motion. These input profiles are shown in Fig. 2.

The compressive load applied to each knee was offset 5 mm medially from the tibial axis, as recommended in the ISO 14243 [7] standard for a knee of the dimensions used in this study. The simulator was run at a frequency of 1 Hz and the lubricant used for testing was 25 % (v/v) newborn calf serum (Harlan Sera-Lab, Loughborough, UK) with 0.1 % (m/v) sodium azide solution in sterile water. The serum solution in each station was replaced at intervals of approximately 330,000 cycles.

Motion profiles for the AMTI simulator testing were adopted from the proposed standard for displacement control (ISO 14243–3 [7]). This resulted in anterior-posterior sliding translation of 0–5.2 mm and internal-external rotation of +2°/–6° (Fig. 3).

The applied load was offset so that 60 % and 40 % of the compressive force was applied to the medial and lateral condyles, respectively, and the simulator was cycled at a frequency of 2 Hz. The test lubricant was a solution of 90 % (v/v) bovine serum (HyClone, Logan, Utah, USA) with 0.2 % (w/v) sodium azide in 20 mM EDTA and was filtered through a 0.2 μm filter prior to use. This lubricant was replaced at intervals of one million cycles. All kinematic input profiles used in the Leeds and AMTI simulator testing are summarized in Table 1.

Components were tested in the knee simulators for up to five million cycles, which is equivalent to approximately five years service in vivo. Gravimetric measure-

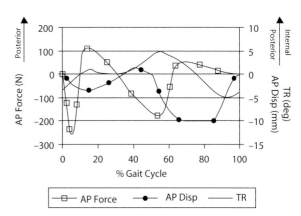

Fig. 2. Leeds knee simulator input profiles for anterior-posterior (AP) force, AP sliding displacement and internal-external tibial rotation (TR)

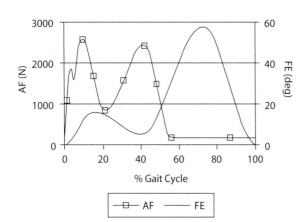

Fig. 1. Knee simulator input profiles for axial force (AF) and flexion-extension (FE)

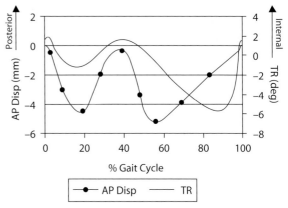

Fig. 3. AMTI knee simulator input profiles for anterior-posterior (AP) sliding displacement and internal-external tibial rotation (TR)

Table 1. Inputs for standard and reduced kinematics testing on the Leeds and AMTI knee simulators

Kinematics	TKR Design	Maximum Axial Force (N)	Flexion-Extension (°)	Anterior-Posterior Translation	Internal-External Rotation (°)
Leeds Standard	PFC Sigma	2600	0–58	0–10 mm	±5
	LCS RP	2600	0–58	–262 N to 110 N	±5
Leeds Reduced	PFC Sigma	2600	0–58	0–5 mm	±2.5
AMTI Standard	PFC Sigma	2600	0–58	0–5.2 mm	+2/–6
	LCS RP	2600	0–58	0–5.2 mm	+2/–6
AMTI Reduced	PFC Sigma	2000	0–58	0–2.6 mm	0/–3

ments of the tibial inserts were obtained before testing and at half million or million cycle intervals. Unloaded soak controls in serum solution were used to monitor moisture uptake. Volumetric wear of the bearings was calculated from the weight loss of the inserts during testing and using density of 0.934 mg/mm^3 for the 1020 GVF polyethylene. The wear rate under each set of conditions was defined as the slope of the linear regression line for cumulative volumetric wear versus the number of cycles completed in the test. Digital images of the wear scars on the superior surfaces of the UHMWPE bearings were obtained after completion of testing. The area of each wear scar from the Leeds simulator was quantified and then expressed as a percentage of the intended articulating area. In addition, femoral and tibial tray surface damage was analyzed using a Form Talysurf stylus profilometer.

3.2 Kinematics

The effect of kinematic input conditions on UHMWPE wear in fixed bearing TKR was examined at both test centers using the PFC Sigma knee design. Six PFC Sigma knees were tested under "low" kinematic conditions on a Leeds knee simulator for three million cycles. During this testing, the internal-external rotation and anterior-posterior sliding translation motions were reduced to half the values used for the standard condition studies, that is ±2.5° and 0–5 mm, respectively.

Reduced kinematic testing was also completed on the AMTI knee simulator. Six PFC Sigma TKR were subjected to eight million cycles with reduced inputs for axial force (maximum 2000 N), AP sliding displacement (0–2.6 mm) and internal-external rotation (0/–3°).

3.3 Femoral Counterface Damage

The influence of femoral counterface damage on TKR wear was investigated using the Leeds simula-

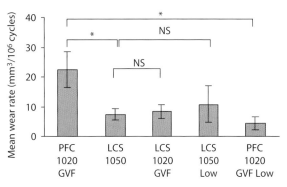

Fig. 4. Mean wear rates with 95% confidence limits for PFC Sigma and LCS Rotating Platform TKR components with the Leeds simulator using standard conditions (PFC 1020 GVF, LCS 1020 GVF) and reduced kinematics (PFC 1020 GVF Low). Note: * significant difference (p<0.05)

tor. One scratch (mean Rp = 1.69±0.50 μm, mean Rv = 2.96±0.51 μm) was inscribed on the center of each condyle of the PFC Sigma femoral components parallel to the flexion-extension direction using a conical diamond stylus (50 μm diameter). Similar scratches (mean Rp = 1.73±0.56 μm, mean Rv = 2.72±0.37 μm) were positioned on the LCS RP femoral components. Each set of knee components was tested for one million cycles while subjected to the standard kinematic input conditions.

4 Results

4.1 Standard Conditions

The PFC Sigma fixed bearing knees exhibited a mean wear rate with 95% confidence limits of 22.75±5.95 cubic millimeters per million cycles (mm^3/MC) when subjected to high rotation kinematics in the Leeds simulator testing (Fig. 4).

In contrast, a mean wear rate of 10.85±2.39 mm^3/MC was observed for the LCS Rotating Platform mobile bearing components. This twofold reduction in wear of the rotating platform mobile bearing knees in com-

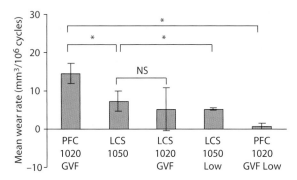

Fig. 5. Mean wear rates with 95% confidence limits for PFC Sigma and LCS Rotating Platform TKR components with the AMTI simulator using standard conditions (PFC 1020 GVF, LCS 1020 GVF) and reduced kinematics (PFC 1020 GVF Low). Note: * significant difference (p<0.05)

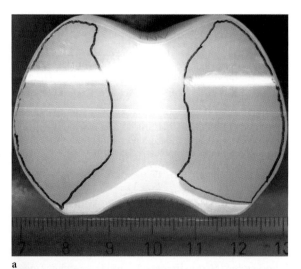

a

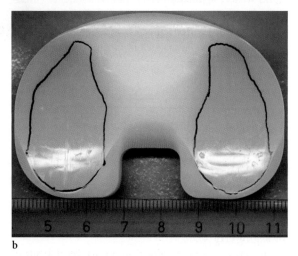

b

Fig. 6a,b. Example wear scars for **a** LCS Rotating Platform mobile bearing; and **b** PFC Sigma fixed bearing TKR after standard testing in the Leeds simulator. Note: Anterior towards top and medial towards left of images

parison to the fixed bearing knees was highly significant (p<0.01). Displacement-controlled testing on the AMTI simulator similarly revealed a highly significant (p<0.01) two-fold reduction in wear for the mobile bearing knees with mean wear rates of 14.57±2.63 mm³/MC and 5.19±5.61 mm³/MC observed for the PFC Sigma and LCS RP inserts, respectively (Fig. 5).

The large error bars reported for the AMTI simulator test with LCS RP components resulted from the small sample size included in the study. Differences in the absolute wear rates obtained at each center may be attributed to differences in test conditions, such as serum concentrations and cycle frequencies.

The mean wear scar areas with 95% confidence limits on the femoral articulating surfaces of the Leeds PFC Sigma and LCS RP tibial inserts, expressed as a percentage of the total articulating area, were 48±3% and 70±7%, respectively (Fig. 6).

This difference in wear area was highly significant (p<0.01) and confirms the low contact stress design principle of the LCS Rotating Platform TKR.

Deep scratches with no obvious lips were observed on the Leeds PFC Sigma femoral components parallel to the flexion-extension motion. Significant fretting wear was observed on the superior surfaces of the PFC Sigma tibial trays in the direction of tibial rotation and was located primarily towards the rim on both the medial and the lateral condyles, indicating a lack of wear resistance of the titanium alloy surface. Microscopic examination revealed large pits where particles had been plucked out of the titanium alloy surface. It is postulated that these particles were removed from the tray-insert articulation by the entraining motion of the lubricant and subsequently caused the scratching observed on the femoral components.

Scratches were observed on the LCS femoral components in a similar direction to those present on the PFC Sigma components but these tended to be shallower. The LCS tibial trays exhibited severe scratching in the direction of tibial rotation with the counterface damage worsening towards the medial and lateral edges of the trays. Similar scratching and wear patterns were observed on the PFC Sigma and LCS RP components tested using the AMTI simulator.

4.2 Kinematics

When subjected to low kinematic inputs on a Leeds simulator, the wear rate exhibited by the PFC Sigma components was only 4.36±2.12 mm³/MC (see Fig. 4). This five-fold wear reduction, in comparison to the wear observed under high kinematics, was highly significant (p<0.001).

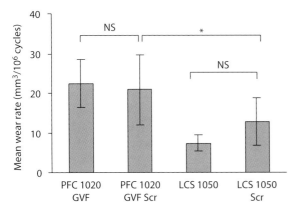

Fig. 7. Mean wear rates with 95% confidence limits for PFC Sigma and LCS Rotating Platform TKR components with the Leeds simulator using standard conditions (PFC 1020 GVF, LCS 1020 GVF) and with femoral scratching (PFC 1020 GVF Scr, LCS 1020 GVF Scr). Note: * significant difference (p<0.05), *NS* no significant difference

The AMTI knee simulator testing also revealed a highly significant (p<0.001) decrease in UHMWPE wear for the PFC Sigma knees when the AP displacement, IE rotation and axial force inputs were reduced (see Fig. 5).

4.3 Femoral Counterface Damage

No significant increase in UHMWPE wear rate was observed when the PFC Sigma femoral components were intentionally scratched parallel to the direction of flexion-extension and subsequently subjected to high rotation kinematics on the Leeds simulator (p>0.05; Fig. 7).

Similarly, the wear rate of the rotating platform bearings did not increase significantly after the femoral components were intentionally scratched (p>0.05). However, when each TKR design was articulated against intentionally scratched femoral components, the PFC Sigma knees still exhibited a significantly greater wear rate than the LCS RP components (p<0.05).

5 Discussion

5.1 Effect of TKR Design

The LCS Rotating Platform TKR has significantly greater conformity between the polyethylene insert and the femoral component in comparison to the PFC Sigma knee, as evidenced by the larger wear scars on the superior surfaces of the polyethylene bearings. However, despite increased contact areas on both the tibial and femoral counterfaces of the inserts, the LCS RP mobile bearing knees produced a significantly lower mean volumetric wear rate of polyethylene than the PFC Sigma fixed bearing components when subjected to high internal-external rotation kinematic inputs. This trend was observed on the knee simulators at both test centers despite use of different test frequencies and serum lubricant concentrations, thereby revealing that TKR design was the dominant factor affecting UHMWPE wear.

We postulate that the rotating platform mobile bearing design decouples the motions between the femoral-insert and tray-insert articulating surfaces. Most of the rotation occurs at the distal tibial articulating surface of the UHMWPE insert, which is simply a unidirectional rotation motion that is known to produce low wear [11, 15]. Since the majority of the rotation occurs at the distal interface, the proximal femoral articulating interface experiences very low rotation. Therefore, at the femoral-insert articulation the motion is also preferably unidirectional and similarly has a low wear rate. Hence, the unique design of the rotating platform mobile bearing knee translates complex input motions into more unidirectional motions, thus benefiting from a reduced wear rate due to decreased cross shear on the molecularly oriented UHMWPE.

In contrast, rotation of the knee with the PFC Sigma fixed bearing TKR occurs entirely at the femoral-insert articulation. The resulting multidirectional wear path at this interface increases the amount of cross shear on the polyethylene articulating surface and, therefore, produces a greater polymer wear rate when subjected to high rotation kinematic inputs.

5.3 Effect of Kinematics

In vitro wear of fixed bearing TKR components in knee joint simulators is highly dependent on kinematic inputs for AP translation and IE rotation [8]. Using a Leeds ProSim knee simulator, Barnett et al. [2] revealed that a twofold reduction of IE rotation and AP displacement inputs to PFC (DePuy) knees produced a fivefold reduction in UHMWPE wear. This phenomenon was further evidenced, as described in this chapter, by the fivefold reduction in wear of the PFC Sigma fixed bearing components on the Leeds simulator when subjected to the low kinematic inputs and also by the substantial reduction in PFC Sigma wear on the AMTI simulator with reduced kinematic inputs. This has potential consequences for highly active patients.

The greater wear of the PFC Sigma fixed bearing components under high kinematics in comparison to low kinematics may be attributed to the increased cross shear on the polyethylene when subjected to greater internal-external rotation. UHMWPE becomes molecularly oriented in the principal direction of sliding (anterior-posterior), producing a strain hardened effect which increases the wear resistance [13, 15]. Consequently, the polyethylene strain softens along the axis transverse to the sliding motion and exhibits less wear resistance in that direction. Introducing a motion such as internal-external rotation, which produces a friction force in the direction transverse to sliding, increases the polymer wear rate. Therefore, the cross shear, which results from increased rotation when fixed bearing knees are subjected to high kinematic input conditions, accelerates polyethylene wear.

5.3   Effect of Femoral Counterface Damage

Total hip replacement retrieval studies and laboratory tests have revealed that discrete scratches on the metallic counterface, located perpendicular to the principal direction of sliding, can increase UHMWPE wear rates by a factor of two to three [1, 14]. However, in vivo scratches observed on knee retrievals primarily occur on the femoral component in the anterior-posterior direction, which is parallel to the principal sliding direction [4]. Whilst the primary direction of sliding in the knee is anterior-posterior as a result of flexion-extension motion, there is also a degree of multidirectional motion produced by internal-external rotation of the joint. This has the potential to accelerate the wear of UHMWPE in the presence of scratched femoral components. However, in both the fixed bearing and the rotating platform mobile bearing knees tested in this study, no significant increase in UHMWPE wear was observed after deliberate scratching of the femoral components parallel to the principal direction of sliding. This supports the postulate that scratches positioned parallel to the principal direction of motion have less effect on UHMWPE wear than scratches located perpendicular to the direction of sliding. However, a significant reduction in wear was still observed with RP mobile bearing knees in comparison to PFC Sigma fixed bearing TKR when articulated against scratched counterfaces.

6   Conclusions

The potential for long term osteolysis necessitates minimization of the number of particles generated due to TKR surface wear, particularly for implantation in younger, more active patients. Despite increased contact areas on both the tibial and femoral counterfaces and the presence of two articulating surfaces, the LCS Rotating

Platform mobile bearing knees produced a significantly lower volumetric wear rate of polyethylene than the PFC Sigma fixed bearing knees when subjected to high kinematic inputs. The unique design of the rotating platform mobile bearing knee translates complex input motions into more unidirectional motions, thus benefiting from a reduced wear rate due to decreased cross shear on molecularly oriented UHMWPE. This tribological advantage of reduced polymer wear in rotating platform TKR has been evidenced in simulator studies completed at two independent test centers with different cycle frequencies and lubricant concentrations. Therefore, patients with higher activity levels may benefit from the implantation of a rotating platform mobile bearing knee.

The wear of fixed bearing TKR decreased significantly when kinematic inputs were reduced, which has implications for highly active patients. Femoral counterface scratching parallel to the principal direction of sliding did not significantly affect UHMWPE wear rates in the PFC Sigma fixed bearing or LCS Rotating Platform mobile bearing knees. However, the significant reduction in wear provided by RP mobile bearing TKR in comparison to fixed bearing knees still remained when articulated against scratched counterfaces.

Thus, the design of TKR chosen for implantation is an important factor that influences UHMWPE surface wear and may affect the long-term success of total knee replacements.

References

1. Barbour PSM, Stone MH, Fisher J (2000) A hip joint simulator study using new and physiologically scratched femoral heads with ultra-high molecular weight polyethylene acetabular cups. Proc Instn Mech Engrs Part H 214: 569–576
2. Barnett PI, Auger DD, Stone MH, Ingham E, Fisher J (2001) Comparison of wear in total knee replacements under different kinematic conditions. J Mats Sci Mats In Med 12: 1039–1042
3. Fisher J (1994) Wear of ultra high molecular weight polyethylene in total artificial joints. Current Orthopaedics 8: 164–169
4. Hailey JL, Fisher J, Dowson D, Sampath SA, Johnson R, Elloy M (1994) A tribological study of a series of retrieved Accord knee explants. Med Eng Phys 16: 223–238
5. Howling GI, Barnett PI, Tipper J, Stone MH, Fisher J, Ingham E (2001) Quantitative characterization of polyethylene debris isolated from periprosthetic tissue in early failure knee implants and early and late failure Charnley hip implants. J Biomed Mater Res (Appl Biomater) 58: 415–420
6. Ingham E, Fisher J (2000) Biological reactions to wear debris in total joint replacement. Proc Instn Mech Engrs Part H 214: 21–37
7. ISO 14243 (1999) Implants for surgery – Wear of total knee joint prostheses – Parts 1, 3
8. Johnson TS, Laurent MP, Yao JQ, Gibertson LN (2000) The effect of displacement control input parameters on tibiofemoral prosthetic knee wear. In: Trans 6th World Biomat Cong, p 56

9. Lafortune MA, Cavanagh PR, Sommer HJ, Kalenak A (1992) Three-dimensional kinematics of the human knee during walking. J Biomech 25: 347–357

10. Liao Y, McNulty D, Swope S (2001) Effects of sterilization method, load input and kinematic input on mobile bearing knee wear. Proc 47th Ann Mtg Orth Res Soc, p 222

11 Marrs H, Barton DC, Jones RA, Ward IM, Fisher J, Doyle C (1999) Comparative wear under four different tribological conditions of acetylene enhanced cross-linked ultra high molecular weight polyethylene. J Mats Mats In Med 10: 333–342

12. McEwen HMJ, Goldsmith AAJ, Auger DD, Hardaker C, Stone MH, Fisher J (2001) Wear of fixed bearing and rotating platform mobile bearing knees subjected to high internal and external tibial rotation kinematics. J Mats Sci Mats In Med 12: 1049–1052

13. Pooley CM, Tabor D (1972) Friction and molecular structure: the behaviour of some thermoplastics. Proc R Soc Lond A 329: 251–274

14. Tipper JL, Ingham E, Hailey JL, Besong AA, Fisher J, Wroblewski BM (2000) Quantitative analysis of polyethylene wear debris, wear rate and head damage in retrieved Charnley hip prostheses. J Mats Sci Mats In Med 11: 117–124

15. Wang A, Stark C, Dumbleton JH (1996) Mechanistic and morphological origins of ultra-high molecular weight polyethylene wear debris in total joint replacement prostheses. Proc Instn Mech Engrs Part H 210: 141–155

8.2 Retrieval Analysis of Mobile Bearing Prosthetic Knees Devices*

J. P. Collier, I. R. Williams, M. B. Mayor

1 Introduction

The success of total knee arthroplasty is influenced by a large number of factors related to surgical technique, patient characteristics, and implant design and, as described in this paper, polyethylene wear and oxidation. The examination of failed retrieved devices offers an opportunity to assess design elements which are beneficial to implant longevity as well as those which may contribute to implant failure. This study focuses on the effectiveness of bearing mobility as a design parameter and whether it offers potential for increased implant longevity. It must be recognized that this is a study of devices which have all failed for a variety of reasons and have been sent to us for examination. These components are a tiny subset and are almost certainly less than 0.01 % of the implanted population of each specific type and are likely to represent much less than 1 % of the failures of any given design. However, we believe that the phenomena observed in this small subset are representative of those occurring clinically and it is with this perspective that this study has been carried out.

The prosthetic knee replacements in this study all have a tibial bearing of ultra high molecular weight polyethylene (hereafter referred to as polyethylene) that is fixed in place against a metal backing. Mobile bearing devices interpose the polyethylene bearing between the femoral component and a smooth surfaced polished tibial component upon which the bearing slides with knee motion.

The New Jersey low-contact stress (LCS) knee system (DePuy, Warsaw, Indiana) was introduced clinically in the late 1970s by F. Buechel and M. Pappas and is available in either a meniscal bearing or rotating platform

design [8, 10]. Although other mobile bearing designs are in use clinically, the LCS is the most widely used mobile bearing system in the world today and the only one extensively used in the United States. It is the only mobile bearing design for which we have a population of retrievals suitable for a study.

Buechel and Pappas and others have noted the advantages of a mobile bearing knee system [1, 9, 14, 23, 24, 37]. They propose that bearing mobility addresses two major long term problems of knee arthroplasty. First, implant loosening may result if torsional stresses are resisted at the articular interface and transferred to the implant fixation interface. Mobile bearings, however, are free to move so as to minimize stresses transferred. Second, polyethylene wear has been shown to be related to the level of contact stress [2, 3, 11, 17, 22, 31, 32, 41]. Fixed bearing prostheses will generally have some nonconformity at the bearing/condyle interface to address the aforementioned issue of loosening due to constraint. These non-matching geometries will generally yield higher contact stresses than if the interfaces were fully conforming. The LCS design is fully conforming in extension and has been shown to have comparatively low levels of contact stress compared to fixed bearings.

In contrast to studies of the prosthetic hip, wear in the prosthetic knee has rarely been measured quantitatively. The difficulty arises from non-uniform bearing geometries, the range of possible wear patterns within the geometries, the prevalence of fatigue damage, and the challenge of determining the initial unworn thickness. This study attempts to overcome those obstacles and provide a rate of linear wear for the LCS meniscal bearing. The difficulties are overcome with the assistance of the device manufacturer who provided the design drawings for the meniscal bearings and by having a large enough retrieval collection to study a significant number of properly aligned bearings with long duration and without detrimental fatigue damage.

The long-term success of both mobile bearing [7, 9, 10, 19, 35] and fixed bearing [13, 29, 34, 39] designs are

* The authors acknowledge and thank the many surgeons who supplied the retrieved components for this study. This research was supported by the Veteran's Administration Research and Rehabilitation Service through grant 3A-473-3DA; DePuy, a Johnson & Johnson Company; Smith & Nephew Inc.; and Zimmer, Inc.

well documented. However, there are concerns regarding mobile bearings expressed in the literature. For example, dual surface articulation has the potential to generate increased polyethylene wear debris which could lead to a greater incidence of osteolysis. Also, the surgical technique is challenging since the bearings' position needs to be dictated by ligamentous tensioning. This may result in the need for greater rigor in implant positioning and a higher potential for implant malposition and instability, possibly resulting in a higher incidence of dislocation or subluxation of the bearings [5, 6, 16, 19, 38].

This retrieval analysis was undertaken to assess the LCS mobile bearing design, and determine the impact of the aforementioned advantages and disadvantages on wear of the tibial bearing. It should be noted, however, that data gathered from retrievals does not necessarily reflect the clinical arena as a whole and caution should be used when making extrapolations.

2 Materials and Methods

An implant retrieval collection containing 206 mobile bearing knee devices (144 meniscal bearing, 62 rotating platform) and 619 fixed bearing knee devices was assembled across a span of 10 years. All of the polyethylene components had been sterilized using gamma radiation in air. This collection was provided by nearly 300 surgeons from across the United States and represents 12 different manufacturers. All mobile bearings were produced by one manufacturer (DePuy, a Johnson & Johnson Company; Warsaw, IN). In most cases, the surgeon provided clinical information such as the duration of the implant's service life and why it was retrieved.

All implants were evaluated and scored for wear by one of the authors (MBM). The bearings were examined with a Nikon binocular dissecting microscope (Nikon, Inc., Tokyo, Japan) at magnifications from 10 to 63X. A modification of the method of Hood et al. [15] was used to assign overall wear scores to the articular polyethylene bearing surfaces. They were rated for the following modes of wear: burnishing, scratching, abrasion, pitting, delamination, cracking, and cold flow. The following ratings were assigned: 0 – not present, 1 – visible to mild presence, 2 – moderate damage, 3 – severe damage. If the polyethylene thickness had been penetrated completely by wear and/or fatigue damage it was rated as being worn through. Thin cross sections were cut from a subset of the polyethylene bearings (34 mobile, 273 fixed). These bearings were selected to represent various manufacturers, designs, materials, and ages. A band saw was used to cut transversely from anterior

to posterior through the bearing. Two hundred micron thick sections were removed from the exposed flat surface using a Jung microtome (Jung, Heidelberg, Germany). Thin sections were examined at a magnification of 10X and the presence or absence of a subsurface white band was noted. The white band is an artifact of the microtome slicing through an embrittled oxidized region and can take the form of polyethylene grain separation, grain cracking, and macrocracking.

For the linear wear analysis, a subset of bearings was assembled which included bearings in vivo for greater than 3 years, that were not obviously malaligned, and had no evidence of fatigue damage in the region to be measured. In most cases, it was not known if a bearing was medial or lateral. Both bearings from a LCS-MB device were included in the dataset except in those cases where one bearing was excluded due to fatigue damage. The dimension measured was the distance between the nadir of the articular dished surface and the opposing point on the back surface. The minimum measured thickness of retrieved bearings was compared with the original bearing thickness as determined from design drawings. The difference between these values measures a combination of wear and creep, but since they are inseparable this study refers to them together as "linear wear". Machining tolerances also lend some variability to the measurements. This study offers wear measurements based upon the worst case scenario which assumes that the bearing thickness was originally at the upper limit for acceptable thickness. This point was near the outside edge of the dovetail track. Measurement was accomplished with a 0.001 "dial indicator" (B. C. Ames Co., Waltham, MA).

The single wear measurement includes the wear of both the top and bottom articular surfaces. A series of unimplanted bearings provided by the manufacturer were measured to provide confidence that bearings are manufactured to the intended tolerances.

Statistical analyses were used to compare the performance of mobile and fixed bearings. Contingency tests between these groups were performed regarding the presence (scored 2 or 3) or absence (scored 0 or 1) of the following articular and back surface wear modes: burnishing, scratching, abrasion, pitting, delamination, cracking, and cold flow. Reasons for retrieval of the implants, as noted by the surgeon, were also compared.

3 Results

3.1 Circumstances of Retrieval

The average in vivo duration of the mobile bearing set and the fixed bearing set were comparable (47 months

Reasons for Retrieval

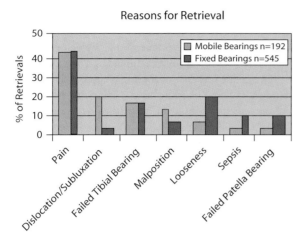

Fig. 8. These were the most commonly cited reasons for implant retrieval. Highly significant differences were found in the incidence of dislocation/subluxation and loosening. Dislocation/subluxation was primarily a problem associated with the mobile meniscal bearing

vs. 45 months). Both sets had a range in service life duration from 1 month to 170 months. In most cases, multiple reasons for retrieval were noted. Care should be exercised not to consider this retrieval data as a mirror of actual retrieval rates. The most common notation for both mobile and fixed bearings was the presence of pain (42% and 43%) which most of the time is not due to implant failure (Fig. 8).

"Looseness" was given as the second most common reason for a fixed bearing device to be retrieved. There was a 19% incidence in fixed bearings compared to an 8% incidence for mobile bearings. This was a significant difference (p<0.01).

Dislocation or subluxation was significantly more common (p<0.01) for mobile bearings (20%) than fixed bearings (4%). Meniscal bearings were at greatest risk for this complication. Twenty-nine of 137 meniscal bearing devices experienced either partial or complete extrusion of a bearing over the edge of the metal tray. In nearly half of these instances the bearing fractured (12/29). An additional 6 meniscal bearing devices were removed for dislocation unrelated to bearing extrusion. The incidence of dislocation/subluxation for the rotating platform design was comparable to that of fixed bearings (5%, 3/55). Three rotating bearings were noted to have twisted into a transverse orientation in vivo.

Malposition was more frequently reported for mobile bearings than with the fixed bearing designs (13% vs. 7%). The difference in incidence was significant (p<0.05).

Wear-through or fracture of the tibial and patellar bearings was also a major contributor to device failure

Articular Damage Modes

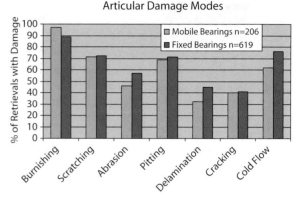

Fig. 9. Clinical wear damage of the articular surfaces of mobile and fixed bearings. "S" designates differences that are significant (p<0.01)

of both mobile and fixed bearings. The incidence of tibial wear through and/or fracture was 18% for both mobile bearings and fixed bearings. However, mobile patellar bearings had significantly fewer (p<0.01) occurrences of wear through and/or fracture than metal-backed fixed bearings (4% and 10% respectively).

3.2 Clinical Wear Analysis

3.2.1 Articular Damage

Polyethylene wear and damage was prevalent in both fixed and mobile bearing knee designs. In vivo durations of just one month were seen to result in evident burnishing of the articular surface. Implants retrieved after 3 years in vivo generally demonstrated wear dominated by the mechanisms of delamination and/or cracking. These fatigue modes were present in 75% of both mobile bearings and fixed bearings retrieved after 3 years. The incidence of burnishing was significantly greater in mobile bearings (p<0.01). Fixed bearings were found to have a significantly greater incidence of abrasive wear, delamination, and cold flow (p0<.01). There were no apparent differences in regard to the incidence of articular scratching, pitting, cracking, or wear through (Fig. 9).

Burnished surfaces that lacked the wear modes that generate macro particles, i.e. delamination, pitting and scratching, often revealed a striated pattern of wear. Various sized groups of very small depressions or pits usually no more than 2 mm in length and 0.5 mm wide were observed scattered about the non-fatigued burnished areas of some of the LCS meniscal bearings. They were generally oriented in an anterior/posterior direction. Of the 50 LCS meniscal bearings measured for linear wear, 36 (72%) had evidence of these striations (Fig. 10).

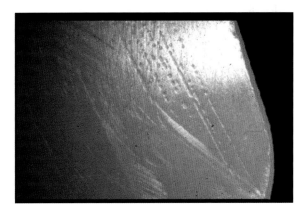

Fig. 10. Appearance of striated pattern of wear on a meniscal bearing that was in vivo for 118 months

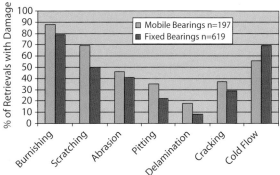

Fig. 11. Clinical wear damage of the back surfaces of mobile and fixed bearings. "S" designates differences that are significant (p<0.01)

3.2.2 Back Surface Damage

Nearly all (97%) fixed bearings presented visible fretting of the polyethylene back surface. Fretting was manifested as burnishing and/or scratching. Fretting of the metal counterface occurred in 67% of the set. While the fretting could be extensive at this fixed bearing interface, it was generally mild in nature with minimal removal of material.

The vast majority (97%) of the mobile bearings presented some back surface fretting. Scratches concentric to the direction of bearing travel were a common observation. Due to the consistent observation that machining lines remained visible on the mobile bearings back surface, it is surmised that back surface wear did not result in appreciable removal of material even in those bearings of longest duration. The mobile bearings had a significantly greater (p<0.01) incidence of backside burnishing, scratching, pitting, and delamination than the fixed bearing designs. Fixed bearings had significantly more creep (p<0.01). There was no difference in the incidence of abrasion or cracking (Fig. 11).

The metal counterfaces of mobile bearings had a significantly higher incidence of fretting (83%); the pattern corresponded to the rotational motion of the bearings.

3.2.3 Linear Wear

Fifty retrieved mobile meniscal bearings from 27 patients were measured for linear wear. The method accounted for wear on both the top and bottom surfaces. The majority (82%) of the measured bearings had an original thickness of less than 8 mm at the bottom of the articular dish. The average in vivo duration for the bearings was 82 months. At the time of retrieval the average patient age was 70 years and their average weight was 184 pounds.

Assuming a worst case scenario where each bearing was machined to the high end of the tolerances, the worn meniscal bearings had an average total linear wear of 0.560 mm and an average rate of wear of 0.092 mm/yr. In a best case scenario assuming each bearing was machined to the low end of the tolerances, the bearings had an average total linear wear of –0.024 mm and an average rate of wear of –0.008 mm/yr. The appearance of negative wear is a result of 34 bearings (68%) having a measured thickness within the allotted machining tolerances. The true rate of wear falls somewhere within that range perhaps approximating 0.05 mm/yr. The amount of wear did not correlate with in vivo duration. Twenty unimplanted mobile meniscal bearings had their thicknesses measured in the same location as for the retrieved bearings. These bearings were all found to have been machined within the allotted tolerances of +/– 0.2921 mm.

3.3 Thin Section Oxidation Analysis

The presence of a white band in a thin section (Fig. 12) is a positive indicator for the presence of accelerated bearing oxidation [12, 40]. Oxidation proved to be more prevalent in mobile bearings (85%, 29/34) than in fixed bearings (64%, 174/273). The difference in incidence was found to be significant (p<0.05).

4 Discussion

A successful total knee arthroplasty is dependent on an array of factors. When considering how best to optimize design factors, a number of different approaches have been undertaken. Arguably the most distinct design variation is the addition of mobility to the polyeth-

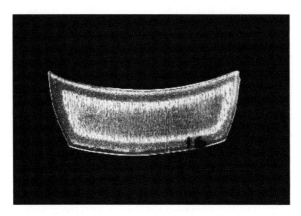

Fig. 12. Sterilization with gamma-irradiation-in-air has been shown to accelerate the oxidation of polyethylene bearings. As shown here, the oxidation is frequently manifested as a subsurface white band in thin section. Creation of this subsurface embrittled region may lead to delamination and cracking of a tibial knee bearing. This LCS –RP bearing was in vivo for 75 months and was badly damaged by fatigue

yleneplastic bearing. This implant retrieval analysis addresses what failure mechanisms are at work and how they compare to those observed for fixed bearings.

Complications arising from polyethylene bearing wear and implant loosening are two common reasons for retrieving prosthetic knee implants. These failure mechanisms are considered in many cases to be interdependent. Loosening may lead to a release of cement, porous coating, or bony particles from the fixation interface which may then infiltrate the articular and nonarticular surfaces and cause damage to the polyethylene. Wear of the polyethylene will produce debris which may lead to osteolysis which in turn may lead to loosening. The mobile bearing knee prosthesis addresses both these concerns by limiting stress at the fixation interface while concurrently reducing and diminishing stress on the polyethylene bearing surface.

The data collected in this retrieval analysis lends support to these assertions. Loosening, for example, was noted less frequently for mobile bearings as a reason for retrieval. However, it should be recognized that this could be due to a number of different factors unrelated to mobility. For example, most of the LCS trays in this set had a beaded porous coating and had a large, robust central peg. This has been shown to be a stable and efficient construct. Mobile bearings do not have screw holes and this would be advantageous in limiting the migration of debris from a bearing's back surface to the fixation interface and thus may limit the initiation of loosening due to osteolysis. These factors may have contributed to a reduced incidence of loosening, in addition to the probable conclusion that bearing mobility diminished the amount of stress at the fixation interface.

Important differences in the wear of polyethylene between mobile and fixed bearings were observed. Of greatest note is the observation that mobile bearings had a lower incidence of abrasion. Abrasion is the removal of material by a grinding or rubbing process and may generate a notable topographic relief in relation to adjacent unworn areas. It is arguably the best indicator that bearing material had been steadily removed by the motion of the femoral condyles upon the bearing. The abrasion factor is important since with the advent of sterilization methods that limit bearing oxidation and its accompanying fatigue mechanisms, abrasion will likely become the wear mode of greatest concern in knee devices. Currently the fatigue mechanisms of cracking and delamination dominate. Mobile bearings were found to have significantly less incidence of delamination than fixed bearings. The comparative deficit of abrasion and delamination fatigue damage in LCS bearings could be attributed to their lower contact stress regime. Reduced stress could also explain the lower incidence of polyethylene cold flow observed for mobile bearings.

Burnishing is a similar process to abrasion, but material is removed to a lesser extent and on a fine enough scale to develop a polished surface. A higher incidence of burnishing may indicate that the polyethylene of the LCS was either more abrasion resistant or that stress upon the polyethylene was comparably less. In addition, an interesting feature was observed in many of the burnished areas of mobile and fixed bearings. Small depressions or pits forming a striation pattern were observed scattered about the non-fatigued burnished areas. The relationship of these to the oxidation of polyethylene was not determined.

Researchers have demonstrated that the LCS has very low contact stress in extension and extrapolated that this would lead to reduced wear damage in vivo [11, 12, 21, 26, 36]. The wear damage observed in this study seems to corroborate what other researchers have surmised with in vitro testing and finite element analysis of tibial bearing designs of varying conformity.

The material quality of the polyethylene was mentioned as one possible explanation for the differing incidences of abrasion and burnishing between mobile and fixed bearings. However, the thin sectioning data does not indicate that the LCS bearing material possessed an advantage. In fact, the LCS bearings may have been at a disadvantage based on the greater incidence of oxidation seen in the subset of bearings that were thin sectioned. Oxidation has been shown to result in embrittlement of the polyethylene which predisposes it to fatigue damage such as delamination and cracking [4, 12, 18]. Because the mobile bearings demonstrated a higher incidence of oxidation, it would be expected that they would have a correspondingly higher incidence of delamination and cracking. In fact, the incidence of cracking is equivalent to that of fixed bearings and the incidence of delamination is significantly less than that found in fixed bearings. From this data it might be postulated that a low contact stress knee bearing is less likely to delaminate, or will take longer to delaminate, even when it has been embrittled due to oxidation.

The LCS bearings in this study demonstrated a higher level of oxidation than the set of fixed bearings. All of the Polyethylene bearings in this study were sterilized with gamma irradiation in an air environment and then stored in air. It is clear from our earlier research that this will result in degradative oxidation which will increase with time in inventory before implantation [12, 27, 30, 33, 36, 40]. The oxidation level is also potentially influenced by the choices of bearing material, fabrication process and, the amount of radiation dosage.

The embrittlement of the bearing due to oxidation may lead in some cases to catastrophic implant failure in some of the retrieved knee components. The polyethylene bearing may crack apart or have regions completely worn through due to delamination and pitting. These modes of fatigue damage were present in more than half of the knee implant retrievals analyzed. All fatigue-damaged components showed evidence of considerable oxidation. If polyethylene oxidation fatigue is removed from the equation, as is hoped will occur now that gamma irradiation in air is no longer utilized, the frequency of fatigue damage should be drastically reduced and should no longer be the most frequent type of damage in polyethylene knee bearings.

The knee motion is primarily linear while the hip includes a crossing pattern. It has been theorized that wear rates are lower in the knee than in the hip, however, the lack of quantitative wear measurements for knee retrievals has made this a difficult contention to support. A review of the literature found four other studies that reported quantitative wear measurements for knee bearings. The authors have previously reported an average wear rate of 0.09 mm/yr for twenty ethylene oxide gas (EtO) sterilized unicompartmental bearings. These were of a high contact stress design and included bearings with an original thickness of less than 6 mm [33]. Two studies of the highly conforming Oxford unicompartmental meniscal knee bearing derived rates for bearing wear. Psychoyios et al. reported 0.036 mm/yr [28] and Argenson and O'Connor reported 0.026 mm/yr [1]. Plante-Bordeneuve and Freeman reported on 22 posterior cruciate ligament sacrificing total knee replacements with a high degree of tibiofemoral conformity in the sagittal plane. They measured an average wear rate of 0.025 mm/yr [25]. The analysis provided here indi-cates that a low contact stress prosthetic knee design with a linear wear pattern can be expected to have a rate of wear less than 0.09 mm/yr. The actual wear rate may be considerably less as this measurement included creep and assumes that the original thickness is at the low end of the tolerance range.

This study illuminated some concerns regarding mobile bearings. Most notably, the incidence of dislocation/subluxation and that of malposition were higher for mobile bearings than for fixed bearings. These failures may come as a result of the demanding surgical technique that is required to ensure that an LCS prosthesis is properly inserted and aligned and that the soft tissues are optimally balanced.

Meniscal mobile bearings are additionally at risk for subluxation due to the possibility that they may travel beyond the edge of the metal tray. This mechanism contributed to the failure of 21% of the retrieved meniscal bearings in this study. Some bearings became trapped on the metal edge and others fractured. Rotating platform bearings were less frequently observed less frequently to have complications as a result of alignment/laxity issues. Three of the 55 were retrieved due to subluxation of the condyles causing the bearing to twist and become trapped in a transverse orientation.

The concern that mobile bearings have a dual articulation and therefore the potential for increased debris generation appears to be mitigated by the observation that even fixed bearings fret against their metal counterfaces and produce backside wear debris. The wear data indicate very low wear rates for the dual articulation mobile bearing system.

Total knee arthroplasty is now in a new era. With the elimination of gamma in air sterilization severe oxidation of polyethylene bearings leading to fatigue should be dramatically reduced if not eliminated. With the potential elimination of bearing fatigue as a concern, mobile bearings would still appear to offer a range of advantages. This study has indicated that mobile bearing devices are less likely to experience loosening and have a reduced incidence of abrasive. Concern for greater debris generation due to dual articulation appears unfounded, linear wear of these bearings was found to be almost immeasurable. Of the 50 meniscal bearings measured for wear (avg. duration 82 months), 34 were found to be still within the original machining tolerances.

References

1. Argenson JN, O'Connor JJ (1992) Polyethylene wear in meniscal knee replacement. A one to nine-year retrieval analysis of the Oxford knee. J Bone Joint Surg 74B: 228–232
2. Bartel DL, Bicknell VL, Wright TM (1986) The effect of conformity, thickness, and material on stresses in ultra-high

molecular weight components for total joint replacement. J Bone Joint Surg 68 A:1041–1051

3. Bartel DL, Rawlinson JJ, Burstein AH et al. (1995) Stresses in polyethylene components of contemporary total knee replacements. Clin Orthop 317: 76–82

4. Bell CJ, Walker PS, Abeysundera MR et al. (1998) Effect of oxidation on delamination of ultrahigh-molecular-weight polyethylene tibial components. J Arthroplasty 13: 280–290

5. Bert JM (1990) Dislocation/subluxation of meniscal bearing elements after New Jersey low-contact stress total knee arthroplasty. Clin Orthop 254: 211–215

6. Bert JM (1996) Delayed failure of meniscal bearing elements in total knee arthroplasty. J Arthroplasty 11: 611–612

7. Buechel FF (1994) Cementless meniscal bearing knee arthroplasty: 7 to 12 year outcome analysis. Orthopedics 17: 833–836

8. Buechel FF, Pappas MJ (1986) The new jersey low-contact-stress knee replacement system: Biomechanical rationale and review of the first 123 cemented cases. Arch Orthop Trauma Surg 105: 197–204

9. Buechel FF, Pappas MJ (1989) New Jersey low contact stress knee replacement system. Ten-year evaluation of meniscal bearings. Orthop Clin North Am 20: 147–177

10. Buechel FF, Pappas MJ (1990) Long-term survivorship analysis of cruciate-sparing versus cruciate-sacrificing knee prostheses using meniscal bearings. Clin Orthop 260: 162–169

11. Collier JP, Mayor MB, McNamara JL, Surprenant VA, Jensen RE (1991) Analysis of the failure of 122 polyethylene inserts from uncemented tibial knee components. Clin Orthop 273: 232–242

12. Collier JP, Sperling DK, Currier JH et al. (1996) Impact of gamma sterilization on clinical performance of polyethylene in the knee. J Arthroplasty 11: 377–389

13. Font-Rodriguez DE, Scuderi GR, Insall JN (1997) Survivorship of cemented total knee arthroplasty. Clin Orthop 345: 79–86

14. Goodfellow JW, O'Connor J (1986) Clinical results of the Oxford knee. Surface arthroplasty of the tibiofemoral joint with a meniscal bearing prosthesis. Clin Orthop 205: 21–42

15. Hood RW, Wright TM, Burstein AL (1983) Retrieval analysis of total knee prostheses: A method and its application to 48 total condylar prostheses. J Biomed Mater Res 17: 829–842

16. Huang CH, Young TH, Lee YT, Jan JS, Cheng CK (1998) Polyethylene failure in New Jersey low-contact stress total knee arthroplasty. J Biomed Mater Res 39: 153–160

17. Ishikawa H, Fujiki H, Yasuda K (1996) Contact analysis of ultrahigh molecular weight polyethylene articular plate in artificial knee joint during gait movement. J Biomech Eng 118: 377–386

18. Jahan MS, Stovall JC, Davidson JA, Hines G (1995) Long-term effects of gamma-sterilization on degradation of implant materials. Appl Radiat Isot 46: 637–638

19. Jordan LR, Olivo JL, Voorhorst PE (1997) Survivorship analysis of cementless meniscal bearing total knee arthroplasty. Clin Orthop 338: 119–123

20. Keblish P (1991) Results and complications of the LCS (Low Contact Stress) knee system. Acta Orthopaedica Belgica 57 (Suppl 2): 124–127

21. McNamara JL, Collier JP, Mayor MB, Jensen RE (1994) A comparison of contact pressures in tibial and patellar total knee components before and after service in vivo. Clin Orthop 299: 104–113

22. Morra EA, Postak PD, Greenwald AS (1997) The effects of articular geometry on Delamination and pitting of UHM-WPE tibial inserts: A finite element study. Scientific Ex-

hibit, 64th Annual Meeting of the American Academy of Orthopaedic Surgeons, Feb 13–17, San Francisco, CA

23. Morra EA, Postak PD, Greenwald AS (1998) The influence of mobile bearing knee geometry on the wear of UHM-WPE tibial inserts: A finite element study. Scientific Exhibit, 65th Annual Meeting of the American Academy of Orthopaedic Surgeons, Mar 19–23, New Orleans, LA

24. O'Connor JJ, Goodfellow JW (1996) Theory and practice of meniscal knee replacement: designing against wear. Proceedings Inst of Mech Eng. Part H – J Eng Medicine 210: 217–222

25. Plante-Bordeneuve P, Freeman MA (1993) Tibial high-density polyethylene wear in conforming tibiofemoral prostheses. J Bone Joint Surg Br 75(4): 630–636

26. Postak PD, Steubben CM, Greenwald AS (1993) Tibial plateau surface stress in TKA: A factor in clinical failure. Scientific Exhibit, 60th Annual Meeting of the American Academy of Orthopaedic Surgeons, Feb 18–23, San Francisco, CA

27. Premnath V, Harris WH, Jasty M, Merrill EW (1996) Gamma sterilization of UHMWPE articular implants: An analysis of the oxidation problem. Biomaterials 17: 1741–1753

28. Psychoyios V. Crawford RW. O'Connor JJ. Murray DW (1998) Wear of congruent meniscal bearings in unicompartmental knee arthroplasty: a retrieval study of 16 specimens. J Bone Joint Surg Br 80(6): 976–982

29. Ranawat CS, Flynn WF, Saddler S et al. (1993) Long-term results of the total condylar knee arthroplasty. A 15-year survivorship study. Clin Orthop 286: 94–102

30. Ries MD, Weaver K, Rose RM et al. (1996) Fatigue strength of polyethylene after sterilization by gamma irradiation or ethylene oxide. Clin Orthop 333: 87–95

31. Rose RM, Goldfarb EV, Ellis E, Crugnola AM (1983) On the pressure dependence of the wear of ultra-high molecular weight polyethylene. Wear 92: 99–111

32. Rostoker W, Galante JO (1979) Contact pressure dependence of wear rates of ultra-high molecular weight polyethylene. J Biomed Mater Res 13: 957–964

33. Sauer WL, Weaver KD, Beals NB (1996) Fatigue performance of ultra-high-molecular-weight polyethylene: Effect of gamma radiation sterilization. Biomaterials 17: 1929–1935

34. Schai PA., Thornhill TS, Scott RD (1998) Total knee arthroplasty with the PFC system. Results at a minimum of ten years and survivorship analysis. J Bone Joint Surg 80B: 850–858

35. Sorrells RB (1996) The rotating platform mobile bearing TKA. Orthopedics 199: 793–796

36. Szivek JA, Anderson PL, Benjamin JB (1996) Average and peak contact stress distribution evaluation of total knee arthroplasties. J Arthroplasty 11: 952–963

37. Tsakonas AC, Polyzoides AJ (1997) Reduction of polyethylene wear in a congruent meniscal knee prosthesis. Experimental and clinical studies. Acta Orthop Scand 275 (Suppl): 127–131

38. Verhaven E, Handelberg F, Casteleyn PP, Opdecam P (1991) Meniscal bearing dislocation in the Oxford knee. Acta Orthop Belg 57:430–432

39. Whiteside LA (1994) Cementless total knee replacement. Nine-to 11-year results and 10-year survivorship analysis. Clin Orthop 309: 185–192

40. Williams IR, Mayor MB, Collier JP (1998) Impact of sterilization method on wear in knee arthroplasty. Clin Orthop 356: 170–180

41. Wright TM, Bartel DL (1986) The problem of surface damage in polyethylene total knee components. Clin Orthop 205: 67–74

Clinical

Chapter 9
Indications

9.1 Mobile Bearing Unicompartmental Knee Replacement

P.A. KEBLISH, J.L. BRIARD

1 Historical Background (Metallic Femoral or Tibial – Without Cement)

The concept of unicondylar resurfacing was developed by McKeever and Elliot [27] in the 1950s and utilized through the 1960s. Cemented hemiarthroplasty (femoral and tibial surfaces) was first reported in the early 1970s in North America by Gunston. Marmor [25] utilizing the fixed-bearing knee with different geometry (Fig. 1).

The Gunston failed early because of the straight tracks that failed to allow rotation. During this development period (late 1970s), a few negative reports on unicompartmental knee arthroplasty (UKA) [10, 11, 18] appeared and proved to be damaging to the concept. Most centers abandoned UKA (and its teaching) as a viable treatment option. Therefore, many "trained orthopedists", especially in the United States have little to no exposure with the procedure. Many centers around the world, especially in Scandinavians. [21–23] continued to have a satisfactory experience with hemiarthroplasty. They and others [7, 8] have continued to teach and recommend the procedure as an excellent treatment option in angular knee deformity. Mobile-bearing uni-condylar arthroplasty was introduced by Goodfellow and O'Connor (Oxford knee) in 1975 [6] and subsequently enhanced by Buechel and others (New Jersey LCS) [1, 3] to improve contact stress kinematics and wear (Fig. 2).

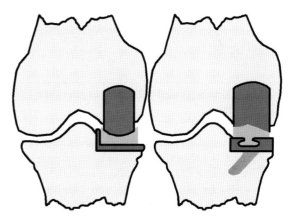

Fig. 2. Mobile bearing UKA: Oxford design fully congruent without track (left). LCS design with dovetail radial track and cementless option (right)

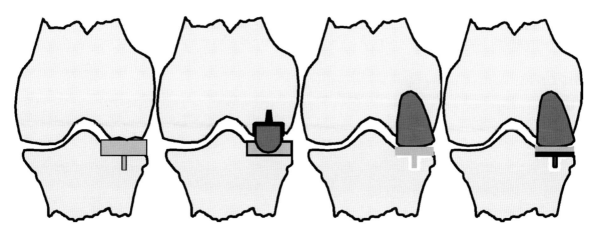

Fig. 1. Fixed bearing UKA designs (left to right): McIntosh partial hemicondylar replacement, Gunston straight track (cemented), highly constrained, Marmor type cemented non-metal backed, constrained, metal backed tibial – flat to slightly dished with different models

Why the difference in approach? Is there a variable population base? Are expectations different? These questions and others are of interest since results and opinions regarding successful UKA varies from surgeon to surgeon, center to center, and country to country. There is renewed interest in UKA with "minimally invasive" techniques and newer instrumentation, which is reviewed in another chapter.

We have always favored a minimally invasive technique (mid- or subvastus), but one adequate to perform the procedure accurately. Caution must be noted to surgeons jumping on the "minimally invasive" approach bandwagon for the wrong reasons. UKA is a technically demanding procedure and patient selection is critical. Small incisions, poor patient selection with "oversell", and small technical errors can lead to less than ideal results. Early to intermediate results are now being reported for the "minimally invasive" approach [29]. However, the procedure is being hyped by many centers previously not familiar with UKA, and caution remains. Is a smaller incision better if it compromises any aspect of the procedure?

2   Introduction: Surgical Options for Angular Knee Deformity

When angular knee deformity with unicompartment involvement is present, surgical options include total knee arthroplasty (TKA), osteotomy, and UKA. Indications for TKA are well established. High tibial osteotomy (HTO) for genu varum deformity has proven to be effective and remains a well-accepted procedure [12]. Supra-condylar varus osteotomy for genu valgum is performed less commonly, but is also effective, especially in the young, obese female. Literature reviews report satisfactory results of HTO ranging from 28 % [26] to 77 % [4], with a general consensus that the procedure is 60 % to 70 % successful. Technical problems, need for immo-

bilization, longer rehabilitation, and other factors have dampened the enthusiasm for the procedure (if other options are available) and emphasized the more strict criteria (Table 1) required in selecting the best procedure for a given patient.

UKA provides an alternative to HTO and TKA for angular knee deformity. Criteria and selection factors in the literature to date have been conservative [8, 24, 33]. The procedure is usually recommended for relatively inactive, elderly patients. An increasing number of patients, however, are more youthful, more active, will live longer, and desire to maintain an active lifestyle, including recreational athletics such as tennis, skiing, etc. These patients may be too young for TKA and may not meet the treatment criteria for HTO or newer approaches such as autologous cartilage autotransplantation and allograft (bone-cartilage-meniscal) transplantation, which remain experimental from intermediate term regarding durability. Improvement in prosthetic design, materials, instrumentation, and surgical technique have renewed interest in UKA for this patient group.

The philosophy of UKA is to realign minimal, correctable angular deformity while preserving normal kinematics. The procedure entails a resurfacing to re-establish the normal ligament environment (cruciates, collaterals) and the mechanical axis to the pre-morbid alignment, which is dictated by collateral ligament tension. Flexion-extension balancing must be accomplished without lengthening releases, subtle elevation of the joint line, overloading the opposite compartment, overcorrection, or creating patellofemoral impingement.

The advantages for unicompartmental knee arthroplasty (UKA) include preservation of:

- bone stock,
- normal articulating surfaces of the uninvolved compartments,
- near-normal kinematics, and
- normal or near normal range of motion.

Table 1. Patient selection factors for angular knee deformity

Factors	Osteotomy	UKA
Deformity	Fixed	Correctable (without releases)
ROM	Near normal; age-diagnosis dependent	Normal
Disease process	Osteoarthritis, Post-traumatic arthritis, Selective inflammatory arthritis (Juvenile RA – hemophilia)	Osteoarthritis Post-traumatic arthritis Osteonecrosis
Opposite compartment Patellofemoral compartment	Variable near normal; age dependent	Peripheral osteophytes acceptable; Normal/near normal
ACL/PCL	Variable; age dependent	Normal; intact and functional
Weight	No limit	Reasonable height/weight ratio
Activity level	No limit	Active with reasonable limits

In addition, surgical trauma is minimal, blood replacement is not required, rehabilitation is rapid, hospitalization is shorter, and the procedure is cost-effective.

3 Factors Influencing TKA Outcomes

Patient selection. Patient selection is perhaps the most important factor, followed by prosthetic design and surgical technique if consistent results are to be achieved. All authors have stressed that UKA patient selection is most important, including proper diagnosis, age, activity level, weight, and at times appropriate imaging studies (MRI, CT) to confirm non-inflammatory single compartment disease. The patient should be well motivated with a good understanding of the philosophy of the procedure. Many patients have had previous arthroscopic surgery with well-documented compartment pathology and overall joint assessment. Patient permission for conversion to TKA at surgery, if felt indicated, should be agreed upon since more extensive disease may be present than had been anticipated.

Selection factors for UKA, based on 30 years of personal experience and supporting literature, the most important criteria for selecting UKA are:

- a correctable deformity with minimal to no ligament releases,
- an intact ACL,
- avoiding over-correction and subsequent overload of the opposite compartment, and
- the surgeon's experience (Fig. 3).

The operating surgeon must be a "believer" in UKA and be familiar with the technique and system being utilized.

He/she must communicate the controversial but conservative nature of the procedure to the patient and family if UKA is not commonly performed in the community. Patients must be well-informed and give preoperative consent in all cases to allow conversion to TKA at the time of surgery. Conversion to TKA may be necessary if factors listed above prove to be less than ideal, except perhaps in younger patients who understand the risk and are willing to accept discomfort with increased activity.

4 Prosthetic Design

Prosthetic design is another key factor in achieving successful UKA and must allow for unconstrained motion without mechanical (translational or rotational) blocks [9]. Designs that have attempted to introduce increased stability without allowing for mobility have resulted in premature mechanical failures [16, 21], while designs with high contact stress have led to failures secondary to polyethylene wear [5, 21, 23]. Two basic designs have stood the test of time: round-on-flat or slightly dished fixed-bearing and meniscal bearing with more congruent geometry. Fixed-bearing designs include all polyethylene tibial components (Marmor prototype) and metallic-backed polyethylene tibial components (Brigham prototype) which have been modified to allow for cementless fixation and modularity. Fixed bearing devices that have attempted to add increased congruity may lead to increased torque and tensile forces, high contact stresses with potential loosening and/or subluxation (Fig. 4). Meniscal bearing designs include the Oxford (Goodfellow/O'Connor) cemented straight track constant radius and the Low Contact Stress (LCS; DePuy, Leeds, UK) radial track with decreasing radius of curvature.

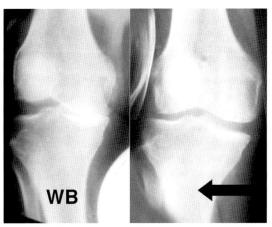
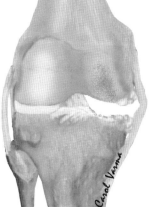
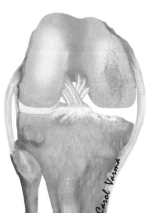

Fig. 3. Ideal patient for UKA. Note correctable varus instability with stress X-rays. Ideal anatomic candidate for UKA with isolated compartment disease, a correctable deformity and intact ligaments

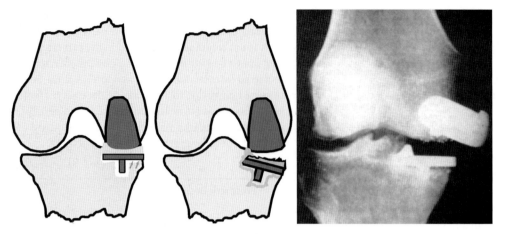

Fig. 4. Fixed bearing UKA with built in constraint on left. Rotational forces can lead to failures in the femoral and/or tibial side

Fig. 5. Generation 1 LCS with single femoral stem and unsupported lateral poly lip. Note long-term follow-up with bearing movement posterior in flexion and anterior in extension. There is natural kinematic rollback of the femur

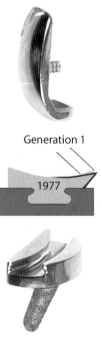

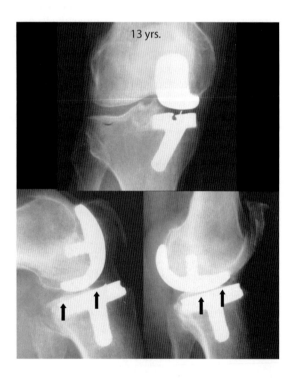

Mobile bearing rational. Consequences of polyethylene wear have been the initiating causes of TKA and UKA. Mobile bearing UKA addresses problems of wear with improved congruent mobility, kinematics stability and potentially normal ROM. The LCS provides the option of cementless fixation. Biomechanics of the original and second generation modifications that have a 25-year follow-up (with no change in articulating geometry) are shown in Fig. 5, 6, and 7. The ability to exchange polyethylene bearings is a major advantage that allows the active young patient an option for longer term success with minimal operative downtime. Conversion TKA has not been a problem and is less challenging than HTO conversion in this authors opinion.

Fixed and meniscal bearing knees have been used successfully for over 25 years and provide options for the orthopedic surgeon who believes in the concept of UKA. Both fixed and meniscal bearing knees present the surgeon with the challenge of proper implantation. More precise instrumentation and improved prosthetic design have enhanced the surgeon's ability to achieve a better outcome.

Fig. 6. Generation 2 LCS with additional femoral peg and supportive polyethylene edges. Eleven year cementless follow-up showing no polyethylene wear/osteolysis and normal kinematics in flexion and extension

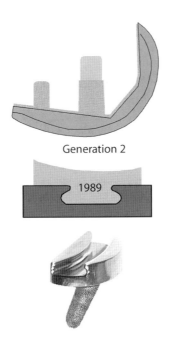

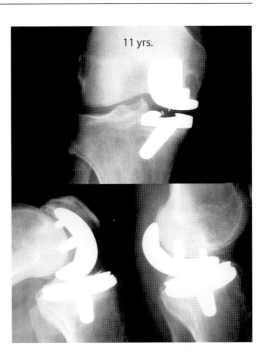

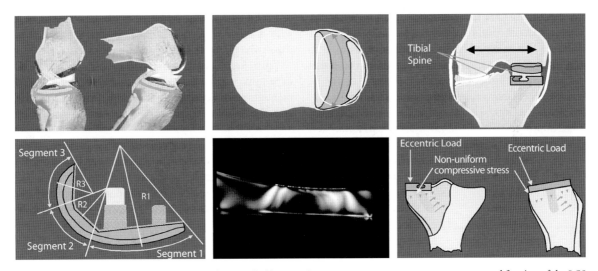

Fig. 7. Summary of design and biomechanical rational of kinematics, movement, geometry, contact stress, and fixation of the LCS unicompartment arthroplasty

4.1 Surgical Approach

Surgical technique and principles of accurate surgical alignment in UKA are important factors that are basic to satisfactory outcomes. The technique of UKA is more challenging, and experience with operative techniques is frequently limited in residencies and/or fellowships. Basic surgical principles apply to all design systems and will be addressed with the LCS system.

Medial UKA. A midline anterior skin incision is preferred. The incision is angled distally to the medial side of the tibial tubercle. Minimal undermining is required. The arthrotomy incision can be performed via the standard parapatellar, subvastus, or a short midvastus variation, which is the current approach of choice. The midvastus approach, popularized by Engh et al. [5], splits the medial quadriceps and capsule from the anteromedial attachment of the patella proximally along a natural cleavage plane. A limited medial sleeve release of the upper tibia enhances the exposure. The status of the lateral and patellar femoral compartments can be assessed without everting the patella. Patella eversion and extensive exposure are not required in UKA. However, if the surgeon is more comfortable with a more extensive exposure, it is easily accomplished with the midvastus approach. The advantages of patella translocation (rather than eversion) include minimizing the external tibial rotation, which improves rotational positioning and protecting the normal articular cartilage. Maintaining the bulk of the medial quadriceps to the central tendon allows for better patella control intraoperatively, less postoperative pain, and more rapid rehabilitation.

Lateral UKA. Lateral compartment replacement for valgus instability is best performed via a modified direct lateral approach, which accomplishes the lateral release with the exposure. The skin incision is proximal midline ending distally at a point between Gerdy's tubercle and the tibial tubercle. The arthrotomy incision splits the retinaculum (superficial layer) at the medial border of Gerdy's tubercle and extends proximally, one to two centimeters lateral to the patella. The deep capsular layer is released from the patellar rim. The proximal arthrotomy can be completed by splitting the vastus lateralis, sub-vastus, or a limited lateral parapatellar incision made obliquely through the central tendon.

The direct lateral approach allows for direct soft tissue release, adequate exposure without everting the patella, improved patellofemoral tracking, minimal soft tissue trauma, and rapid rehabilitation. The approach can be extended if TKA is required, as described in the chapter on the lateral approach and previously by others [12, 13, 15].

4.2   Technique Principles

The technical principles of UKA are similar to but subtly different from TKA. Re-establishing the joint line of the diseased compartment and restoring the altered anterior cruciate ligament, posterior cruciate ligament, and collateral (medial and lateral) kinematics are key goals of implantation. When proper indications exist, normal knee function is possible. Instrumentation systems plus surgical expertise must provide for accurate compartment resurfacing of the femoral condyle and tibial plateau. Technical errors of malposition (rotational, varus-valgus, flexion-extension) and gap imbalance (depth of resection) will negatively affect stability, mobility, wear, and fixation with less than satisfactory clinical outcomes. Since few UKA are performed, even by so-called

experts, more attention to detail is required. Excellent long-term results can be appreciated when patient selection, prosthetic design, and surgical technique are optimal. This section addresses the key technical aspects of UKA that will affect clinical results [14].

4.3   Bone Resections

Position and Orientation Variables. Effective instrumentation should reliably establish the correct size, position, and orientation of the femoral and tibial components. The variables of axial rotation, varus-valgus tilt, flexion-extension orientation, anteroposterior (A-P) position, and joint line level must be correctly defined by the surgeon using instruments designed for these purposes. Proper flexion-extension gap balancing should allow for unimpeded motion with normal kinematic control. Bone resections are the key element in preparing implantation surfaces and dictate final positioning. The potential for mal-resection exists on both femoral and tibial sides and will be described in more detail. Errors are compounded if instrument malposition (mal-resection) is made on both sides and are more common with anatomic variations such as flared femoral condyles, which may be a contradiction to UKA (Fig. 8).

Tibial first or femoral first approaches can be utilized, depending on the UKA system [2, 18, 31] and instrumentation philosophy/rationale. Most implantation systems, however, have similar guidelines which include:

- referencing off the sub-chondral bone, which is more consistent, or a fixed point such as the ACL insertion maintaining the proper joint line,
- correct tibial rotation to reproduce a perpendicular mediolateral plane with a 5° to 7° posterior slope,
- extramedullary instrumentation for the tibial resection,
- mating the femoral resection to the tibial resection plane via appropriate resection blocks.

Femoral orientation can employ either extramedullary or intramedullary instrumentation. An intramedullary system requires a more extensive approach and violation of the femoral canal, both potential disadvantages.

Exposure of the tibial plateau is enhanced by a sleeve elevation that is adequate enough to allow for exposure and removal of peripheral osteophytes to normal anatomy. Preservation of the outer meniscal rim is recommended to maintain the integrity of the medial sleeve, preserve optimal stability, and avoid geniculate vessels.

Tibial and femoral osteophytes are best removed with a reciprocating saw and/or rongeurs to re-establish pre-

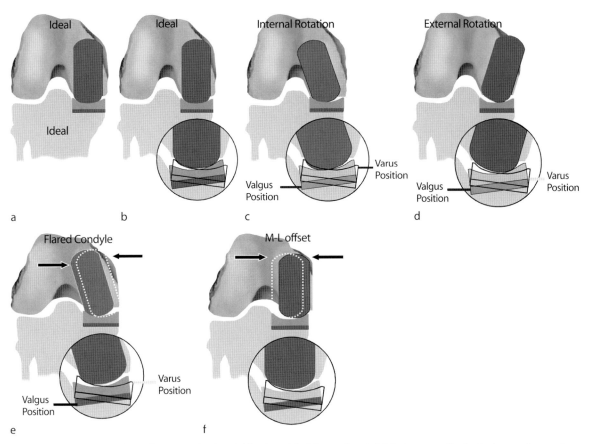

Fig. 8a–f. Bone resection (prosthetic position) variables from ideal femoral and tibial placement (in flexion), to mal-resection potentials. Mal-resection are compounded if 1) femoral geometry is atypical, 2) gaps unequal, and become less than ideal as the knee ranges from flexion to extension

morbid anatomy. External tibial rotation will improve access to the posterior corner. Loose bodies or remaining posterior osteophytes are removed. Anatomic variants, pathological erosions, the tibial slope, and bone quality are assessed. Articular (cartilage and bone) high points or irregularities should be removed to subchondral bone, since referencing is more accurate and the bone surfaces are more accessible for instrumentation.

4.4 The Tibial "L" Resection

General Principles. Accuracy of the tibial resection is critical and will be determined by proper instrument positioning for variables of rotation (coronal plane), varus-valgus tilt, flexion extension (A-P slope), horizontal limit (sizing), and depth of resection (Fig. 9).

Rotational orientation influences varus-valgus and the A-P positions (posterior slope) and, therefore, should be established first. Malposition of the rotational setting can lead to subtle or obvious changes in the varus-valgus and A-P slope cuts which may lead

to less than ideal resections. Malresections will result in higher contact stress at the articulating surface and increased torque forces at the bone (cement) prosthetic interface, especially in fixed-bearings with round-on-flat or dished geometries.

Tibial resection guide positioning. Extramedullary guide systems are the norm. Lower profile UKA tibial resection guides, as utilized in the LCS system, allow for instrumentation with more limited compartment exposure as recommended. The resection guide should allow for small adjustments of the alignment rod to fine-tune rotation, varus-valgus, and A-P positions. The guide should allow for an adjustable resection block to accommodate the depth of resection changes.

Rotation alignment. The sagittal plane of the "L" resection dictates the rotational orientation of the tibial component; therefore, this setting is critical. Internal or external positioning will result in rotational mal-alignment that will be accentuated with the knee in extension.

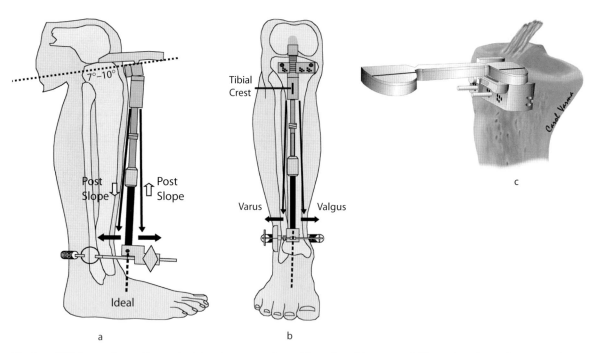

Fig. 9a–c. Tibial resection guide emphasizing the proper AP and lateral position. Central illustration shows the proper depth, plane and rotation of the L-resection, which re-establishes the normal joint line (at the ACL insertion) to allow an 8 mm polyethylene bearing

Varus-valgus alignment. The mediolateral resection should be made perpendicular to the anatomic (mechanical) axis of the tibia. The alignment rod is best referenced distally (ankle level) to the tibialis anterior tendon. The lateral border of the tibialis anterior tendon is easily palpable and centers over the midpoint of the talus. This point is slightly medial to the midpoint of the malleus and centers over the second metatarsal when the foot is normal. Medial rod placement will result in a valgus position, and lateral rod placement, which is more common, will result in a varus position. An ideal (perpendicular) resection is critical; therefore, the alignment rod should be re-checked prior to final resection.

Flexion-extension (A-P) alignment. Reproducing the patient's normal posterior slope (5° to 10°) is the goal and is important for restoration of normal kinematics of the ACL/PCL and the so-called four-bar linkage. Alignment systems should allow for A-P adjustment. The LCS resection block is set for a 7° posterior resection when the alignment rod is parallel to the tibial crest and/or fibular shaft as viewed from the lateral side. Anterior placement of the rod will increase the posterior slope while posterior rod alignment will decrease the posterior slope. Some "eye-balling" may be required if external landmarks are obscured. Remember that a neutral or decreased posterior slope will limit roll back and

flexion, increase contact stress on the posterior bearing surface, increase polyethylene wear, and increase the potential for prosthetic lift off and prosthetic fixation failure (Fig. 10).

Depth of resection. The depth of resection is best determined after having confirmed the other variables. The goal is to resect enough bone to allow space for the "total tibial prosthetic thickness" without elevating the joint line (femoral-tibial articulating surface). The most consistent landmarks for establishing the proper depth of resection are the ACL insertion and the upper slope of the tibial spine. The final joint line (articulating interface) should be located at this level to allow for optimal kinematics. The space is more finite in UKA (ACL-PCL controlled) and relates most critically to the normal opposite compartment. Final selection of the tibial component size is determined following completion of the "L" resection. Optimal peripheral bony rim contact should be obtained with abutment of the sagittal tibial surface against the vertical arm of the "L" resection. The ACL insertion must be preserved and the final tibial articulating surface adjusted to the original tibial plateau surface. The spacer block of appropriate size and depth is inserted to check all tibial resection variables. A drop rod attached to the guide rechecks the varus-valgus and the A-P slope. Ranging the knee from 90° to full exten-

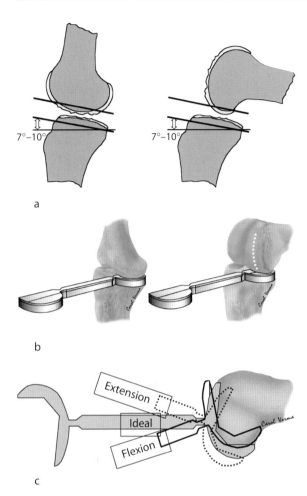

7°–10°   7°–10°

a

b

c

Fig. 10a–c. Spacer block placement following tibial resection. Mapping the tibial from flexion to extension confirms the rotational position and flexion/extension gaps

sion rechecks the level and orientation of the tibial resection and maps the rotational tracking to the femoral surface before instrumentation of the femoral side. The tibial resection should be re-checked when the femoral resections are referenced from the tibia, and vice versa if a femoral first approach is used.

4.5   Femoral Preparation and Size Selection

The femoral condyle is frequently irregular, with bony and/or articular cartilage high spots. Referencing from the subchondral bone is more consistent and is recommended with use of most instrument systems, whether a femoral first or tibial first approach is utilized. Removal of irregular high spots, from the femoral condyle surfaces is accomplished utilizing an oscillating saw. Smoothing of the subchondral surface allows for better seating of alignment shells or cutting jigs.

Femoral size selection which best approximates the existing bony geometry is initially estimated by use of an A-P template and mediolateral sizing shells (Fig. 11).

It is important to keep in mind that it is the shape of the subchondral bone and not the articular cartilage that is to be re-established. Rotational (coronal and sagittal) planes are checked. Care must be taken to avoid overcorrection and over-sizing, which increases the risk of soft tissue and/or patella impingement. The medial and lateral prosthetic borders should lie flat or just within the femoral condyles. The most superior medial edge is often flush with the condyle in the typical medial UKA. Overhang must be avoided. Flared condyles may present a problem.

4.6   Flexion-Extension Gap Balancing

The A-P femoral position (resection) dictates the flexion gap, and the distal position dictates the extension gap. Condylar resections (thickness) must accommodate the prosthetic mass. Checking the flexion and extension gap with a shell positioner assures that the proper amount of bone is resected. If the flexion gap is tight, the sizing template can be moved anteriorly to, but not beyond, the limiting point previously described. Downsizing the femoral component may be required if the flexion gap is too tight or there is impingement anteriorly. It is important to recognize this potential error prior to femoral resection, although it can be corrected following trial component placement. Re-attachment of the resection block, however, may be less exact, re-cuts less precise, and the final fit compromised if previous fixation holes need to be re-done.

4.7   Femoral Rotation Considerations

The femoral component can be placed correctly, too far medially or laterally, internally or externally rotated (coronal plane), and flexed or extended in the sagittal plane. Malrotation will be exacerbated if these resections are additive and/or combined with tibial malpositioning. As noted above, recognition of these potential errors, by mapping the rotation plane from 90° to 0°, will avoid the initial mal-resections as previously illustrated. Internal malrotation of the femoral component will result in:

- high contact stress on the more central articulation,
- increased torque on the prosthetic component,
- flexion gap instability, and
- rotational incongruence in extension.

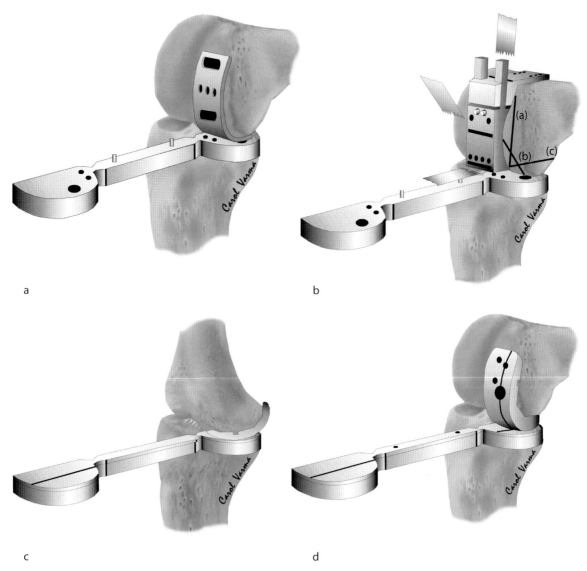

Fig. 11a–d. The femoral shell/drilling guide is set and the cutting gig is impacted to the subchondral surface to establish the proper depth and plane of the distal campher and posterior cuts (top and bottom left). Drilling templates are secured and rotation and flexion/extension gap stability re-checked. Anchoring holes are made for trial and final prosthetic insertion (top and bottom right)

External malrotation will result in:

- high contact stress on the peripheral articulating surface,
- increased torque,
- flexion gap instability, and
- increased potential for soft tissue impingement due to proximal overhang of the prosthesis.

Flexion positioning of the femoral component will result in bearing impingement anteriorly in extension. Conversely, extension positioning of the femoral component will result in bearing impingement posteriorly in flexion. Lateral (central) positioning will result in impingement

on the tibial spine whereas medial (peripheral) component positioning will result in medial tibial component overload. Both will increase the potential for patella and/or medial soft tissue impingement. These malrotations (malresections) may lead to increased wear and loosening, the primary cause of failure in UKA.

4.8   Femoral Resection

Coronal plane orientation (axial positioning) of the femoral component must align to the tibial component in flexion and extension. Resection blocks should be oriented to the femoral axis and allow for proper flexion-extension position (referencing parallel to the anterior femoral cortex). Take care to set the resection block flush to the subchondral bone. If the block is proud (setting on high points), the distal resection will be inadequate and/or rotationally malaligned. These malpositions will result in a tight extension gap with overcorrection and overload of the opposite compartment and/or an abnormal articulation at the prosthetic interface. Femoral referencing is accomplished with the LCS resection block as an extramedullary approach. Systems using an intramedullary approach also reference the anatomic femoral axis and the anterior femoral cortex. Both systems work. Understanding the principles is most important because anatomical variances may require fine adjustments, which are more technically subtle with UKA than TKA.

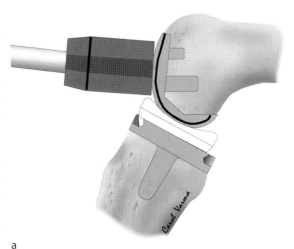

a

4.9 Final Positioning and Trial Reduction

The trial tibial component should be inserted first, followed by the bearing and the femoral component (Fig. 12).

Final impaction will position the tibial component against the sagittal resection. A stemmed unit, such as the LCS, may require rotational maneuvering. External rotation of the tibia will aid in exposure and insertion of the tibial component. The bearing is inserted by placing a valgus stress from flexion to extension and back to extension in order to clear the femoral condyle. The femoral component is then impacted, beginning at 100° and completed with the knee at 60° to 70°. The patella is then reduced and the knee ranged from extension to maximum flexion. Normal, natural range of motion with meniscal bearing movement, anterior in extension and posterior in flexion, confirms normal kinematic control. There should be no patella impingement and no component lift off from either tibial or femoral sides with extremes of motion. The most common cause of lift off or a tight flexion block is failure to slope the A-P resection 7° to 10° as recommended. Fine-tuning of any resection variables should be completed before permanent prosthetic placement.

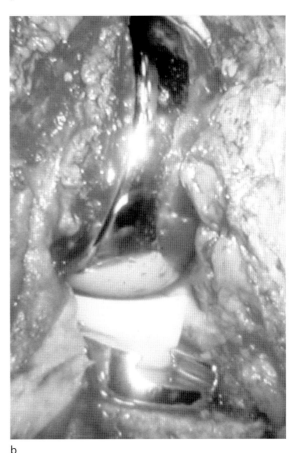

b

Fig. 12a,b. The permanent components are driven to the bone surfaces with or without cement. Final clinical result in deep flexion, excellent contact with posterior bearing movement allows for ideal kinematics

5 Clinical Results of UKA

Surgical outcomes of UKA have varied from the dismal failure rate reported by Insall and Walker [11], Insall and Aglietti,[10], Swank et al. [32], and Laskin [18], to the more optimistic reports of Lewold et al. [20], Marmor [24], Kozinn et al. [17], Scott et al. [30], Buechel and Pappas [1], Goodfellow and O'Connor [6], and others. Why are reported results so variable? Critics of the negative papers highlight patient selection, surgical technique, and prosthetic design as major causes of failure. The Insall and Walker report [11] of 24 UKAs is faulted for having a poor design (blunted anterior flange causing patellar abutment), producing overcorrection with thick tibial components and having 15 patellectomies in their series. The Insall and Aglietti report [10] of 32 knees included the original 24 patients with 10 lost to follow-up. The Laskin report [18] of 37 knees included 35 obese patients with a high incidence of subsidence and failure of the opposite compartment (probable overcorrection and overload). Swank et al. [32] reported poor results (cementless design) with failure due to dissociation, fixation and medial subluxation. The issue of prosthetic design and ACL competence must be raised in these series.

The positive UKA experience in the literature addresses the factors summarized above and reports satisfactory (good/excellent) results between 85% to 90% [1, 2, 13]. Perhaps these results can be improved with more strict selection criteria, [2, 5, 13] surgical technique, and improved prosthetic design.

Personal experience with cemented Marmor modular UKA (1972–1980) and the LCS meniscal-bearing UKA (1980 up to present) at the Lehigh Valley Hospital has been very positive. Prospective evaluation of 109 LCS UKA followed for a mean of 5.2 years has shown 93% good/excellent results. There were 96 medial and 13 lateral replacement performed with cemented (49) and cementless (65) fixation. A longer term study, being prepared for publication, suggests that cementless and cemented LCS meniscal-bearing UKA in a more active population is equal to or better than previous UKA reports and comparable to current TKA results. Prosthetic design, fixation, and future materials improvement are also factors that may improve outcome.

6 Discussion/Conclusion

UKA remains controversial and its application varies from country to country, region to region, and within orthopedic training centers. Literature reports have been variable, ranging from negative studies of Insall and Aglietti [10], Laskin [18], and Swank et al. [32] to multiple positive studies [2, 3, 6, 13, 17, 33]. Advocates of UKA cite the multiple advantages which include:

- restoration of normal kinematics,
- preservation of normal structures,
- avoidance of major problems reported with TKA,
- maintaining and/or improving functional range of motion which is frequently decreased following TKA,
- lower morbidity with no need for blood transfusions, less soft tissue damage, etc., and
- lower prosthetic costs and shorter hospitalization.

Non-advocates of UKA cite higher failure rates, problems of selection and technique, and difficulty in revision to TKA. Conversion of UKA, however, is reported to be less difficult than revision TKA [19], which has also been this author's personal experience.

All authors agree that patient selection and prosthetic design can influence outcomes. Grelsamer and Cartier [7] stressed that UKA is not «half a total knee», with major differences mostly related to technical factors which have been discussed and illustrated. The Swedish knee study [20, 21] reported improved results of a large series (1969 cemented Marmor fixed-bearing) of UKAs relative to the time of implant. Five-year cumulative revision rates were reduced from 11% (1975–83 cases) to 5% (1983–89 cases), suggesting that experience, patient selection, and surgical techniques are major determinants of clinical results.

Materials, improved fixation, and design improvements such as meniscal bearings, which combine controlled motion with matching spherical geometry and are illustrated in this section, provide potential for improved results [3, 13] and early bearing exchange without component removal in the extremely active, younger patient population. Results of the Oxford [6] and LCS [1] UKA compare with or exceed best results reported in the literature. Improvement in technique and experience should further improve outcomes as UKA becomes a more accepted alternative in correctable angular knee deformity. Surgical technique of UKA is more demanding but should not be a deterrent to learning and offering this conservative option to patients who meet the selection criteria.

A philosophy of the UKA concept, good judgment, and understanding of the surgical principles and instrumentation systems of a proven prosthetic design, along with exacting surgical technique, should decrease failures in UKA that are due to surgeon-dependent technical factors. However, slightly higher failure rates must be anticipated if the procedure is extended to the younger, more active patient. The LCS, with potential for bearing exchange, offers an excellent option in this difficult patient group.

References

1. Buechel FF, Pappas MJ (1989) New Jersey low contact stress knee replacement system. Ten-year evaluation of meniscal bearings. Orthop Clin North Am 20:147–177
2. Cartier P, Sanouiller JL, Grelsamer RP (1996) Unicompartmental knee arthroplasty surgery. 10-year minimum follow-up period. J Arthroplasty 11:782–788
3. Cohen M, Buechel F, Pappas MJ (1991) Meniscal-bearing unicompartmental knee arthroplasty. An 11-year clinical study. Orthop Rev 20:443–448
4. Coventry MB (1987) Proximal tibial varus osteotomy for osteoarthritis of the lateral compartment of the knee. J Bone Joint Surg [Am] 69A:32–38.

5. Engh GA, Holt BT, Parks ML (1997) A midvastus muscle-splitting approach for total knee arthroplasty. J Arthroplasty 12: 322–331
6. Goodfellow JW, O'Connor JJ (1982) The Oxford knee: A clinical trial. J Bone Joint Surg [Br] 64-B: 620
7. Grelsamer RP, Cartier P (1992) A unicompartmental knee replacement is not «half a total knee»: Five major differences. Orthop Rev 21: 1350–1356
8. Heck DA, Marmor L, Gibson A et al. (1993) Unicompartmental knee arthroplasty. A multicenter investigation with long-term follow-up evaluation. Clin Orthop 286:154–159
9. Hodge WA, Chandler HP (1992) Unicompartmental knee replacement: a comparison of constrained and unconstrained designs. JBJS [Am] 74: 877–883
10. Insall J, Aglietti P (1980) A five to seven-year follow-up of unicondylar arthroplasty. JBJS [Am] 62-A: 1329–1337
11. Insall J, Walker P (1976) Unicondylar knee replacement. Clin Orthop 120: 83–85
12. Insall JN, Scott WN, Keblish PA et al. (1994) Total knee arthroplasty exposures and soft tissue balancing. In: Insall JN, Scott WN (eds), VideoBook of Knee Surgery. Lippincott, Philadelphia
13. Keblish PA (1994) The case for unicompartmental knee arthroplasty. Orthopedics 17: 853–855
14. Keblish PA Jr (1998) Surgical techniques in the performance of unicompartmental arthroplasties. Operative Techniques in Orthopaedics 8: 134–145
15. Keblish PA (2002) Surgical approaches: lateral approach. In: Scuderi GR, Tria JA (eds) Surgical techniques in total knee arthroplasty. Springer, Berlin Heidelberg New York Tokyo
16. Knight JL, Atwater RD, Guo J. Early failure of the porous coated anatomic cemented unicompartmental knee arthroplasty. Aids to diagnosis and revision. J Arthoplasty 1997; 12:11–20.
17. Kozinn SC, Marx C, Scott RD (1989) Unicompartmental knee arthroplasty: A 4.5–6-year follow-up study with a metal-backed tibial component. J Arthroplasty 4 (Suppl): S1-S10
18. Laskin RS (1976) Modular total knee-replacement arthroplasty. A review of eighty-nine patients. JBJS 58: 766–773
19. Levine WN, Ozuna RM, Scott RD et al. (1996) Conversion of failed modern unicompartmental arthroplasty to total knee arthroplasty. J Arthroplasty 11: 797–801
20. Lewold S, Knutson K, Lidgren L (1993) Reduced failure rate in knee prosthetic surgery with improved implantation technique. Clin Orthop 287: 94–97
21. Lindstrand A, Stenstrom A, Lewold S (1992) Multicenter study of unicompartment knee revision. PCA, Marmor, and St. Georg compared in 3,777 cases of arthrosis. Acta Orthop Scand 63: 256–259
22. Lindstrand A, Stenstrom A, Ryd L, Toksvig-Larsen S (2000) The introduction period of unicompartmental knee arthroplasty is critical: a clinical multicentered and radiostereometric study of 251 Duracon unicompartmental knee arthroplasties. J Arthroplasty 15: 608–616
23. Lindstrand A, Stenstrom A (1992) Polyethylene wear of the PCA unicompartmental knee. Prospective 5 (4–8) year study of 120 arthrosis knees. Acta Orthop Scand 63: 260–262
24. Marmor L (1990) Patient selection for osteotomy, unicompartmental replacement, and total knee replacement. Am J Knee Surg 3: 206–213
25. Marmor L (1988) Unicompartment arthroplasty of the knee with a minimum ten-year follow-up period. Clin Orthop 228: 171–177
26. Matthews LS, Goldstein SA, Malvitz TA, Katz BP (1988) Proximal tibial osteotomy. Factors that influence the duration of satisfactory function. Clin Orthop 229: 193–200
27. McKeever DC, Elliot RB (1960) Tibial plateau prosthesis. Clin Orthop 18: 86–95
28. Robertsson O, Borgquist L, Knutson K, Lewold S, Lidgren L (1999) Use of unicompartmental instead of tricompartmental prostheses for unicompartmental arthrosis in the knee is a cost-effective alternative. 15,437 primary tricompartmental prostheses were compared with 10,624 primary medial or lateral unicompartmental prostheses. Acta Orthop Scand 70: 170–175
29. Romanowski MR, Repicci JA (2002) Minimally invasive unicondylar arthroplasty: eight-year follow-up. J Knee Surg 15: 17–22
30. Scott RD, Cobb AG, McQueary FG, Thornhill TS (1991) Unicompartmental knee arthroplasty. Eight- to 12-year follow-up evaluation with survivorship analysis. Clin Orthop 271: 96–100
31. Stulberg SD (1990) Unicompartmental knee replacement. Tech Ortho 5: 1–74
32. Swank M, Stulberg SD, Jiganti J et al. (1993) The natural history of unicompartmental arthroplasty. An eight-year follow-up study with survivorship analysis. Clin Orthop 286: 130–142
33. Van Dalen J, Krause BL (1991) Medial unicompartment knee replacement. Minimum five year follow-up. Aust NZJ Surg 61: 497–500

9.2   Bicruciate Ligament Retention

K. J. HAMELYNCK

1   Introduction

Bicruciate ligament retention Total Knee Arthroplasty (TKA) has never become popular with the majority of orthopedic surgeons. Many surgeons have never seen or learned how to perform bi-cruciate ligament retention TKA. Most surgeons are either satisfied with their results of posterior cruciate ligament (pcl) preserving or pcl-sacrificing posterior stabilizing TKA or when not satisfied, do not consider anterior cruciate ligament (acl) retention as a possible method to improve the results. What is more, in most knees they may notice that the acl is absent or not functioning.

Most total knee designs need the central part of the tibia for the introduction of a stem, which is part of the tibial component and contributes considerably to its fixation. As a consequence resection of the acl is necessary even when it is well functioning, because the insertion of the ligament is located in the central part of the tibia (Fig. 13).

This is an important reason why retention of both cruciate ligaments is not considered by most surgeons. The surgeon will need strong arguments to change his or her routine and consider retention of both cruciate ligaments.

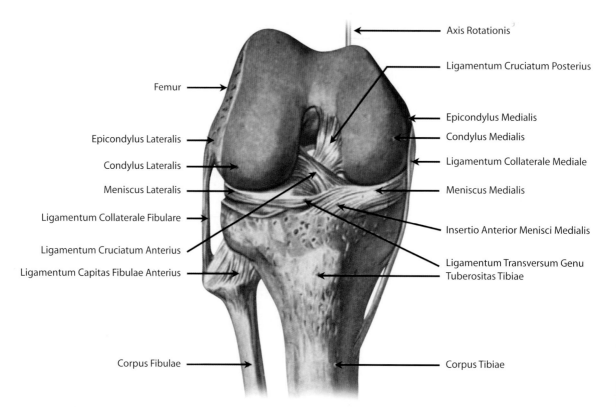

Fig. 13. The insertion of the acl in the centre of the tibia

2   Advantages of Bicruciate Ligament Retention

The advantage of bicruciate ligament retention is a better overall functional performance after TKA. Bi -cruciate ligament retention provides the knee with a near-anatomic range of motion and optimal extrinsic stability. Bicruciate retaining knee arthroplasties demonstrated a good performance in gait studies and with stair climbing [1, 6, 14], where pcl-retaining arthroplasties showed extensor moment weakness with forward leaning and decreased stance phase knee flexion so typical for the acl-deficient knee [1].

Natural anatomic kinematics of the knee are possible only if knee motion is guided by close to normal geometry of the components and isometric tension of the recruited ligaments. The recruited ligaments are all of the ligaments including acl and pcl. If one ligament, e.g. the acl, is absent, normal kinematics are out of the question. The motion pattern of the knee is changed in such a manner that sometimes rather bizarre movements may be demonstrated during fluoroscopic examination, like anterior translation of the femur when the knee is flexed [15]! If the acl is absent, the rollback mechanism is destroyed however many surgeons-examiners try and prove the contrary.

Anatomic motion is not just an ideal. Anatomic motion leads to optimal function of the muscles about the knee joint. The effectiveness and efficiency of the extensor mechanism is very much dependent on the position of the femur relative to the tibia. In the absence of the acl, the position of the femur is posterior to the middle of the tibia in the extended knee [15].

Mahoney et al. [10] found that normal pcl strain levels are produced in only 37 % of cruciate-retaining arthroplasties and femoral rollback is decreased by an average of 36 %. This was associated with a 15 % loss in extensor efficiency! To induce rollback in the absence of the acl the tibial component may be provided with a post. In Mahoney's experiments cruciate substitution resulted in a 12 % loss in rollback and an 11 % decrease in extensor efficiency. Post and cam mechanisms used to induce rollback have a drawback. Whenever a movement is forced by the configuration of a component more forces will be conducted to the bone-prosthesis interface with possible negative consequences for fixation. If there is no acl the surgeon has no choice, but many young patients do in fact have intact acl's. When preserving the acl such a post is not needed as the normal anatomical structure supporting rollback is already present. As far as kinematics are concerned, preservation of both cruciate ligaments is the only way to create close to normal knee motion without negative consequences for lifelong fixation.

The cruciate ligaments play an important role in stabilising the knee. The role of the ligaments in maintaining anterior-posterior stability is well known. Much attention is given to the reconstruction of the ligaments after traumatic rupture of one or both ligaments in order to restore anterior-posterior stability. The significance of the cruciate ligaments in medial-lateral stability or control of varus-valgus rotation however well documented [8], does not get sufficient attention. Both cruciate ligaments may, according to W. Mueller [11], be considered as the collateral ligaments of the compartments: the pcl being the lateral collateral ligament of the medial compartment and the acl being the medial collateral ligament of the lateral compartment. Important is the observation that as in a-p stabilization, the cruciate ligaments in m-l stabilization work best if both ligaments are present and functioning [8].

In the absence of the acl, the pcl is less efficient. The pcl, already not being able to function normally in the absence of the acl, will be overloaded. It is questionable if the ligament can sustain these loads.

One should realize that in the absence of or by removing the cruciate ligaments the forces normally being conducted through these ligaments do not disappear. A redistribution of forces will take place and the remaining ligaments will have to sustain forces higher than in the normal situation. Most ligaments may sustain forces up to 2–3 times the peak force of activities of daily life [16]. Therefore, In the absence of the cruciate ligaments the collateral ligaments may easily be overloaded. This is of particular interest in young and active patients. For the extrinsic stability of the knee, preservation of both cruciate ligaments is of great importance for these patients in particular.

There is no unanimity about the role of the ligaments in providing propriocepsis [5, 13]. It is certain however that the motion and stabilization of the knee only partly result from will power. Most of the activity is stimulated by reflexes and guided by information gathered from muscles, capsule and ligaments. All ligaments contain neuroreceptors, which, depending on the amount a ligament recruited, send out signals. The quality of the proprioceptive activity does not remain at the same level throughout life but diminishes with age [2]. This may easily be noticed when the walking pattern of the elderly is observed. The level of deformity of the joint plays a role as well [9, 13]. Fortunately the elderly are usually not very active so their need for proprioceptive information may be limited. Young and active humans on the contrary are very much dependent on proprioceptive information to function normally, so removing structures containing mechanoreceptors, which are important for propriocepcis, has negative implications for the dynamic stabilization of the knee.

While discussing the need for bi-cruciate ligament retention in TKA it needs to be clear that this procedure must be confined to patients with intact well functioning ligaments for whom cruciate ligament preservation may make sense. These patients are the young and active ones.

In this patient category it is also important to perform conservative TKA. In the young and active patient the surgeon must be aware that one day this knee replacement will have to be revised. To be conservative during the first implantation offers a good possibility for a successful revision arthroplasty later. The best way to be conservative is to retain all healthy well functioning structures and to preserve the joint space. By retaining the cruciate ligaments, the joint space will not be altered. If instead of retaining, the cruciate ligaments are resected, a larger joint space is created and a thicker spacer is needed to tension the collateral ligaments. Most forces will be guided through only the collateral ligaments (which may be right in the elderly but not in the young and active patient). The tibia will also be moved distally which includes distalisation of the tibial tuberosity and patella. This may result in sub-optimal function of the extensor mechanism. If after primary cruciate ligament sacrifairy TKA, revision is required. Revision components will become necessary which would not be needed after a cruciate retaining TKA. Retention of the cruciate ligaments also plays a role in maintaining fixation of prosthetic components. If ligaments are retained, most forces will be conducted through the ligaments. The need for intrinsic stability to stabilize the knee is therefore minimal. Too much intrinsic stability of prosthetic components is detrimental for their lifelong fixation. Free rotational and translational movements are restrained and the forces are directly conducted to the interface. In this situation, mechanical loosening is more likely to occur [7]. Whenever a ligament is sacrificed, more intrinsic constraint of components is needed to stabilize the joint. It is better to retain the ligaments, the natural conductors of forces, to minimize the transmission of forces to the interface and so to protect the fixation of components.

Wear of polyethylene plays an important role in the long term outcome of total joint prostheses. In the knee, wear of polyethylene causes a painful synovitis or after several years of use, aseptic loosening of components as a result of osteolysis. Wear of polyethylene is multi-causal. Mechanical factors play an important role. It has been demonstrated that gliding of two relatively small contact area's causes delamination of polyethylene [3]. This situation is particularly seen in knee replacement systems with fixed polyethylene bearings and pcl-retention. In bicruciate ligament retention TKA, with intact rollback

mechanism, this gliding caused by the tension of the pcl does not occur. So bi-cruciate ligament retention may also play a role in minimizing polyethylene wear (?).

3   Disadvantages of Bicruciate Ligament Retention

Bicruciate ligament retention in TKA offers some difficulties for the surgeon, which are not encountered during routine pcl-retaining or substituting TKA. Anterior subluxation of the tibia, a familiar procedure for exposure, is not possible. While performing the osteotomy of the tibial surface the bony attachment of the acl may be easily undercut. Cleaning the posterior part of the knee, removing the posterior osteophytes and performing a posterior capsule release is difficult.

In bicruciate ligament retention a central medullary stem cannot be used for fixation of the tibial component. This is an important disadvantage. The use of a central medullary stem has proven to be an effective method of fixation. The fixation of the bicruciate ligament retaining tibial component will be dependent on cortical rim contact and screws or fins in the subchondral tibial bone. These screws and fins cannot be longer than 2–2.5 cm because there is no place for a longer screw or fin. The fixation of these tibial components is presumably not as good as the fixation of tibial components with central medullary stems.

To tension the ligaments correctly is difficult if not impossible as the original anatomy of the femoral condyles has been changed. It is possible however to tension the cruciate ligaments close to normal using a tensor [4]. Only after a careful reconstruction of the original tibial height and the inclination of the tibial surface, is it possible to create the required tension on the ligaments. Any difference in joint level or inclination may cause the rupture of the acl. The acl may also be pulled out of the tibial surface.

Bicruciate retaining TKA may be successful only in the hands of the experienced surgeon, who is regularly performing TKA and takes the time necessary to perform this more difficult arthroplasty. This arthroplasty is done however in young patients who demand a long lasting good result. There is a good reason to try and perform the best possible surgery in these patients, even when it is time consuming!

4   Surgical Technique of Bicruciate Ligament Retaining TKA

There are three possible ways to retain the cruciate ligaments in knee arthroplasty:

- implantation of two unicondylar prostheses,
- implantation of a total knee prosthesis with a tibial component designed for bicruciate ligament retention,
- implantation of a femoral component and two unicondylar tibial components.

The implantation of two unicondylar prostheses is an interesting option in osteoarthritic knees with intact cruciate ligaments and limited patellofemoral arthritis. When patients are suffering from serious patellofemoral complaints, replacement of at least one side of the articulation is necessary. The use of a femoral component and two unilateral tibial components is an interesting option as well. The risk of fracturing the place of insertion of the acl, the tibial eminentia, is avoided.

The use of the LCS total knee system with a tibial component designed for bicruciate ligament retention (BCR) is the subject of this chapter (Fig. 14).

The surgical technique for bicruciate ligament retention is based on the normal LCS surgical technique using the Milestone or API instruments. The placement of the tibial component is crucial. The surgeon needs to care for the correct level, the right inclination and perfect anterior-posterior direction of the osteotomy of the tibial articular surface:

- The tibial surface must be resected at such a level that after implantation of the BCR tibial component and the use of the 10 mm meniscal bearing, the joint line is not raised. Under-resection of the tibia will surely lead to raising the joint line and causing too much tension on the acl when the knee is brought in full extension. There is no instrument to measure the correct amount of bone to be resected. Starting with minimal resection, the right amount of bone may be measured with the help of an osteotome of the same

height as the tibial component and a 10 mm insert (Fig. 15 and 16).

- The resection of the tibial surface must be done with the correct inclination, that is the original inclination of the knee to be replaced. This inclination may vary from 5 to 15 degrees of flexion. A wing should be used to check the inclination angle by eye.
- It is of great importance that the osteotomy is done in perfect anterior-posterior direction. A slight deviation of the slope, e.g. from 10 degrees anteromedial to 10 degrees posterolateral may seriously affect the tension in the acl in the full range of motion. To be sure about the anterior-posterior direction the author uses a pin which is placed in the tibial head in the a-p direction. The pin is placed prior to the use of any other instrument while the knee is fully extended and placed in correct rotational alignment taking the patella or rather the fovea of the femur as a reference.
- The tibial template must be placed parallel to this a-p pin. The template must cover the whole tibial surface in such a manner that the tibial component will have

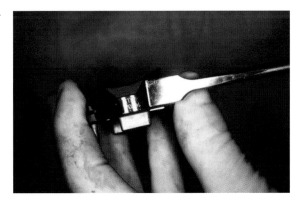

Fig. 15. The osteotome is indicating the height of the tibial component with a 10 mm meniscal bearing

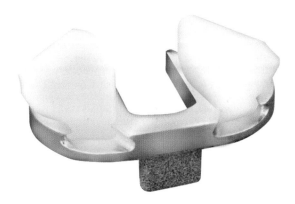

Fig. 14. The LCS bi-cruciate ligament retaining tibial component with three short fins for fixation

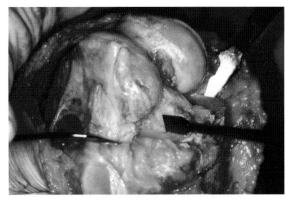

Fig. 16. The amount of bone resected measured at the eminential bony bridge

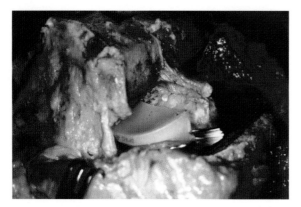

Fig. 17. Tibial component and meniscal bearing in situ showing that the original joint level has been reconstructed

cortical contact after implantation. It is wise to keep the eminential bony bridge relatively large. The tibial component may help and maintain the fixation of the bridge. The anterior part of the bridge should be resected at the last moment to protect the fixation of the bony bridge during surgery. There is a considerable risk to undercut the eminentia while performing the osteotomy of the tibial surface.

- No trial prosthesis is used. The use of a tibial trial component will unnecessarily widen the holes prepared for fixation of the fins. The definitive BCR tibial component may be placed directly by compressing the prosthesis into soft bone, which is usually seen in rheumatoid arthritis, or into the prepared holes when the tibial bone is normally hard (Fig. 17).

- To tension the ligaments, firstly 10 mm meniscal bearings are used together with the trial femoral component. Stability is checked in flexion and extension. The surgeon should know that the acl may be rather slack in flexion and tight in extension, so tension needs to be checked in extension especially. A thicker component may be used when needed but care must be taken not to stretch the acl too much in extension. When in doubt about the correct tension of the acl, a meniscal bearing should be chosen with good tension of the acl in extension and somewhat slack in flexion. This acl will still be able to induce some rollback and will certainly prevent the bizarre motion pattern of knees without an acl.

5 Outcome of Bicruciate Retaining TKA Using the LCS BCR Tibial Component

The outcome of the world wide experience in bicruciate ligament retaining TKA using the LCS BCR tibial component will be reported in chapter 11 of this book.

6 Summary

Bicruciate ligament retaining TKA is indicated in young active patients with intact sufficient cruciate ligaments. Bicruciate ligament retention will provide the knee with near to normal motion and optimal extrinsic stability. This is done whilst propriocepsis is preserved in the best possible manner.

The surgical technique is demanding. Bicruciate ligament retaining TKA should be performed only by surgeons willing to take the time to achieve a better result.

References

1. Andriacchi TP, Galante JO, Fermier RW (1982) The influence of total knee replacements design on walking and stair climbing. J Bone Joint Surg Am 64: 1328
2. Barrett DS, Cobb AG, Bentley G (1991) Joint proprioception in normal, osteoarthritic and replaced knees. J Bone Joint Surg Br 73: 53
3. Blunn GW, Joshi AB, Minns RJ et al. (1997) Wear in retrieved condylar arthroplasties. J Arthroplasty 12: 281
4. Cloutier JM, Sabouret P, Deghrar A (1999) Total knee arthroplasty with retention of both cruciate ligaments. J Bone Joint Surg Am 81: 697
5. Fuchs S, Thorwesten L, Niewerth S (1999) Proprioceptive function in knees with and without total knee arthroplasty. Am J Phys Med Rehabil: 78: 39
6. Goodfellow JB, O'Connor JJ (1988) Retention of the anterior cruciate in arthroplasty of the knee. J Bone Joint Surg Br 70: 333
7. Greenwald AS (1989) Stability characteristics of total knee replacements. AAOS 56th Annual Meeting (Scientific Exhibit) in Las Vegas, Nevada
8. Grood ES, Noyes FR, Butler DL, Suntay WJ (1981) Ligamentous and capsular restraints preventing straight medial and lateral laxity in intact human cadaver knees. J Bone Joint Surg Am 63: 1257
9. Koralewicz LM, Engh GA (2000) Comparison of proprioception in arthritic and age-matched normal knees. J Bone Joint Surg Am 82: 1582
10. Mahoney OM, Noble PC, Rhoads DD, Alexander JW, Tullos HS (1994) Posterior cruciate function following total knee arthroplasty. A biomechanical study. J Arthroplasty 9: 569
11. Mueller W (1982) Das Knie. Form, Funktion und ligamentäre Wiederherstellungschirurgie, Springer, Berlin Heidelberg New York
12. Nelissen RG, Hogendoorn PC (2001) Retain or sacrifice the posterior cruciate ligament in total knee arthroplasty, a histopathological study of the cruciate ligament in osteoarthritic and rheumatic disease. J Clin Pathol 54: 381
13. Pap G, Meyer M, Weiler HT, Machner A, Awiszus F (2000) Proprioception after total knee arthroplasty: a comparison with clinical outcome. Acta Orthop Scand 71:153
14. Pritchett JW (1996) Anterior cruciate retaining total knee arthroplasty. J Arthroplasty 11:194
15. Stiehl JB, Komistek RD, Dennis DA et al. (1995) Fluoroscopic analysis of kinematics after posterior-cruciate-retaining knee arthroplasty. J Bone Joint Surg Br 77: 884
16. Viidik A (1980) The mechanical properties of parallel fibered collagenous tissue. In: Viidik A, Vuust J (eds) Biology of collagen. Academic Press, London, pp 237–255

9.3 Posterior Cruciate Ligament Retention

W. Mueller, N. F. Friederich

1 Ligaments in Total Knee Arthroplasty (TKA)

Total knee arthroplasty requires bone resections as well as careful appreciation of the soft tissues. This includes judgement of both active and passive structures such as extensor and flexor mechanisms, collateral ligament complexes and cruciate ligaments. The collateral ligament complexes play a major role in determining a balanced flexion and extension gap throughout the entire range of motion and knee kinematics close to a normal knee joint. This chapter addresses special attention to the question whether or not the cruciate ligaments should be retained or sacrificed. Most current knee systems used worldwide are designed for ACL sacrifice with or without PCL retention.

Kinematics vary in healthy and arthritic knee joints, however the durability of any modern prosthetic design (fixed or mobile bearing) decreases with non-physiologic motion and lack in stability. Healthy knee joints have six degrees of freedom within a soft tissue envelope, which includes limited physiological translation, rotation, lateral lift-off and femoral roll-back. These motions are controlled by both active and passive structures as well as proprioception. In general, the collateral ligament complexes control varus-valgus stability, whereas both cruciate ligaments predominantly control anteroposterior and rotational stability of the knee joint. Any total knee system and surgical technique, that implements these kinematic issues, will increase stability and conformity, ultimately reducing polyethylene wear. One important goal of prosthetic design is to partially compensate for anteroposterior stability, femoral roll-back, and lateral lift-off without increasing contact stresses above a critical value (usually five to ten MPa). On the one hand every TKA will lack stability if the complex soft tissue sleeve of the knee is not individually appreciated throughout the entire range of motion, on the other hand sacrificing both cruciate ligaments during surgery does not necessarily create generally unstable TKA. Much depends on the pre-morbid condition, the integrity of the soft tissues, the components used, and the surgical technique. In summary, there appears to be no general right or wrong with respect to the cruciate ligament treatment in TKA.

1.1 Normal Function of Healthy Cruciate Ligaments

Both, anterior and posterior cruciate ligaments form an inconsistent (moving) central pivot of the knee joint, which can be described as a four bar linkage chain. This four bar linkage chain defines the individual roll-back (gliding) pattern of the femoral condyles as well as the anatomic features of both the femoral and the tibial metaphyses. This results in a considerable interpersonal variation of anatomic and kinematic features. The physiological central pivot is variable and moves a certain amount in all three dimensions allowing antero-posterior and medio-lateral translation combined with tibiofemoral rotation and lift-off (Fig. 18a,b).

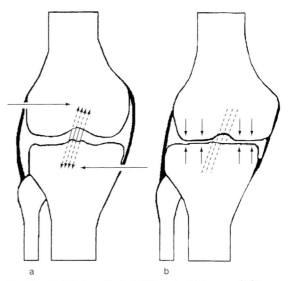

Fig. 18. a Stabilizing effect of PCL against latero-medial translation. **b** Increased compression forces on joint surfaces with translation after the loss of PCL

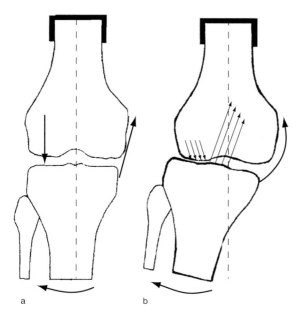

Fig. 19a,b. Stabilizing effect of PCL against valgus rotation and distraction. Its short fibers act even before the longer peripheral ligament fibers which have more elastic elongation reserve because of their length. b shows by the short arrow at the medial side also the stabilization force of the meniscal rim.

The cruciate ligaments lever arm is short, and therefore has a limited ability to control tibiofemoral rotation. Further rotational and translational stability of the normal knee joint is guided by both menisci and their meniscofemoral ligaments (Wrisberg, Humphry) as well as all collaterals including LCM, POL medially and LCL, popliteus tendon and iliotibial band (ITB) laterally (Fig. 19a,b).

1.2 Ligament Function in TKA

Passive stability such as anatomical shape, menisci, cruciate ligaments and at times collateral ligament function in TKA may be partially compensated by the prosthetic design, particularly with mobile bearings. However, stability is not defined by passive structures alone but by active knee joint muscle forces and proprioception. Rotational and anterior stability of the ACL can be compensated by prosthetic congruency. A healthy PCL controls posterior and medio-lateral translation as well as lift-off, which may partly be controlled by either design and/or a posterior post and cam mechanism. Due to these concerns, it appears to be logical that prosthetic knee designs in the past were usually "over-constrained" with, at times huge stems [10, 16, 19], axes, bars and links.

The main problem with these designs were increased constraint forces at the implant-bone interface, which ultimately lead to early aseptic (mechanical) loosening. The ideal prosthetic design should accommodate all demands in an optimal fashion: minimal contact stress, minimal constraint forces and maximum stability.

2 Key Function of PCL in Healthy Knees

- Reduces posterior tibial translation,
- controls mediolateral translation,
- reduces lift-off,
- maintains some effect of RB,
- centres the longitudinal rotational axis,
- limits varus-valgus deviation,
- reduces patellofemoral loads and shear forces,
- defines tibial slope angle.

There is no doubt that osteoarthritic knee joints differ from normal knees in many respects. Soft tissue changes are often underestimated, particularly in degenerative diseases with varus/valgus or fixed deformities. Before retention of the PCL is considered one must assure that the PCL is of good quality, since most osteoarthritic knee cases are associated with a poor condition of the PCL. A weak and degenerated PCL of poor quality is likely to fail the forces in TKA. Multiple reports in the literature address the insufficient quality and strength of PCL in elder or arthritic knee joints [3, 9]. Macroscopically abnormal PCL showed more than 50% degeneration in histology with loss of mechanoreceptors as demonstrated by Franchi et al. [7].

Therefore, PCL of insufficient properties are not recommended for retention independent of surgeons preferences and prosthetic design. Perfect tension and positioning of all components is mandatory for acceptable and long-term function of the PCL. Sensitive deviation from perfect positioning and compromise in blood supply will ultimately result in PCL failure.

Surgeons with preference to retain the PCL must keep the option to sacrifice as a back-up. When retention of the PCL is desired (and possible) the knee design must be selected, but. Key requirements of such a prosthesis include: anatomical multiradial shape of the femoral component with patellar groove, congruent (mobile bearing) polyethylene bearing with sufficient space posteriorly (impingement), tibial resection with posterior slope, and balanced flexion and extension gaps (nut cracker effect). PCL retention defines the joint line and the tibiofemoral distance, which is less forgiving, since the healing process of TKA offers little biological adaptation («intelligence of tissues»).

3   PCL and Co-Restraints in TKA

- PCL retention requires precise tibial and femoral resections to preserve vascularity.
- The posterior capsule and the rim of the medial meniscus wall provide further stability.
- Gaining length in fixed flexion deformity may be achieved by blunt means or posterior capsule pie crusting (transverse/oblique).
- Posterolateral stability includes preservation of the popliteus tendon, lateral meniscus rim, and Wrisberg-PCL complex, which sends its fibres from the PCL into the posterior rim of both the lateral meniscus and popliteus tendon. This forms a stable posterolateral corner in TKA improving rotational stability as well as lift-off.
- PCL and popliteus tendon form a direct reciprocal system (as does the popliteus tendon and the LCL) with regards to the direction of the forces applied. With voluntary incisions of the fascicles, the extension and flexion gap opens step by step. The lateral rim absorbs the major part (up to 75 %) of the posterior forces from 0 to 30° flexion [15]. Main posterior stabilizing force from 30° flexion is the isometric posterior bundle of the PCL followed by the ACL [8].

4   PCL and Implant Design

Decreased tibial slope and a tight flexion gap in PCL retention increase the risk of a lever effect (nut cracker), which leads to increased contact stresses with polyethylene wear, over-stretching of the PCL and lack of flexion (Fig. 20a,b).

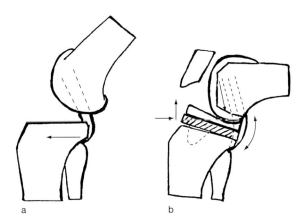

a   b

Fig. 20. a Non anatomometric overtightened PCL pushes the tibial plateau forward into anterior subluxation. **b** Posterior plateau elevation limits RB and flexion, tightens the PCL, creates excessive pressure on the posterior tibial plateau and lifts up the anterior edge of the tibial component

Increased tibial slope and a lose PCL increase anterior tibial subluxation in extension and posterior subluxation in flexion. This will ultimately cause shear forces and increased polyethylene wear. Joint line elevation or lowering has considerable consequences when the PCL is retained, since the biokinematics of the TKA, the PCL tension, and extensor mechanism alter significantly by a difference as little as two to four mm [1, 4, 17]. This can result in reduced extensor mechanism function as demonstrated in the literature [1]. Independent of PCL preferences it is essential to preserve a proper joint line in TKA. Two healthy cruciate ligaments provide best kinematics. That is true for healthy knees, but is different in osteoarthritic knees joints. In most current knee systems, however, the ACL is sacrificed and retention of the PCL alone does not provide the above mentioned four bar linkage system. PCL retention or sacrifice will always be a compromise in TKA. There are excellent clinical long term data with over 13 years track record without PCL retention (Sorrels) as there excellent results with PCL retention (Hamelynck). The question of PCL management in TKA is certainly multifactorial and may work either way if biomechanical aspects, surgical technique and prosthetic design are well chosen.

5   Literature

Sorger and the Grood group 1997 [17] demonstrated experimentally that the preserved PCL in TKA is able to maintain femoral RB. When the PCL was cut, significant changes in kinematics were observed. Levandowski et al. 1997 [11] compared LCS meniscal bearing «A» and LCS rotating platform «B» and found anterior translation greater in «A» than in «B». The extension gap in «A» was 2 mm greater than in the normal knee and in «B» it was 4 mm more. The required quadriceps force for full extension was 30 % more in «A» than in the normal knee and 50 % more in «B». This may have an impact on activities such as rising from a chair. Mahoney et al. 1994 [12] looked at three groups of TKA; «A» PCL retaining, «B» PCL excised and «C» posterior stabilized: In «A» only 37 % demonstrated a normal PCL strain, femoral RB was reduced by an average of 36 % and there was 15 % loss of extensor efficiency. In «B» RB was decreased by 70 % and there was 19 % loss of extensor efficiency. In «C» RB was decreased by 12 % and there was an 11 % loss of extensor efficiency. Montgomery et al. 1993 [13] reported on 2 % of late ruptures of the PCL leading to chronic instability and disabling pain in a series of 150 PCL retaining TKA. Yasuda and Sasaki 1986 [21] found that in TKA with PCL retention there were significantly smaller moments and a better and more regular distribution of stresses in the proximal and posterior parts of the tibia than in the posterior stabilized TKA in which there were large local concentrations of von Mises stresses in front of the stem under the plateau. They recommended PCL retention when ever possible. Emodi et al. l999 [6] demonstrated the beneficial effect of the PCL on extensor function. They emphasized how important it is to restore the preoperative joint line and to avoid an overly lax PCL with loss of its function. Wasielewski et al. 1998 [20] found early incapacitating instability of PCL retaining TKAs secondary to early PCL deficiency. Typical symptoms and complaints were: persistent swelling, effusions, anterior knee pain and giving way with episodes of instability related to activities of daily living. It is very interesting to note that in the same series of patients those who did not have PCL deficiency had on average only a 5 mm rise in joint line as compared to the PCL deficient knees where the average rise was 10.3 mm.

Takatsu et al. 1998 [18] demonstrated that PCL strain and RB were significantly influenced by the posterior tilt of the tibial component as well as by the external rotation of the femoral component. Ten degrees of tilt as compared to 0° clearly decreased the PCL strain, and RB was decreased in the medial compartment but increased in the lateral one. Pereira DS et al. 1998 [14] evaluated the functional outcome of 143 TKAs with the same Kinemax prosthesis implanted between 1988 and 1992. They compared «A» 93 knees with sacrifice and «B» 50 knees with preservation of the PCL and did not find any difference in clinical or early radiological outcome between «A» and «B». They recommend that the PCL should be sacrificed in cases where extensive release and complex ligamentous balance are required. Fluoroscopic kinematic studies by Komistek of the rotating platform with a sacrificed PCL demonstrated similar roll-back and lift-off pattern compared with the normal knee joint.

6   Discussion

Retaining the PCL seems to be desirable provided the ligament is of a good quality and the surgery is optimally performed. This means placing the tibial component with an anatomical slope and recreating the original joint line. The design of the prosthesis must allow for near normal kinematics. A good functional PCL may give near normal kinematics and better gait with more power when climbing stairs. This good functional PCL may be seen in young patients requiring TKA, especially in those patients who also have an intact ACL. In the elderly, most cruciate ligaments are degenerated or weakened by disease [2]. In those patients cruciate ligament

retention should not be considered as instability may develop in the years after surgery. As fixation of components is no longer a serious problem, it is important during surgery to think not only about the present but also about the future. Fortunately the activity level of elderly patients is usually very different from that of younger and more active patients. So most probably these elderly patients will function well with the support of the collateral ligaments only and some more intrinsic constraint of the components, e.g. the rotating platform. When retaining the PCL the surgeon should not only think about control of AP-translation, but defining translations, rotations, and condylar lift-off as well [5]. In this respect retention of the PCL may be beneficial for active and younger patients.

7   Conclusion

The mobile bearing principle with the LCS system offers all possibilities with regards to cruciate ligament management. There is a bi-cruciate retaining meniscal bearing device, an PCL retaining device with combined rotation and AP glide bearing, and a bicruciate substituting device (the classic rotating platform used since the late 1970s. The bicruciate retaining meniscal bearing device is a technically demanding prosthesis, which gives good results in the hands of an experienced surgeon. The PCL retaining AP glide device may cause anterior impingement problems, therefore, it is not generally recommended in all cases. The classic rotation platform bicruciate substituting LCS implant is the most frequently used and successful knee prosthesis of all LCS knees, which has shown to provide excellent results for the majority of knee deformities even in the lesser experienced hand. Retention of the PCL may beneficial in active and younger patients, however there are no hard data in the current literature to prove that hypothesis, except in cases with insufficient PCL, they should not be retained. With the LCS system the surgeon has all options and preferences with regards to the PCL management.

References

1. Andriacchi TP, Galante JO, Fermier RW (1982) The influence of total knee replacement design on walking and stair climbing. J Bone Joint Surg [Am] 64 A: 1328–1335
2. Barrett DS, Cobb AG, Bentley G (1991) Joint proprioception in normal, osteoarthritic and replaced knees. J Bone Joint Surg Br 73: 53
3. Caton J, Boulahia A, Patricot LM (1998/1999) Natural history of the posterior cruciate ligament in osteoarthritis, Communication ESSKA Nice 1998 and SICOT, Sidney 1999
4. Chatain F et al. Influence du positionnement de l'interligne articulaire sur la cinématique du genou prothèse et sur le comportement des ligaments collatéraux. 9es Journées Ly-

onnaises de chirurgie du genou La chirurgie prothétique du genou (Chambat, Neyret, Deschamps) Ed. Sauramps médical Montpellier France,

5. Dennis DA, Komistek RD, Walker SA, Cheal EJ, Stiehl JB (2001) Femoral condylar lift-off in vivo total knee arthroplasty. J Bone Joint Surg 83B: 33–39

6. Emodi GJ, Callaghan JJ, Pedersen DR, Brown TD (1999) Posterior cruciate ligament function following total knee arthroplasty. The effect of joint line elevation. Jowa Orthop J 19: 82–92

7. Franchi A, Maccherotti G, Aglietti P (1995) Neural system of the human PCL in osteoarthritis. J Arthroplasty 10: 679–682

8. Friederich N et al. (1992) Klinische Anwendung biomechanischer und funktionell anatomischer Daten am Kniegelenk. Orthopäde 21: 41–50

9. Goutallier D, Allain J, Le Monel S, Voisin MC (1998) Evaluation de l'état histologique du ligament croisé postérieur en fonction de l'état macroscopique du ligament croisé antérieur. Intérêt pour l'indication des prothèses conservants le où les ligaments croisés. Communication à la 73 me réunion de la SOFCOT, Paris

10. Gunston FH (1971) Polycentric knee arthroplasty. J Bone Joint Surg 53-B(2) : 272–277

11. Lewandowsky PJ, Askew MJ, Lin DF, Hurst FW, Melby A (1997) Kinematics of posterior cruciate ligament retaining and sacrificing mobile bearing total knee arthroplasties. An in vitro comparison of the New Jersey LCS meniscal bearing and rotation platform prosthesis. J Arthroplasty 12(7): 777–784

12. Mahonney OM, Noble PC, Rhoads DD, Alexander JW, Tullos HS (1994) Posterior cruciate function following total knee arthroplasty. A biomechanical study J Arthroplasty 9(6): 569–578

13. Montgomery RL, Goodman SB, Csongradi J (1993) Late rupture of posterior cruciate ligament after total knee replacement. Jowa Orthop J 13: 167–170

14. Pereira DS, Jaffe FF, Ortiguera C (1998) Posterior cruciate ligament – sparing versus posterior cruciate ligament sacrificing arthroplasty. Functional results using the same prosthesis J Arthroplasty 13(2): 138–144

15. Race A, Amis AA (1996) Loading of the two bundles of the posterior cruciate ligament: an analysis of bundle function in A-P drawer. J Biomechanics 29(7): 873–879

16. Shiers LGP, Exerpta medica (1954) Arthroplasty of the knee Preliminary report of a new method. J Bone Joint Surg 36-B: 553

17. Sorger JI, Federle D, Kirk PG, Grood E, Cochran J, Levy M (1997) The posterior cruciate ligament in total knee arthroplasty. J Arthroplasty 12(8): 869–879

18. Takatsu J, Itokazu M, Shimizu K, Brown TD (1998) The function of posterior tilt of the tibial component following posterior cruciate ligament retaining total knee arthroplasty. Bull Hosp Jt Dis 57(4): 195–201

19. Walldius B (1957) Arthroplasty of the knee using endoprosthesis Acta Orthop Scand 23 (Suppl): 121

20. Waslewski GL, Marson BM, Benjamin JB (1998) Early, incapacitating instability of posterior cruciate ligament – retaining total knee arthroplasty. J Arthroplasty 13(7): 763–767

21. Yasuda K, Sasaki T (1986) Stress analysis after total knee arthroplasty with posterior cruciate ligament resection type and retention type prosthesis with special reference to the significance of retaining the posterior cruciate ligament. Nippon Seigeigrka Gakkai Zasshi 60(5): 547–562

9.4 Cruciate Ligament Substitution

B. Sorrells, D. E. Beverland

The development of total knee arthroplasty (TKA), one of the most frequently performed orthopedic surgical procedures today, has occurred in only the last thirty years. Evolution of design and technique has been characterized by steady and significant change.

Early TKA designs utilized hinges which, although providing flexion and extension, frequently loosened on both the femoral and tibial sides as a result of over-constraint. Later designs with a highly congruent femoral-tibial articulation but without provision for axial rotation, experienced a high complication rate of tibial loosening resulting from excessive torque exerted on the tibia. Subsequently, curved-on-flat geometry TKA's appeared. These are still common today, and although offering axial rotation and less tibial loosening, they have resulted in a high incidence of polyethylene wear and failure secondary to point loading and resultant high contact stress exceeding the polyethylene yield strength.

Newer condylar design TKA's that simulate the natural knee now share many common features. The advent of mobile bearing TKA in the late 1970s has allowed the incorporation of axial rotation much as in the normal knee. This has resulted in a low occurrence of component loosening. The mobile bearing TKA reduces torque and allows for greater femoral-tibial and patella-femoral congruency. This concept functions to increase contact area, reduce contact stress, and leads to a great reduction of polyethylene wear [13].

While great progress has been made in TKA development and similarity of design has emerged, considerable controversy still exists concerning the role of the posterior cruciate ligament (PCL). Should this structure be retained or substituted at the time of surgery? It seems that few surgeons question the sacrifice of the anterior cruciate ligament (ACL). This structure is routinely removed in the TKA procedure as though unimportant, yet these same surgeons labor to arthroscopically reconstruct or replace this ligament in their injured patients. Perhaps the fact that it is technically difficult to preserve the ACL during TKA has determined its fate. On the other hand, the PCL can often be surgically retained and although resulting in a more difficult and lengthy procedure, many surgeons still extol the virtues of its preservation. At the time of surgery it is often found to be stretched, worn, or contracted. It may be partially released surgically, and it is usually less than a normal structure that often is incapable of sustaining the loads imposed by a prosthetic knee.

Conversely, PCL substitution (PCS), with a biomechanically sound prosthesis devised especially for this application has proven not only easier and faster, but it has also demonstrated an outstanding long-term outcome [18]. Many reports indicate substitution superior to PCL retention (PCR). This has been especially true with the rotating platform design of the LCS TKA [2, 17].

Since implant designs both retaining the PCL and substituting the PCL have demonstrated excellent long-term clinical results [14], the decision often comes down to the surgeon's preference. Most surgeons prefer a procedure that is easier, faster, more predictable and successful. Hence, a great trend towards the use of PCL substitution has developed, especially in recent years.

In the early years of implantation of the LCS TKA about 85 percent were of the meniscal bearing, PCR design. Later experience has resulted in an approximate reversal of these percentages. The rotating platform PCS design of the LCS TKA has become the choice of the great majority of surgeons using mobile bearings worldwide.

The LCS rotating platform is uniquely designed for the substitution of both ACL and PCL functions. It is of a highly congruent sphere-and-trough geometry and is inherently stable in the anteroposterior direction (Fig. 21).

It is fully congruent and sagittally constrained from 0 degrees to 35 degrees flexion (similar to the natural knee). This flexion range is the weight bearing arc in which the ACL and PCL function in order to produce

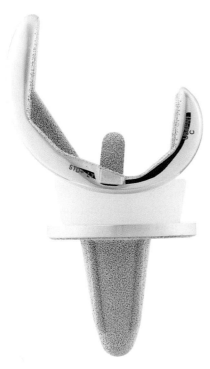
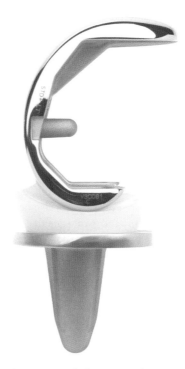

Fig. 21. Sagittal plane view of LCS rotating platform TKA demonstrating femoral-tibial congruence and anteroposterior stability

Fig. 22. Sagittal plane view of LCS rotating platform TKA in flexion demonstrating anteroposterior mobility

knee stability. The rotating platform design nicely substitutes for the ligaments in this range.

As further flexion past 30 degrees is attained, the lesser posterior radius of the femoral component allows for decreased congruency and therefore greater freedom of anteroposterior translation, a concept which facilitates range of motion without sacrifice of stability (Fig. 22).

The authors take the position that to substitute for the PCL is an easier, safer, and better method. There are numerous clinical factors that influence this conclusion. Some of these are the following.

1   PCL is not Spared in the Arthritic Process

The arthritic knee has abnormal synovium, cartilage, bone and synovial fluid. It seems reasonable that the cruciate ligaments might be pathologically affected as well. To depend on these abnormal structures for prosthetic support is risky. Several studies have histologically evaluated the posterior cruciate ligaments taken from knees at the time of TKA and compared them with age-controlled non-arthritic specimens. These studies have confirmed that marked histological degeneration exists in the majority of the arthritic PCL's as compared to minimal degeneration in the non-arthritic specimens.

Kleinbart et al. conclude that "the PCL is not spared degenerative changes in involved arthritic knees" [8]. Nelissen and Hogendoorn state that "because of extensive architectural and probably functional damage of the PCL in patients with grade five radiologic knee joint destruction, retention of the PCL in knee prostheses should not be advocated ..." [9].

2   The PCL May Fail in the Post-Operative Period

To depend upon a weakened PCL to stabilize a prosthetic construct, even more so when the ligament has been partially released, is potentially fraught with complications. Many surgeons have observed late rupture of a PCL post-operatively when using a PCR prosthesis with resultant instability in the knee. It is recommended that only minimal tibial resection be carried out when attempting to retain the PCL ligament. To excise greater amounts can result in further weakening of the PCL insertion on the tibia. Oschner concludes that "proximal tibial resections should be limited to 5–6 millimeters of bone when performing TKA" [10]. Fontanesi estimates that approximately 30 percent of PCL's saved are not functional due to the weakening effect of the tibial cut on the PCL insertion [5]. And Pagnano states that "delayed rupture of the PCL and an unbalanced flexion space can lead to symptomatic flexion instability after PCR TKA" [10]. This conclusion has also been confirmed by Kadoya et al. who demonstrated an average 3 mm increase in the flexion gap with resection (and presumably rupture) of the PCL [7].

3   The PCL May Accelerate Polywear

Several authors have described the difficulty of adequately balancing a retained PCL in attempt to simulate normal knee kinematics. Excessive contact stress can result, especially posteriorly, and premature polywear has also been described in the literature. Swany and Scott state that "an incorrectly tensioned PCL – too tight or too loose – may exaggerate the disadvantages of the retaining design and lead to early catastrophic failure" [20]. Dennis et al. note that "the abnormal anterior femoral translation observed in PCL retaining knees may be a factor in premature polyethylene wear observed in retrieval studies" [4].

4   Suggested Advantages of Posterior Cruciate Retaining (PCR)

Some surgeons feel that retaining the PCL is desirable simply to avoid sacrificing a major ligament in the knee; yet the ACL is routinely sacrificed and the desirable four bar linkage immediately destroyed. Furthermore, if retaining the PCL results in subsequent rupture and instability, this obviates this theoretical advantage.

Some observers claim that proprioception is better in the PCR knee but, Simmons and Associates reporting in the Journal of Arthroplasty, recently concluded that "retaining the PCL in TKA did not result in improved performance in proprioception testing" [15].

It is proposed by some surgeons that retention of the PCL enhances femoral roll-back. This has been proven to the contrary by Dennis, Stiehl and Komisteck. They have shown that cruciate retaining designs in their cineradiographic studies frequently demonstrate paradoxical anterior translation with knee flexion [3]. They observe that "greatly abnormal kinematics are produced in cruciate retaining TKA's". Finally, Stiehl concludes that "the rotating platform LCS design demonstrates the best overall kinematics compared to posterior cruciate retaining designs" [19].

Some authors claim a theoretical advantage of PCL retention is the enhancement of collateral stability. The PCL has even been referred to as the LCL of the medial compartment of the knee. No such benefit has been seen with the LCS TKA. In fact, the bearing dislocation rate as a result of instability has been greater using the PCR meniscal bearing variant than with the PCS rotating platform. As yet there are no comparative figures for the new PCR AP glide design.

In an attempt to further investigate their patients' perception, Becker and Dorr each treated a series of patients with a PCR design in one knee and PCS design in the other. These patients when evaluated several years later were evenly divided as to which knee they preferred. Clinical outcomes were similar in both groups. Becker concludes that there was "no clinical advantage of one type TKA over the other" [1].

In 1993, one of the authors (Sorrells) compared 461 PCR LCS TKA's with 256 rotating platform PCS TKA's performed by fifteen surgeons over a six year period, data that are part of an FDA Investigational Device Exemption (IDE) [16]. Complications were infrequent in both groups, but bearing problems were a bit more common in the meniscal bearing PCR design. Patella problems were rare in both groups (less than one percent) and good and excellent scores were present in greater that 97 percent of both groups from years 2 through 6. There was no statistical difference in total score, pain, flexion or function in the two groups.

When survivorship analysis was constructed for these PCR and PCS patients, the end results were similar. The PCR meniscal bearing patients had a six year survivorship of 95.3 percent. The PCS rotating platform patients had a bit better survivorship at 96.6 percent. While survivorship was outstanding in both groups, the actual survivorship curve was quite different (Fig. 23 and 24).

The PCR group was noted to have failures occurring over the six year period, some of these thought to be the result of late posterior cruciate ligament failure, instability and revision. On the other hand, the rotating platform group which tended to be in the more severely diseased knees had all failures occur in the first eighteen months. Thereafter, the knees proved stable without revision to year six. It is thought that survivorship in the posterior cruciate substituting group will continue to prove superior over the long term.

5   Potential Advantages of Posterior Cruciate Substitution (PCS)

- An easier soft tissue balancing procedure when the cruciates are removed,
- a faster procedure with limitation of tourniquet time and a lessened chance of infection,
- permits use of a more congruent prosthesis with less chance of developing post-operative anteroposterior instability,
- complications less frequent (18),

Fig. 23. Kaplan-Meier Survival Estimate. PCL retaining LCS TKA

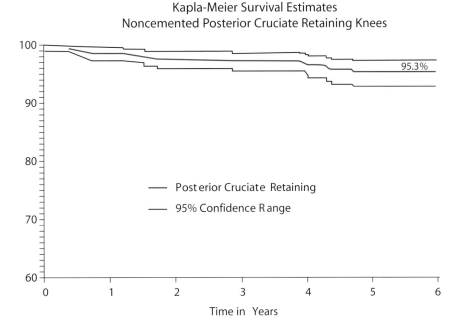

Fig. 24. Kaplan-Meier Survival Estimate. PCL substituting LCS TKA

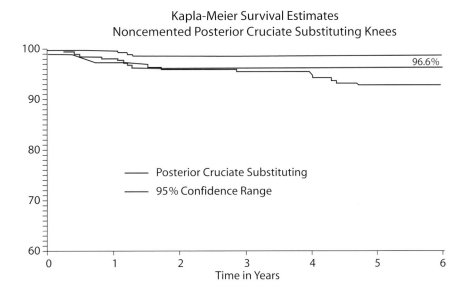

- yields decreased bearing wear and other bearing problems compared to PCR knees,
- a better procedure for the post proximal tibial osteotomy patient,
- allows better correction of severe deformities,
- preservation of the joint line is less critical,
- allows more normal kinematics,
- greater prosthetic survivorship (18).

So the debate goes on. But it appears that the tide is turning. In 1972 Insall said "preservation of the cruciate ligament is not only unnecessary, but may be detrimental in that this ligament imposes a gliding motion and dictates an arc of movement that may be incompatible with the prosthetic geometry" [6]. Pagnano, writing in the JBJS twenty-six years later, responds that "early claims that retention of the PCL in TKA would allow better range of motion, better stability, more normal gait, and enhance prosthetic longevity compared with PCL substituting designs have not been supported by subsequent clinical and basic science research" [12]. In the authors' opinion, Pagnano's conclusion sums up the PCL debate. We have concluded that to substitute for the PCL is an easier, faster and better procedure.

Refererences

1. Becker et al. (1991) Bilateral TKA. One cruciate retaining and one cruciate substituting. Clin Orthop 271: 122–124
2. Callaghan et al. (2000) Cemented rotating platform total knee replacement. J Bone Joint Surg 82 A: 705–711
3. Dennis DA et al. (1996) In vivo kinematics derived using an inverse perspective technique. Clin Orthop 331: 107–117
4. Dennis DA et al. (1998) In vivo anteroposterior femorotibial translation of TKA: a multicenter analysis. Clin Orthop 356: 47–57
5. Fontanesi G et al. (1991) Retentionof the PCL in TKA. Ital J Orthop Traumatol 17(1): 65–71
6. Insall JN, Burstein AH (1972) Hospital for Special Surgery white paper.
7. Kadoya Y et al. (2001) Effects of cruciate ligament resection on the tibiofemoral gap. Clin Orthop 391: 207–210
8. Kleinbart FA et al. (1996) Histological comparison of posterior cruciate ligaments harvested from arthritic and age-matched knee specimens. J Arthroplasty 11: 726–731
9. Nelissen PC, Hogendoorn PCW (2001) Retain or sacrifice the PCL in TKA? A histopathological study of the cruciate ligament in osteoarthritic and rheumatoid disease. J Clin Pathol 54: 381–384
10. Oschner JL (1993) Rupture of the PCL after TKA. Presented at Mid-America Orthopedic Association meeting
11. Pagnano MW et al. (1997) Flexion instability after primary total knee arthroplasty. Clin Orthop 356: 39–46
12. Pagnano MW et al. (1998) Role of the posterior cruciate ligament in total knee arthroplasty. J Amer Acad Orthop Surg 6(3): 176–187
13. Pappas MJ, Buechel FF (1995) Biomechanics and design rationale: New Jersey LCS® knee replacement system. Biomedical Engineering Trust Publication: 1–32
14. Scuderi GR, Insall JN (1992) Total knee arthroplasty, current clinical perspectives. Clin Orthop 276: 26–32
15. Simmons S et al. (1996) Proprioception following total knee arthroplasty with and without the posterior cruciate ligament. J Arthroplasty 11(7): 763–768
16. Sorrells RB et al. (1993) Comparison of the clinical results and survivorship of noncemented cruciate substituting versus cruciate retaining TKA's. AAOS Scientific exhibit, San Francisco, CA, and white paper DePuy, Inc. Warsaw, In.
17. Sorrells RB (2001) The rotating platform mobile bearing total knee arthroplasty. Surg Technol Intl IX: 245–256
18. Stern SH, Insall JN (1994) Cruciate-substituting knee arthroplasty. In: Scott WN (ed) The knee. Mosby, St. Louis, pp 1179–1198
19. Stiehl JB et al. (2000) The cruciate ligaments in total knee arthroplasty: a kinematic analysis of 2 TKA's. J Arthroplasty 15(5): 545–550
20. Swany MR, Scott RD (1993) Posterior polyethylene wear in PCL retaining TKA (1993) J Arthroplasty 8(4): 439

9.5 Patella Options in TKA

P. A. Keblish

1 Introduction

Patella management in total knee arthroplasty (TKA) remains controversial. Tricompartmental TKA (with resurfacing of the patella) is performed most commonly, especially in the United States, primarily because of the potential for postoperative pain and early failure when the patella is left unresurfaced. However, since patella-femoral complications with resurfacing have resulted in major and, at times, catastrophic failures, the option of not resurfacing the patella has gained more popularity. If patella non-resurfacing (retention) is to be recommended, clinical outcomes must be equal or better than those of routine patella resurfacing in the specific prosthesis utilized. Different philosophies exist in different countries, regions, and centers regarding the treatment of the patella. Specific selection criteria for optimal treatment of the patella in TKA have not been clearly defined, therefore, options remain. The surgeon should understand patella biomechanics and characteristics of the prosthesis being used.

The patella has been analyzed in many excellent studies, from normal to diseased states, as well as in TKA. The patella is an integral part of knee joint movements and plays a prominent role in total knee kinematics, whether retained or resurfaced. It acts as a guide for the quadriceps-patella-tendon (QPT) mechanism in centralizing the vector forces to the trochlear groove, protects the joint, and enhances the efficiency of the soft tissues of the extensor mechanism and the distal femur throughout the range of motion. Control of these forces is influenced by many factors, including quadriceps-hamstring balance, the biomechanical axis (extremity), cruciate competence, bone quality, disease process, and others.

The patella-femoral (PF) joint is a highly complex articulation and requires equal attention in design as the femoral-tibial joint during total knee replacement surgery in terms of design, biomechanical, and physiological interaction. Patellar relationships (to the PF joint) change after TKA, even in an ideal situation. Component position placement (medial vs. lateral, superior vs. inferior), thickness, tilt, pre-existing "baja", design geometry, etc. can influence patella tracking, often in subtle ways. The success of patella retention is, therefore, multifactorial and dependent upon many factors including:

- "patella-friendly" femoral prosthetic design,
- correct rotational positioning of the femoral component prosthetic design,
- patella size and quality,
- patella position (alta/baja),
- soft tissue balancing,
- surgical approach, and
- patella bed management.

Many TKA designs appear to treat the femoral patellar relationship as a secondary thought, requiring patella resurfacing of various dimensions (usually dome-shaped) in order to adapt to different non-anatomical (patella-unfriendly) femoral designs.

2 Patella Resurfacing Options

Patella resurfacing in TKA was developed in the 1970 s at the Hospital for Special Surgery because of a high rate of patella pain with early condylar designs [1, 12]. The cemented all polyethylene dome-type patellae became the standard, but poor femoral trochlear designs lead to other problems, primarily because of high contact stress and edge loading. The development of metal backing to dome patellae, to allow for cementless fixation (in the 1980s), lead to an increasing number of wear failures. Many of these failures were catastrophic because of poly "wear through" and metallosis. Failure rates of 5–15% were often reported, usually with poor or "unfriendly patella" designs. Subsequently many fixed bearing design changes were made to address the patella problem. A "second look" at patella retention was reported with

Fig. 25. Comparisons of contact type with various fixed bearing patellofemoral articulations as compared to the LCS rotating design

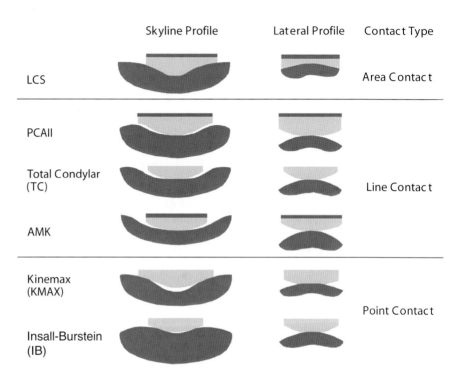

Surface Geometry of Patello-Femoral Articulations
(30 Degrees Flexione)

	Skyline Profile	Lateral Profile	Contact Type
LCS			Area Contact
PCAII			
Total Condylar (TC)			Line Contact
AMK			
Kinemax (KMAX)			
Insall-Burstein (IB)			Point Contact

many designs, but failure rates were often unacceptable. Femoral design and poor understanding of femoral rotation alignment were common factors in fixed bearing designs, with or without patella resurfacing. Incongruence and contact stress were looked at with renewed interest concerning design [10, 12], and most designs are becoming more accommodating to the patella femoral articulation.

3   Patella Designs

The all-polyethylene cemented dome-shaped patella has remained the norm for most tricompartmental knee systems. The surfaces geometries and contact stresses of the dome vary depending on the femoral trochlear anatomy, sizing, positioning etc. The majority of designs produce line or point contact as shown as in Fig. 25.

Figure 26 shows computed contact stresses in various TKA designs that are frequently above the manufacturer's limit for ultra-high molecular weight polyethylene (UHMWPE) [5, 6]. These high-contact areas are accentuated with metal backing and less than ideal femoral rotation alignment, which is addressed in another chapter.

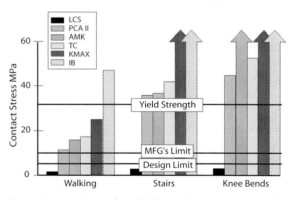

Fig. 26. Comparisons of patellofemoral contact stresses with various fixed bearing as compared to LCS mobile bearing prosthetic design

Dome patella results in most modern design TKA have improved significantly with the improved understanding of soft tissue balancing, femoral tibial positioning, flexion-extension gap balancing and more recently with mobile bearing TKA designs (other than the LCS). The dome patella has been used successfully with the LCS rotation platform by Johnston in an early experience (as a surgeon's choice) [8], before the all-polyethylene anatomic LCS design was available. Personal experience using a dome patella with the LCS meniscal and rotating platforms, for technical reasons (mainly spin-out with trial reduction), and in revision cases, supported the use of a dome-type patella with the LCS femoral flange, which was prior to the development of the all poly anatomic patella. The compromise (less than perfect contact) appears to be tolerated because of the excellent patella tracking and deep sulcus of the LCS femoral flange that will be discussed in the next section.

4   LCS Patella Femoral Joint

The LCS patellofemoral and femoral tibial articulations were designed by Pappas to accommodate interfaces that require absorption of high loads with angular torque forces. The patella articulates with an area of the femoral surface in deep flexion, which is the same surface the tibia «sees» in near full extension. To accommodate this articulation overlap, the LCS femoral component is designed as a common generating curve for the patella and tibial articulations and a common radius of curvature for most of the patellar articulation and part of the tibial articulation [5–7]. The femoral component design, from its inception, was also felt to be most accommodating to an unresurfaced patella. The natural patella always articulates against the same surface shape (except near full extension) and therefore can more easily accommodate (with less remodeling) most other designs that have non-anatomical, varying shapes. This femoral design concept has proven effective for patella function with the LCS moveable and fixed bearing patellar components as well as without resurfacing [4, 18]. Understanding these design principles are important and allow the operating surgeon patella options with the LCS system not available with any other design; namely

- metal-backed rotating,
- all poly-modified anatomic, and
- patelloplasty without resurfacing.
  These three options will be discussed in more detail.

4.1   LCS Metal-Backed Rotating Patella

As noted in the chapter on the LCS design, the rotating patella has been part of the original system and has proven to be effective in multiple reported series [11, 13, 17, 23]. The unique design of a metal-backed rotating anatomic unit added a very different and controversial option in addressing the patellofemoral joint [5] as noted in the previous chapter on design. The coronal plane rotation allows for optimal congruent contact in

keeping with the LCS principles. The base plate with the original cruciform and current 3-peg configuration has been successful from a fixation and mobile articulation standpoint (Fig. 27).

The trunnion bearing assembly allows for ease of exchange at the time of revision surgery, an option not available with other knee systems, and allows for upgrading with improved polyethylene at the time of revision for tibial or bearing problems that are the most common indication for revision TKA (Fig. 28).

The same polyethylene component replacement is available from the original design.

The design allows for options of cemented or cementless fixation, both of which have proven successful in long-term follow-up studies [13, 23] porous-coated backside (Porocoat, DePuy Orthopaedics, Inc., Warsaw, IN) has been modified from the original cruciform to a 3-peg base-plate for both cement and cementless fixation. The 3-peg design allows for easier insertion and less bone removal. Both designs have proven successful. Cementless fixation has been extremely effective and failures are rare. Retrieval specimens have shown excellent osseous integration. Personal experience with fixation (cemented and cementless) over 20 years has shown no bone fixation failures with the metal-backed components. Other studies have shown under 1% failure rates [6, 11, 13, 17, 23], most commonly related to patella mal-tracking. The LCS 3-peg fixation system has been available for the past 5–6 years, without any reported changes in outcomes regarding fixation.

The downside of any metal-backed patella is the potential for wear secondary to abnormal tracking (under 1% problem). Rotation of the LCS design adds another potential complication, namely spin-out or edge-loading of the poly insert. Therefore, polywear (due to a multitude of factors) can be addressed by replacement with superior materials and the same prosthetic design in revision TKA. Large series are not available since failure rates have been low for most LCS series, and patella-femoral complications under 1%.

The rotating patella complications have been low, but problems of spin-out and edge wear have a «potential complication» with a different dimension. Spin-out and/or metallic wear is a serious complication which has been observed and reported [11, 13, 17, 23]. This complication can be avoided by careful trial testing of all component articulations prior to permanent implantation.

Complications of the LCS rotating anatomic patella have been under 1% in previously cited series and remains a treatment option in LCS tri-compartmental replacements. However, potential risks presented by any metal-backed patella, mal-tracking/wear issues and subsequent metal damage has not been totally elimi-

Fig. 27. Illustration of the LCS metal-backed rotating patella. Note the original cruciform and more current 3-peg base plate (available for cement or cementless application)

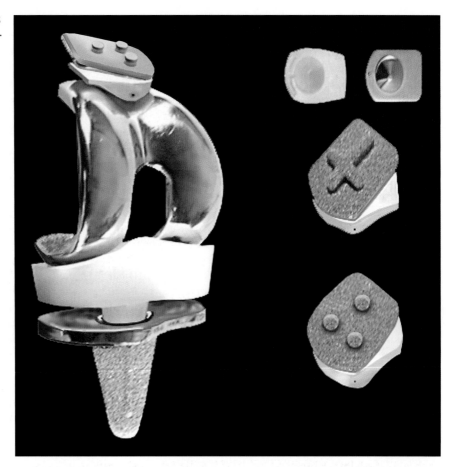

nated. Many surgeons prefer options of an all poly resurfacing or not resurfacing. As noted previously, personal experience with patella-femoral mal-tracking and a less than ideal patella-femoral articulation (at trial reduction) lead to the use of an all poly dome patella with the LCS system [15, 18], with no known failures to date. The recent report by Callahan et al. [8] in primary LCS rotating platforms and success with well fixed dome patellae in LCS revisions suggests that use of a all poly dome patella (although a minor compromise) is another option in both primary and revision TKA.

4.2   LCS Anatomic All Poly

Because of the above stated issues, a 3-peg anatomic patella was designed by Dr. Pappas in the early 1990 s and has had increasing use over the past 5 years. The design (Fig. 29) follows the principles of the LCS, namely optimizing area contact against the generating curve of the femoral sulcus (Fig. 30).

The deep sulcus of the femoral component and soft tissue compliance allow for excellent/near congruent

contact throughout the range of motion. Personal experience with the component in over 100 (unpublished) cases has been excellent, with no failures over a 6- to 7-year time period. This option is being selected as the preferred treatment with many surgeons who routinely resurface the patella and are fearful of metal backing for the reasons stated.

4.3   Patella Non-Resurfacing

The other option regarding patella management is retention or not resurfacing the patella bone. Key factors in patella outcomes include femoral component design and rotational positioning, femorotibial positioning and treatment of the extensor mechanism and patella (if left unresurfaced). Multiple designs exist varying from extreme non-anatomic designs that are too flat to others that are too constrained and are not favorable for patella retention. The LCS femoral component was designed to the natural patella shape and contour with a common generating curve and deep trochlear groove, which best accommodates the un-resurfaced

Fig. 28. Clinical example of revision surgery with simple trunnion polyethylene bearing exchange. Note excellent congruent tracking (of new bearing) in deep flexion

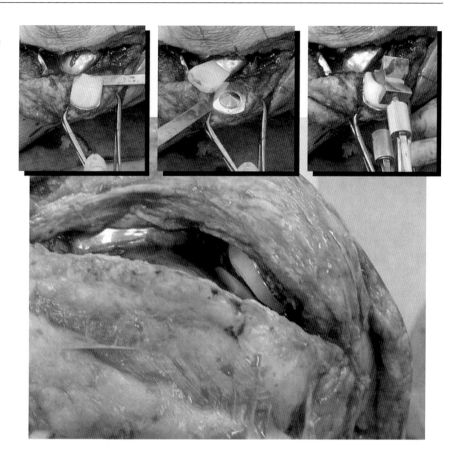

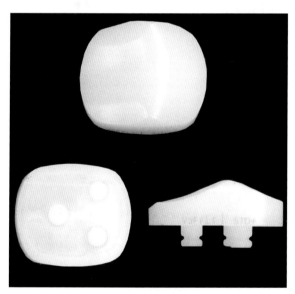

Fig. 29. Articulating, backside, and tangential projections of all-polyethylene LCS anatomic patella design

patella. These design parameters contribute to patella tracking and stability, which allow for optimum contact with the retained patella or anatomic patella (rotating or non-rotating).

Biomechanical studies on cadaver knees published by Matsuda et al. [19] demonstrated no change in contact stress independent of patella resurfacing. However, several biomechanical studies of the knee show significant alteration of forces following TKA, including the extensor mechanism and patella. Reuben et al. [21] have shown that patella thickness reduced in less than 14 mm can decrease tensile strength by as much as 50 %, which definitively increases the likelihood of patella avulsions and fractures. Multiple problems of patella resurfacing such as fracture, quadriceps-patella-tendon (QPT) rupture, component loosening, dislocation, bearing edge wear, increased incidence of heterotopic ossification starting at the patella poles, etc. have been reported in 5 to 20 % of metal-backed resurfaced patellae. Kinematic studies of the normal, ACL-deficient, fixed-bearing resurfaced and mobile bearing resurfaced and unresurfaced patellofemoral joint have shown that the unresurfaced patella with the LCS system best simulates normal (regarding patella tilt, tracking, and separation). The LCS metal-backed rotating patella was second best and fared better than all fixed bearings compared [26].

Patelloplasty. When the patella is left unresurfaced, assessment of the size, shape, remodeling deformities,

Fig. 30. Intraoperative views of preparation, fixation, insertion, and contact areas of the all-polyethylene anatomic design in deep flexion

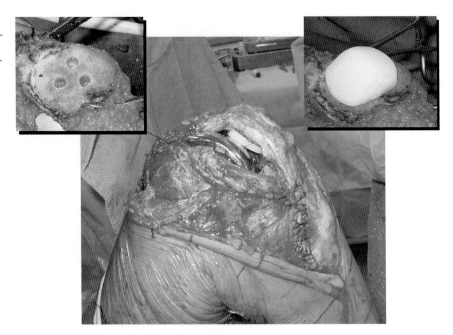

Fig. 31. Demonstration of patelloplasty procedure to include detilting with lateral rim release, circumferential cauterization, and osteophyte removal contouring which allows for anatomic patella tracking. Formal lateral releases (seldom required), are performed preferably via the outside-in method as shown

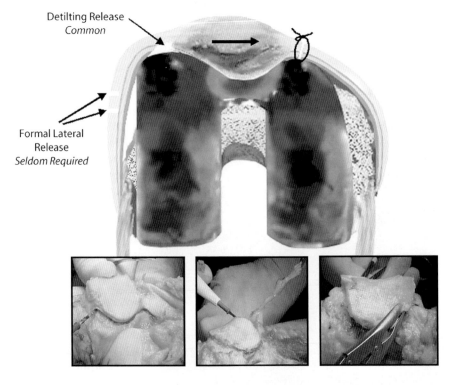

position and surface defects may be of importance. A method of treatment of the extensor mechanism including the patella bed has evolved [4]. It includes:

- lateral rim release to include "filet" expansion of the vastus lateralis tendon,
- circumferential rim cautery for partial denervation [2, 27],
- osteophyte removal, and
- downsizing/contouring to original anatomy (Fig. 31).

A formal lateral release (if required) can be made from outside-in (preferred) or inside-out as advocated by other authors. The patelloplasty method/steps are modified when the direct lateral approach is utilized, since lateral releases and medial patella mobilization are per-

Table 2. Summary of indications for patella nonresurfacing vs. resurfacing

	Patelloplasty (Nonresurfaced)	Patella Resurfacing
Strong	Small patellae Poor bone quality Vascular compromise-extensive release Complex QPT tracking Minimal patellar pain (preop) Patella baja	Wide and/or thick patellae Deformed/non-conforming patellae Severe preop. patellar pain Multiply operated knee Complex knee pain pattern RSD type personality Poor patient compliance
Relative	Younger/higher demand patient Rheumatoid – poor bone stock Good patient compliance	Well-informed patient Rheumatoid – good bone stock Poor patient compliance

formed with the arthrotomy (as noted in the chapter on the valgus knee) [6, 16, 17].

Recent publications have suggested that results of TKA without patella resurfacing can be equally satisfactory. Freeman et al. [10] advocated the importance of improved patellofemoral design as early as 1973. Shoji et al. [22] reported excellent to good results in rheumatoid patients with and without resurfacing of the patella in the same patient, did not advocate routine resurfacing in RA, since there were similar results in the contralateral knee. Boldt et al. [4] found no significant difference between resurfaced and non-resurfaced patellae (bi-lateral) in a prospective study of LCS knees. Key advantages for clinical outcome of patellofemoral function, such as good tracking, improved range of motion, and higher level of activities, were described by those authors who did not find a benefit with patella resurfacing in their studies [3, 14, 18, 22].

Indications and contraindications for patella resurfacing. Setting absolute criteria for patella resurfacing vs. non-resurfacing is difficult. In an attempt to establish some guidelines, strong and relative indications for patella resurfacing are suggested (Table 2).

These criteria represent a combination of the subjective and objective. A near-normal appearance and contour of the patella theoretically favors patella non-resurfacing, and is the most commonly cited criteria advocating selective non-resurfacing. However, no published study has shown that a near-normal macroscopic appearance of the patella is related to better functional outcome. Dye et al. [9] have shown that the majority of patella pain is present primarily at the peripheral tendon insertions and fat pad, supporting the concept of patelloplasty with appropriate prosthetic designs. Our personal histologic evaluation of patella rim tissue has confirmed a rich nerve supply in the peripheral patella rim tissue which is also supporting evidence that the majority of patella pain emanates from soft tissue attachments (Fig. 32).

Long-term evaluation of nonresurfaced patellae frequently demonstrates a neomeniscus-like fibrocartilidge rim devoid of nerve supply (Fig. 33).

If patella nonresurfacing is favored (or contemplated), patients should be advised of the advantages and potential risk factors (primarily anterior knee discomfort) which is slightly higher in nonresurfaced patellae. Therefore, the potential of informed consent/legal implications for patients with less than ideal outcomes are obviated. It has been shown that anterior knee pain is similar with resurfaced or nonresurfaced in our personal study and others as previously noted.

Intraoperatively, patella options should be deferred until trial tibial and femoral reduction has been accomplished. Anatomic alignment and kinematic testing through the full flexion/extension arc will allow for more accurate evaluation of the patella-femoral articulation and influence the decision of whether to resurface or not. Patella options in revision TKA can be simple (debride, leave alone), resurfaced, reconstructed with autograft, allograft, or newer materials such as tantalum mesh attachments for a polyethylene patella resurfacing. This topic is well covered in Dr. Buechel's chapter on revision TKA.

5   Conclusions

Surgeons should evaluate the pros and cons of patella management and options of non-resurfacing or resurfacing with various types of prosthetic designs. Key determinants of patellofemoral tracking and ultimate out-

Fig. 32. Histologic appearance of extensive nerve supply with routine H&E stained patella rim tissue

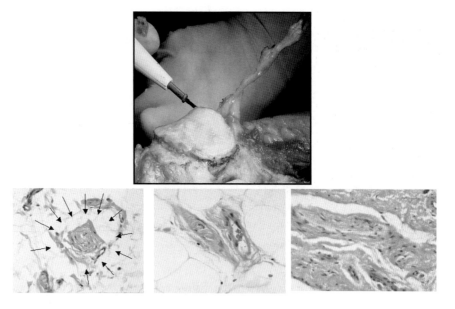

Fig. 33. Clinical example of nonresurfaced patella at 10-year follow-up for femoral-tibial bearing exchange. Patella was left unresurfaced. Histologic studies revealed an absence of nerve tissue

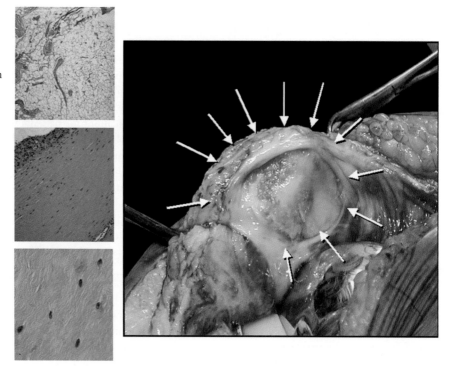

comes include attention to proper soft tissue balancing of the extensor mechanism and femoral rotational alignment [24] which is also addressed in another chapter. The surgeon's goal is to improve the risk/reward ratio and minimize potential complications that lead to less than optimum results and/or need for re-operation. Options presented in this chapter are generic to all TKAs, and also specific to the unique aspects of the LCS design that has proven favorable to long-term patella outcomes with and without resurfacing (Fig. 34).

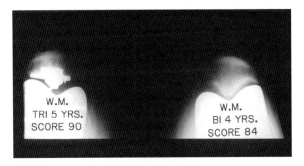

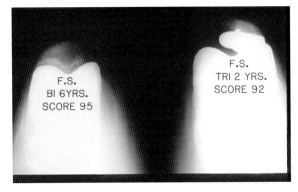

Fig. 34. X-ray examples of resurfaced and nonresurfaced patellae at 7- and 10-year follow-up

References

1. Aglietti P, Insall JN, Walker PS, Trent P (1975) A new patella prosthesis. Design and application. Clin Orthop 107: 175–187
2. Badalamente MA, Cherney SB (1989) Periosteal and vascular innervation of the human patella in degenerative joint disease. Semin Arthritis Rheum 18: 61–66
3. Barrack RL, Wolfe MW, Waldman DA, Milicic M, Bertot AJ, Myers L (1997) Resurfacing of the patella in total knee arthroplasty. A prospective, randomized, double-blind study. J Bone Joint Surg [Am] 79-A: 1121–1131
4. Boldt J, Keblish P, Drobny T, Munsinger U, Varma C (2001) Patella non-resurfacing in low-contact-stress (LCS) mobile-bearing total knee arthroplasty (TKA): results of 1,777 TKAs with 2- to 15-year follow-up. Presented at AAOS 68th Annual Meeting, San Francisco, CA, February 28-March 4
5. Buechel FF, Pappas MJ, Makris G (1991) Evaluation of contact stress in metal-backed patellar replacement. A predictor of survivorship. Clin Orthop 273: 190–197
6. Buechel FF, Pappas MJ (1989) New Jersey low contact stress knee replacement system. Ten-year evaluation of meniscal bearings. Orthop Clin North Am 2: 147–177
7. Buechel FF, Rosa RA, Pappas MJ (1989) A metal-backed, rotating-bearing patellar prosthesis to lower contact stress. An 11-year clinical study. Clin Orthop 248: 34–49
8. Callaghan JJ, Squire MW, Goetz DD, Sullivan PM, Johnston RC (2000) Cemented rotating-platform total knee replacement. A nine- to twelve-year follow-up study. JBJS [Am] 82: 705–711
9. Dye S et al. Cause of pain in the patella
10. Freeman MA, Samuelson KM, Elias SG, Mariorenzi LJ, Gokcay EI, Tuke M (1989) The patellofemoral joint in total knee prostheses. Design considerations. J Arthroplasty 4 (Suppl): S69–74
11. Hamelynck KJ (1998) The total knee prosthesis: indications and complications. Ned Tijdschr Geneeskd 142: 2030–2034
12. Insall JN, Aglietti P, Tria AJ Jr (1983) Patellar pain and incongruence. II. Clinical application. Clin Orthop 176: 225–232
13. Jordan LR, Olivo JL, Voorhorst PE (1997) Survivorship analysis of cementless meniscal bearing total knee arthroplasty. Clin Orthop 338: 119–123
14. Kajino A. Yoshino S. Kameyama S. Kohda M. Nagashima S (1997) Comparison of the results of bilateral total knee arthroplasty with and without patellar replacement for rheumatoid arthritis. A follow-up note. J Bone Joint Surg [Am] 79: 570–574
15. Keblish P (1991) Results and complications of the LCS (Low Contact Stress) knee system. Orthopaedica Belgica 57 (Suppl 2): 124–127
16. Keblish PA (2002) Alternate surgical approaches in mobile-bearing total knee arthroplasty. Orthopedics 25: 257–264
17. Keblish PA (1991) The lateral approach to the valgus knee. Surgical technique and analysis of 53 cases with over two-year follow-up evaluation. Clin Orthop 271: 52–62
18. Keblish PA, Varma AK, Greenwald AS (1994) Patella resurfacing or retention in total knee arthroplasty: A prospective study of patients with bilateral replacements. J Bone Joint Surg [Br] 76: 930–937
19. Matsuda S, Ishinishi T, Whiteside LA (2000) Contact stresses with an unresurfaced patella in total knee arthroplasty: the effect of femoral component design. Orthopedics 23: 213–218
20. Reilly DT, Martens M (1972) Experimental analysis of the quadriceps muscle force and patellofemoral joint reaction force for various activities. Acta Orthop Scan 43: 126–137
21. Reuben JD, McDonald CL, Woodward PL, Hennington LJ (1991) Effect of patella thickness on patella strain following total knee arthroplasty. J Arthroplasty 6: 251–258
22. Shoji H, Yoshino S, Kajino A (1989) Patellar replacement in bilateral total knee arthroplasty. A study of patients who had rheumatoid arthritis and no gross deformity of the patella. J Bone Joint Surg [Am] 71-A: 853–856
23. Sorrells RB (1996) The rotating platform mobile bearing TKA. Orthopedics 19: 793–796
24. Stiehl JB, Cherveny PM (1996) Femoral rotational alignment using the tibial shaft axis in total knee arthroplasty. Clin Orthop 331: 47–55
25. Stiehl JB, Komistek RD, Dennis DA, Keblish PA (2001) Kinematics of the patellofemoral joint in total knee arthroplasty. J Arthroplasty 16: 706–714
26. Stiehl JB, Komistek RD, Dennis DA, Keblish PA (2001) Kinematics of the patellofemoral joint in total knee arthroplasty. J Arthroplasty 16: 706–715
27. Wojtys EM, Beaman DN, Glover RA, Janda D (1990) Innervation of the human knee joint by substance-P fibers. Arthroscopy 6: 254–263

Chapter 10
Surgery

10.1 Surgical Technique of the LCS

F. F. Buechel

1 Surgical Concepts

Total knee arthroplasty represents a major advance in the management of severe, crippling arthritis of any kind. Both cemented and non-cemented implants have been developed in the New Jersey Low-Contact-Stress (LCS) Knee System of components [5, 8].

Textured implants use polymethylmethacrylate for primary fixation of the femoral, tibial and patellar components, while the porous coated components can be used without cement, relying on tissue ingrowth stabilization into the micro-porous coated (275 micron pore size) fixation surface of each component [1–3, 12].

1.1 Stabilizing Unconstrained Mobile Bearings

Since meniscal or rotating bearings are unconstrained in axial rotation, subluxation or dislocation can occur if contact pressure is removed from the bearing surface during any phase of motion. With this in mind, surgical placement of these mobile bearings depends upon balanced flexion and extension tension of the collateral and cruciate ligaments. This tension in the ligamentous apparatus maintains contact pressure on the bearing surfaces to maintain their position in the knee. If one tibiofemoral compartments is too loose, then the femoral component can pivot on the tight compartment and allow the loose compartment bearing to sublux or dislocate.

1.2 Flexion-Extension Gap Adjustment

To assure proper tension in both compartments, spacer blocks are used during the procedure to determine the specific flexion and extension surgical gaps used for the implants. In well-aligned (neutral) knees, no specific releases are needed to ensure equal compartment tension because an axial positioner is used to orient the femoral resection guide to give equal medial and lateral compartment tension in flexion. In neutral knees, the distal femoral cut is also balanced by the same spacer block to maintain contact pressure in both compartments in full extensions. Thus in the neutral knee, balanced compartment tension in flexion and extension assures good contact pressure and bearing stability throughout the arc of motion.

1.3 Varus or Valgus Deformities

In fixed varus or fixed valgus knees, subperiosteal soft tissue sleeve releases [4, 9] must be performed to align the knee prior to bony resection. These soft tissue sleeves are stretched in full extension by use of a spacer block when an intramedullary distal femoral resection guide is used. The flexion gap is determined following sleeve release using a spacer block. Subperiosteal sleeve releases stabilize mobile bearings in the same way as fixed bearings and allow the correction of fixed deformities. Once healed, these corrected deformities maintain their alignment as if they were neutral knees.

1.4 Tibia-Cut-First Approach

A tibia-cut-first approach similar to the successful total condylar procedure was chosen to provide a logical, time-tested method of establishing a stable, reproducible flexion-gap which can then be easily balanced by an equal and stable extension-gap. This provides total knee stability throughout the range of active and passive motion. Such stability maintains contact pressure on mobile bearings and prevents subluxation or dislocations. The technique incorporates the basic surgical philosophy of balanced flexion and extension gaps developed by Michael Freeman, MD and John Insall, MD [13].

This surgical technique can be used for either cemented or cementless application of the implants, since the resection surfaces are designed for press-fit stability of all components.

1.5   Femoral Reference Points

Primary femoral bone cuts preserve a maximum of bone stock using the anterior femoral shaft, epicondyles and center of the femoral canal for surgical reference points. Slight external rotation of the femoral component allows for a perpendicular resection of the proximal tibia in the frontal plane, while providing equal medial and lateral compartment tension in flexion, as well as providing a more stable tracking position for the patella.

Posterior inclination of the proximal tibial cut, parallel to the anatomical inclination angle during this procedure, provides compressive loading of tibial components and avoids the shearing effects associated with perpendicular lateral plane resections.

Resection of the patellar articulating surface at the level of the quadriceps and patella tendons, respectively, allows sufficient bone stock and blood supply [14] to implant a cruciate fixturing element(and more recently a 3-peg component), which stabilizes a rotating-bearing patella replacement.

1.6   Instrument Development

The use of mobile bearing elements in the new jersey LCS System, combined with the precise use of instruments for insertion should provide the surgeon with a superior alignment and placement of all components with bearing elements designed for maximum wear resistance without mechanical restrictions to movement. These implants have now been in clinical use in their present articulating geometry for more than 25 years, a testimony to their acceptance and durability [8, 10, 11].

1.6.1   Original New Jersey Knee Instrumentation

Our original New Jersey Knee instruments were developed in 1977 [6] as what Dr. Pappas and I perceived to be "user friendly" modifications of the total condylar instruments (Fig. 1). A unique feature of this early instrument system, still important today, was the femoral guide positioner. This patented U-shaped device simplified positioning the femoral resection guide by anatomically creating a rectangular space between the femoral resection guide and the perpendicular tibial cut in the frontal plane [7]. This ideal femoral resection guide position was based upon collateral ligament tension, which could be titrated in case of varus or valgus contracture. The linking of axial femoral alignment position to the proximal tibial cut and collateral ligament tensions

Fig. 1. Original New Jersey Knee Instruments which were designed to be user friendly versions of the total condylar instruments

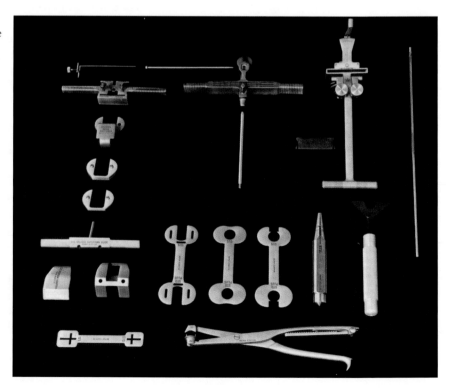

also gave automatically correct patellofemoral tracking alignment, a feature still desired by all surgeons.

1.6.2 Advanced Performance Instrumentation

By the end of the FDA multicenter clinical trial in 1985 [1], the more complex extension-tension-femoral alignment guide of the original instruments was replaced by an intramedullary distal femoral resection guide at the advice of many of the participating surgeons. This newer instrument system, called API™ (Advanced Performance Instrumentation), also initiated the use of more convenient spacer blocks to measure the flexion and extension gaps during surgery (Fig. 2).

1.6.3 Milestone Instrumentation

In the early 1990's a better femoral intramedullary guide was developed to give a fixed 5°, 4° or 3° valgus cut on the distal femur based upon the patient's height, namely height <5'11"=5°, 5'11" to 6'1"=4°, >6'1"=3°. This simplified the distal femoral cut significantly and became part of the Milestone Instrumentation. Additionally, a 2 degree varus-valgus correction block was developed in response to surgeons complaining of many varus cuts on the tibia, despite following the technique. It seems that tibial varus placement errors were becoming common, while trying to drill and pin the tibial resection guide. These errors were in the 2-degree range, thus and easy to slide on "cheater block" saved the surgeon from

going through all the tibial guide alignment steps, while still correcting the error.

Another Milestone instrument was developed to simplify and combine the recessing and chamfer guides into the finishing guide, thus saving the surgeon the time for removal and repositioning a second instrument. This modified guide was useful and well-received by most surgeons.

1.6.4 Conical Tibial Reamer

In the early 1990s, Dr. Pappas and I developed a conical tibial reamer and tibial reamer guide template to eliminate the need for the tibial centering punch, pilot punch and tibial punch, which were responsible for numerous proximal tibial fractures. The new conical reamer made tibial preparation accurate and easy while eliminating the risk of fracture, see Fig. 29. Despite our insistence on using this new device early on DePuy has only recently incorporated this instrument into the Milestone set because of cost containment issues.

1.6.5 Patella Resection

Patella resection instruments have come and gone during the 25 years history of the New Jersey LCS knee. Current instruments still require cumbersome set-up time without a guarantee of the exact cut desired. The difficulty lies in the peripatellar tissue upon which most guides rest. If the guide is tilted slightly or uneven with

Fig. 2. API™ Instrumentation

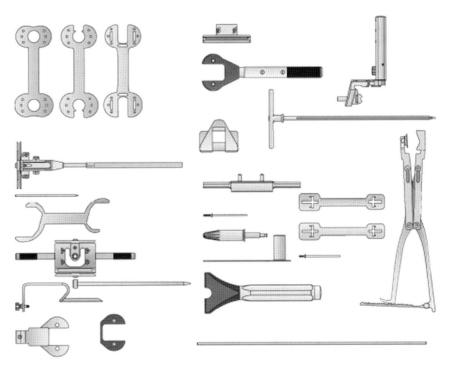

the quadriceps tendon, then the patellar resection will be incorrect. I still prefer the freehand technique that cuts the patella surface from above, using the exposed quadriceps tendon as the reference for the depth of cut while maintaining a parallel articular surface border. This technique, once mastered, is quick, easy and reproducible.

1.6.6   Rotation and the cruciate ligaments

The concept of axial knee rotation is constantly being challenged. In the normal knee, the majority of rotation occurs laterally with less motion seen medially; both condyles pivot about the intercondylar eminence as the center of rotation. Our surgical technique is based on the principle that reproducing normal knee rotation is desirable when the anterior and or posterior cruciate ligaments are intact.

If the posterior cruciate is absent or sacrificed, the axis of rotation remains central and equally shared by both compartments. The design of this implant allows for this and eliminates the need for right and left tibial components or bearings. In this technique, the objective is to produce a knee that has equal soft tissue tension medially and laterally in both flexion and extension. This results in a stable total knee throughout the range of active and passive motion. Such stability maintains contact pressure on the mobile bearing and protects against subluxation and dislocations.

The philosophy of mobile bearing knee replacement has not changed over the past quarter century even though some instrument improvements have eased the surgical burden of prosthetic insertion [9]. For this reason, it is useful to briefly illustrate the current concepts and instrumentation for implanting the New Jersey LCS knee.

2   Surgical Technique

2.1   Incision and Exposure

With the knee slightly flexed, make a straight mid-line incision form 3–4 inches above the patella, over the patella, and ending at the tibial tubercle (Fig. 3a). With neutral alignment or with varus deformity, make a median parapatellar incision though the retinaculum, capsule and synovium (Fig. 3b). The subvastus ("Southern") approach may be used. If significant valgus deformity exists, a lateral parapatellar deep incision as part of a lateral release may be preferred (Fig. 3c).

Excise hypertroptic synovium and a portion of the infrapatellar fat pad to allow access to the medial, lateral and intercondylar spaces. Excise redundant synovium to prevent possible impingement or postoperative over-

growth. Some surgeons prefer a complete synovectomy. Evaluate the condition of the cruciate ligaments to determine the appropriate tibial component use [15].

2.2   Ligament Balancing

Remove femoral and tibial osteophytes, especially any deep to the collateral ligaments. Lateral soft tissue release and, occasionally, osteotomy and removal of the fibular head will enable correction of valgus contracture (Fig. 4a) [4]. Medial release may be necessary for fixed varus deformity (Fig. 4b). An extensive medial tibial subperiosteal sleeve may be necessary in severe varus angulation.

2.3   Tibial Resection

Proper rotational alignment is established by positioning the appropriate malleoli wings parallel to the transmalleolar axis (Fig. 5). Place the alignment rod proximally over the center mark on the tibia, usually slightly medial to the tibial tubercle. It should be directly over the longitudinal mark distally, just lateral to the tibialis anterior tendon (Fig. 6).

When the rod is parallel to the intramedullary axis of the tibia as viewed laterally, the posterior slope of the tibia should parallel the chosen resection block (7 to 10 degrees). Impale the second spike. The slope may be further adjusted by loosening the ankle clamp knob and sliding the rod anteriorly or posteriorly. When proper positioning is achieved, lock the ankle clamp knob.

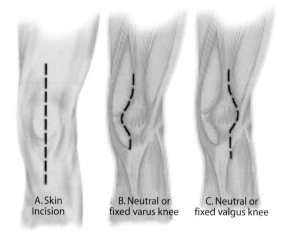

Fig. 3. a Skin incision centered on the knee joint. b Medial parapatellar incision for neutral or fixed varus knees, and c lateral parapatellar incision for fixed valgus knees

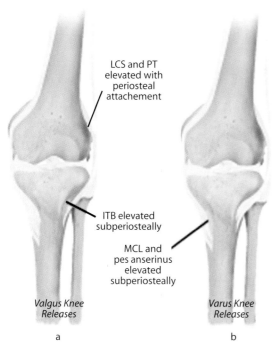

Fig. 4. a Ligament balancing and releases for valgus knees, and b for varus knees

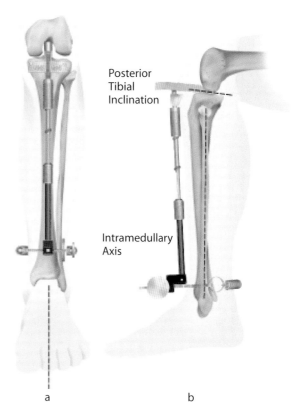

Fig. 6. a Alignment of the tibial resection guide in the frontal and b sagittal planes

Remove the stylus, (a 6 mm stylus is also provided. The 6 mm measurement is used when referencing the unaffected plateau.)

Check alignment by attaching the alignment tower and rod to the tibial cutting block. The distal end of the rod should lie over the longitudinal ankle mark, in line with the second toe and just lateral to the anterior tibialis tendon insertion (Fig. 7a). If alignment is found to be in variance, the cutting block can be removed from the pins and the special two-degree varus/valgus block applied to the pins for correction (Fig. 7b). Use corresponding holes. Since the fixation pin holes of all tibial cutting block s are parallel to the cutting surface, this block will only alter the varus/valgus angle by two degrees and will not affect the posterior slope.

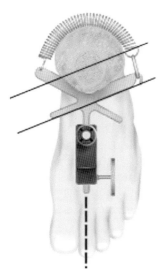

Fig. 5. Alignment of tibial resection guide centered on ankle joint shown from the transverse plane

Attach the stylus (0 or 2 mm) to the tibial cutting block on the side of the lower tibial compartment. Lower the cutting block and stylus by turning the knurled cylinder to the left until the top of the stylus contacts the tibial plateau. Determine what the level of the tibial resection is satisfactory, then predrill and place two 3 inch long 1/8 inch fixation pins in the marked row of holes.

Apply the saw capture (Fig. 8), resect the proximal tibia (Fig. 9) and remove the block. Leave the fixation pins in place. Once the proximal bone has been removed, further ligament balancing becomes easier. With pre-existing flexion contracture, preliminary removal of the tibial plateau usually allows full extension of the knee to facilitate ligament balancing.

Before proceeding further, assure that the extremity can be brought into normal medial-lateral alignment in

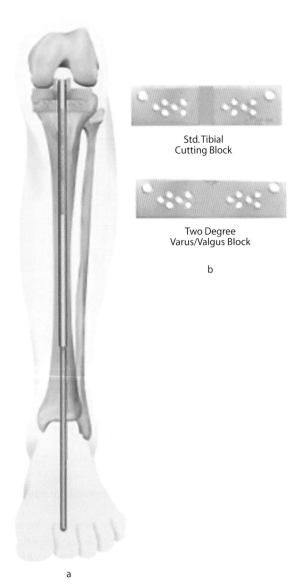

Std. Tibial
Cutting Block

Two Degree
Varus/Valgus Block

b

Fig. 7. a Alignment tower used to check frontal alignment after resection block is pinned, **b** differences between standard cutting block and correction block

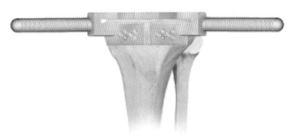

Fig. 8. Capture plate is applied to the resection block

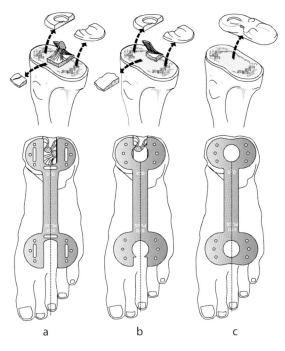

Fig. 9a–c. Tibial cuts required for **a** bicruciate retaining platform, **b** posterior cruciate retaining platform, **c** rotating platform

extension. Place traction on the foot and perform additional soft tissue balancing until the normal mechanical axis is obtained. The electrocautery cord of suction tubing can be stretched from the center of the femoral head (approximately two finger breadths medial to the ASIS) to the center mark on the ankle. The line should pass through the center of the knee joint. This confirms that the ligaments are balanced in extension.

2.4 Femoral Sizing

Select a femoral sizing template. The inside of each template corresponds to the inside geometry of the selected size of femoral component. The outside of the template corresponds to the outside surface of the femoral component. When sizing, it is important to keep the anterior flange of the femoral component in the same plane as the anterior cortex.

With the knee in flexion, place the femoral template against the lateral condyle to visually determine the best fit. Check to assure the bony resection depths look reasonable (Fig. 10). This will determine the best AP component fit and should be the primary sizing method.

2.5   Femoral Preparation

Attach the guide yoke to the appropriate size AP femoral resection guide (Fig. 11). Slip the yoke beneath the muscle anteriorly on the periosteum. Establish the center of the IM canal by positioning the yoke centrally on the an-

terior femoral shaft (Fig. 12) and centering the guide between the epicondyles (Fig. 13).

The centering mark that was previously drawn will be helpful. In this position, the only contact between the resection guide and the distal femoral condyles may be on the posterior medial condyle. The position of the femoral guide hole is generally 3 to 5 mm medial to the apex of the intercondylar notch (Fig. 14). Place one temporary pin in any of the femoral resec-

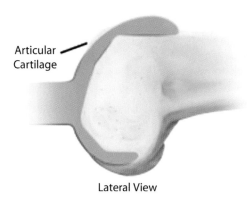

Articular Cartilage

Lateral View

Fig. 10. Femoral template used to size the femur on the lateral border to the bony, not cartilage surface

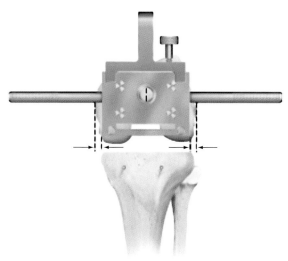

Fig. 13. Placement of AP Resection Guide on distal femur (frontal plane)

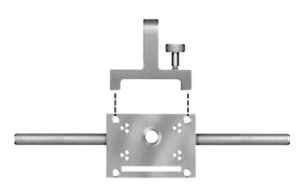

Fig. 11. Assembly of anterior guide yoke to the AP resection guide

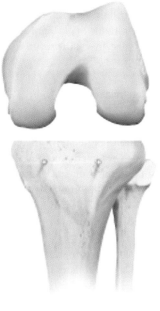

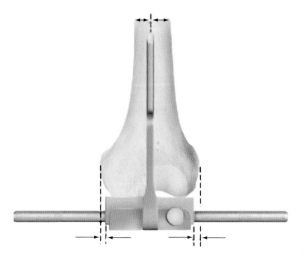

Fig. 12. Placement of AP Resection Guide on anterior femur

Fig. 14. Location of drill hole, usually 3–5 mm medial to the intercondylar notch

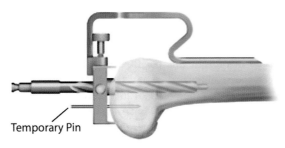

Fig. 15. Insertion of stabilizing temporary pin and drilling of distal femur

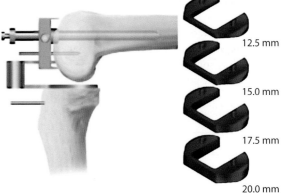

12.5 mm

15.0 mm

17.5 mm

20.0 mm

Fig. 17. Spacers or thickness adaptors used to provide proper soft tissue tensioning

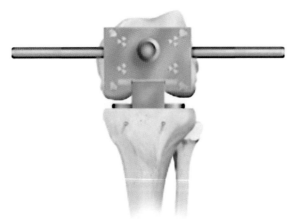

Fig. 16. Femoral positioner used to make the anterior and posterior femoral resections parallel to the tibial resection

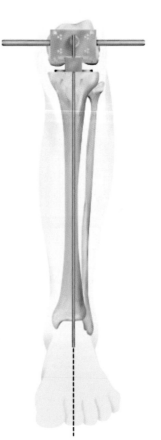

tion guide holes for stability Drill the femoral IM guide hole using a 9 mm diameter initiator drill (Fig. 15). Remove the temporary pin and yoke. Insert the seven-inch, 9 mm diameter rod.

2.5.1 Femoral Rotation Determination

Slide the femoral guide positioner into the joint space engaging the slot of the femoral AP resection guide (Fig. 16). Slightly flex or extend the knee until the positioner lies flat on the previously resected proximal tibia. If the positioner will not fit into the joint space, use the tibial fixation pins to realign the tibial resection block, by selecting a more proximal row of holes on the block, lowering the block and removing additional proximal tibial bone.

If the space is to lax add tibial spacer shims and reassess until equal medial and lateral collateral ligament tension is achieved (Fig. 17). Evaluate the tibial alignment once more by sliding the external alignment rod through the femoral positioner (Fig. 18).

Evaluate femoral rotation prior to pinning the resection guide in place. It is customary to implant the femo-

Fig. 18. Long rod placed through the positioner showing proper frontal plane alignment of the resection guide

ral component in relative external rotation. In this system, however, specific external rotation is defined by the femoral guide positioner, which also establishes equal compartmental tension. The goal is to establish a quadrilateral space with the resected posterior femoral condylar surfaces parallel to the resected tibial surfaces when the collateral ligaments are tensioned. Pin the femoral AP resection guide in two places, using the middle holes in the lower set of holes. Remove the femoral guide positioner and the tibial fixation pins, if they are still in place.

2.5.2   AP Femoral Resection

Attach the saw capture and cut the anterior and posterior femoral condyles. The anterior resection is flush with the anterior cortex of the femur (Fig. 19).

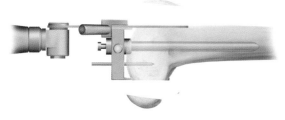

Fig. 19. Osscilating saw used to make anterior and posterior femoral resection

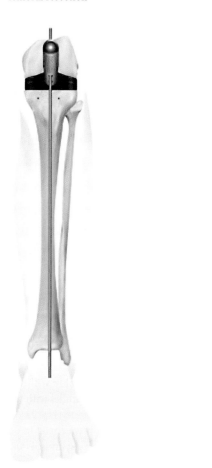

Fig. 20. Spacer block employed to check flexion gap and assure alignment

Once the resections are completed, remove the guide and pins. Insert the spacer block assembly into the flexion gap. The assembly mimics the thickness of the femoral, tibia and 10 mm bearing components. Assure equal medial and lateral compartmental tension. If necessary add a tibial shim to the spacer block to fill the gap (Fig. 20).

The fixation pin hole pattern on the AP femoral resection guides is the same distance from the anterior cuffing surface regardless of component size. Thus, the anterior femoral resection will remain flush with the shaft if downsizing is performed. Therefore, resection of additional posterior condylar bone is simplified.

2.5.3   Checking Flexion Gap

If one compartment is still too tight in flexion, release additional soft tissue to achieve equal compartmental tension. Insert the external alignment rod through the spacer block handle to again check the frontal and lateral plane alignment on the tibia (see Fig. 20). Make note of the thickness of the spacer block utilized to fill the flexion gap. This will subsequently determine the extension gap.

2.5.4   Distal Femoral Resection

With the cuffing block locked into place, insert the 8 mm diameter femoral IM rod into the distal femoral cutting guide assembly (Fig. 21a). The rod is fluted and 1 mm smaller than the pilot hole to minimize pressure build-up in the canal and to allow the isthmus to dictate rod placement. Slowly advance the femoral IM rod into the distal femur Full seating is not necessary as the rod may

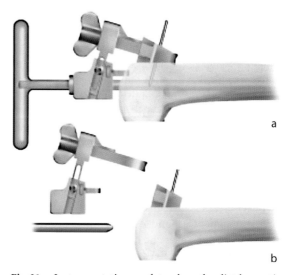

Fig. 21. a Instrumentation used to place the distal resection guide at the proper location. **b** Distal guide locator removed leaving the resection block alone

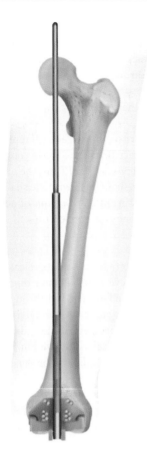

Fig. 22. Alignment tower is used to check the varus/valgus alignment of the distal cut before resection. It should be centered on the femoral head

reach the isthmus. The blunt tip will easily pass into the IM canal while minimizing the chances of perforation.

The modular cuffing block should rest flush on the anterior femoral cut. Secure it in place by predrilling and inserting two pins through the marked center row of holes. Disengage the alignment guide from the cuffing block by turning the wing nut to the neutral position. Remove both the IM rod and the alignment guide, leaving the block in place (Fig. 21b).

Verify varus/valgus alignment by using the external alignment tower (Fig. 22). With the femur in extension and in neutral rotation, correct alignment is indicated when the proximal end of the external alignment rod is centered over the head of the femur or approximately two finger breadths medial to the anterior superior iliac spine. If alignment is found to be other than desired, the valgus angle can be altered by two degrees with the use of a two degree varus/valgus cutting block. If more correction is necessary then choose another cuffing block, mount it on the IM guide and reposition it off the anterior cut.

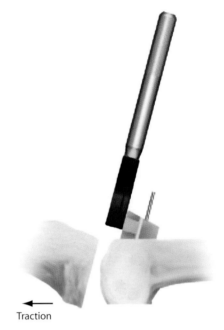

Traction

Fig. 23. The spacer block is used to sight the resection before it is made

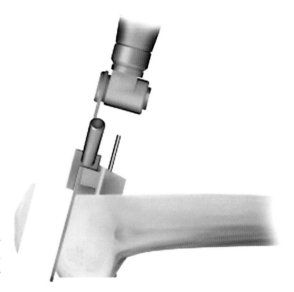

Fig. 24. After application of the capture plate, the distal resection is made

To ensure the correct depth of the distal femoral cut, have an assistant place traction on the ankle with the knee in extension. Place a spacer block parallel with the tibial cut and the anticipated femoral cut (Fig. 23). A shim is applied to the spacer block if it was used in determining the flexion gap. The extension gap must equal the flexion gap. If the spacer block is parallel and clears the tibial cut the distal femoral cuffing block is correctly located. The cuffing block can be positioned in a different row of holes(2.5 mm apart) to resect a greater or lesser amount of distal femur to assure the spacer block will fit in the extension gap.

Before proceeding, it is necessary to correct either the distal femoral or proximal tibial cut to assure equal flexion and extension gaps. The distal femoral cut will affect the extension gap; the tibial resection will affect both flexion and extension. The extension gap must equal the flexion gap.

Attach the saw capture and cut the distal femur (Fig. 24). Extend the knee and insert the spacer block (with the shim if it was used for the flexion gap). It should fit snugly in the gap with equal MCL and LCL tension (Fig. 25a,b). Remove the spacer block and fixation pins.

2.5.4 Femoral Finishing Resection

Flex the knee. Center the finishing guide between the epicondyles and impact it until fully seated. The finishing guide is the exact width of the corresponding femoral component size. Two anterior fixation pins will secure the guide to the femur (Fig. 26). Ensure the anterior and distal surfaces are flush. Using the 1/4 inch diameter stop drill, create two 3/4 inch deep holes through the distal guide holes (Fig. 27). Cut the anterior and posterior chamfers with the oscillating saw (Fig. 28a). Using an osteotome or a narrow oscillating saw make the recessing cut from the proximal end of the finishing guide. Save this bone to fashion a cone to plug the femoral IM hole. Use the power saw to resect the posterior femoral condyle remnants to assure and equate flexion clearance (Fig. 28b). Remove the finishing guide.

2.5.5 Final Tibial Preparation

Where a bicruciate retaining tibial plateau is used, align the appropriate size bicruciate retaining tibial template, and pin in place using the Fixation Pins. Then burr the three fixation fin channels using the tibial burr (Fig. 29a).

For the remaining type tibial plateaus align the correct size tibial reamer guide template where a posterior

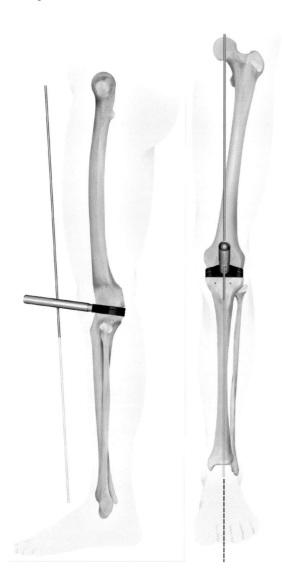

Fig. 25a,b. Spacer block used to check both alignment and extension gaps

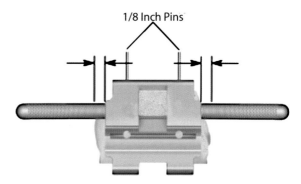

Fig. 26. The finishing guide is fully seated and centered on the femur

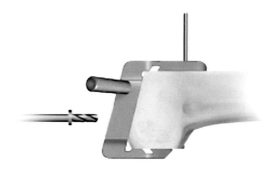

Fig. 27. The fixation pins holes are created with a stop drill to make them the proper depth and diameter

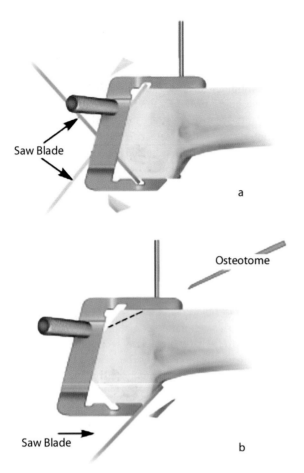

Saw Blade

Osteotome

Saw Blade
b

Fig. 28. a An oscillating saw is used to created the anterior and posterior chamfers, and **b** to create a relief cut for improved flexion and to create a rescessing cut on the anterior femur

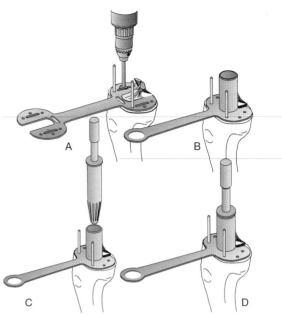

A

B

C

D

Fig. 29. a For the bicruciate tibial tray, fixation fins are created with a power burr through the template. **b,c,d** A conical reamer is used to fashion the tibial fixation hole in the proximal tibia

cruciate tibial plateau is used, and for best boney coverage where the cruciate sacrificing, or revision, tibial plateau is employed. Pin the guide in place using the fixation pins. Ream the hole for the plateau stem using the conical tibial reamer (Fig. 29b–d).

2.6 Patellar Preparation

Resect the patellar surface, at and parallel to, the level of the quadriceps tendon using an oscillating saw. Ensure that the resected surface is flat and that the patella thickness is uniform. This thickness should generally be 12–14 mm (Fig. 30a). Take care not to resect below the level of the tendon, as this will excessively weaken the patellar bone bed.

Reduce the resected patella and orient the patella template corresponding in size to the femoral size chosen against the resected surface. Place the patella template perpendicular to the tibial axis (Fig. 30b).

Evert the patella and the patella template on the resected surface with the plate centered on the bone bed. The handle will usually lie approximately 30° downward from the perpendicular to the tibial axis (Fig. 30c). Mark this position with a cautery or a marking pen.

Align the appropriate size and type patellar template with the marking on the resected patellar surface representing proper patella placement. Ensure that the template is flush. A hard bone patella template for sclerotic bone, and a soft bone patella template for osteoporotic bone, is available. Prepare the cruciate channels using the patella burr through the slot in the template. Insure that the channels are sufficiently deep to avoid any "hang up" of the fixturing fins (Fig. 30d).

2.7 Trial Reduction

Insert and impact the appropriate size and type trial tibial component using the impactor (Fig. 31a). Ensure that the tibial surface is properly covered and aligned. If not, adjust the position of trial tibial component. The tibial components are aligned for the best bony coverage as shown below. The cruciate retaining tibial components must also be aligned in the direction of normal gait (Fig. 31b,c). The alignment of these latter com-

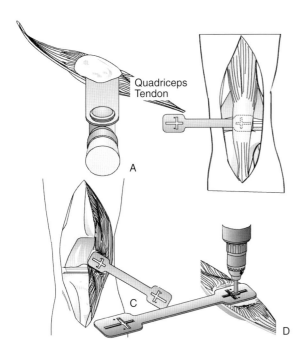

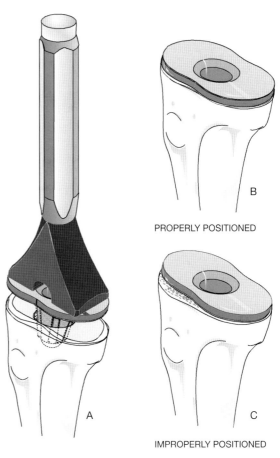

Fig. 30. a The patellar is resected using a power saw. b The patellar template is placed at 90° to the patellar tendon, keeping superior traction on the extensor mechanism. c The patella is everted and the proper size template is centered on the resected patella. d A power burr is used to created the cruciate fixation channel

PROPERLY POSITIONED

IMPROPERLY POSITIONED

Fig. 31 a Tibial impactor used to impact the trial tibial component. b Malrotation of the tibial trial. c Proper rotation of the tibial trial

ponents will be checked after completion of the trial reduction and adjusted if needed.

Axial alignment of the cruciate sacrificing tibial plateau with respect to the direction of normal gait is unnecessary. Such misalignment is accommodated by the rotating bearing.

Insert the trial meniscal or rotating bearing(s). Flex the leg to about 120° to allow the posterior trial femoral condyles to clear the anterior lip(s) of the bearing(s), and digitally insert the trial femoral component on the distal femur (Fig. 32a). In tight knees, hold the bearing(s) in place and bring the knee into extension to allow the bearing(s) to reduce under the posterior femoral cut. Then flex the knee to insert the femoral component. Extend the leg to about 80° so that the posterior trial femoral condyles will clear the posterior lip(s) of the trial bearing(s). Fully impact the trial femoral component at less than 90° of flexion to avoid rocking the trial tibial component (Fig. 32b).

Check the range of motion of the knee, while looking for free bearing motion and absence of impingement. If these are not present, correct at this stage. At full extension the trial meniscal bearings should be for-

ward in their tracks and should be approximately equidistant from the anterior edge of the trial tibial component. If they are not, correct the rotational position of the trail component.

2.8 Component Implantation

Implant the appropriate tibial component, bearing(s) and femoral component, using cement, and/or impaction, as appropriate, in the same order and manner as the trials (Fig. 33). Insert the fixation fins of the rotating patella component into the cruciate channels in the resected patellar surface (Fig. 34a).

Press the patella anchoring plate flat against the resected bone surface using the patella clamp. Reduce the patella and evaluate the implants (Fig. 34b). Ensure that an unrestricted range of motion, free bearing movement and proper patella tracking are present.

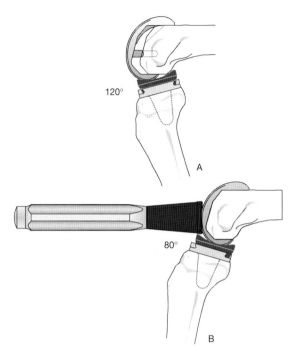

Fig. 32 a After insertion of the proper trial meniscal or rotating bearing(s). Flex the leg to about 120° to allow the posterior trial femoral condyles to clear the anterior lip(s) of the Bearing (S). **b** The leg is extended to about 80° so that the posterior trial femoral condyles will clear the posterior lip(s) of the trial Bearing(s) and the trial femoral component is impacted at less than 90° of flexion to avoid rocking the trial tibial component

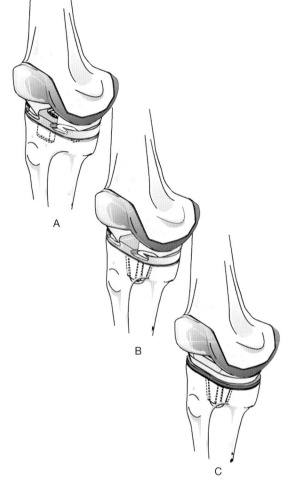

Fig. 33. a Bicruciate retaining tibial component implanted; **b** posterior cruciate retaining tibial component implanted; **c** rotating platform tibial component implanted

2.9 Closure and Post-Operative Management

Release the tourniquet and copiously irrigate the wound with antibiotic saline solution. Check motion with the tourniquet down. Close the deep retinacular tissues using #1 absorbable suture, the subcutaneus tissue with a 2–0 absorbable suture and the skin using staples or a vertical mattress suture. A suction drain may or may not be used (Fig. 35). Apply a Robert Jones compression dressing to the extremity followed by a long leg knee immobilizer. If pressure is needed to gain full extension, apply a long leg cast to hold full extension for 48 hours, then remove the cast and begin routine post-operative rehabilitation.

The patient may be out of bed on the first post-operative day and may begin isometric quad setting exercises of at least ten per hour. Remove suction drains, if used, after 48 hours whereupon an anticoagulation, prophylactic protocol may be instituted. The patient may transfer with weight-bearing to tolerance on the first post operative day and may begin gravity-assist and active-assistive range of motion. Should wound healing be a problem, then defer flexion until the wound quality appears satisfactory.

Perform physical therapy, consisting of progressive ambulation with weight bearing to tolerance, daily for the first two weeks and then three times weekly over the next four weeks. Knee swelling may persist consistent with the rehabilitation status of the quadriceps mechanism. Post operative swelling with a well-functioning quadriceps generally subsides within 6–12 weeks following knee replacement. Isometric quad setting exercises should be continued until knee effusion (swelling) has subsided. Once this effusion has subsided, progressive resistive quadriceps exercises should begin to improve strength and endurance necessary for normal gait.

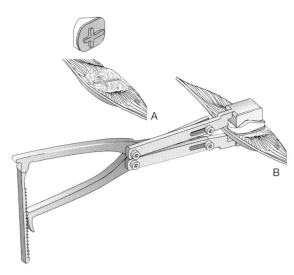

Fig. 34. a Patellar implant is aligned, and **b** the patellar clamp is used to fully seat the component

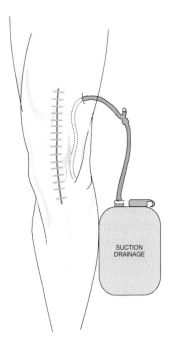

SUCTION
DRAINAGE

Fig. 35. Routine closure with or without suction drainage

References

1. Bobyn JD, Engh CA (1983) Biologic fixation of hip prostheses: review of the clinical status and current concepts. Adv Orthop Surg: 137–150
2. Bobyn JD, Engh CA (1984) Human histology of the bone - porous metal implant interface. Orthop 7: 1410–1427
3. Bobyn JD, Pilliar RM, Cameron HU, Weatherly GC (1980) The optimum pore size for the fixation of porous-surfaced metal implants by the ingrowth of bone. Clin Orthop 150: 263–270
4. Buechel FF (1990) A sequential three-step lateral release for correcting fixed valgus knee deformities during total knee arthroplasty. Clin Orthop 260: 170–175
5. Buechel FF, Pappas MJ (1984) New Jersey integrated total knee replacement system: biomechanical analysis and clinical evaluation of 918 cases. FDA Panel Presentation, Silver Springs, Maryland
6. Buechel FF, Pappas MJ (1986) The New Jersey low-contact-stress knee replacement system: biomechanical rationale and review of the first 123 cemented cases. Arch Orthop Traum Surg 105:197–204
7. Buechel FF, Pappas MJ (1988) Positioner for surgical instruments. U.S. Patent No. 4,738,254
8. Buechel FF, Pappas MJ (1990) Long term survivorship analysis of cruciate sparing vs cruciate-sacrificing knee prostheses using meniscal bearings. Clin Orthop 260: 162–169
9. Buechel FF, Sorrells RB (1994) New Jersey LCS® total knee system surgical technique using Milestone Instruments. DePuy Inc.
10. Buechel FF Sr, Buechel FF Jr, Pappas MJ, D'Alessio J (2001) Twenty-year evaluation of meniscal bearing and rotating platform knee replacements. Clin Orthop 388: 41–50
11. Buechel FF, Rosa RA, Pappas MJ (1989) A metal-backed, rotating-bearing patellar prosthesis to lower contact stress: an 11 year clinical study. Clin Orthop 248: 34–49
12. Engh CA, Bobyn JD (1986) Principles, techniques, results, and complications with a porous-coated sintered metal system. In: Anderson LD (ed) Instructional course lectures, vol 35. CV Mosby, St Louis, pp 169–183
13. Insall JW (1984) Surgical approaches to the knee. In: Insall JN (ed) Surgery of the knee. Churchhill Livingston, New York, pp 4–54
14. Kayler DE, Lyttle D (1988) Surgical interruption of patellar blood supply by total knee arthroplasty. Clin Orthop 229: 221–227
15. Keblish PA, Pappas MJ (1992) Rationale and selection of mobile bearing knee prosthesis, AAOS Scentific Exhibit

10.2 Why the Tibial Cut First?

J. B. Stiehl, R. B. Sorrels

1 Introduction

There are three major objectives of surgical technique in total arthroplasty. First is the need to achieve anatomical alignment of 50° to 70° valgus angulation to the mechanical axis. Second is to establish ligamentous balance by achieving careful balance of the flexion and extension gaps within 2 to 3 millimeters of physiological. Finally, is the desire to optimize the potential kinematics of the chosen prosthetic implant. The basic technique of the LCS method is a tibial cut first approach, which followed the original idea of Dr John Insall that establishing the flexion gap was the most important variable in successful total condylar arthroplasty [5]. We will discuss why this approach has become so important to the LCS system and why others should consider the technique for successful of mobile bearing prosthetics.

2 Rationale

2.1 Insall Method

The goals of surgical technique of the LCS total knee arthroplasty are the same as those originally established by Insall for inserting the total condylar prosthesis including balancing the ligaments and resecting the ends of the femur and tibia so that the spaces between the cut ends were the same when the knee was in flexion and in extension. The classic Insall method required resecting the anterior and posterior femoral condyles with a degree of external rotation to the anatomical axis of the femur. Then resecting the proximal tibia at 900° flexion, with the plane of resection perpendicular to the long axis of the tibia. Then resecting the distal femur using the spacer that fits the flexion space dimension with a long rod to determine correct valgus angulation of the knee [8]. The particular innovations of this approach were to preferentially determine the flexion space, to use a perpendicular cut on the proximal tibia, and to cut the extension space

based primarily on a tension spacer that matched the flexion space. The principles of flexion/extension spacing and utilizing bone cuts to balance the ligaments as opposed to the opposite became well established.

2.2 Measured Resection of the Distal Femur

From a different point of view, surgeons sought to preserve the cruciate ligaments or at least the posterior cruciate ligament, and the concept of spacer tensioning and cutting the tibia before the femur, became secondary to anatomical preparation of the distal femur. In other words, the focus of the technique was measured resection of bone cuts with the goal of recreating the normal shape and alignment of the knee. With the preservation of the posterior cruciate ligament, the primary ligamentous issue was recreating a neutral or 0° mechanical axis in the frontal plane. Balancing of the flexion space was a secondary issue and centered more on recognizing tightness or looseness of the posterior cruciate ligament. If too tight, the posterior cruciate ligament would hold the femur posterior on the proximal tibia causing anterior tibial liftoff. If too loose, there would be flexion space laxity and potential clinical instability. Numerous authors have endorsed balancing the ligaments *after* all bone cuts have been made focusing on the ligaments that affect primarily extension such as the superficial medial collateral, pes tendons, iliotibial tract and lateral collateral ligament. The posterior cruciate ligament could be recessed off the tibia at the end of the procedure.

More recent improvements of the measured resection technique have been to precisely determine the amount of distal femoral rotation for the posterior condyle cuts such that they parallel the axis of knee rotation. These have included posterior condylar reference with cuts of 3° to 5° external rotation, the Whiteside intercondylar line which utilizes a line from the center of the intercondylar groove bisecting the intercondylar space,

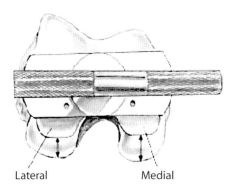

Fig. 36. Distal femoral measured resection with external rotation using the Whiteside line, transepicondylar axis, or a 30–40 external rotation

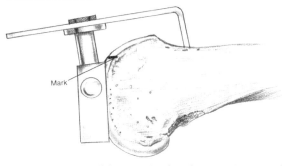

Fig. 37. Posterior condylar resection based on anterior cortical reference with appropriate measured external femoral rotation

and the transepicondylar axis reference which roughly parallels the knee flexion axis (Fig. 36).

Stiehl et al. developed the tibial shaft axis method which uses a long rod attached to a femoral intramedullary rod which centers on the ankle mortise [9, 10]. The goal of these methods was to create a bone resection resulting in a rectangular flexion space based on the principle that the transepicondylar axis is parallel the knee flexion rotation axis and is the target anatomical structure for prosthetic placement (Fig. 37).

2.3   LCS Method

The LCS surgical technique that has evolved from the outset chose the Insall method with "tibial cut first" resection. Early on, flexion space instability was implicated as a primary cause for complications including mobile bearing "spin out" and dislocation which ranged from 0.5 % for the rotating platform to over 3 % for meniscal bearings. Perhaps this was best demonstrated by the experience of Bert et al. who through surgical misadventure had a dislocation rate of nearly 50 % [3]. The problem was so severe that bearings were nearly falling out in the recovery room. Appropriately, focusing on stability of the flexion gap became the primary premise of the

surgical technique. We, of the LCS camp, feel so strongly about this that we believe little can be gained by resorting to a measured distal femoral resection or other similar methods unless they purposefully provide perfect flexion space balance every time.

3   The LCS Tibial Shaft Axis Method

The LCS tibial shaft axis method determines the proximal tibial cut utilizing an extramedullary guide system and the cut of the tibia is made perpendicular to the mechanical axis of the leg (Fig. 38). An intramedullary femoral rod is placed with the anterior/posterior condylar cutting block. Flexion spacing is then done using the horse-shoe spacer to precisely balance and create a rectangular flexion space (Fig. 39, 40). The exact dimension of the flexion space is determined with a block which is then used to cut the distal femoral surface or extension space (Fig. 41, 42).

An important step with the LCS method is that primary extension ligamentous balancing must be established before the flexion space is created. This is because any ligamentous balancing done after these cuts are made can result in the creation of a trapezoidal flexion space. Such a problem often results in bearing dislocation or "spinout". The surgeon must have the knee balanced as his primary step though some releasing, such as the posterior capsule may be made after the proximal tibial cut. This can be advantageous as the posterior capsular origin on the distal femur becomes more accessible. With the knee in full extension, the ligaments should be balanced and tense. If not, additional release should be done. An interesting evolution has been the development of the lateral or valgus approach to the knee joint. For LCS surgeons, the apparent utility of the valgus ap-

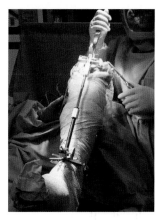

Fig. 38. LCS tibial shaft axis method uses extramedullary guide to cut tibia perpendicular to the limb mechanical axis

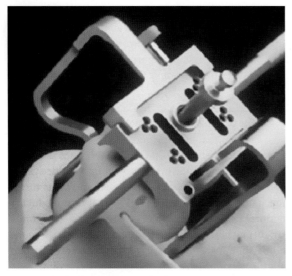

Fig. 39. LCS flexion spacer attached to anterior/posterior cutting block fixed with intramedullary rod and anterior cortical reference with saw bones model

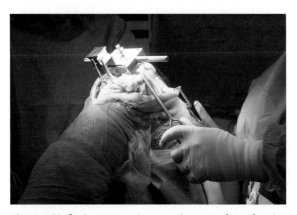

Fig. 40. LCS flexion spacer in operative procedure showing horseshoe spacer used to balance flexion space

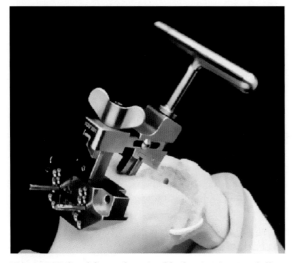

Fig. 41. LCS distal femoral cutting block using intramedullary based to cut extension space

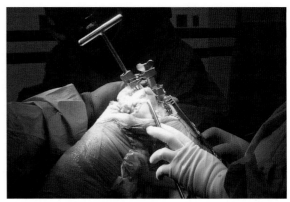

Fig. 42. LCS distal femoral cutting block in operative procedure

proach is that easy access to the posterolateral corner and lateral ligaments is allowed early for primary ligament balancing. A further evolution has been the rod/plate device developed Pony firer. This device has a flat plate fixed to an intramedullary rod at 6° valgus angle. When placed in the intramedullary canal, this device can be used to assess ligament tension in extension.

4   Discussion

The distinct disadvantage of a measured distal femoral resection is the inability to deal with certain outliers such as lateral femoral condylar hypoplasia or severe angular deformities such as proximal tibia vara with a varus joint line. In these patients, ligamentous imbalance occurs commonly and can lead to chronic instability. Berger et al. found the posterior condylar axis to the surgical transepicondylar axis (point of lateral epicondyle to the sulcus of the medial epicondyle) to be 3.5° for males and 0.3° for females which was a highly statistical difference. However, the clinical angle using the prominence of the medial epicondyle was 4.7° for males and 5.2° for females. Significantly, the variance could range from 1° to 9.3° [1]. Mantas et al. found in normal femurs that the range of posterior condylar axis reference to the transepicondylar axis ranged from 0.1° to 9.7° [6].

Fehring compared the Insall method with the measured resection method of distal femur resection using a fixed posterior condylar reference guide finding that the measured resection technique resulted in rotational errors of at least 3° in 45 % of knees [4]. This means that well balanced flexion gaps would have been distorted to trapezoidal gaps in 45 % of cases with potential flexion instability.

Similarly, Olcott and Scott found that the transepicondylar reference most readily determined a balanced flexion space while using 30° rotation off the posterior condyles was least consistent [7].

Berger et al. has shown that internal rotation of the femoral component from the transepicondylar reference combined with tibial internal rotation from the center of the tibial tubercle was a substantial cause of patellofemoral complications. In other words, a group of patients with patellar subluxation, tile, dislocation, and prosthetic loosening, all demonstrated the presence of combined femoral-tibial prosthetic internal rotation of up to 17°.

Boldt et al. has studied the tibial shaft axis method with the LCS total knees comparing the resultant posterior condylar axis with the transepicondylar axis. He found the posterior condylar reference of implanted LCS components paralleled the transepicondylar axis (mean 0.3°). Lateral patellar subluxation was seen in two knees where there was femoral component internal rotation of 40° and 60°. In another study, Boldt found a consistent relationship of femoral component internal rotation (average 5° internal to the transepicondylar axis) and arthrofibrosis from a variety of causes [2].

While the flexion space cuts depend primarily on ligamentous tension, one must avoid certain pitfalls that may occur. For example, if the leg is fixed in a leg holder, it is possible for the weight of the leg to place an artificial tension on the lateral side of the joint, distorting the appropriate ligament tension. Also if an unusual amount of medial or lateral condyle will be resected, the surgeon must check the primary extension balance to make certain that all is correct.

5 Conclusion

The LCS experience has led to the evolution and refinement of a predictable surgical technique to provide sat-

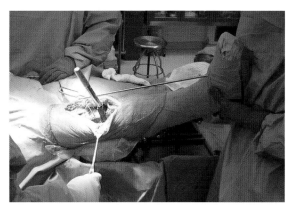

Fig. 44. LCS extension space assessment measures both rectangular space and alignment

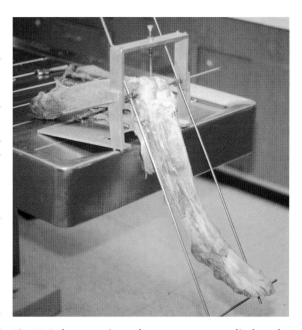

Fig. 45. Cadaver specimen demonstrates perpendicular relationship of tibial shaft axis to the transepicondylar axis with transecting pin

isfactory prosthetic knee kinematics with the elimination of bearing dislocation. The senior author, (JBS) has personally done over 500 LCS rotating platform inserts without a single problem. Experience and careful attention to detail can explain this result with a conscious effort of achieving perfect knee flexion/extension balancing and mechanical alignment (Fig. 43 and 44). The tibial shaft axis method developed for the LCS surgical technique relies on the anatomical relationship of the mechanical axis of the tibia shaft being virtually perpendicular to the transepicondylar axis in both flexion and extension (Fig. 45).

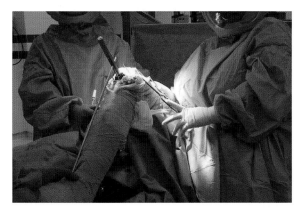

Fig. 43. LCS flexion space assessment measures both rectangular space and alignment

References

1. Berger RA, Rubash HE, Seek MJ, Thompson WH, Crossett LS (1993) Determining the rotational alignment of the femoral component in total knee arthroplasty using the epicondylar axis. CORR 286: 40–47
2. Boldt J, Munzinger U, Beverland D, Stiehl JB, Keblish PA (2001) CT evaluation of femoral rotational alignment post TKA: Comparison of the tibial shaft axis method to the transepicondylar line. Proceedings of the AAOS
3. Bert JM (1990) Dislocation/subluxation of meniscal bearing elements after New Jersey low-contact stress total knee arthroplasty. CORR 254: 211–215
4. Fehring TK (2000) Rotational malalignment of th femoral component in total knee arthroplasty. CORR 380: 72–79
5. Insall JA, Binazzi R, Soudry M. Mestriner LA (1983) Total knee arthroplasty. CORR 192: 13–17
6. Mantas JP, Bloebaum RD, Skedros JG, Hoffmann AA (1992) Implications of reference axes used for rotational alignment of the femoral component in primary and revision knee arthroplasty. J Arthroplasty 7: 531–535
7. Olcott CW, Scott RD (2000) A comparison of 4 intraoperative methods to determine femoral component rotation during total knee arthroplasty. J Arthroplasty 15: 22–26
8. Scott WN, Rubinstein M, Scuderi G (1998) Results after knee replacement with a posterior cruciate substituting prosthesis. JBJS 70 A: 1163–1173
9. Stiehl JB, Abbott BD (1995) Morphology of the transepicondylar axis and the application in primary and revision total knee arthroplasty. J Arthroplasty 10: 785–789
10. Stiehl JB, Cherveny PM (1996) Femoral rotational alignment using the tibial shaft axis in total knee arthroplasty. CORR 331: 47–55

10.3 Approaches to the Varus Knee

R. WINDHAGER, CH. AIGNER

1 Introduction

1.1 Incidence

Varus deformity of the knee joint is one of the most frequent malalignments that orthopedic surgeons are faced with when treating an arthritic knee joint with a total knee arthroplasty. Usually in these cases the varus deformity is a contributory factor and not the cause. The disease process follows a typical pathophysiological sequence and in the case of habitual genu varum may lead to severe deformity with values ranging from 15 to 25 degrees of varus deviation from the mechanical axis. In our patient population varus deformity accounts for more than 60 % of osteoarthritis of the knee.

1.2 Natural History of the Disease – Pathophysiology

Even in the physiologically aligned knee joint distribution of contact forces is known to be asymmetrical. It is estimated that 60 to 75 % of the forces are transmitted through the medial compartment of the knee joint [4, 7, 12]. By definition varus deformity of the knee joint describes a lateral deviation of joint center from the mechanical axis of the leg in the frontal plane or a decrease of the femorotibial angle below the physiological femorotibial valgus of 6 to 7 degrees. There is considerable variation due to anatomical factors such as the pelvic width, femoral neck varus and femoral and tibial bowing as well as femoral length. As a consequence an exact analysis has to be performed to determine whether the deformity is intraarticular or near the articular joint space or extraarticular. This chapter will deal only with intraarticular varus deformity.

The pathophysiological sequence follows a typical pattern starting with loss of cartilage in the medial compartment, which depending on the amount of cartilage destruction as well as the leg length leads to a varus deviation of up to 4 or 5 degrees. This results

in an increased stress on the medial compartment. Initially bone loss typically occurs on the medial tibial plateau but with progress of the disease the femur may also become involved. As a consequence of varus deformity the medial collateral ligament (MCL) undergoes shortening and contracture. This may be worsened by medial osteophytes on the tibia and later also on the femur, which result in a relative shortening of the ligament. On the other side lateral structures like the lateral collateral ligament and the capsule undergo adaptive changes by stretching resulting in an asymmetric varus instability (Fig. 46 a,b).

Unicompartmental knee replacement is only indicated when the deformity is correctable, which means that the MCL must not be contracted.

1.3 Functional Anatomy

Although with increasing deformity and instability it becomes more difficult and almost impossible to restore the physiological function of different structures a basic knowledge of the functional anatomy of these medial structures is important. Up to now there has been no technique, which has enabled release of the medial contracted structures in a selective manner with respect to flexion and extension. In other words it seems almost impossible to restore the physiological function of these structures in a pathological situation [23]. The best compromise we can hope to achieve is a rough balance between the medial and lateral structures in flexion and extension with respect to the functional anatomy of the medial collateral ligament [8, 11, 13, 20].

The MCL can be divided into a superficial and deep layer which are both attached proximally to the medial epicondylar area of the femur as a broad band. On the tibia the anterior portion of the superficial layer of this complex ligament is attached approximately one handbreadth distal to the joint line along the medial tibial flare. This portion is tight in flexion and loose in exten-

Fig. 46a,b. Asymmetric varus instability in the AP (**a**) and lateral (**b**) view. Loss of cartilage and bone at the medial surface of the tibia leads to shrinkage of the medial and elongation of the lateral ligamentous structures and tendons

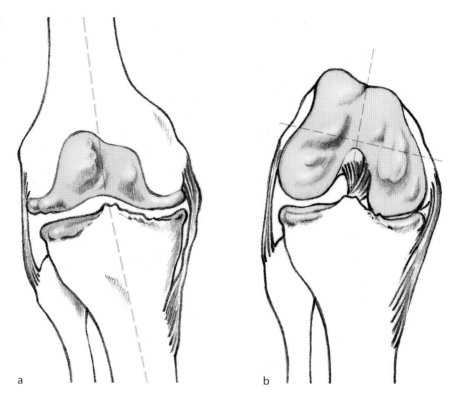

a   b

sion. In contrast the posterior portion of the superficial layer which runs posteriorly in an oblique fashion to attach to the medial tibial flare is tight in extension and loose in flexion [1, 16–18] (Fig. 47).

The deep layer of the medial collateral ligament lies, as the name implies deep to the superficial layer and has a very proximal attachment to the tibia it also blends with the semimembranosis tendon and the posteromedial capsule of the knee. The semimembranosis tendon is divided into five parts. The main part which represents the commonly known tendon crosses between the tibia and the superficial collateral band to insert on the medial proximal tibia. A second strong part inserts on the dorsomedial tibia just below the joint line. But the semimembranosis tendon also forms the posterior oblique ligament and blends with the posterior capsule to insert into the medial meniscus. The posterior capsule itself is only tight in full extension. With this information in mind release of the medial structures can be approached more systematically although due to the difficulties of exact intraoperative evaluation and thus correlation to postoperative result no exact recommendations regarding the amount of release of each of these structures can be made. Consequently repeated intraoperative clinical examination is mandatory in order to achieve an excellent clinical result for each patient.

2   Rationale for Deformity Correction

It has long been recognized that a varus malalignment after total knee arthroplasty predisposes to loosening [10, 15, 21]. These authors observed that the most favorable outcome occurred with a femorotibial angle of between 3 and 7 degrees, the tibial component in neutral and the femoral component in 4 to 6 degrees of valgus. In severely deformed varus knees Teeney et al. [14] stated that 40% of the knees with preoperative varus tended to remain in varus. As a result the medial compartment is more overloaded than in the physiological condition which is exaggerated by the contracture of the insufficiently released medial structures resulting in an increased posteromedial polyethylene wear [19]. Inadequate posterior release especially of the posterior cruciate ligament may lead to additional stress in the posterior part of the tibial component and thus to elevation anteriorly ("booking" according to Insall [6]). We are indebted to John Insall for providing a standardized surgical technique, which has enabled surgeons not only to implant total knee arthroplasties in correct axial alignment but also to stabilize a knee in neutral alignment through staged ligament releases. The effect of different steps in soft tissue release has to be integrated into the

Fig. 47. Anatomy of the medial structures: Deep and oblique layer of the medial collateral ligament (MCL), semimembranosus muscle inserting into the deep MCL, the posterior capsule and the pes anserinus

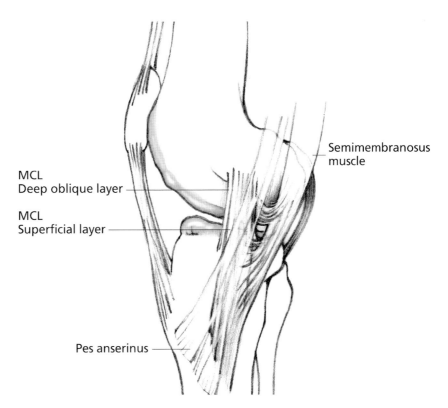

MCL
Deep oblique layer

MCL
Superficial layer

Semimembranosus
muscle

Pes anserinus

approach to allow proper implantation of the prosthetic components. This needs to take into account bony reference marks and has to be completed via a final fine-tuning release of the soft tissues after the trial components have been inserted.

3 Preoperative Assessment and Surgical Planning

Exact preoperative assessment of axial deformity and stability as well as bone loss is mandatory in order to achieve a satisfactory outcome with normal alignment and stability of the knee joint. Clinical evaluation should include a status on the stability of the knee ligaments and an exact assessment of the range of motion with special respect to rotational deviations during flexion and extension. Radiographic evaluation should include full length radiographs showing the hip, knee and ankle joints as well as a lateral view of the knee joint. Care has to be taken in full length radiographs to properly position the patella in the frontal plain in order to avoid miscalculation of alignment values due to incorrect rotation. However in rotational deformity of the tibia, for instance after incorrect high tibial osteotomy, even proper positioning of the patella does not exactly match the clinical situation. In these complex cases repeated intraoperative assessment even with an image intensifier may be necessary.

The femoral and tibial cuts are planned perpendicular to the corrected mechanical axis. This means that the proximal tibia is resected perpendicular to the long axis of the tibia and the distal femoral cut is made perpendicular to the mechanical axis of the femur. The latter is defined by a line drawn from the center of rotation of the hip to the center of the knee joint. This means that in non deformed femurs the resection plane will be in 6 to 7 degrees of valgus in relation to the anatomical axis of the femur which however has to be increased in case of excessive varus bowing of the femur. Preoperative planning is completed by templating the femoral and tibial components and drawing the resection line as well as the entry points for the intramedullary rods onto the radiographs. Especially with severe bone loss of the medial tibial condyle it has to be decided preoperatively how the defect will be reconstructed in order to avoid excessive bone resection of the tibial plateau on the lateral side. Usually the resected lateral part of the tibial plateau can be used as an autograft for the medial side.

After thorough clinical and radiological assessment the deformity is categorized as to whether it is a symmetric varus deformity or an asymmetric varus instability. Whereas symmetric habitual varus deviation usually lacks ligament instability, asymmetric varus instability results from cartilage and bone loss in the medial compartment with or without adaptive changes of the ligaments thus allowing or inhibiting full correction of the mechanical axis. Soft tissue release in these early cases of medial osteoarthritis is not usually indicated and standard surgical techniques and positioning of total knee arthroplasty seems sufficient to balance the ligaments. On the other hand asymmetric instability characterized by soft tissue contracture can not be restored by bone cuts alone and represents an absolute indication for either controlled ligament release on the contracted side or ligament advancement on the elongated convex side. Whereas the later one may be applied in excessive valgus deformity usually an extensive soft tissue release allows adequate balancing even of severe varus deformities without ligament tightening on the lateral side.

4 Surgical Technique

4.1 Positioning of the Patient

Draping of the whole leg including the iliac spine significantly improves the intraoperative judgment of alignment. In obese patients as well as in cases where the femoral neck is deformed an image intensifier helps in defining the center of rotation of the hip. If an Esmarch tourniquet is to be used it can be applied preferably as a sterilized device. A leg holder may help in stabilizing the leg in a flexed position, however larger devices might have disadvantages in defining the center of the ankle joint as well as assessing the stability of the knee joint intraoperatively. The personal preference of the authors is a simple sandbag fixed on the operation table to retain the foot and keep the knee joint in more than 90 degrees of flexion.

4.2 Surgical exposure

Irrespective of whether a medial parapatellar, transpatellar, subvastus or midvastus approach is chosen a 20 to 25 cm long midline skin incision is made over the patella. Distally this should be located 1 cm medial to the tibial tubercle. After splitting the subcutaneous tissue the fascia should be carefully prepared from the midline of the patella to the line of the arthrotomy in order to guarantee sufficient blood supply to the detached skin flap. In the distal part the arthrotomy should proceed directly to the periosteum 1 cm medial to the tibial tubercle. In order to facilitate preparation of an intact sleeve of tissue this step of preparation is more important in severe varus deformities where the contracted and lengthened tissues often retract posteriorly and thus impair a secure

wound closure. Especially in cases with malrotation after failed high tibial osteotomy detachment and retraction of the medial structures leaves a gap, which often causes prolonged swelling and wound drainage.

Proximally the arthrotomy is parapatellar but is made as straight as possible in order to avoid transection of longitudinal fibers of the extensor mechanism. More proximally it is extended along the medial margin of the vastus medialis. Further exposure can be achieved by making a small periosteal detachment of the patellar tendon from the medial part of the tibial tubercle. This significantly reduces the tension on the patellar tendon after eversion thus protecting it from detachment during exposure. Further lateral mobilization of the patella is facilitated by dividing the lateral patellofemoral ligament. There is still some disagreement as to whether the Hoffa fat pad should be excised totally some surgeons consider that a residual fat pad might cause anterior knee pain. We routinely only split the fat pad in the frontal plane to the amount which is necessary to visualize the tibial plateau. By splitting the fat pad at the lateral side even more lateral mobilization of the patella can be gained. After the patella has been everted and the knee flexed to 90 degrees medial exposure is carried on by subperiosteal stripping the medial soft tissue sleeve to the posterior aspect of the proximal medial tibia including the medial capsule, the deep collateral ligament and the semimembranosus tendon. With sufficient external rotation the posteromedial corner of the proximal tibia is visualized and the dorsal insertion of the semimembranosus tendon released with a scalpel.

In stiff or ankylosed knees as well as in revision cases with varus deformity other exposures like quadriceps turndown, the rectus snip or a tibial tubercle osteotomy may be necessary. In long standing ankylosis of the knee joint or for implantation after infection a subperiosteal peel of the femur may be indicated to gain sufficient exposure.

4.3 Stepwise Medial Release

As a first step the osteophytes of the femur and tibia are removed, which diminishes the relative shortening of the MCL and leads to some opening of the medial joint space. During this stepwise procedure it is advisable to reassess the medial stability after each step both in flexion and extension of the knee joint. If the knee cannot be realigned to the physiological valgus position release has to progress to subperiosteal detachment of the MCL (Fig. 48).

If the knee can be realigned in extension and is still tight medially in flexion the anterior portion of the su-

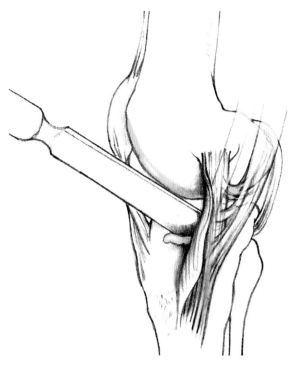

Fig. 48. Before the extensor apparatus is everted the medial release is started by removing all the osteophytes at the medial side of the femur and tibia. The deep layer of the medial collateral ligament is detached subperiostealy together with the joint capsule, the semimembranosus tendon and part of the pes anserinus using a chisel or elevator until the mechanical axis can be corrected. to the physiologic value

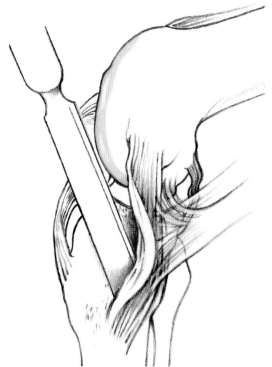

Fig. 49. After eversion of the extensor apparatus and removal of the menisci and the ACL the tension of the medial collateral ligament is checked in flexion of the knee by a laminar spreader and compared to the lateral side. Tightness in the medial compartment is balanced by subperiosteal detachment of the superficial portion of the medial collateral ligament with the help of an elevator directed along the medial side of the tibia more than 8 cm distal to the joint line

perficial MCL has to be released by subperiosteal stripping along the medial side of the tibia with a chisel or an elevator (Fig. 49).

The extent of the release can also be checked by repeated insertion of a lamina spreader or a similar device [22], which not only allows assessment of the alignment but also of the tension in the medial and lateral compartments. However in the flexed position the higher tension in the lateral compartment caused by the everted patella tendon has to be taken into account when determining knee balance. In some cases of severe varus deformity it may be necessary to strip the periosteal sleeve medially up to 15 cm distal to the line of arthrotomy to achieve ligament balance in flexion. Even if an extreme release is necessary this may be possible without discontinuity between the medial soft tissue structures; however beyond the insertion of the superficial MCL thinning of the periosteal layer may be observed. This medial sleeve consists of periosteum, deep medial ligament, superficial medial ligament, insertion of the pes anserinus tendons and more posteriorly the posterior capsule with the semimebranosus insertion.

4.4   Preferred Release Technique with LCS Preparation

After the knee has been realigned as described, tibial resection is performed in the standardized way. Care has to be taken in rotational deformities of the tibia to properly position the tibial cutting guide. With a posterior slope of 7 or 10 degrees in the tibial cutting block external rotation of the device results in a posteromedial slope which results in a varus cut and varus alignment of the tibial component. Conversely internal rotation produces a posterolateral slope resulting in valgus malalignment and overcorrection. As the tibia is rotated externally by the extensor apparatus there is a tendency to position the cutting device in internal rotation. However guarding against this by orientating the device relative to the second toe may be often misleading as the foot tends to drop into a valgus position with increasing dorsiflexion consequently leading to an external positioning of the tibial cutting block.

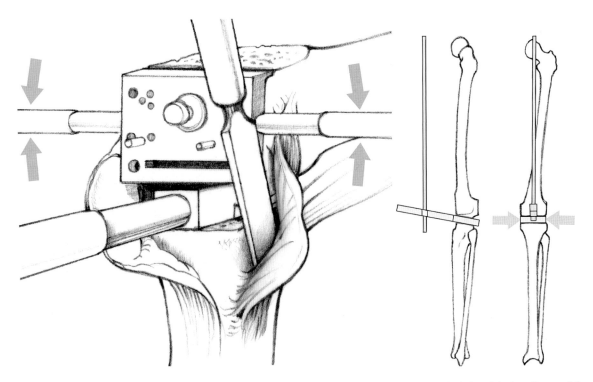

Fig. 50. When the AP femoral cuts have been performed the spacer block is inserted and with the help of the handles at of the femoral resection guide the tension of the collateral ligaments is compared by moving the tibia into varus and valgus or by rotating the resection guide. Additional release of the superficial MCL is carried out until the same stability has been achieved at the medial and lateral side. After distal femoral resection and insertion of the spacer block stability is checked in the frontal plane and corrected by additional release of the deep MCL mainly in the dorsal region

In our practice the decision as to whether a cruciate retaining or sacrificing component will be used mainly depends on the severity of the deformity. Whereas moderate flexion contractures of up to 10 degrees can be managed by a posterior release and retention of the PCL more severe deformities are better treated by resection of the PCL and implantation of the rotating platform cruciate sacrificing component.

With a concomitant flexion contracture the medial release has to be extended posteriorly by detaching the posterior capsule from the tibia with the semimembranosus tendon and if necessary part of the PCL. This part of the release has to be done until muscle fibers are revealed.

Having defined the size of the femoral component the AP femoral cutting block, fixed only by the intramedullary rod is placed on the end of the femur. The flexion gap is then created by inserting the femoral guide positioner into the AP femoral cutting block and onto the resected proximal tibia. The stability of the knee in flexion can again be checked by fixing the femur with the handles of the femoral resection guide and putting valgus and varus stress on the tibia. If the medial side is

still tighter than the lateral one the release of the superficial MCL has to be continued until balance is achieved (Fig. 50).

Balancing the ligaments in flexion can be done much more easily at this stage than after the trial components have been inserted as the handles of the AP resection guide allow for more exact tuning of ligament tension. Also it is very important to try and complete the release of the MCL before the AP femoral cuts are performed as subsequent release can distort the flexion gap thus risking flexion instability. Furthermore if the MCL is tight this tilts the AP femoral cutting block into external rotation. If the AP cuts are performed at this stage, then as well as removing too much bone from the posteromedial femoral condyle there is excessive external rotation of the femoral component. The epicondylar axis should also be used during this step as a further check on the rotational alignment of the femoral component.

Following resection of the AP femoral cuts the flexion gap is measured with the spacer block and the ligament balance is reassessed. Then attention can turn to the distal femoral resection. It is important to ensure that any fixed flexion has been corrected before remov-

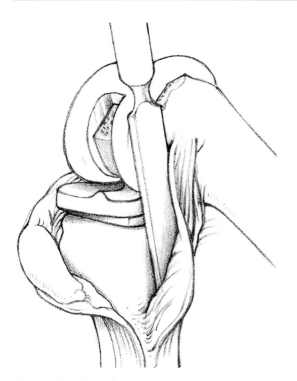

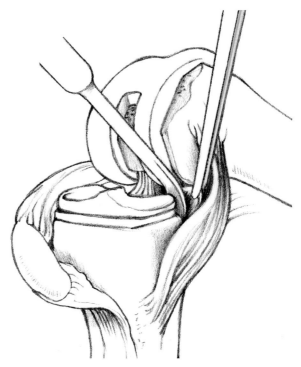

Fig. 51. After the trial components have been inserted additional fine-tuning may be necessary by increasing the release medially and change to a higher bearing component. Attention has to be paid finally to the dorsal posterior release if there is an extension lag or a dislocation of the bearing in maximum flexion. Further detachment of the superficial MCL may be necessary

Fig. 52. Fine-tuning is completed by advanced further release of the posterior capsule, the semimembranosus tendon and the PCL until the bearing moves without friction

ing more bone from the distal femur. The aim is to have equal flexion and extension gaps after all soft tissue releases have been completed.

After completion of all bone cuts the trial components are inserted with the appropriate bearing component. The selection of the latter depends largely on the depth of the tibial resection but can be influenced by the stability achieved during the preparation. Again the balance of the medial and lateral structures are assessed in extension and flexion; additional minor release may be necessary on the medial side if the MCL is still tight in extension resulting in a lateral instability. Remember that any significant release at this stage will distort the flexion gap. This additional release may require a thicker tibial insert to restore the correct tension. When assessing the knee in flexion attention should be drawn to the movement of the tibial bearing in full flexion; if the bearing tends to dislocate laterally while remaining tight medially then release of the superficial MCL (Fig. 51) and the dorsal structures i.e. the capsule and the PCL (Fig. 52) has to be performed until the bearing is stable. However as discussed above it is important

to try and avoid the above scenario by releasing the MCL and balancing the knee in flexion before the AP cuts are performed.

4.5   Patellar tracking

The correction of patellar tracking in the varus knee usually does not offer a great problem, but may require a lateral release (see chapter 10.6 "Technique for not resurfacing the patella").

There is a type of varus knee however where the patella is in lateral luxation. In this condition it is virtually impossible to correct patellar tracking by lateral release only. The patella may stay laterally luxated. In these knees a lateral (!) approach may be advised. The benefits of this approach are: optimal patellar tracking after TKA and better preserving of the blood supply of the patella as only one parapatellar incision is needed as opposed to medial approach and lateral parapatellar release. The lateral approach may necessitate a tibial crest osteotomy (see chapter 10.5). The varus release may well be done by this approach (see chapter 10.4 "Approaching the valgus knee").

5   Rehabilitation

The main aims of rehabilitation are to reduce pain and to preserve the ROM achieved intraoperatively. It has to be kept in mind that in most of the knees proprioception has been lost by resection of the cruciate ligaments and that an ACL deficient knee can demonstrate paradoxical kinematics with the femur moving forward during flexion [2].

So the patient has to be trained on patterns of motion which enable him to compensate for the loss of proprioception and it has to be considered that pain and ongoing scarring hampers the progress of rehabilitation. Operative mismatches may lead to pain, stiffness and instability and will become evident during rehabilitation.

5.1   Pain relief

TKR is a painful procedure, so the application of opioid and antiinflammatory drugs has to be planned in advance and has to be continued in the first days after surgery until active motion can be done without pain related restrictions. In a combined spinal and epidural anesthesia the application of the drug via lumbar epidural catheter allows pain free passive and active motion. This should be continued until at least 90° of flexion are reached. Then the drug can be reduced stepwise.

The application of kryotherapy is recommended from the very beginning and should be continued until there is no prominent swelling of the knee joint.

5.2   Mobilization

The first tension exercise of the quadriceps muscle can be done on the afternoon of surgery and mobilization starts on the next day with crutches for the first 6 weeks. There is an ongoing discussion as to whether a patient with a cementless TKR should be encouraged to be partially or fully weight bearing. Up to now there has been no final conclusion, therefore that decision has to be left to the individual surgeon.

Flexion exercises [5] aim at preventing fibrosis and scarring as well as reaching at least 90° flexion within the first two weeks after surgery. Whenever possible a physiotherapist should help the patient with mobilizing the quadriceps muscle, optimizing the flexion extension circle and keeping the patellar movement free. There is evidence that the maximum achievement from rehabilitation occurs in the first two months after surgery, whereas after three months there are only small improvements.

The use of continuous passive motion (CPM) can give the patient an early feeling of confidence in the function of their new joint but it is not a stand-alone therapy and should only be used as part of a rehabilitation program [9].

5.3   Postoperative stiffness

Manipulation of the knee joint has to be considered when intensive physiotherapy has failed to increase flexion to more than 80 degrees [3] particularly in a knee with a good pre-operative ROM. The goal of a closed manipulation under anesthesia is the release of adhesions, whereas an arthroscopy may eliminate a haematoma and fibrous bundles. Both procedures have to be followed by immediate flexion exercises.

References

1. Burks RT (1990) Gross anatomy. In: Daniel D, Akeson W, O'Connor J (eds) Knee ligaments: structure, function, inquiry and repair. Raven Press, New York, pp 59–76
2. Dennis DA, Komistek RD et al. (1996) In vivo knee kinematics derived using an inverse perspective technique. Clin Orthop 331: 107–117
3. Esler CH, Lock K, Harper WM, Gregg PJ (1999) Manipulation of total knee replacements. Is the flexion gained retained? JBJS (Br) 81(1): 27–29
4. Harrington IJ (1976) A bioengineering analysis of force actions at the knee in normal and pathologic gait. Biomed Engin 11(5): 167
5. Hewitt B, Shakespeare D (2001) Flexion vs. extension: a comparison of post-operative total knee arthroplasty mobilisation regimes. Knee (4): 305–309
6. Insall JN, Easley ME (2000) Surgical techniques and instrumentation in total knee arthroplasty. In: Surgery of the knee. Churchill Livingstone, Edinburgh, pp 1553–1620
7. Johnosn F, Leitl F, Waugh W (1980) The distribution of load across the knee. J Bone Joint Surg Br 62: 346
8. Krackow KA, Mihalko WM (1999) The effect of medial release on flexion and extension gaps in cadaveric knees: implications for soft tissue balancing in total knee arthroplasty. Am J Knee Surg 12(4): 222–228
9. Lachiewicz PF (2000) The role of continuous passive motion after total knee arthroplasty. Clin Orthop 380: 144–150
10. Lotke PA, Ecker ML (1977) Influence of positioning in total knee replacement. J Bone Joint Surg Am 59: 77–79
11. Matsueda M, Gengerke TR, Murphy M, Lew WD, Gustilo RB (1999) Soft tissue release in total knee arthroplasty. Cadaver study using knees without deformities. Clin Orthop 366: 264–273
12. Morrison JB (1968) Bioengineering analysis of force actions transmitted by the knee joint. Biomed Engin 3: 164
13. Saeki K, Mihalko WM, Patel V, Conway J, Naito M, Thrum H, Vandenneuker H, Whiteside LA (2001) Stability after medial collateral release in total knee arthroplasty. Clin Orthop 392: 184–189
14. Teeny SM, Krackow KA, Hungerford DS et al. (1991) Primary total knee arthroplasty in patients with severe varus deformity: A comparative study. Clin Orthop 273: 19–31

15. Vince KG, Insall JN, Kelly MA (1989) The total condylar
    prosthesis: 10–12-year results of a cemented knee replace-
    ment. J Bone Joint Surg Br 71: 793–797
16. Wagner M, Schabus R (1982) Funktionelle Anatomie des
    Kniegelenkes. Springer, Berlin Heidelberg New York
17. Warren LM (1979) The supporting structures and layers of
    the medial side of the knee: An anatomical analysis. J Bone
    Joint Surg AM 61: 56–62
18. Warren LF, Marshall JL, Girgis F (1974) The prime static
    stabilizer of the medial side of the knee. J Bone Joint Surg
    A 56: 665–674
19. Wasiliewski RC, Galanta JO, Leighty RM et al. (1994) Wear
    pattern on retrieved polyethylene tibial inserts and their
    relationship to technical considerations during total knee
    arthroplasty. Clin Orthop 299: 31
20. Whiteside LA, Saeki K, Mihalko WM (2000) Functional
    medial ligament balancing in total knee arthroplasty. Clin
    Orthop 380: 45–57
21. Windsor RS, Moran MC, Insall JN (1989) Mechanisms of
    failure of the femoral and tibial components in total knee
    arthroplasty. Clin Orhop 248: 15–19
22. Winemaker NJ (2002) Perfect balance in total knee arthro-
    plasty: The elusive compromise. J Arthroplasty 17(1): 2–
    10
23. Yagashita K, Muneta T, Yamamoto H, Shinomiya K (2001)
    The relationship between postoperative ligament balance
    and preoperative varus deformity in total knee arthro-
    plasty. Bull Hosp Jt Dis 60(1): 23–28

10.4 Surgical Approaches: Lateral Approach

P.A. Keblish

1   Introduction

Surgical approaches in total knee arthroplasty (TKA) should allow the surgeon to access the knee in the safest, most direct manner that allows for achievement of predictable stability at the patellofemoral and the femorotibial interfaces. Fixed contractures in valgus TKA require sequential releases that include the capsule, ilio-tibial band (I-TB), vastus lateralis (VL) tendon, lateral collateral ligament (LCL), and at times, the popliteus, lateral gastrocnemius, and inner aspect of the fibular head (preserving and lengthening the LCL). These releases are best addressed by the direct access using the lateral approach. The direct lateral approach [2, 6, 7] is a technique that offers many advantages in correction of fixed valgus, as well as other challenges that confront the knee surgeon, primarily patella alignment and soft tissue considerations. It is less commonly used (and understood) than the standard medial approaches, but has been shown to improve stability and patella results in fixed valgus TKA [4, 10, 14, 15].

The lateral approach may also be indicated in several other pathologic conditions without valgus deformity:

- Many, if not all knees with a lateral orientation and/ or patella (sub-)luxation. By performing a lateral approach the lateral release by a second incision is avoided, the blood supply of the patella better preserved and patellar tracking optimally restored.
- Multiply operated knees with scars of the previous surgeries. In those knees a lateral skin incision is preferred giving the best prognosis for wound healing. Why not continue with a lateral approach after a lateral skin incision? This situation may be found in revision surgery and after high tibial osteotomy.

This chapter will:

- define the pathologic anatomy of the valgus knee,
- define the technical problems and disadvantages of the medial approach in fixed valgus deformity,
- illustrate the technique specifics and advantages of the direct lateral approach in fixed valgus deformity, and
- discuss other indications for the lateral approach.

2   Pathologic Anatomy – Valgus Knee

Fixed valgus deformity is usually associated with femoral-tibial mal-rotation, resorption of the lateral femoral condyle and a relatively large, more distal medial condyle (Fig. 53).

Lateral structures are tight and the patella is frequently deformed and subluxed over the deformed lateral condyle. Valgus is most prevalent in females (9:1), and rheumatoid arthritis is more common and associated with flexion contracture. Prosthetic cover and joint seal can be a problem since the skin and soft tissue are often deficient. Excessive undermining, increased tension, or lack of a soft tissue layer between skin and prosthesis can lead to skin necrosis, a potentially devastating complication of TKA. Understanding the anatomy is important.

3   Extra-Articular Layer

The fascia lata extension envelops the quadriceps with attachment to the posterior aspect of the femur. The distal lateral confluence becomes the Ilio-Tibial Band with distinct insertion into Gerdy's tubercle and the lateral tibial plateau. Transverse and oblique fibers extend to the patellar mechanism (lateral retinaculum), and longitudinal fibers attach to bone via Sharpey's fibers and extend to the fascia of the anterior compartment. The I-TB and the lateral retinaculum are deforming factors in the fixed valgus knee. The I-TB attachment to the upper tibia produces a valgus moment with external rotation (and sometimes flexion deformity), and the oblique and transverse extensions produce a lateral (subluxing)

Fig. 53a–c. Valgus deformity involves bone and soft tissue. Deformities are graded from mild (<15°) to severe (>30°) and may be fixed, correctable or partially correctable. Type II valgus deformity implies incompetence of the medial collateral sleeve

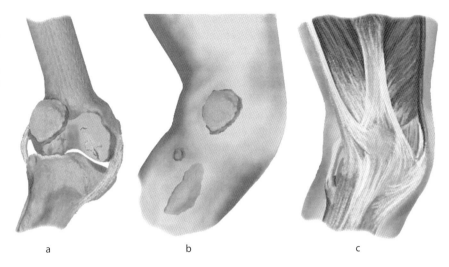

a   b   c

Fig. 54. Deep posterolateral structures are illustrated. Some or all are contracted, or abnormal with fixed valgus deformity

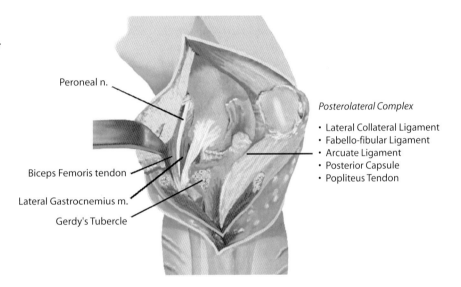

Peroneal n.

Biceps Femoris tendon

Lateral Gastrocnemius m.

Gerdy's Tubercle

Posterolateral Complex

- Lateral Collateral Ligament
- Fabello-fibular Ligament
- Arcuate Ligament
- Posterior Capsule
- Popliteus Tendon

moment to the patella. The extra-articular (superficial) layer also includes the lateral hamstring, the fabellofibular ligament, the lateral head of the gastrocnemius, and the popliteus (Fig. 54).

These structures may be contracted secondary to long-standing valgus. Bony deformity may further increase concave side contractures.

The lateral superficial layer differs from the (compliant) medial oblique retinaculum of the vastus medialis in that the lateral retinaculum is relatively noncompliant. This noncompliant lateral fascial extension to the patellar mechanism, coupled with contractures of the deeper layer, becomes a major determinant of the soft tissue deformity in the valgus knee.

4   Intra-Articular (Deep Layer)

The popliteus tendon, LCL, fabellofibular ligament, arcuate ligament, and capsule form the posterolateral complex. Anteriorly, the vastus lateralis inserts at the proximal patellar facet. The tendon of the vastus lateralis is usually of substantial thickness and joins the lateral aspect of the central quadriceps (rectus tendon). This structure is covered by a capsular and/or synovial layer in the joint. The muscles, by definition, have an extra-articular origin. The LCL differs from the medial collateral ligament (MCL) in that its distal insertion is at the fibular head. The deep anterior and posterior lateral soft tissue layers are usually contracted to different degrees, depending on factors such as the underlying pathology, longevity of the deformity, bony pathology, and others. Management of superficial and deep layer contractures in valgus TKA must be understood, and represents a key to correction of tibial rotation, centralization of the patella, and achieving proper flexion/extension gap balancing. In either case, the direct lateral approach enhances exposure and provides other advantages that will be discussed in the technique section.

5   Medial Approach

The standard medial parapatellar and subvastus/midvastus variations are the most commonly used approaches in TKA [5]. There is a general consensus that sequential releases should be performed from the femoral side prior to or after prosthetic insertion in fixed valgus [4, 5, 9, 14, 12, 15]. However, the medial approach in valgus TKA fails to address the pathologic anatomy directly and releases may be overdone since exposure is limited following patella re-location and trial testing. Patella mal-tracking is more common [11], and there is increased potential for inaccurate flexion-extension gap balancing and less than optimum femoral-tibial stability. Other technical disadvantages include:

- external rotation of the tibia is increased,
- access to the posterolateral corner is more difficult,
- an extensive lateral release is still required,
- joint seal and prosthetic soft tissue coverage is difficult,
- vascularity to the quadriceps patella tendon (QPT) mechanism and lateral skin (beneath the extensive lateral release) is decreased [13],
- it does not allow for optimal correction of the external rotation contracture of the tibia, and
- it may encourage over-release of deep soft tissues.

6   Lateral Approach – Rationale

The lateral approach in valgus deformity, by contrast, addresses the pathologic anatomy in a rational and sequential manner. The approach

- is direct,
- accomplishes the extensive "lateral release" with the exposure,
- decreases skin undermining,
- internally rotates the tibia with improved access to the pathologic posterolateral corner,

- allows for better titration of sequential releases based on flexion-extension gap balance requirements
- preserves vascularity because the medial side is untouched,
- allows for planned soft tissue gap and prosthetic coverage,
- centralizes the QPT mechanism which optimizes patella tracking,
- improves femoral-tibial alignment stability, and
- rehabilitation is unimpeded because the medial quadriceps remains intact.

This approach has not gained widespread use because it is less familiar and more demanding. The patella tendon/tibial tubercle presents an obstacle, and many surgeons associate tubercle osteotomy as a requirement for safe exposure. An in depth illustration of the anatomy and approach (without tubercle osteotomy in the vast majority of cases) is presented to assist the TKA surgeon in addressing this most challenging deformity.

7   Surgical Technique

The surgical technique of the direct lateral approach differs substantially from the standard medial parapatellar approach. The surgeon is less familiar with the lateral side of the knee; orientation is reversed, and more careful handling of the soft tissues is required. The recommended skin incision in the virgin knee follows the Q-angle and is slightly lateral to the patella, lateral border of the patellar tendon, and the tibial tubercle. Long incisions are preferred, especially in short, large legs. It is important to avoid unnecessary undermining and the surgeon must respect layer 1 (superficial layer) and avoid dissecting between the skin and layer1 as much as possible. In previously operated knees, the existing incision should be incorporated and extended proximally and distally. If multiple incisions are present, select the most direct or latest. A sham incision may be performed and consultation of a plastic surgeon considered since any lateral skin necrosis may be devastating

The approach will be described and illustrated. The skin incision should be atraumatic with identification of layer 1 in the plane of the prepatellar bursa medially. The lateral retinaculum is exposed with careful dissection to allow for the initial superficial (retinacular) incision. Six major steps, as guidelines for the surgeon are suggested:

Step I   Superficial longitudinal concave release: I-TB Release/Lengthening
Step II   Lateral Arthrotomy: transverse release – Coronal Plane Z-plasty

Step III Patella Dislocation – Joint Exposure
Step IV Deep Concave Releases (Options)
　　　　 – Tibial Sleeve Release – Osteoperiosteal
　　　　 – Distal LCL Lengthening (Keblish)
　　　　 – Proximal LCL Lengthening: sleeve or osteo-
　　　　　　periosteal, sliding lateral condyle osteotomy
　　　　　　(Briard)
Step V   Instrumentation/Prosthetic Insertion
Step VI Soft Tissue Closure Deep to Superficial Layer

7.1 Technique Points

I-TB Release/Lengthening. The I-TB is exposed proximally by separating the inner fascial sleeve from the VL muscle (Fig. 55).

The vastus lateralis is carefully retracted up to the Linea Aspera. The band is released from the posterior femur (Linea Aspera) and "finger stripped" to the posterolateral corner. A varus stress at the knee joint will "bow-string" the tight fascial bands, allowing for a multiple puncture "pie-crusting" lengthening (under visual and digital control) while paying attention to the most posterior fibers. The release is performed approximately 10 cm proximal to the joint line. The peroneal nerve can be palpated or explored, but this is seldom required and not recommended except in very severe cases.

Lateral Retinacular Incision (superficial layer). The course of the lateral parapatella incision begins 2–4 cm lateral to the patella and extends distally into the midportion of Gerdy's tubercle (Fig. 56a), preserving the fibrous layer which joins with the patellar tendon sheath anteriorly.

Proximally, the incision extends into the central quadriceps tendon. The lateral arthrotomy separates

the superficial from the deep layers; therefore, proceed cautiously through the outer layers.

Lateral Arthrotomy (deep layer). The superficial layer of the retinaculum is separated from the deep layer with a coronal plane Z-plasty, from superficial lateral to deep medial. Proximally, an oblique arthrotomy incision from

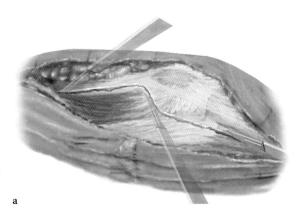

a

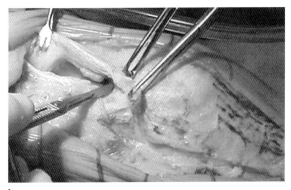

b

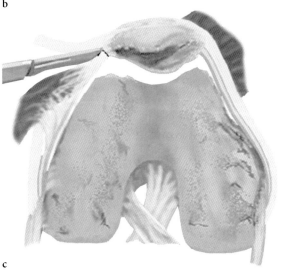

c

Fig. 56a–c. Lateral arthrotomy is performed by separating the superficial and deep layers (coronal plane Z-plasty technique) to prepare the expanded soft tissue sleeve

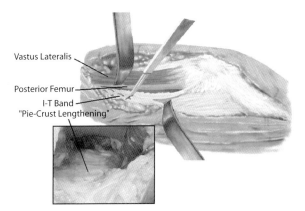

Vastus Lateralis
Posterior Femur
I-T Band
"Pie-Crust Lengthening"

Fig. 55. Iliotibial band release is performed by stripping from the posterior femur and a "pie-crust lengthening" (while a varus stress is applied)

the lateral to medial takes advantage of the laminated anatomy of the central quadriceps tendon. The VL tendon is non-yielding but substantially thick and allows for a horizontal (coronal) plane expansion release as well as a longitudinal expansion as shown. The VL tendon incision begins near the musculotendonous junction and ends distally at the mid-coronal plane of the patella insertion. The mid-portion (lateral retinaculum) separates naturally from the deep capsule and fat pad. The capsule is incised from the patella rim. The fat pad incision continues obliquely to the intermeniscal ligament, retaining about 50 % of the fat pad with the patella tendon and 50 % with the lateral sleeve, which includes the lateral meniscus rim for increased soft tissue stability (Fig. 56b,c).

Distal Tubercle Elevation or Osteotomy [16]. The distal extension of the retinacular incision splits Gerdy's tubercle and continues distally into the anterior compartment fascia (Fig. 57).

The osteoperiosteal sleeve release (utilizing a sharp osteotome), begins at mid-Gerdy's tubercle and extends anteriorly to, but stops at, the tibial tubercle. As the osteoperiosteal sleeve is elevated, muscle fibers of the tibialis anterior are included and preserved in their natural plane. The elevation stops at the lateral border of the patella tendon, protecting the tendon insertion and dissipating stresses to the anterior compartment sleeve. A formal, lateral to medial tibial tubercle osteotomy can be performed to enhance exposure in difficult cases or as the surgeon's choice.

Patella Dislocation – Joint Exposure. The patella is dislocated/everted medially as the knee is flexed with a varus stress. Grasping the patella with a towel clip may be helpful. Following patella eversion, a cobra-type retractor is placed medially through the periphery of the medial meniscus and over the medial cortical rim. Patella dislocation can be performed at this step or after the tibial sleeve release. Medial dislocation/eversion of the patella is more difficult than lateral dislocation. Methods to enhance exposure include: a long proximal incision to include a lateral to medial rectus snip (if indicated), osteophyte removal/downsizing of the patella/femur/tibia to normal peripheral anatomy, pre-cuts (measured) of the larger posterior medial and, at times, the distal medial femoral condyles, and pre-cuts of the tibial spine, including the PCL. These maneuvers are usually adequate to allow for satisfactory exposure.

Tibial Sleeve Release. Tibial Sleeve Release is routinely performed: Osteoperiosteal release from mid-Gerdy's tubercle to the posterolateral tibia begins in extension

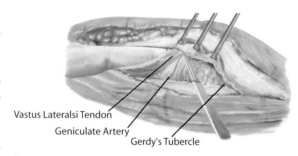

Vastus Lateralsi Tendon
Geniculate Artery
Gerdy's Tubercle

a

Vastus Lateralis Tendon   Lateral Retinaculum

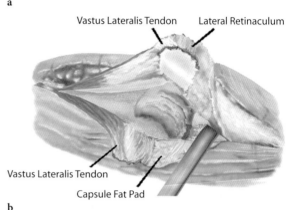

Vastus Lateralis Tendon
Capsule Fat Pad

b

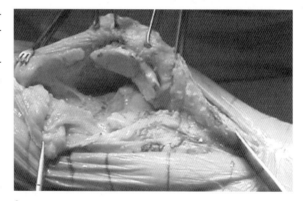

c

Fig. 57a–c. The distal elevation from mid-Gerdy's tubercle can be performed with an osteoperiosteal technique or a formal tibial tubercle osteotomy from lateral to medial

(before joint exposure) and is completed in flexion as shown in Fig. 58.

Osteophytes and posterior capsule are released and flexion/extension correction is checked with lamina spreaders. The posterior cruciate ligament (PCL) can be released at this time (if required because of non-correctable contractures) or by surgeon's choice for PCL-substituting prostheses. If initial releases appear adequate, proceed with instrumentation, bone resection, and prosthetic insertion. In more severe fixed valgus and/or in case of extraarticular deformity, it may be necessary to lengthen or to slide the deep lateral structures and

Fig. 58a,b. Lateral tibial sleeve release begins from mid-Gerdy's tubercle to the posterolateral corner. The release can begin in extension and is completed in flexion. Proximal and distal ligament integrity is preserved

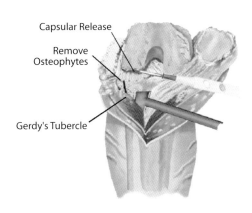

Capsular Release

Remove Osteophytes

Gerdy's Tubercle

a

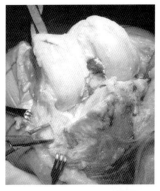

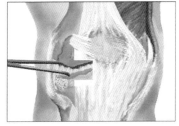

b

Fig. 59a–c. Deep concave side release– distal option: if gap imbalance persists following appropriate level bone cuts, distal LCL lengthening is accomplished by excavating the fibular head and preserving the distal LCL insertion with the periosteum and outer fibular cortex. Note fibular fragmentation and excellent balance on postoperative X-ray

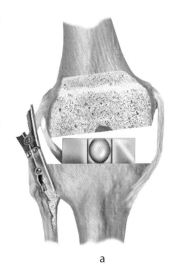

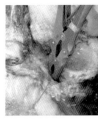

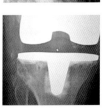

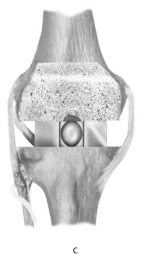

a   b   c

subsequently the posterior structures. Proximal and/or distal lengthening techniques can be used:

Distal LCL Release. When required, direct exposure and removal of the inner proximal fibula (with retention of the outer periosteum and ligament attachments) allows for medial translation and a relative lengthening of the lateral collateral ligament, without the need for fixation. Enough length may be obtained by this maneuver, avoiding the need for femoral side releases. Distal LCL lengthening by the method illustrated in Fig. 59.

This is the preferred method to accomplish mild to moderate correction and can be performed before or after bone resections and trial implants.

Buechel [2] has described a lateral exposure with a 3-step release that varies somewhat, but shares the same basic principles.

Instrumentation (fine-tuning)/Trial Reduction. Instrumentation with a flexion gap/femoral positioner allows for fine-tuning of soft tissue balancing (Fig. 60).

Flexion and extension gaps are checked with appropriate spacer blocks. The distal femoral resection angle may vary from 4–6° and should relate to the hip-knee-ankle axis. Some valgus is tolerable since patients' soft tissues and cosmetic appearance have adapted to this position over time. If stable gap balancing (in all planes) and/or failure to achieve full extension is not accom-

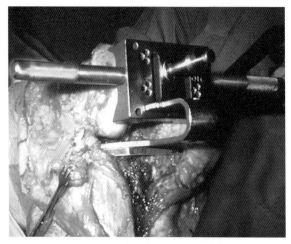

a

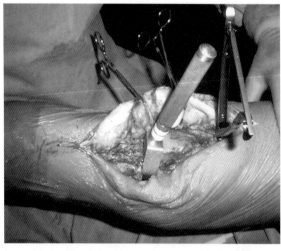

b

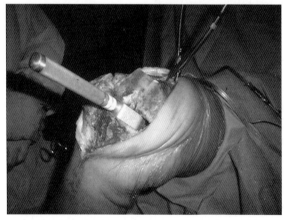

c

Fig. 60a–c. Instrumentation with flexion/extension gap balancing. The deep distal concave lengthenings can be made prior to this step. However, the more extensive proximal osteotomies should be made following prosthetic insertion

plished at this time, the more extensive femoral side releases will be required and are described below.

Femoral Sleeve Release. If required. If severe contractures are present, and large lateral extension space is required, two techniques are available. Osteoperiosteal release (limited osteotomy) or soft tissue sleeve release (preferably without the popliteus insertion) extends proximally (Fig. 61). The sleeve release is the more commonly recommended method, but it can lead to compromised ligament attachment and resultant instability. A proximal periosteal sleeve or limited osteotomy may not be very strong due to the absence of continuous soft tissue attachments.

The sliding lateral condyle osteotomy has been described by Briard to overcome the potential for lateral instability. The osteotomy allows for a strong/stable retention of femoral soft tissue (LCL and popliteus) attachments with correction of soft tissue contractures and achievement of an adequate extension gap. The osteotomy steps are outlined in Fig. 61. The initial cut is performed in the sagittal plane (just outside the anchoring hole that preserves a large bone segment (with ligament attachments) which can be inset into the lateral condyle of the femoral implant and securely fixed. Extension of the knee allows the osteotomy fragment to migrate distally to the appropriate position, achieving the correction of the coronal deformity. Resection and contouring of the distal bony fragment (preserving the ligament attachments of the popliteus and LCL) allows the large bony fragment to self-adjust (at the proper tension). The fragment is then inset and fixed with one or two screws inside the housing of the lateral condyle of the prosthesis, which insures stability.

Trial Component Insertion. Reduction with trial components is recommended in order to check position, stability, and mobility prior to permanent prosthetic insertion (Fig. 62) shows an intraoperative example of trial reduction using a rotating-platform prosthesis. Note the medial position of the tibial tubercle with correction of tibial rotation and natural patella tracking. The rotating bearing allows for self-adjustment at the femoral tibial interface.

Soft Tissue Sleeve Closure. Closure is accomplished in flexion. The expanded soft tissue closure is completed using sutures of choice proximally. The distal (bony) portion of the I-TB is re-attached with trans-osseous sutures. Prosthetic joint seal can be accomplished in all cases (Fig. 63). The use of the fat pad may be required, especially in soft-tissue deficient rheumatoid knees [7, 8].

Clinical Case Examples: X-ray example of severe valgus correction in a 63-year-old white female. Patella

Osteoperiosteal
Small Sleeve

Sliding Lateral
Condylar Osteotomy

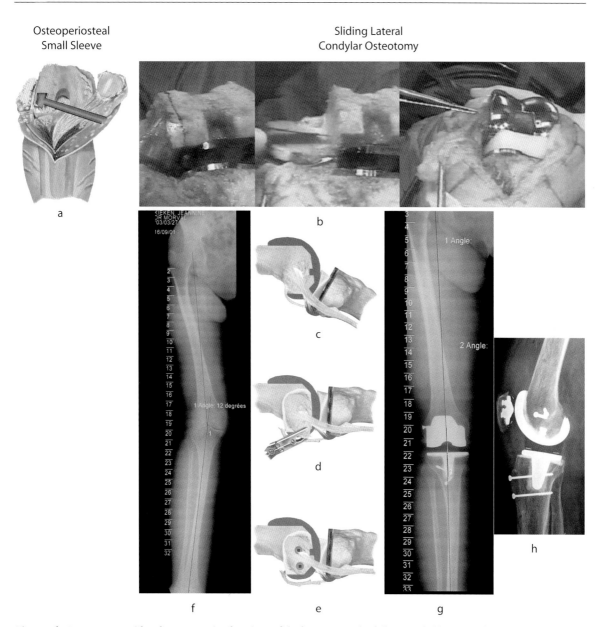

Fig. 61a–h. Deep concave side release – proximal options: If the knee cannot be fully extended because of severe lateral contractures, proximal femoral release options include: 1) the more commonly performed soft tissue or small osteoperiosteal sleeve release with/without reattachment (especially with the medial approach); or 2) sliding lateral condyle osteotomy that preserves soft tissue attachments and allows for extensive correction without loss of stability. X-ray example of severe valgus correction with lateral and tibial tubercle osteotomy

femoral tracking and femoral-tibial stability is excellent at 3 years. The patella was left unresurfaced (Fig. 64).

7.2   Tips and Pearls – Lateral Approach

• The VL tendon must be carefully incised through the mid-coronal plane to accomplish the lengthening release and subsequent closure at this most critical

point. If the expansion release cannot be performed because of inadequate VL tendon thickness, the more compliant capsule/fat pad and/or hypertrophic (proximal) capsule can be mobilized to achieve the joint seal [7].

• The quadriceps tendon incision should proceed from superficial lateral to deep medial at an angle of approximately 30–45°, which allows for a natural expansion of the laminated central quadriceps tendon

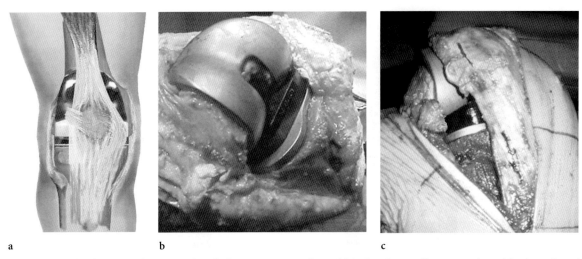

Fig. 62a–c. Trial reduction with LCS rotating platform components in position showing excellent correction with adaptation of femoral-tibial and patella-femoral joints

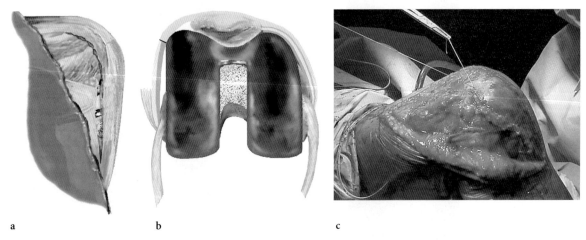

Fig. 63a–c. Soft tissue sleeve closure from superficial to deep layers. The IT band is reattached with proper tension utilizing transosseous sutures

fibers. If a thick, hypertrophic supra-patellar pouch is present, incising the capsule more medially will allow for a well-vascularized tissue mass that can be mobilized for incorporation into the lateral sleeve closure.

- The main technical (instrument) problem is "working around" the prominent tibial tubercle when using an extra-medullary tibial resection guide. A surgical option (to the osteoperiosteal technique) is the "formal" tibial tubercle osteotomy (lateral to medial), which allows for improved exposure, protection of the patella tendon, avoidance of proximal snip procedures, and ease of prosthetic removal in revision cases [1, 3]. The osteotomized fragment must be large and long and the soft tissues must be preserved medially to allow the tubercle to rotate around this soft tissue hinge.

- The depth of the medial tibial resection is less than usual in the valgus knee, especially in type II appearing (real or pseudo-laxity) deformities, which allows for presentation of the MCL complex and improves stability.

- The lateral tibial release from mid-Gerdy's tubercle to the posterolateral corner can be performed before or after joint exposure. An osteoperiosteal technique with a sharp osteotome and/or electrocautery allows for exposure/release of the posterolateral corner and the posterior capsule. Release of the lateral gastrocnemius with the posterolateral capsule may also be required to achieve adequate lateral compartment space in extension.

- If satisfactory correction is accomplished following the tibial sleeve, capsular/PCL releases, and downsiz-

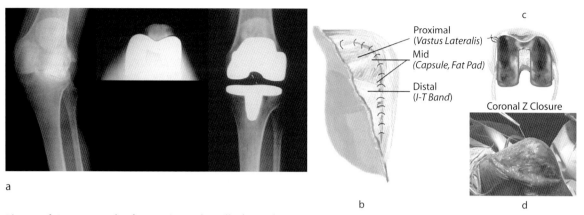

Fig. 64a–d. X-ray example of correction and patella-femoral tracking in severe valgus deformity

ing maneuvers, proceed with bony resections and fine-tune the ligament releases at time of trial reduction. If the lateral structures remain tight and do not allow for satisfactory varus/valgus balance, proceed with distal LCL lengthening (fibula or proximal lengthening femoral side).

- When concave side releases of the LCL, popliteus, and secondary structures are required, they can be performed prior to or following trial reduction. Keep in mind that the LCL affects both the flexion and extension gap stability, while the popliteus tendon affects flexion and rotation stability. The more commonly recommended technique (with the medial approach) is a soft tissue release of the ITB and posterolateral complex from the femur. The sliding lateral condyle osteotomy with a more extensive bone segment is a newer concept that has the advantage of maintaining a strong proximal soft tissue ligament attachment.

- When correcting a valgus deformity, distal femoral resection of 6–7° is often acceptable because it allows for improvement of extension gap balancing and tensioning of "intact" medial structures. "Slight" residual valgus is cosmetically acceptable in the patient with long-standing valgus deformity.

- Type II valgus with stretch-out of the medial structures can create instability in the M-L and rotational planes. Most pre-existing instabilities represent pseudo-laxity and are corrected with the direct lateral approach (when the medial side is left untouched) and a minimal medial tibial resection. True medial instabilities due to incompetent soft tissue structures can be treated with a combination of prosthetic implants such as the posterior stabilized (PS) or varus/valgus constrained (VVC) and/or proximal medial collateral ligament (MCL) advancement.

- When using fixed bearing tibial implants, rotation position of the tibial tray is critical. Rotating bearings, with or without PS or VVC options, are pref-

erable, since they self align to allow for optimum femoral-tibial interface positioning.

- Patella bone bed treatment is important. The lateral facet is often flattened, thin, and/or distorted. If a severely distorted patella is not seating well but has adequate bone stalk, resurfacing is favored. However, if any question exists regarding viability, tracking, bone-bed quality, the patella is best left unresurfaced.

- Patella alta is more common in congenital/developmental valgus. Therefore, raising the joint line is less critical and iatrogenic (problematic) patella baja is not usually a problem.

- Autograft enhancement of lateral defects, when present, is preferred over deeper resections, which may compromise the flexion/extension gap stability. Referencing from the medial femoral condyle is recommended.

- Long-standing posterolateral contractures with severe rotation deformities require more prospective releases and concern for peroneal nerve stretch and/or compression injury. The peroneal nerve can be exposed and decompressed proximally and/or a partial proximal fibulectomy performed as described previously. It is advised to maintain the knee in some flexion postoperatively to avoid tension on the peroneal nerve.

- When performing extensive soft tissue dissection in a high-risk rheumatoid type (thin-skinned) patient or after some MCL tightening procedures, splinting for 2–3 days should be considered. In general, the rehabilitation is less intensive in this high-risk group, since achieving good range of motion (ROM) with the lateral approach is seldom a problem.

8   Conclusions: Indications for Lateral Approach

Fixed valgus deformity presents a major challenge in TKA. Literature suggests that correction of fixed valgus deformities via the standard medial parapatella approach leads to higher failure rates, primarily at the patellofemoral joint. A common factor in all reports is the medial surgical approach. Therefore, the surgeon should be familiar with and consider the direct lateral approach in challenging total knee replacements which include:

- fixed valgus deformity with patella subluxation,
- partially correctable valgus with lateral orientation and/or patella subluxation,
- varus knee with severe tibial rotation, increased Q-angle, tight retinaculum, and I-TB with patella tilt and/or subluxation,
- grossly unstable knee in a rheumatoid with expanded supra-patellar pouch,
- previous lateral incisions in multiply operated knee-when skin at risk (with undermining),
- lateral uni-compartmental replacement, and
- high tibial osteotomy (HTO) conversion to TKA, especially if lateral incision and/or retained metal.

References

1. Arnold MP, Friederich NF, Widmer H, Muller W (1998) Patellar substitution in total knee prosthesis– is it important? Orthopäde 27: 637–641
2. Buechel FF (1990) A sequential three-step lateral release for correcting fixed valgus knee deformities during total knee arthroplasty. Clin Orthop 260: 170–175
3. Burki H, von Knoch M, Heiss C, Drobny T, Munzinger U (1999) Lateral approach with osteotomy of the tibial tubercle in primary total knee arthroplasty. Clin Orthop 362: 156–161
4. Fiddian NJ, Blakeway C, Kumar A (1998) Replacement arthroplasty of the valgus knee. A modified lateral capsular approach with repositioning of vastus lateralis. JBJS [Br] 80: 859–861
5. Insall JN, Scott WN, Keblish PA et al. (1994) Total knee arthroplasty exposures and soft tissue balancing. In: Insall JN, Scott WN (eds) VideoBook of Knee Surgery. JB Lippincott, Philadelphia
6. Keblish PA (1985) Valgus deformity in TKR: The lateral retinacular approach. Orthop Trans 9: 28
7. Keblish PA (1991) The lateral approach to the valgus knee: Surgical surgical technique and analysis of 53 cases with over two-year follow-up evaluation. Clin Orthop 271: 52–62
8. Keblish PA, Boldt J, Varma C, Briard JL (2002) Soft-tissue balancing in fixed valgus TKA: methods of achieving concave side releases. Presented at AAOS 2002 Scientific Exhibit, Dallas, Texas
9. Krackow KA, Jones MM, Teeny SM et al. (1991) Primary total knee arthroplasty in patients with fixed valgus deformity. Clin Orthop 273: 9–18
10. Lootvoet L, Blouard E, Himmer O, Ghosez JP (1997) Complete knee prosthesis in severe genu valgum. Retrospective review of 90 knees surgically treated through the anterio-external approach. Acta Orthopaedica Belgica 63: 278–286
11. Merkow RL, Soudry M, Insall JN (1985) Patellar dislocation following total knee replacement. J Bone Joint Surg [Am] 67: 1321–1327
12. Ranawat CS (1988) Total-condylar knee arthroplasty for valgus and combined valgus-flexion deformity of the knee. Tech Orthopaedics 3: 67–76
13. Scapinelli R (1967) Blood supply of the human patella. J Bone Joint Surg 49B: 563
14. Tsai CL, Chen CH, Liu TK (2001) Lateral approach without ligament release in total knee arthroplasty; new concepts in the surgical technique. Artificial Organs 25: 638–643
15. Whiteside LA (1993) Correction of ligament and bone defects in total arthroplasty of the severely valgus knee. Clin Orthop 288: 234–245
16. Wolff AM, Hungerford DS, Krackow KA et al. (1989) Osteotomy of the tibial tubercle during total knee replacement. J Bone Joint Surg [Am] 71: 848–852

10.5 Tibial Crest Osteotomy

T.K. Drobny, U.K. Munzinger

1 Introduction

The standard surgical approach in TKA at the Schulthess Klinik is the medial Para patellar retinacular approach. To date there have been more than 3500 mobile bearing TKA implanted using this technique. However, some difficult knee arthropathies such as valgus knee deformities, arthrofibrosis, previously osteotomized knee joints, patella baja (infera) and revision situations require a more sophisticated surgical management, which includes a lateral approach with or without a tibial tubercle osteotomy (TTO). This technique has been used with slight changes for over 15 years in this center with satisfactory results. Refixation of the tibial tubercle has been altered from wires to cancellous screws, but the principle of this approach remains unchanged.

Lateral retinacular releases are frequently performed after medial arthrotomy, particularly in cases with patellar maltracking, lateral subluxation, or tilt. These problems are frequent in fixed valgus knees as well as in varus knees with substantial external tibial rotation. A lateral release improves patella maltracking. When the standard medial approach is used in combination with a lateral release, the vascularity of the patella and extensor mechanism might be compromised. Thus, the lateral approach to the knee, popularized by Keblish in the eighties and published in 1991 uses a lateral release that forms an integral part of the surgical approach, and the vascularity is preserved because the medial side remains untouched.

Mechanical compromise of the tibial tendon insertion is a catastrophic complication in TKA. In our experience, a liberal and preoperatively planned tibial tubercle osteotomy is a safe method to avoid this complication in total knee arthroplasty. An alternative osteoperiosteal elevation of the tubercle insertion has a higher risk of detachment and was, therefore, not used. Approaching the knee joint laterally with a tibial tubercle osteotomy gains safe and wide access to the knee joint (open book) without stressing the entire extensor mechanism (Fig. 65).

With this approach flexion of the knee joint is facilitated especially in knees with considerable fixed valgus and varus deformities, fixed flexion deformities, or other causes that may lead to a stiff and fibrosed joint. In these cases the patellar tendon insertion may be prone to spontaneous avulsion, when the knee is forcefully flexed during surgery (Fig. 66).

Another advantage of this method is a reduced external rotation of the tibia, which facilitates further soft

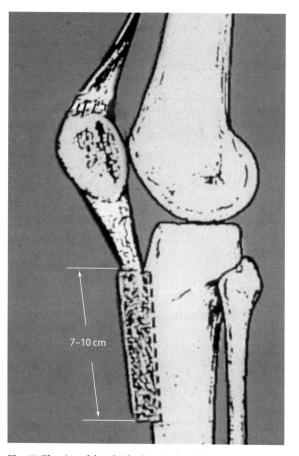

Fig. 65. The size of the tibial tubercle should be ideally 8–10 cm by 2–3 cm as demonstrated

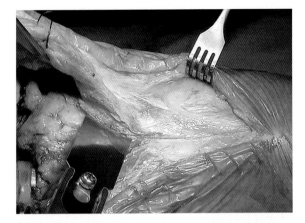

a

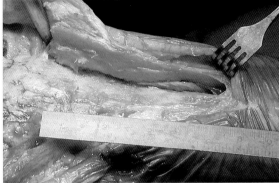

Fig. 67. Intraoperative view of the tubercle, which is carefully reverted. Care must be taken throughout the operation to preserving the medial periosteal sleeve

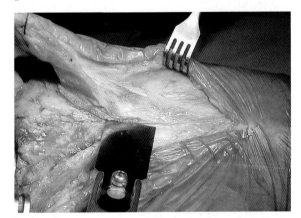

b

Fig. 66a,b. Sharp osteotomes are preferably used creating a hockey club type shape of the tibial tubercle. The distal cut is prepared prior to the proximal cuts in order to protect the middle third tibial from fracturing

tissue releases and proper positioning of the tibial component. Patients with rheumatoid arthritis benefit from this procedure in particular, because of increase incidence of valgus deformities, excessive synovitis, osteopenic bone stock and vulnerability of the extensor mechanism. Although Whiteside reported a tibial fracture post TTO, we could not confirm this complication in our series.

The rate of non-union or mal-union of the tibial tubercle after osteotomy is reported in the literature, but did not occur in our series. It appears vital for the success of this method to avoid under sizing of the osteotomized fragment. We recommend a length of no less than 7 cm and width of no smaller than 2 cm at the proximal aspect. This leaves a large surface for comfortable handling and allows for sufficient refixation and vascularity of the avulsed tubercle with two or three cancellous lag screws. The medial periosteal tether should be carefully preserved throughout the entire operation. Us-

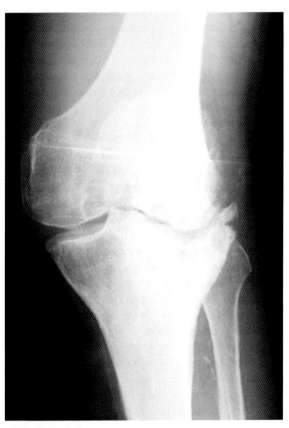

a

Fig. 68a–c. Radiographs of a typical valgus knee deformity, which was approached using a lateral tibial tubercle osteotomy. After implantation of an unconstrained mobile bearing LCS total knee arthroplasty, the quest was reattached with three cortical lag screws

ing an osteotome instead of an oscillating saw is a less traumatizing and devitalizing and is therefore preferred (Fig. 67). An illustration of a typical valgus knee is shown in (Fig. 68).

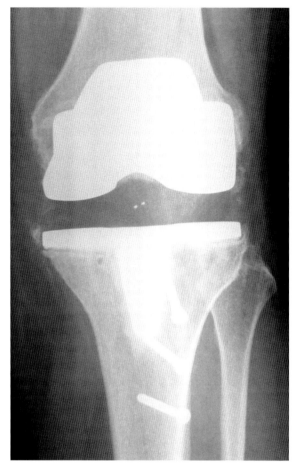

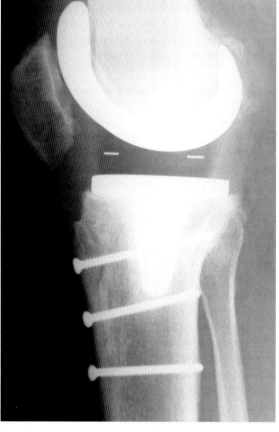

Fig. 68 b.   **Fig. 68 c.**

Postoperative hematoma can develop in some cases and may be avoided with meticulous hemostasis. Compartment syndrome is another complication that is very hazardous. We, therefore, recommend routine anterior tibial fascia release by using several long incisions, when tibial tubercle osteotomy has been performed.

Keblish reported that approaching the knee laterally is advantageous since it includes the lateral release that becomes mandatory in most cases with valgus knee, patella subluxation, external tibial rotation, or arthrofibrosis. Proper patellofemoral tracking as well as patella baja or alta can be alternatively achieved with lateral soft tissue releases or alteration of the tubercle refixation. The procedure of moving the position of the tubercle proximally prior to fixation allows also for extensor mechanism lengthening in cases with limited flexion.

In order to evaluate the success of this method we performed a prospective study, in which a conventional lateral approach was combined with an additional osteotomy of the tibial tuberosity in valgus knees and knees that had previous non-arthroplasty surgery. Between January 1993 and December 1995 there were 61 primary TKA performed in 51 patients at the Schulthess Klinik. In all cases a direct lateral approach with tibial crest osteotomy from lateral to medial was performed. In a published prospective study we evaluated both clinical and radiographical results of TKA that included valgus knee deformities, high tibial correcting osteotomies and other non-arthroplasty procedures. The preoperative diagnosis was osteoarthritis in 78% and rheumatoid arthritis in 12%, the mean age was 63 years with 73% being female. Valgus knee deformity was the predominant pathology with 73% in this study. The preoperative score was 59.2 on a 100-point maximum scale (modified HSS score) and the mean preoperative range of motion was 92 degrees. All surgery was performed by two very experienced consultant orthopedic surgeons using unconstrained mobile bearing LCS components. Different bearing devices were utilized: in 40 cases a rotating platform with cruciate substituting function, in two cases PCL retaining anteroposterior glide bearing, and in nine cases PCL retaining meniscal bearings. The postoperative rehabilitation followed a standard protocol that was similar to patients without osteotomy and included criterion based closed chain exercises with early weight bearing, except straight leg raise for 8 weeks postoperatively. All patients were assessed both clinically and radiographically after 2, 6, and 12 months.

2   Surgical technique

The skin incision is made 5 to 10 mm more lateral than the standard midline incision aiming towards Gerdy's tubercle distally and 1 to 2 cm lateral to the tibial tendon insertion. The lateral arthrotomy is begun along the lateral border of the quadriceps tendon. The incision is made approximately 2 cm lateral of the patellar and is carried trough to Gerdy's tubercle 7 to 10 cm distal to the tibial tendon insertion with preservation of the fat pad. Mobilization of the fat pad and the lateral synovial layer is essential. Lateral releases of various forms include the ilio-tibial band, the posterolateral corner (arcuate complex), the lateral head of the gastrocnemius or the inner border of the fibula head. The osteotomy is performed using sharp and broad osteotomes rather than an oscillating saw in order to preserve viability. The size of the osteotomy should be at least 7 cm long and 2 cm wide proximally. It is re-fixed using two or three counter sunk 3.5 mm lag screws (Fig. 69).

Alternatively wire can be used but this is not preferred in this center. Fixation and patellofemoral tracking is checked in 90 degrees flexion. Expansion of the lateral retinaculum is performed as advocated by Keblish using a coronal Z-plasty. A method described in this book. Fascia and skin is closed in routine fashion with metal clips to skin. In cases with patella baja (infera), the tibial tubercle can be proximalized by up to 1.5 cm, filling the distal gap with autologous bone graft (Fig. 70).

After 12 months the mean score in this group improved significantly from 59.2 to 84.4 points with 88% of the cases scoring excellent or good results, 8% had fair results and 4% poor results. The mean postoperative range of motion was 101 degrees (range: 35–30). Radiographic analysis showed primary healing of all osteotomy sites without signs of mal-union or nonunion. The mean time for healing of the osteotomy was 2 months in all but one case, which took 4 months for complete union. The average length of the osteotomy was 79±16 mm. No lag screw required removal for anterior knee pain or loosening. After one year there was no evidence of patella osteopenia or avascular necrosis. Complications that occurred included four cases with subcutaneous hematoma, five cases with partial skin demarcation, one compartment syndrome of the ante-

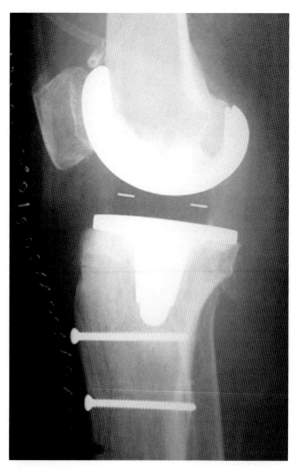

Fig. 69. An example of sufficient tibial tubercle osteotomy using two cortical screws only. The surgeon must evaluate both bone quality and stability of the tibial quest

rior tibial compartment and one case with arthrofibrosis. All these complications required a second operation that was successful in all cases without removal of prosthetic components.

3   Summary

Tibial tubercle ostetomy in difficult total knee arthroplasty is a safe, predictable and advantageous procedure that delivers a wide exposure, facilitates soft tissue management, and preserves viability of the extensor mechanism. This technique addresses problematic knee pathologies, which include the valgus knee, stiff knees and any type of patella mal-tracking or patella baja situation. The clinical results, as shown, are similar or better than those without osteotomy. However, this procedure should be planned preoperatively and is best performed from lateral to medial creating a large tubercle

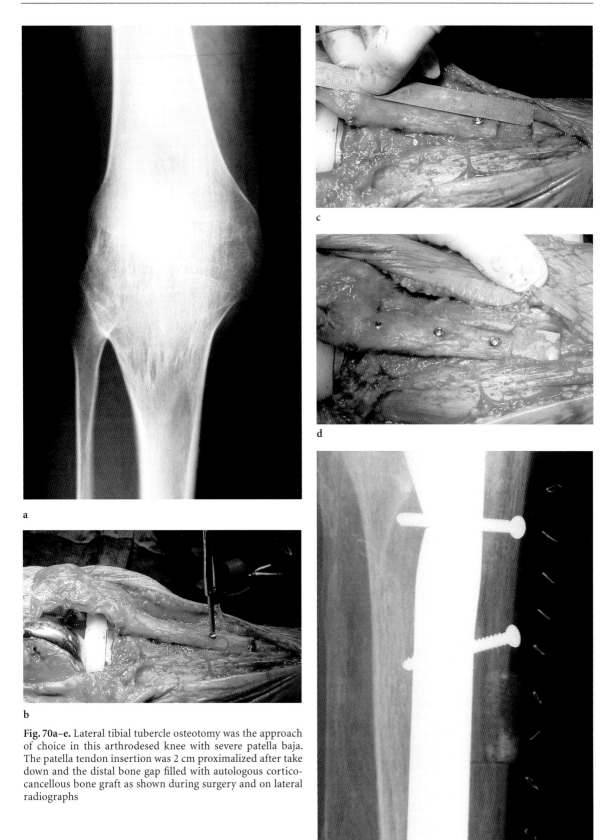

Fig. 70a–e. Lateral tibial tubercle osteotomy was the approach of choice in this arthrodesed knee with severe patella baja. The patella tendon insertion was 2 cm proximalized after take down and the distal bone gap filled with autologous cortico-cancellous bone graft as shown during surgery and on lateral radiographs

(7□2). The use of cortical lag screws for refixation of the tubercle allows for a postoperative rehabilitation that is similar to conventional TKA except forceful knee extension and straight leg raise in the first 8 weeks. Therefore, tibial tubercle osteotomy has become the method of choice at the Schulthess Klinik in all cases that present with valgus knee deformity, arthrofibrosis, patella mal-tracking and revision cases.

Acknowledgements: Hubert Burki MD for clinical data, Jens G. Boldt MD for review of manuscript.

References

1. Arredondo J, Worland RL, Jessup DE (1998) Nonunion after a tibial shaft fracture complicating tibial tubercule osteotomy. J Arthroplasty 13(8): 958–960
2. Barrack RL, Smith P, Munn B, Engh G, Rorabeck C (1998)The Ranawat Award. Comparison of surgical approaches in total knee arthroplasty. Clin Orthop 356: 16–21
3. Buechel FF (1982) A simplified evaluation system for the rating of the knee function. Orthop Rev 11(9): 97–101
4. Burki H, von Knoch M, Heiss C, Drobny T, Munzinger U (1999) Lateral approach with osteotomy of the tibial tubercle in primary TKA. Clin Orthop 362: 156–161
5. Cosgarea AJ, Freedman JA, McFarland EG (2001)Nonunion of the tibial tubercle shingle following Fulkerson osteotomy. Am J Knee Surg 14(1): 51–54
6. Davis K, Caldwell P, Wayne J, Jiranek WA (2000) Mechanical comparison of fixation techniques for the tibial tubercle osteotomy. Clin Orthop 380: 241–249
7. Dolin MG (1983) Osteotomy of the tibial tubercle in TKA. J Bone Joint Surg 65 A: 704–706
8. Engh GA, Parks NL, Ammeen DJ (1996) Influence of surgical approach on lateral retinacular releases in total knee arthroplasty. Clin Orthop 331: 56–63
9. Insall J, Salvati E (1971) Patella position in the normal knee joint. Radiology 101: 101–104
10. Kanamiya T, Naito M, Ikari N, Hara M (2001) The effect of surgical dissections on blood flow to the tibial tubercle. J Orthop Res 19(1): 113–116
11. Kayler DE, Lyttle D (1989) Surgical interruption of patellar blood supply by TKA. Clin Orthop 229: 221–271
12. Keblish PA (1991) Lateral approach to the valgus knee. Clin Orthop 271: 52–62
13. Keblish PA (1994) Patellar resurfacing of retention in total knee arthroplasty. J Bone Joint Surg 76B: 930–937
14. Lonner JH, Pedlow FX, Siliski JM (1999)Total knee arthroplasty for post-traumatic arthrosis. J Arthroplasty 14(8): 969–975
15. Lonner JH, Siliski JM, Lotke PA (2000) Simultaneous femoral osteotomy and total knee arthroplasty for treatment of osteoarthritis associated with severe extra-articular deformity. J Bone Joint Surg Am 82-A(11): 1672–1673
16. Maruyama M (1997) Tibial tubercle osteotomy in revision total knee arthroplasty. Arch Orthop Trauma Surg 116(6–7): 400–403
17. Masri BA, Campbell DG, Garbuz DS, Duncan CP (1998) Seven specialized exposures for revision hip and knee replacement. Orthop Clin North Am 29(2): 229–240
18. Nizard RS, Cardinne L, Bizot P, Witvoet J (1998) Total knee replacement after failed tibial osteotomy: results of a matched-pair study. J Arthroplasty 13(8): 847–853
19. Ries MD, Richman JA (1996) Extended tibial tubercle osteotomy in total knee arthroplasty. J Arthroplasty 11: 964–967
20. Ritter MA, Herbst SA, Keating EM, Farls PM, Meding JB (1996) Patellofemoral complications following total knee arthroplasty. J Arthroplasty 11: 368–372
21. Scapinelli R (1967) Blood Supply of the human patella. J Bone Joint Surg 59B: 563–570
22. Wang CJ (2001) Management of patellofemoral arthrosis in middle-aged patients. Chang Gung Med J 24(11): 672–680
23. Whiteside LA (1995) Exposure in difficult total knee arthroplasty using tibial tubercle osteotomy. Clin Orthop 3211: 32–37
24. Whiteside LA, Ohl MD (1990) Tibial tubercle osteotorny for exposure of the difficult total knee arthroplasty. Clin Orthop 260: 6–9
25. Wolff AM, Hungerford DS, Krackow KA, Jacobs MA (1989) Osteotomy the tibial tubercle during total knee replacement. J Bone Joint Surg 7 1 A: 848–852
26. Younger AS, Duncan CP, Masri BA (1998) Surgical exposures in revision total knee arthroplasty. J Am Acad Orthop Surg 6(1): 55–64

10.6 Technique for Non-Resurfacing of the Patella

D. E. Beverland

1 Introduction

Resurfacing or non-resurfacing of the patella continues to be a major source of controversy. There still is no right answer and persuasive arguments can be found to support either view. I feel at present the conclusion from the literature is best summarized by the following generalized quote: "Authors and speakers often begin with their predetermined conclusions and then find evidence to support only this point of view" [15]. Despite the large literature in this area there are very few prospective randomized controlled trials comparing resurfacing and non-resurfacing with Barrack et al [2, 3] providing a notable exception. They found no significant difference between the two groups.

Irrespective of whether or not the patella is replaced the surgeon must ensure that the patella tracks centrally within the patellar groove and that it is restored to its correct location in all three planes. The patellar groove should be restored to its correct medial to lateral location within the sagittal plane. Also within the sagittal plane the patellar groove should be aligned with the mechanical axis both in extension and flexion. In the coronal plane it should be the correct distance from the anterior femoral cortex and it should have the correct tilt and in the transverse plane the patella should be at the correct height relative to the joint line. In addition the patella needs to track in an appropriately shaped patellar groove such as is provided by the LCS femoral component. Based on the present evidence I feel that if these principles are adhered to then when using the LCS knee whether or not the patella is resurfaced is probably irrelevant.

In my own practice I have used the LCS rotating platform knee since 1993. During that time I have performed over 2,500 rotating platform LCS knees and in over 2,450 of those cases I have not resurfaced the patella. To date as a secondary procedure I have resurfaced 8 patellae (0.33%). For the last 6 years I have not resurfaced any patellae even in the presence of isolated patellofemoral osteoarthritis.

Older patients with isolated patellofemoral osteoarthritis provide an interesting sub-group. This has been reported to occur in approximately 5% of patients with osteoarthritis of the knee [13]. These patients are often severely disabled. I now have a series of 31 such patients (33 knees) with a minimum follow up of 3 years (range 3–6) and an average age of 73 (range, 58–89), in whom I have performed an LCS rotating platform total knee arthroplasty without patellar resurfacing [17]. Other potential options for such patients include isolated patellofemoral resurfacing but results from this procedure have not always been good [18].

Preoperatively all patients had significant knee pain. Sleep disturbance was reported in 21 patients. At latest review, 21 knees are pain-free, the remaining 12 knees describing only occasional knee pain. Two patients continue to have night pain. The results in this particular subgroup of patients have confirmed my prejudice that patellofemoral resurfacing is not required for any patient when using the LCS knee.

2 Pre-operative Assessment

It is important to document symptoms of patellofemoral disease before surgery. These include difficulty ascending or descending stairs, arising from chairs and riding comfortably in a car. We have also found that night pain is generally a more prominent feature [17]. Anterior knee pain and a history of recurrent "giving way" of the knee due to the patella locking or sticking in its groove are also common clinical features [1]. We have found that the Bartlett Patellar score [7] provides a useful measure of patellar pain before and after surgery.

I perform a pre-operative skyline view of all patients before TKA. This gives information about the severity of the patellofemoral disease. Sperner et al [16] provide a useful classification based on 5 grades (0–4). Grade 0, no degenerative changes through to grade 4, which is a tight joint space and large osteophytes with a deformed patella. I refer to this deformity as an 'S' shaped patella as shown in Fig. 78. With grade 4 disease the patella will not track correctly following surgery unless the patellar deformity is corrected – see page 173.

Lateral patellar tilt can be measured according to the method described by Gomes et al. [9] on both the preoperative and postoperative skyline views. Patellar congruency can be measured on both the preoperative and postoperative skyline views using the method described by Keblish et al. [12].

3   Patellar Dislocation and Mobilisation Via a Lateral Arthrotomy

I now approach all primary knees via a medial arthrotomy. In the past I used the lateral approach for all valgus knees but one draw back to the lateral approach is the difficulty that occurs when dislocating the patella over the medial femoral condyle. In my experience in about one third of lateral approaches it is not possible to safely dislocate the patella because of the excessive tension and risk of damage to the extensor mechanism. As a result

some form of release of the extensor mechanism has to be used. Many surgeons use a tibial tubercle osteotomy (see Chapter 10.5) but I used a modification of the modified Coones Adams approach as described by Scott [14]. Scott's technique was based on an initial medial arthrotomy whereas I approached via a lateral arthrotomy and then made a similar incision down the medial side of the quadriceps tendon again leaving a 2–3mm cuff of tendon laterally to aid repair (Fig. 71).

The incision is stopped just above the patella to avoid damage to the superior medial geniculate artery. This should allow the patella to be dislocated over the medial femoral condyle. Thereafter the procedure with regard to the patella is similar to that used with the medial artrotomy.

4   Patellar Dislocation and Mobilisation Via a Medial Arthrotomy

I make my initial incision with the knee flexed to 90 degrees. I use a midline incision except in the obese knee when I make the incision a little more lateral as this

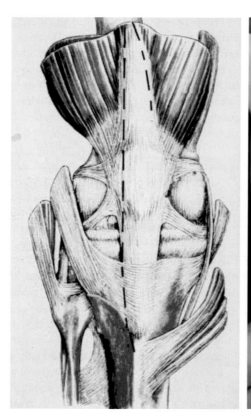
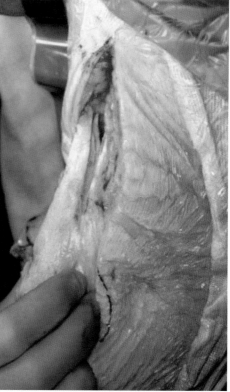

a   b

Fig. 71a,b. Modification of the modified Coones Adams approach. Used to provide proximal quadriceps release in a lateral approach

Fig. 72. Release of infrapatellar fold

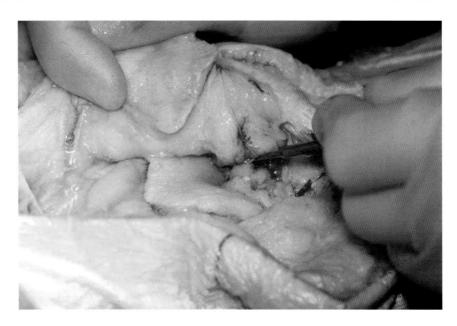

helps with patellar eversion. In this position I perform a complete arthrotomy using a midline capsular incision as described by Insall [10] beginning proximally along the medial edge of the patellar tendon leaving a 2–3mm cuff of tendon on the medial side to aid closure. Distally the arthrotomy is down the medial edge of the patellar ligament and in the middle the incision is carried directly over the medial quarter of the patella. When the arthrotomy is complete I extend the knee and evert the patella. If in the extended position the patella will not easily evert this is usually because of a tight infra-patellar fold (Fig. 72).

This can be palpated as a tight band in the inter-condylar region and can be released using a knife. Once the patella is everted the knee can be flexed and the patella dislocated over the lateral femoral condyle. With a medial approach and in a primary knee I have always been able to dislocate the patella over the lateral femoral condyle without having to use any additional procedure. This is in contrast to the lateral approach discussed above.

Occasionally and particularly in Rheumatoid disease there may be partial fibrous ankylosis between the patella and the underlying trochlea which has to freed to allow patellar eversion and knee flexion.

With the knee still flexed lateral mobility of the patella and extensor mechanism can be improved by release of soft tissues proximally and distally. This also facilitates exposure of the proximal tibia. The structures concerned are put under tension by pulling the patella laterally using a swab. Proximally the lateral patellofem-

oral ligaments are released by cutting them as they insert into the lateral femoral condyle (Fig. 73).

Distally the infra-patellar bursa, which is just above the insertion of the patellar ligament into the tibial tubercle, is opened and released (Fig. 74).

If patellar mobility (particularly eversion) is still poor then a peri-patellar release can be performed. This is done by first extending the knee, everting the patella and cutting along the lateral edge of the patella from the articular surface side. The eversion of the patella required to carry out this manoeuvre is conveniently done using a towel clip. This manoeuvre is also described for patellar release to improve tracking but in my experience a formal lateral patellar release is usually required. The knee is then flexed again to 90 degrees. As discussed earlier in obese knees it helps to make the initial incision more lateral to facilitate patellar eversion. Again in the obese knee patellar eversion can be further improved by making a sub-fascial pocket for the patella to evert into. Although with a more lateral skin incision and a peri-patellar release this has not been required in my experience.

At this stage I excise the fat pad. This is controversial as some surgeons feel it should be left in place. I feel that its removal improves exposure of the antero-lateral proximal tibia. Also there is evidence to suggest that it can be a source of pain within the knee [6]. LCS surgeons who use the AP glide feel that the fat pad, if not excised, can cause impingement and pain post-operatively because of the greater anterior translation of the bearing. This is also a good opportunity to remove any

Fig. 73. Release of patellofemoral ligaments

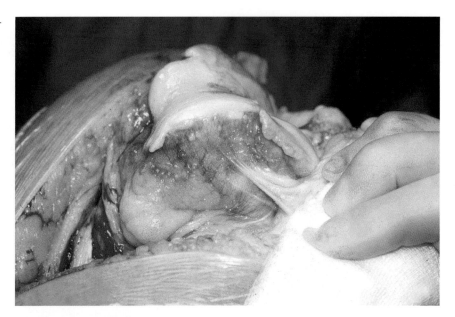

Fig. 74. Release of infra-patellar bursa

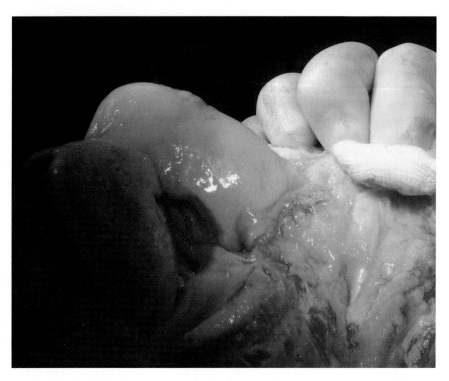

patellar osteophytes using large bone nibblers. Also at
this stage I use the diathermy pencil to mark the patellar groove (Whiteside's line – see Fig. 75a) this provides
a landmark for centering the femoral component. I then
pay no further *direct* attention to the patella until the
components are in place. It is however important to be
aware of the influence that the tibial and femoral bone
cuts and component placement can have on subsequent
patellar tracking and function.

5 Influence of Bone Cuts and Component Placement on the Patellofemoral Joint

5.1 The Q-angle and the Patellofemoral Joint

The Q-angle is the physiological valgus of the lower
limb. It is defined as the angle made between a line
drawn from the anterior superior iliac spine to the centre of the patella and from there to the center of the tibial

Fig. 75a,b. Flexion gap land-marks showing the effect on femoral rotation of over re-lease of the MCL

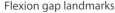
Flexion gap landmarks

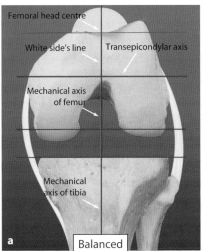

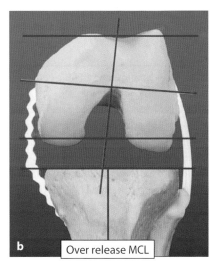

Red lines represent bonecuts

tubercle. In contrast the anatomical valgus of the lower limb is angle between the femoral and tibial anatomical axes. In the normal knee the Q-angle is maximum in full extension because of the 'screw home' mechanism of the tibia which moves the tibial tubercle laterally.

During TKA the normal Q-angle should be restored but any increase in Q-angle increases the lateral vector and will increase the risk of lateral patellar subluxation. The Q-angle is increased if the post-operative mechanical axis is in valgus and therefore care needs to be taken to avoid a valgus cut on the proximal tibia or an excessive valgus cut on the distal femur. Medial placement of either the femoral or tibial component will also increase the Q-angle. On the femoral side the patellar groove of the femoral component should be centered on the previously marked patellar groove (Whiteside's line). At times this may mean that the femoral component may overhang laterally by a few mms and this should be accepted. Whiteside's line was described by Whiteside and Arima [19] as a method of setting femoral rotation thus the patellar groove of the component should parallel Whiteside's line and this will be the case if the AP cuts are at right angles to it (Fig. 75a). The tibial component I place centrally to give edge to edge contact medially and laterally between the component and tibia. If the component is slightly larger than the tibia then the slight over hang should be accommodated laterally. This reduces the Q-angle but also avoids the patient discomfort that can be produced by medial over hang of the tibial component. In fixed bearing knees placing the tibial component in internal rotation relative to the tibia will also increase the Q-angle. In the LCS knee the mobile bearings protect against this, but

bearing rotation is determined by the femur and therefore leaving the femoral component in internal rotation will increase the Q-angle with the knee extended as the bearing will internally rotate thus lateralizing the tibial tubercle.

5.2   Femoral Rotation and the Patellofemoral Joint

Correct femoral rotation is a key factor in achieving satisfactory function of the tibiofemoral joint but it is also important for the patellofemoral joint.

Figure 75a shows the important anatomical landmarks and relationships of the flexion gap. This is where femoral rotation is set. In the LCS knee as with most knees the proximal tibia is cut at right angles to its mechanical axis. With LCS when the knee is balanced and the flexion gap is created using the femoral guide positioner the femur will adopt the correct rotation. As shown in Fig. 75a the proximal tibial cut is at right angles to the mechanical axis of the tibia and the AP cuts are parallel to the proximal tibial cut. If the knee is balanced the AP cuts will then in turn be at right angles to the mechanical axis of the femur (Whiteside's line) and the patellar groove of the femoral component will be in line with the mechanical axis of the lower limb as planned. Also the lateral anterior femoral condyle is more prominent which protects against patellar subluxation. If the AP cuts on the femur are in internal rotation as can happen with over release of the MCL then the AP cuts will not be at right angles to the mechanical axis of the femur. As can be seen in Fig. 75b firstly the lateral anterior femoral condyle becomes less prominent and secondly the trochlear groove of the femoral component will now deviate medially which increases the Q-angle in flexion (internal femoral rotation also increases the Q-angle in extension). Both decrease the lateral stability of the patellofemoral joint.

5.3 The Coronal Plane and the Patellofemoral Joint

One of the biomechanical functions of the patella is to increase the lever arm of the patellofemoral joint by anteriorly displacing the extensor mechanism from the flexion/extension axis of the femur and tibia. In order to restore a normal relationship the anterior rim of the tibial component should be placed flush with the anterior tibial cortex. The femoral component should similarly be placed flush against the anterior cortex of the femur. If the femoral component is left too anterior this can over stuff the patellofemoral joint and may impede flexion. It can also increase the flexion gap which can contribute to patella Baja – see below.

5.4 Restoring the Patellofemoral Joint to its Correct Transverse Plane

This refers to patellar height in relation to the joint line. A patella baja or infera occurs when the lower pole of the patella ends up at or below the joint line. This has been shown to have an adverse outcome following TKA

[8]. The two factors that control the height of the patella above the joint line are firstly the length of the patellar tendon running from the tibial tubercle to the lower pole of the patella and secondly the height of the joint line *relative to the tibia*. Obviously trauma during surgery can lead to contracture of the patellar tendon which will produce a patella Baja and this is felt to be factor compromising results of TKA after high tibial osteotomy [20]. However patella Baja not present before surgery but apparent immediately following surgery can only be as a result of raising the joint line or by moving the tibial tubercle distally following osteotomy. In the absence of tibial tubercle osteotomy too proximal a resection of the distal femur is normally blamed. However over resection of the distal femur on its own does not produce patella Baja because the distance from the tibial tubercle remains constant as illustrated in Fig. 76c.

It is only when the tibial joint line is raised by using a thicker insert that patella baja results as illustrated in Fig. 76d. The need for the surgeon to use a thicker insert normally arises when the flexion gap has been made too big. The common causes for an abnormal increase in the flexion gap are:

- making the AP cuts too anterior such that less bone is removed from the anterior femoral conyles and more from the posterior femoral condyles,
- using too small a femoral component,

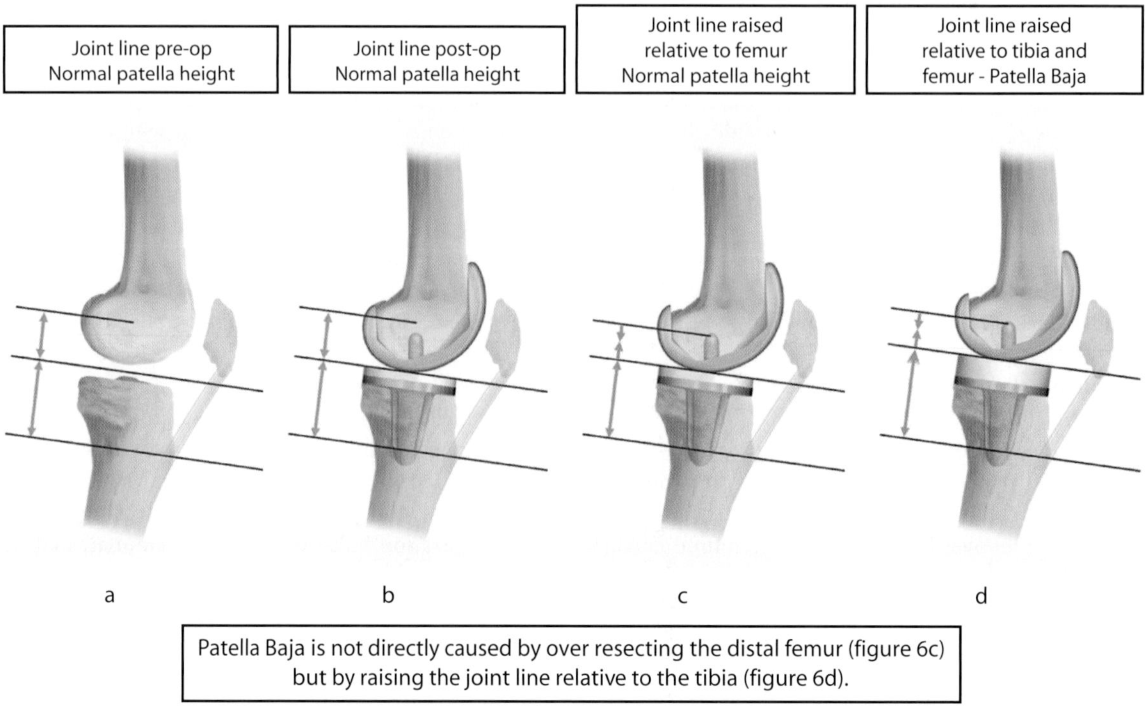

Joint line pre-op Normal patella height	Joint line post-op Normal patella height	Joint line raised relative to femur Normal patella height	Joint line raised relative to tibia and femur - Patella Baja

a   b   c   d

> Patella Baja is not directly caused by over resecting the distal femur (figure 6c) but by raising the joint line relative to the tibia (figure 6d).

Fig. 76a–d. Creating patella baja by raising the joint line relative to the tibia

- over release of the MCL,
- release of soft tissue from the lateral epicondyle in a valgus knee prior to the AP cuts.

To accommodate the increased flexion gap the surgeon has to use a thicker insert and in order to compensate for the latter more bone has to be resected from the distal femur to gain full extension. Therefore although patella baja is associated with excessive distal femoral resection the underlying problem is an increased flexion gap and a raised joint line relative to the tibia.

6   Patella Tracking, Patella Contouring and Patellaplasty

When the components are in place patellar tracking can be checked by bringing the knee from full extension into full flexion. No attempt should be made to restrain the patella during this manoeuvre. The patella should track centrally in the patellar groove and both patellar facets should remain in contact with the femoral component beyond 90 degrees of flexion. If it does not track centrally in the groove this is patellar subluxation. If the medial facet of the patella does not make contact with the medial femoral condyle beyond 90 degrees of flexion then I regard this as patellar tilt. Occasionally mild degrees of tilt are corrected if the tourniquet is momentarily released. It is rare for mal-tracking to be so severe that the patella will dislocate out of the trochlear groove during this manoeuvre but lesser degrees of patellar shift and tilt are common and should be corrected as shown in Fig. 77.

Prior to performing a lateral release it is important to ensure that the patella is the correct keel or 'v' shape. The commonest problem is patellar deformity (Grade 4 Sperner) with lateral osteophyte which if present will prevent the patella from tracking correctly. On the skyline view this produces an 'S' shaped patella (Fig. 78).

Even in cases of quite marked patellar maltracking 'contouring' of the patella by removing this osteophyte can allow the patella to track centrally with no patellar release. This lateral osteophyte is best removed by using the saw. The patella is everted and the saw is used to remove the patellar osteophyte in the coronal plane (Fig. 79).

The peri-patellar release is only effective with a minor degree of tilt and normally a full lateral patellar re-

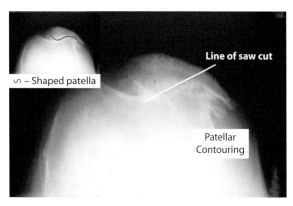

Fig. 78. Patellar contouring for a deformed patella

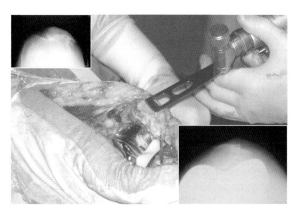

Fig. 79. Patellar contouring using the saw

Fig. 77a,b. Patellar release for mal-tracking

Before lateral release

After lateral release

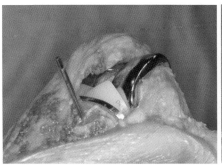

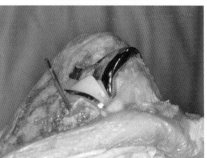

a

b

lease is required. This is performed from within out and extends from just above the level of the tibial tubercle distally to approximately 3 finger-breadths above the patella proximally. The incision should be made at least one fingerbreadth lateral to the edge of the patella. This is made much easier if the assistant holds the leg in full extension as this relaxes the extensor mechanism. The surgeon can then retract the patella anteriorly, which places the lateral retinaculum under tension allowing the release to be done under direct vision from within out using a knife. Care needs to be taken just to cut the capsular layer, cutting diathermy should not be used because of the risk of damaging the overlying skin. It is possible to perform a lateral release and protect the lateral geniculate artery but I find this difficult to achieve and therefore I cut and then use diathermy to seal any vessels. I do not release the tourniquet to do this. An essential part of the lateral release is cutting the tendon of vastus lateralis, which can be recognized as a discrete band about one fingerbreadth in width running obliquely inferiorly and medially to insert into the patellar tendon just above the upper pole of the patella. Once the release has been done the surgeon can place his or her hand in the capsular defect and check for any residual bands. Patellar tracking should then be checked once more to ensure correction.

If the patellar articular surface was eburnated then in the past it was recommended that the eburnated area be drilled with a 2.5 mm drill [11]. This has now been shown to result in patellar cyst formation in between 5 and 10% of patients at 5 years and is therefore no longer recommended [5]. To theoretically reduce the incidence of post-operative patellar pain rim cautery has also been described by Keblish and Greenwald [11]. This is where the soft tissue around the patella is either cut or diathermy is used circumferentially down to the level of the quadriceps tendon. I personally do not do this routinely.

References

1. Amis AA (1999) Patello-femoral joint replacement. Current Orthop 13: 64
2. Barrack RL, Wolfe MW, Waldman DA, Milicic M, Bertot AJ, Myers L (1997) Resurfacing of the patella in total knee arthroplasty. J Bone Joint Surg 79-A: 1121–1131
3. Barrack RL, Bertot AJ, Wolfe MW, Waldman DA, Milicic M, Myers L (2001) Patellar resurfacing in total knee arthroplasty. J Bone Joint Surg 83-A: 1376–1381
4. Berger RA, Crossett LS, Jacobs JJ, Rubash HE (1998) Malrotation causing patellofemoral complications after total knee arthroplasty. Clin Orthop 356: 144–153
5. Boldt J, Munzinger U, Keblish PA (2001) Patella non-resurfacing in LCS mobile bearing TKA. Evaluation of 1777 cases with 2 to 15 year follow-up. Proceedings AAOS
6. Dye SF, Vaupel GL, Dye CC (1998) Conscious neurosensory mapping of the internal structures of the human knee without intraarticular anaesthesia. Am J Sports Med 6: 773
7. Feller JA, Bartlett RJ, Lang DM (1996) Patellar resurfacing versus retention in total knee arthroplasty. J Bone Joint Surgery 78-A: 226–228
8. Figgie HE, Goldberg VM, Heiple KG, Moller HS, Gordon NH (1986) The influence of tibial patellofemoral location on function of the knee in patients with the posterior stabilized condylar knee prosthesis. J Bone Joint Surgery 68-A: 1035
9. Gomes LSM, Bechtold JE, Gustilo RB (1988) Patellar prosthesis positioning in total knee arthroplasty. A roentgengraphic study. Clin Orthop 236: 72
10. Insall JN (1984) Total knee replacement. In: Insall JN (ed) Surgery of the knee. Churchill Livingstone, New York, pp 587–695
11. Keblish PA, Greenwald AS (1990) Comparison of patella retention and patella replacement in LCS mobile bearing TKA: a prospective comparison of 52 knees in 26 patients. Orthop Trans 14: 599
12. Keblish PA, Varma AK, Greenwald AS (1994) Patellar resurfacing or retention in total knee arthroplasty: a prospective study of patients with bilateral replacements. J Bone Joint Surg 76-B: 930
13. Laskin RS, van Steijn M (1999) Total knee replacement for patients with patello-femoral arthritis. Clin Orthop 367: 89
14. Scott RD (1988) Revision total knee arthroplasty. Clin Orthop 266: 65–77
15. Slawson DC, Shaughnessy AF (1997) Obtaining useful information from expert based sources. BMJ 29: 947–949
16. Sperner G, Wantschek P, Benedetto KP, Glotzer W (1990) Spatergebnisse bei Patellafrakturen. Akt Traumatol 20: 24–28
17. Thompson NW, Ruiz AL, Breslin E, Beverland DE (2001) Knee arthroplasty without patellar resurfacing in isolated patello-femoral osteoarthritis. J Arthroplasty 16: 607–612
18. Tauro B, Ackroyd CE, Newman JH, Shah NA (2001) The Lubinus patellofemoral arthroplasty. A five- to ten-year prospective study. J Bone Joint Surgery 83-B: 696–701
19. Whiteside LA, Arima J (1995) The anteroposterior axis for femoral rotational alignment in valgus total knee arthroplasty. Clin Orthop 321: 168–172
29. Windsor R, Insall JN, Vince KG (1988) Technical considerations of total knee arthroplasty after proximal tibial osteotomy. J Bone Joint Surgery 70-A: 547–555

10.7 Femoral Rotation Based on Tibial Axis

J.G. Boldt, J.B. Stiehl, P. Thuemler

Femoral rotation positioning is critical for successful TKA. Three different methods of referencing are generally accepted. These include the transepicondylar axis (TEA), as advocated by Insall, arbitrary external rotation from the posterior condyles, and the so-called Whiteside line. Another less well recognized method, which has been used for over 20 years is referencing femoral component rotation perpendicular to the tibial shaft axis via a balanced flexion tension gap. Placing the femoral component parallel to the TEA leads to a biomechanically sound knee motion in full flexion and extension. However, this method has potential errors that include any anatomical deviations of the distal femur, which may occur in cases with severe varus or valgus angle deformity, condylar dysplasia, or other rotational pathology of the lower extremity.

Clinical outcomes after TKA are dependent upon multifactorial issues; one of which is femoral component rotational alignment. Prosthetic design and implantation of femorotibial components vary with different total knee systems. The surgeon must evaluate and address variables that include varus-valgus alignment, extra-articular deformities, soft tissue contractions, exaggerated Q angle, patella position, size, and shape as well as femorotibial rotation. Intraoperative variables include surgical approach, femorotibial stability, soft tissue management, extensor mechanism and patella treatment, prosthetic selection and positioning. Femoral component rotational alignment has gained more attention in the recent literature, since component malpositioning "negatively" influences knee kinematics, including patellofemoral tracking and range of motion.

The TEA is the most commonly referenced anatomic landmark for rotational positioning of the femoral component in TKA. It is reported as being more predictable than Whiteside's line or the posterior condyle. However, the TEA depends on estimated landmarks and may be altered in both varus and valgus knees and/or other pathological variations that may change lower limb rotational axes. Tibial rotation position, an important consideration in fixed bearing designs, is also a factor that affects gap balance and the patellofemoral joint. Tibial rotational positioning is of lesser concern in mobile-bearing TKA because of the ability (of the bearing) to adapt to tibiofemoral rotation in flexion and extension.

Rotational mal-positioning creates a trapezoidal rather than rectangular flexion gap with an altered patellofemoral articulation and unbalanced femorotibial kinematics. Instability in flexion with a tighter medial and more lax lateral compartment occurs when the femoral component is internally mal-rotated. This is frequently combined with lateral patellofemoral subluxation and instability (lift-off) of the lateral compartment in flexion. In most TKA systems, for a given amount of tibial resection, there is an appropriate amount of posterior condylar resection required to create a symmetric flexion gap. Different opinions of surgical approach exist regarding soft tissue releases, tibia first or femoral first bone cuts, as well as the femoral rotation resection. The most common method of tibial resection is perpendicular to the mechanical axis with some posterior inclination.

The three established methods of determining femoral rotational positioning in TKA consist of: the transepicondylar axis as advocated by Insall (Fig. 80),

Whiteside's line, or a line perpendicular to the anteroposterior femoral axis (Fig. 81), referencing 3 to 4° external rotation from the posterior condyles (Fig. 82). The posterior condylar reference as described by Hungerford (Fig. 83) is seldom utilized since it results in consistent femoral internal rotational positioning, often excessive. The LCS method is based on the tibial shaft axis and balanced flexion gap and has been utilized since 1977 with mobile bearing TKA (Fig. 84). Potential advantages and errors of each method will be discussed.

Olcott and Scott have recently reported that these three widely accepted methods were consistent in yielding a symmetric, balanced flexion gap within 3°. However, significant variable and inconsistencies were noted. The transepicondylar axis failed to yield flexion gap

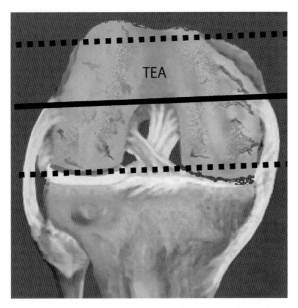

Fig. 80. The transepicondylar axis (Insall) is identified after intraoperative identification of both lateral and medial femoral epicondyles. Potential errors are landmark inconsistencies, previous trauma, femoral rotation, and inability to digitally identify both medial and lateral epicondyles

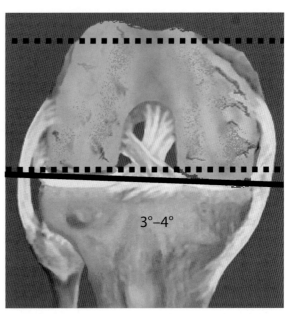

Fig. 82. Referencing femoral rotation in 3–4° external rotation to the posterior condylar line leads to an component positioning that approximates to the transepicondylar line, but has a large angular range. This method is arbitrary, based on estimates with variable reference lines in possibly distorted condyles, particularly in valgus or varus deformities

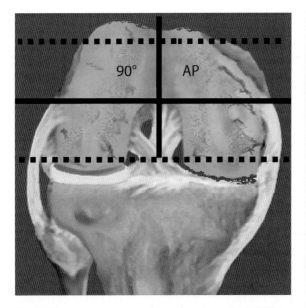

Fig. 81. The anteroposterior femoral axis method (Whitesides's line) references femoral rotation perpendicular to that line, which places the component approximately parallel to the transepicondylar line. Potential errors are femoral rotation variables, previous trauma, or patellofemoral diseases that may hinder anatomical identification

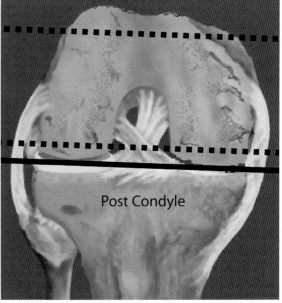

Fig. 83. Referencing femoral rotation from the posterior condylar line leads to an internally mal-rotated component positioning with an average of 4–5° to the transepicondylar axis, which requires varus tibial resection and increased valgus femoral resection to achieve a balanced rectangular flexion tension gap. Internal rotation will also have negative impact to the patellofemoral articulation

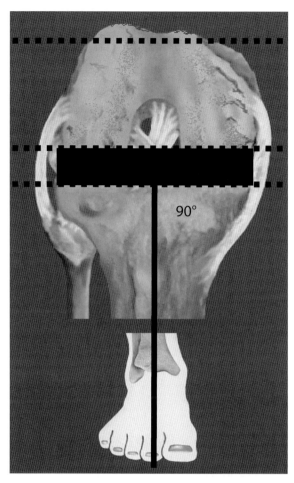

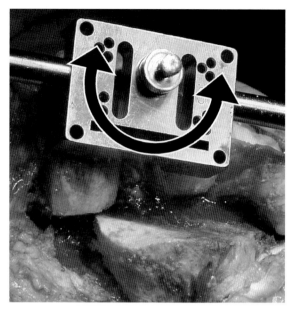

Fig. 85. Free moveable femoral resection guide is attached to an intra-medullary femoral rod

Fig. 84. Referencing femoral rotation perpendicular to the tibial shaft axis and a balanced flexion tension gap (LCS method) leads to prospectively predictable alignment parallel to the transepicondylar axis (mean 0.3°)

symmetry in 10% of neutral varus TKA and 14% valgus TKA, with discrepancies varying from 9° too little to 6° too much external rotation, which is less than desirable. The authors recommended using a combination of these methods to avoid potential mal-resections.

Clinical studies by Stiehl and Cherveny compared the tibial shaft axis method to other methods for determining femoral rotation in four different fixed bearing knee systems utilizing a femoral first approach. With the posterior method, 72% required lateral release with occuence of 7% patella fractures reported. When 4 to 5° of external rotation was used, 28% lateral release of cases used. When the tibial shaft axis method was utilized, femoral component placement was reported within 10° of external rotation compared to the TEA. There were decreased numbers of lateral releases required and no patella complications. Katz et al. [14] showed in a cadaver study of eight knees (a three surgeon evaluation) that de-

termination of femoral component rotational positioning was more reliable using a balanced flexion gap and the anteroposterior axis. A similar study performed by Jerosch emphasized that the inaccuracy of anatomically identifying the TEA of the femur by eight surgeons in three knee cadavers was 23 degrees. Intraoperative evaluation of the femoral epicondyles and the TEA is less predictable and accurate than previously established methods. The method used to define femoral rotation with the LCS system is referenced on a tibial cut perpendicular to the tibial shaft axis and a symmetrical (rectangular) flexion gap. This method automatically defines the position of the free moveable femoral resection guide (Fig. 85), avoiding the need of identifying anatomical landmarks. A rectangular spacer block is then applied to the rotationally unconstrained femoral component and sits flat on the tibial resection. The flexion tension is set and checked for proper balance (Fig. 86, 87).

The extension gap is balanced to the flexion gap with a distal femoral resection, establishing the mechanical axis (Fig. 88).

Comparison of this tibial axis method with the TEA methods adds to our understanding of this most important technique step in TKA. CT scan evaluation is the most accurate method to objectively assessing femoral component rotational placement compared to a known anatomic landmark post TKA. In order to clinically investigate the accuracy of the LCS method with regard to femoral component rotational positioning, we performed a study in which helical CT scan investigation was used referencing the femoral prosthetic placement

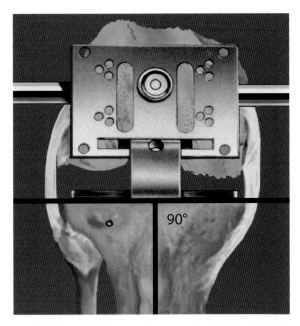

Fig. 86. Spacer block (perpendicular to the tibial shaft axis) is attached to the femoral component and sits flat on the tibial resection for flexion balance check and determination of femoral rotational alignment

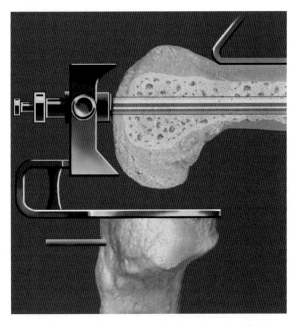

Fig. 87. Tibial resection is perpendicular to the tibial shaft axis and femoral resection block parallel to the tibial resection

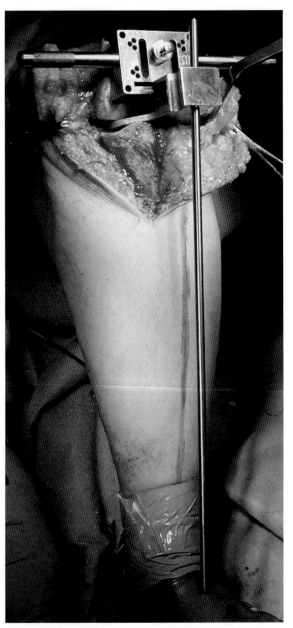

Fig. 88. Spacer block determines rotational alignment of the femoral resection block with a balanced rectangular flexion tension gap setting the guide parallel to the tibial shaft axis

to the transepicondylar axis. From a cohort of 3058 mobile bearing low contact stress (LCS, Depuy Int, Leeds, UK) TKA, 40 (1.3%) clinically well functioning knees were randomly selected for evaluation of femoral component rotational alignment. All patients with TKA in this center underwent routine clinical examination and follow-up radiographs at 1 week, 6 weeks, 1 year, 5 years, or when complications occurred. Mean age in this cohort was 67 years (range 54 to 77). Inclusion criteria for this subset was range of motion (ROM) over 100 degrees, lack of pre- or postoperative complications, and excellent or good clinical results according to a modified HSS 100-point clinical score with a mean of 91.2 points (81 to 100). One patient had to be excluded because of inability to identify appropriate anatomical landmarks on CT scans, and another patient refused CT investigation.

Of the 38 cases available for this study, the patella was left unresurfaced in 36 (95%) cases, one was previously patellectomized, another patella was resurfaced using a metal-backed rotating patella component.

Follow-ups at regular intervals included a clinical evaluation and X-ray protocol. Radiographic analysis was focused on patella tracking, congruency, and patella tilt with comparable pre- and postoperative skyline radiographs. Patella tracking was based on alignment of the femoral trochlear sulcus and the crown of the patella and measured in millimeters of lateral deviation on comparable pre- and postoperative skyline views.

The ultimate 38 cases were randomly selected from patients who were scheduled by a computerized system for 1-, 5-, or 10-year routine follow-up. These patients were invited to participate in the study until the appropriate number was obtained. Of the two cases eliminated one patient refused to participate another was eliminated for technical reason as noted. Of this group all patients had excellent or good clinical results and no patient refused participation. The local university ethics committee approved the study.

All cases were investigated by one of two consultant musculoskeletal radiologists with CT experience of more than fifteen years. Before the start of the examination they examined a few patients not included into the investigation in order to use the same criteria, which were identical to those used for everyday examinations. The radiologists were not aware of the patients'

knee status (single blinded). They were instructed not to talk with the patients about the status of their knees but about technical CT aspects only. All data for femoral component rotational positioning were analyzed using a helical CT scanner. Femoral component rotational alignment was calculated by referencing the two posterior condyles to the transepicondylar axis, which was a line drawn between the spike of the lateral epicondyle and the sulcus of the medial epicondyle as recently recommended by Yoshino et al. [29] (Fig. 89). One case was excluded because of inability to identify the medial sulcus despite 2 mm cuts. Angles were calculated utilizing sophisticated helical CT-implemented software.

An independent statistician analyzed all data. The distribution of angles in each group were analyzed using the one-sample Kolmogorov-Smirnov test which indicates whether the number of cases is sufficient and a normal "bell-curve" distribution is demonstrated. A positive Kolmogorov-Smirnov test validates further parametric statistical analyses.

The subset of 38 cases (follow-up: 12 to 120 months) studied in this series had clinical results comparable to a larger cohort group of over 3000 TKA. All cases were well functioning knees with good or excellent clinical results. The mean ROM was 115° (range 100 to 135). Preoperatively, 3 of 38 cases had documented patella subluxation and tilt of more than 6°. Postoperatively all three achieved perfect patellofemoral tracking. Decreased height and sclerosis of the lateral patella facet was seen in two case without clinical symptoms. There were no fixation failures, no patella failures and no re-operations for any reason in this group.

Mean femoral alignment was near parallel (0.3° internal rotation) to the TEA with a range of 6° internal to 4° external rotation (Fig. 90).

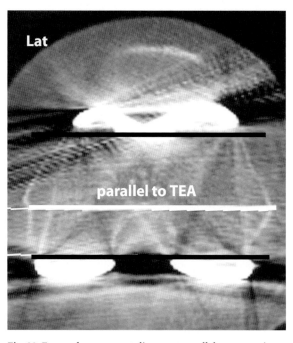

Fig. 89. Femoral component alignment parallel to transepicondylar axis ensures optimum patellofemoral tracking

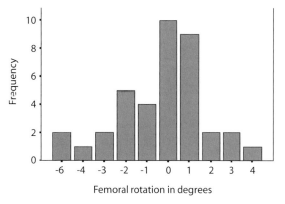

Fig. 90. Transversal CT scans are a practical method for accurate determination of femoral component rotational positioning in TKA best referenced to the transepicondylar axis. Example of a well-aligned femoral component parallel to the TEA

Fig. 91. Graph showing normal distribution of femoral component rotational alignment in the subset group. Mean rotation of the femoral component was parallel (0.3°) to the transepicondylar axis, ranging from 6° internal to 5° external rotation

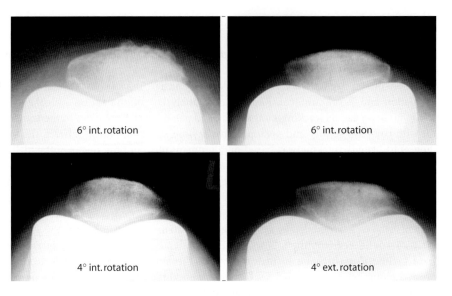

Standard deviation was 2.2 and standard error 0.4. All angles were normally distributed using one-sample Kolmogorov-Smirnov test, which validates a statistical mean value and outliers. Four cases fell outside of the predicted mean value (more than 3° internal or external rotation). Three had internal rotation and one case had external rotation. All four cases with maximum internal and external rotation showed perfect patellofemoral tracking on skyline views (Fig. 91, 92).

A second study was performed at the St Vinzenz Hospital in Dusseldorf, Germany with special focus on femoral rotational alignment in problematic TKA, seen at first follow-up. In contrary to the Swiss study, inclusion criteria here were all TKA seen at one-year follow-up with a moderate or poor clinical outcome using the Knee Society Score. Reduced mobility, pain, and patella problems were most frequent in this group. Infection, trauma, or wound problems were exclusion criteria. Two different mobile bearing knee systems were utilized, the LCS (DePuy Int, Leeds, UK) and MBK (Zimmer, Warsaw, USA). From more than 200 LCS and 70 MBK prostheses 27 cases entered the study, all of which underwent spiral CT investigation for evaluation of femoral component rotational alignment. There was an increased incidence of femoral component internal rotation in this group with poor outcome. Mean internal rotation was 4.2 degrees (0 to 8) in relation to the transepicondylar axis. There was no difference between both groups with regards to femoral rotational alignment. As data in the Swiss center indicates an association of arthrofibrosis with internal rotational alignment of the femoral component, the German data presented a high incidence of patellofemoral problems including maltracking, anterior knee pain, synovial impingement and clinically

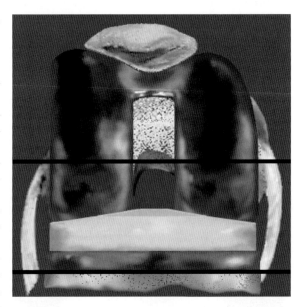

Fig. 92. Perfect patellofemoral tracking can be expected when the femoral component is rotationally aligned parallel to the TEA

unstable knee joints. Particularly internal malrotation does often lead to flexion instability, poor biomechanics, and patellofemoral tracking problems with lateral subluxation as demonstrated in this example (Fig. 93). In this study early postoperative complications in TKA were also associated with femoral component internal malrotation. We, therefore, recommend CT evaluation of component alignment in clinically doubtful knees. Cases that present with internal malrotation should be considered for revision surgery with the view to revise the femoral and/or tibial component.

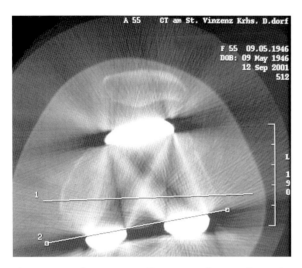

Fig. 93. Femoral component alignment with more than 8 degrees internal malrotation and patella subluxation. Patient presented with anterior knee pain

The data of this German study also emphasized that correct femoral component rotational positioning, utilizing the tibial shaft axis method, results in a high level of consistency for accurate patellofemoral alignment and predictable clinical outcome.

In summary, femoral rotational alignment based on the tibial axis and balanced flexion tension is an instrumented technique that

- avoids relationship to arbitrary landmarks,
- establish a precise flexion gap which allows for a stable relationship to the corrected bio-mechanical axis,
- is patient-specific regarding bone and soft tissue variations,
- is reproducible (especially in severe deformities such as the valgus knee), and
- results in predictable patella outcomes in reported series.

Femoral component rotational alignment is technique- and instrument-dependent and influences patella tracking, gap balance, and soft tissue kinematics. Deviation into internal rotation results in less than ideal patellofemoral tracking and clinical outcomes. Potential complications, such as the painful and/or stiff TKA (arthrofibrosis) has been shown to correlate with significant internal rotation of the femoral component. The tibial shaft axis method as used with the LCS system provides perfect rotational alignment without anatomical landmark identification, and is, therefore, felt to be as or more predictable than all other currently practiced methods.

Acknowledgement: C. Varma BS for illustrations (Allentown, PA, USA), J. Hodler MD and M. Zanetti MD for helical CT data (Zurich, Switzerland), T. Drobny MD for clinical support (Zurich, Switzerland), P. Keblish MD for critical mansucript review

References

1. Akagi M, Matsusue Y, Mata T, Asada Y, Horiguchi M, Iida H, Nakamura T (1999) Effect of rotational alignment on patellar tracking in total knee arthroplasty. Clin Orthop 366: 155–163
2. Arima J, Whiteside LA, McCarthy DS, White SE (1995) Femoral rotational alignment, based on the anteroposterior axis, in total knee arthroplasty in a valgus knee. A technical note. J Bone Joint Surg Am 77(9): 1331–1334
3. Berger RA, Rubash HE, Seel MJ, Thompson WH, Crossett LS (1993) Determining the rotational alignment of the femoral component in total knee arthroplasty using the epicondylar axis. Clin Orthop 286: 40–47
4. Berger RA, Crossett LS, Jacobs JJ, Rubash HE (1998) Rotation causing patellofemoral complications after total knee arthroplasty. Clin Orthop 356: 144–153
5. Buechel FF (1982) A simplified evaluation system for the rating of the knee function. Orthop Rev 11(9): 97–101
6. Churchill DL, Incavo SJ, Johnson CC, Beynnon BD (1998) The transepicondylar axis approximates the optimal flexion axis of the knee. Clin Orthop 356: 111–118
7. Dennis DA, Komistek RD, Walker SA, Cheal EJ, Stiehl JB (2001) Femoral condylar lift-off in vivo in total knee arthroplasty. J Bone Joint Surg Br 83(1): 33–39
8. Eckhoff DG, Piatt BE, Gnadinger CA, Blaschke RC (1995) Assessing rotational alignment in total knee arthroplasty. Clin Orthop 318: 176–181
9. Engh GA (2000) Orienting the femoral component at total knee arthroplasty. Am J Knee Surg 13(3): 162–165
10. Fehring TK (2000) Rotational malalignment of the femoral component in total knee arthroplasty. Clin Orthop 380: 72–79
11. Griffin FM, Insall JN, Scuderi GR (1998) The posterior condylar angle in osteoarthritic knees. J Arthroplasty 13(7): 812–815
12. Griffin FM, Insall JN, Scuderi GR (2000) Accuracy of soft tissue balancing in total knee arthroplasty. J Arthroplasty 15(8): 970–973
13. Hungerford DS (1995) Alignment in total knee replacement. Instr Course Lect 44: 455–468
14. Katz MA, Beck TD, Silber JS, Seldes RM, Lotke PA (2001) Determining femoral rotational alignment in total knee arthroplasty: Reliability of techniques. J Arthroplasty 16(3): 301–305
15. Lonner JH, Siliski JM, Scott RD (1999) Prodromes of failure in total knee arthroplasty. J Arthroplasty 14(4): 488–492
16. Mantas JP, Bloebaum RD, Skedros JG, Hofmann AA (1992) Implications of reference axes used for rotational alignment of the femoral component in primary and revision knee arthroplasty. J Arthroplasty 7(4): 531–535
17. Nagamine R, Miura H, Inoue Y, Urabe K, Matsuda S, Okamoto Y, Nishizawa M, Iwamoto Y (1998) Reliability of the anteroposterior axis and the posterior condylar axis for determining rotational alignment of the femoral component in total knee arthroplasty. J Orthop Sci 3(4): 194–198
18. Nagamine R, Miura H, Bravo CV, Urabe K, Matsuda S, Miyanishi K, Hirata G, Iwamoto Y (2000) Anatomic variations should be considered in total knee arthroplasty. J Orthop Sci 5(3): 232–237

19. Olcott CW, Scott RD (1999) The Ranawat Award. Femoral component rotation during total knee arthroplasty. Clin Orthop 367: 39–42

20. Olcott CW, Scott RD (2000) A comparison of 4 intraoperative methods to determine femoral component rotation during total knee arthroplasty. J Arthroplasty 15(1): 22–26

21. Poilvache PL, Insall JN, Scuderi GR, Font-Rodriguez DE (1996) Rotational landmarks and sizing of the distal femur in total knee arthroplasty. Clin Orthop 331: 35–46

22. Scuderi GR, Insall JN, Scott NW (1994) Patellofemoral pain after total knee arthroplasty. J Am Acad Orthop Surg 2(5): 239–246

23. Stiehl JB, Abbott BD (1995) Morphology of the transepicondylar axis and its application in primary and revision total knee arthroplasty. J Arthroplasty 10(6): 785–789

24. Stiehl JB, Cherveny PM (1996) Femoral rotational alignment using the tibial shaft axis in total knee arthroplasty. Clin Orthop 331: 47–55

25. Stiehl JB, Dennis DA, Komistek RD, Keblish PA (1997) In vivo kinematic analysis of a mobile bearing total knee prosthesis. Clin Orthop 345: 60–66

26. Stiehl JB, Dennis DA, Komistek RD, Crane HS (1999) In vivo determination of condylar lift-off and screw-home in a mobile-bearing total knee. J Arthroplasty 14(3): 293–299

27. Whiteside LA, Arima J (1995) The anteroposterior axis for femoral rotational alignment in valgus total knee arthroplasty. Clin Orthop 321: 168–172

28. Yamada K, Imaizumi T (2000) Assessment of relative rotational alignment in total knee arthroplasty: usefulness of the modified Eckhoff method. J Orthop Sci 5(2): 100–103

29. Yoshino N, Takai S, Ohtsuki Y, Hirasawa Y (2001) Computed tomography measurement of the surgical and clinical transepicondylar axis of the distal femur in osteoarthritic knees. J Arthroplasty 16(4): 493–497

10.8 Alternative Technique of Conservative Distal Femoral Cut First

D. Beverland

1 Introduction

It is generally accepted that creating balanced and equal flexion and extension gaps is a pre-requisite for successful outcome in TKR. This is particularly true for mobile bearing knees where flexion imbalance can lead to bearing instability and spinout. The recommendation in the LCS knee, in common with other knee systems, is that the knee should be balanced before the bone cuts are performed. In order to do this the surgeon has to estimate the line of the mechanical axis of the lower limb in extension. Once balanced a "tibia first" approach is used after which the AP femoral cuts are performed, the operative steps are illustrated in Fig. 94. The AP femoral cuts are a key step because they set femoral rotation and if correct create a rectangular and balanced flexion gap.

The technique used in the LCS is very simple and effective. A femoral guide positioner is used to separate the femur and tibia in flexion and this automatically aligns the AP femoral cutting block parallel to the proximal tibial cut. This ensures that the AP femoral cuts will be at right angles to the mechanical axis of the tibia. Consequently if the soft tissues are balanced the femur

automatically adopts the correct rotation and the AP cuts will also be at right angles to the mechanical axis of the femur and will be parallel to the transepicondylar axis as shown in Fig. 95a.

This "tibial axis" method for setting femoral rotation is very effective and is considered superior to other methods that use anatomical landmarks such as the transepicondylar axis and Whiteside's line. It works provided that the soft tissues are balanced before the AP cuts are performed. A significant problem can however arise if in a varus knee the AP cuts are performed without soft tissue balance. This can occur by either under or over releasing the MCL. In this situation the AP cuts may be parallel to the proximal tibial cut but they will not be at right angles to the mechanical axis of the femur. As a result the flexion gap will not be balanced and femoral rotation will be incorrect (Fig. 95b,c).

The conservative distal femoral cut first (CDFCF) is an alternative technique which adheres to all the principles of LCS but allows the extension gap to be balanced before the AP cuts are made. It is applicable to a varus knee with a pre-operative deformity of greater than 10 degrees especially if associated with a fixed flexion deformity. In a valgus knee the flexion gap is not normally tight in flexion and therefore the AP cuts can be done before the soft tissues are balanced. The order of bone cuts in the conventional LCS technique was illustrated in Fig. 94 and the order of bone cuts for the alternative technique is illustrated in Fig. 96. In this technique the proximal tibia is cut first as with the conventional LCS technique. Thereafter a conservative cut is performed on the distal femur. This then allows the extension gap to be balanced with correction of any fixed flexion. Having balanced the knee, the operation then proceeds as per the conventional technique with the AP femoral cuts followed by the definitive distal femoral cut. This technique can be performed using the basic Milestone instruments.

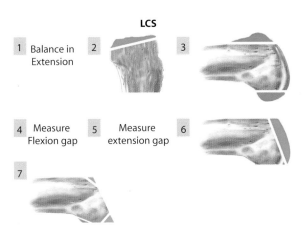

Fig. 94. Basic steps in performing the LCS knee

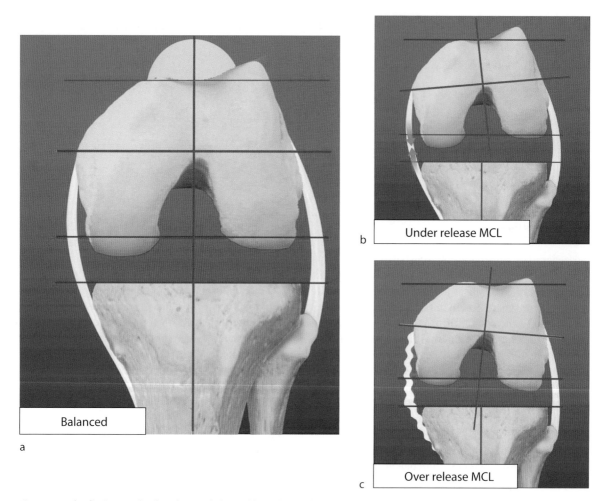

a Balanced

b Under release MCL

c Over release MCL

Fig. 95a–c. The flexion gap landmarks. In a balanced knee the AP femoral cuts are made at right angles to the mechanical axis of the lower limb. **b** When the MCL has been under released the AP femoral cuts are made in excessive external rotation. **c** When the MCL has been over released the AP femoral cuts are made in excessive internal rotation

Classic LCS – alternative new technique

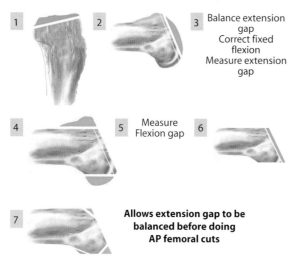

1   2   3 Balance extension
              gap
              Correct fixed
                 flexion
              Measure extension
                 gap

4   5 Measure   6
        Flexion gap

7   **Allows extension gap to be
        balanced before doing
        AP femoral cuts**

Fig. 96. Sequence of steps in the distal conservative cut first technique

2 Making the Conservative Distal Femoral Cut

Having resected the proximal tibia the AP block is used in the usual way to create the IM hole after which the AP block is removed. The trans-epicondylar axis (TEA) is marked using diathermy to give an approximate guide to the rotational alignment of the distal femoral cutting guide. The Milestone distal femoral cutting jig is then assembled using the 5-degree distal femoral cutting block. The rod of the assembled jig is now placed into the IM canal.

Normally this jig is used after the AP cuts and there is a flat anterior cut for the distal femoral cutting block to sit on. This both stabilizes the jig and sets the rotation of the distal femoral cut. When used in this way obviously the AP cuts have not been done and in a large knee the anterior limit of the femoral condyles may have to be trimmed with the saw to allow the cutting block

Fig. 97. Making the conservative distal femoral taking care to ensure correct 15 degree slope and setting approximate rotation

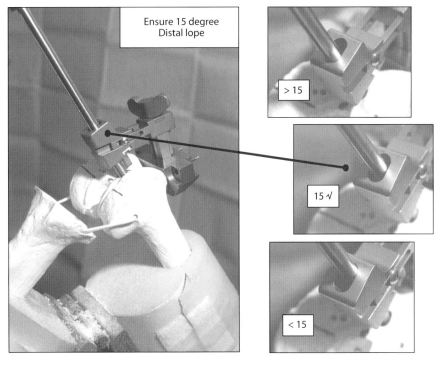

to sit anterior to them. The jig is advanced until it impacts on the femoral notch and its inferior edge is lined up with the TEA to set an approximate rotation. Then in order to create a conservative cut the wing nut on the distal femoral cutting guide is loosened, the calibrated stop is lifted and the block slid distally by at least 2.5 mm. This jig is designed such that when the calibrated stop is down and the cutting guide is sitting against the notch, 10 mm of bone will be resected from the distal femoral condyles. With the modified technique described above only 5 or 7.5 mm are removed.

The locking nut is then tightened again. The final point in positioning is to control the flexion/extension of the jig. The distal femoral cut is made at an extension slope of 15 degrees relative to the anatomical axis of the femur. At the entry point of the IM rod into the distal femoral cutting guide there is an oval opening (Fig. 97). When the rod sits in the middle the angle is 15 degrees when it sits at the top the angle is less than 15 and when at the bottom it is more than 15 degrees. The jig is then pinned using holes 2.5 mm distal to the proximal holes. This allows the block to be moved distally and also avoids capturing the same holes that will be used for the later definitive distal femoral cut.

Once pinned the distal femoral cutting guide jig is unlocked and the assembly is removed leaving only the distal femoral cutting block. The surgeon can then do a visual check that the cut is appropriately conservative, if not the block can be moved proximally or distally. When the

distal femoral cut has been done there should be a ring of cartilage around the distal lateral femoral condyle, which indicates that the cut has been conservative (Fig. 98). Also note that the cortex around the IM hole remains intact. If the definitive distal femoral cut is performed at this stage this cortex can be weakened and with the femoral guide positioner in place the IM rod could more easily migrate anteriorly through the softer bone.

3 Measuring the Conservative Extension Gap

Before measuring the conservative extension gap it is important to have a clear understanding of the spacer blocks and how they are used. The nomenclature is somewhat confusing. First of all if you look at a 10 mm spacer block it is quite clearly more than 10 mm so what is the actual dimension of the spacer block?

Figure 99 illustrates the actual sizes of the components that make up the "10 mm" extension gap in a large/large+ knee. The depth of the femoral component is 9.5 mm and the combined depth of the tray and insert is 11 mm. The same dimensions are true for the flexion gap. This means that when using a 10 mm insert a total of 20.5 mm of bone are removed to create the extension and flexion gaps (Fig. 100). Thus approximately 10 mm of bone are removed from each bone surface.

Remember that our first distal femoral cut has been a conservative one. This means that our total gap will be

Fig. 98. Appearance of distal
femoral cut. Note the intact
cortex anterior to IM hole

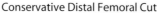

Conservative Distal Femoral Cut

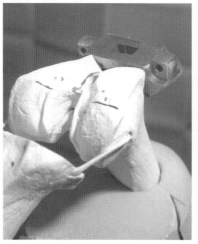
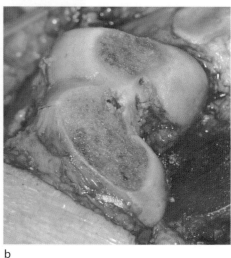

a   b

Fig. 99. Actual dimensions of
the component relative to the
spacer block

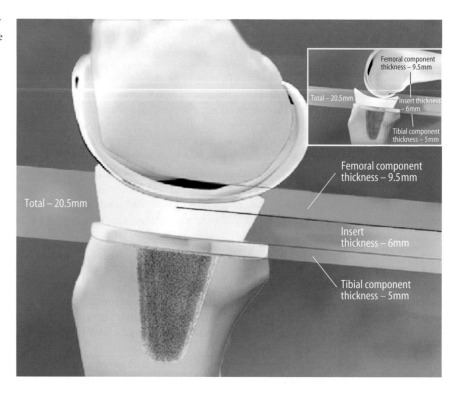

less than 20.5 mm. Hypothetically if we assume that we
removed 7.5 mm of bone from the distal femur instead
of 10 mm then the overall gap in extension will be (20.5–
2.5) 18 mm as illustrated in Fig. 101. This means that
our spacer block instead of being 10 mm now has to be
7.5 mm if we are going to measure the gap. So when using LCS how do we create a smaller spacer block?

Figure 102 shows the standard/standard+ spacer
block with shims. The shims are called 12.5 mm, 15 mm
etc. The actual dimensions of the shims are 2.5 mm, 5 mm

etc. Therefore when a 12.5 mm shim (actual size 2.5 mm)
is added to the 10 mm spacer block it becomes 12.5 mm.

Figure 103 again shows the std/std+ spacer block.
The spacer adapter, which can be removed from the
spacer block, happens to measure 7.5 mm and therefore as can be confirmed from the figure the adapter
is the same size as the 17.5 mm shim. This makes this
block useful for creating gaps smaller than 10 mm (the
adapter for lge/lge+ is 9 mm and therefore is best not
used to create a smaller gap).

Fig. 100. Depth of bone resection required to create a 10 mm extension and flexion gap

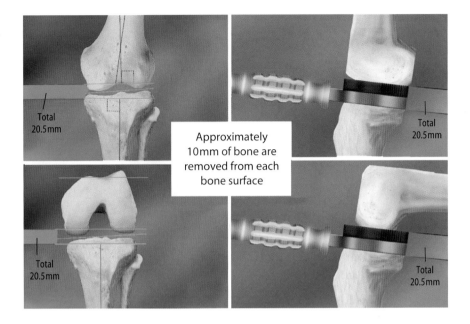

Total 20.5mm

Approximately 10mm of bone are removed from each bone surface

Total 20.5mm

Total 20.5mm

Total 20.5mm

Fig. 101. Dimensions of conservative extension gap

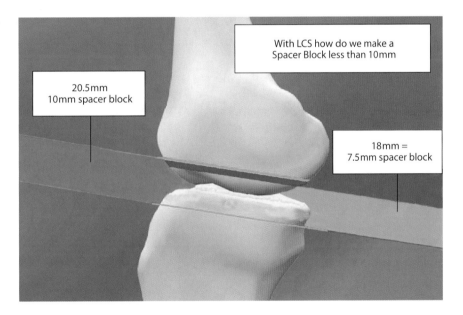

With LCS how do we make a Spacer Block less than 10mm

20.5mm 10mm spacer block

18mm = 7.5mm spacer block

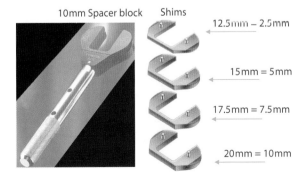

10mm Spacer block   Shims

12.5mm – 2.5mm

15mm = 5mm

17.5mm = 7.5mm

20mm = 10mm

Fig. 102. The Standard/Standard + spacer block with shims

As can be seen in Fig. 104a when the spacer adapter is removed from the std/std+ block then for a std/std+ knee the 10 mm spacer block becomes a (10–7.5) 2.5 mm spacer block (Fig. 104b). If a 12.5 mm shim (actual depth 2.5 mm) is then added the spacer block without the adapter then its size increases by 2.5 mm and it becomes a 5 mm spacer block (Fig. 104c). If a 15 mm shim (actual depth 5 mm) is used the value becomes 7.5 mm (Fig. 104d). It is important to remember that spacer blocks less than 10 mm are not real and are just for measuring purposes. The smallest insert is 10mm!

Fig. 103. With the Standard Standard + spacer block the spacer block adapter measures 7.5 mm

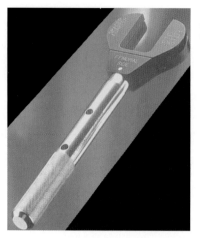

Standard 10mm spacer
- spacer adapter = 7.5mm
- without adapter on = (10–7.5) 2.5mm

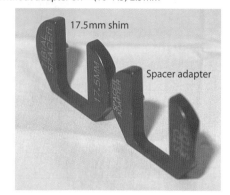

17.5mm shim

Spacer adapter

Fig. 104. Using the Standard/ Standard + spacer block to create 2.5 mm, 5 mm and 7.5 mm spacer blocks in a Standard/Standard + knee

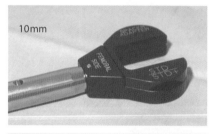

10mm

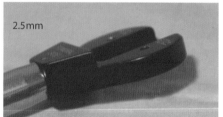

2.5mm

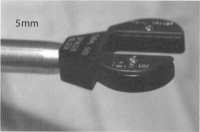

5mm

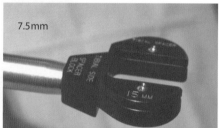

7.5mm

For Standard / Standard +

Fig. 105. Using the Standard/ Standard + spacer block to create 0 mm, 2.5 mm, 5 mm and 7.5 mm spacer blocks in a Large/Large+ knee

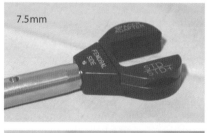

7.5mm

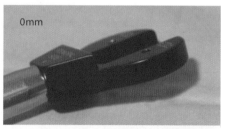

0mm

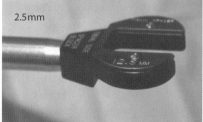

2.5mm

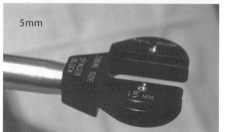

5mm

For Large / Large +

In the case of a lge/lge+ knee the Std/Std+ 10 mm spacer block is 2.5 mm smaller so on its own the 10 mm Std/Std+ spacer block can be used to create a 7.5 mm space as can be seen in Fig. 105a. Consequently when used with a lge/lge+ knee when the spacer adapter is removed the Std/Std+ spacer block becomes (7.5–7.5) = 0 mm (Fig. 105b). When the 12.5 mm shim is added it becomes 2.5 mm (Fig. 105c) and when the 15 mm shim is added it becomes 5 mm (Fig. 105d).

---

4 Balancing the Conservative Extension Gap

With the spacer block in place and in extension the knee can be considered to have 5 constraints 3 soft tissue and 2 bone:

1. the medial complex,
2. the lateral complex,
3. the posterior capsule,
4. the distal femur,
5. the proximal tibia (if it has been under-resected).

For perfect balance and full extension all have to be correct. Each constraint can be too tight or too slack. This can also be thought of in terms of length i.e. the tight side is too "short".

Before measuring the extension gap all osteophytes should be removed from the femur. The tibia should have already been cleared. Clear the femoral notch and ensure the PCL has been completely released. If necessary the saw or an osteotome can be used in advance of the posterior chip cuts to clear any large osteophytes posteriorly.

If the pre-operative deformity included fixed flexion then it should be addressed before the varus deformity as fixed flexion contributes to the varus deformity. This is because when fixed flexion co-exists with varus deformity the posterior capsule is usually tight predominantly on the medial side. Thus when released the varus deformity is also decreased. The same applies to the valgus knee where the posterior capsule tends to be tighter on the lateral side. In order to release the fixed flexion deformity use laminar spreaders to tension the posterior capsule with the knee extended as shown in Fig. 106. The capsule can then be cut under direct vision. The point of the sucker is useful for "palpating" the posterior capsule in order to locate the part of capsule that is tight.

When all osteophytes have been removed and the posterior capsule has been released the dimensions of the extension gap can be assessed. Initially this can be done by applying firm traction to the lower leg with the knee extended. Not only does this give information about the size of the gap it also gives an indication of balance. For example if the MCL is still tight the gap will tend to be trapezoidal and not rectangular. At this stage an appropriately sized spacer block can be placed in the gap. If the MCL is tight, then, when a valgus stress is applied the joint will feel stable but with a varus stress the knee will open laterally as illustrated in Fig. 107. This means that a medial release has to be done to achieve balance. This needs to be done carefully to avoid over release.

Medial release can be performed using a Cobb with the spacer block in situ but sometimes access to the insertion of the superficial MCL is easier when the spacer block is removed and the knee is flexed. Release should be sequential and at each stage the gap should be checked so as not to over release.

If the medial side of the knee is still tight then reconsider the posterior capsule. If the posterior capsule is still tight then there will be some laxity when testing both collaterals albeit more on the lateral side (Fig. 108). With this spacer block in place the knee will fully extend (Fig. 109), but despite the collateral laxity if a larger spacer block is inserted the knee will not extend under its own weight (Fig. 110). In this situation the posterior capsule should be checked again using laminar spreaders with the knee extended. Particular attention should be paid to the posteromedial capsule, which includes the region of the deep MCL. If the posterior capsule is still tight then with the knee flexed use an osteotome and a hammer and release the posterior capsule from the posterior surface of the lower femur (Fig. 111). When the knee is balanced there should be no opening medially or laterally and it should be fully extended (Fig. 112).

At this stage in the operation the dimensions of the conservative extension gap are known. This is useful information that can be used when fine-tuning the dimensions of the flexion gap.

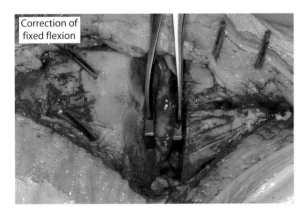
Correction of fixed flexion

Fig. 106. Correction of fixed flexion

Fig. 107. Testing the soft tissue balance of extension gap

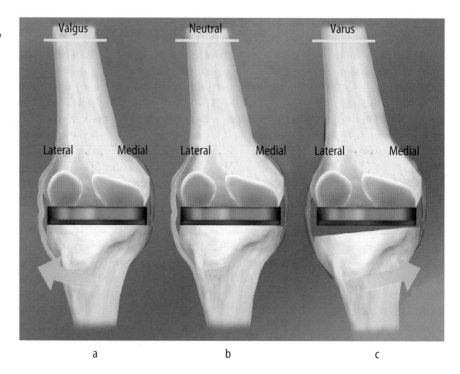

Fig. 108. The appearance of the extension gap with tight posterior capsule

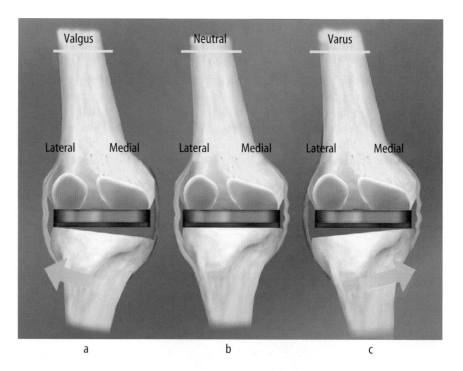

5   AP Cuts with the CDFF Technique

At this stage the appropriately sized AP cutting block is placed on to the femur using the short IM rod. Based on the size of the conservative extension gap the surgeon should have a good estimate for the expected size of the flexion gap. For example if the distal femoral cut was conservative by 5 mm and the conservative extension gap was 7.5 mm then the flexion gap should be (7.5+5) 12.5 mm. If in this situation with the femoral guide positioner in place the flexion gap was 15 mm as shown in Fig. 113 then it is possible that the AP block is sitting too anteriorly. The more anterior the AP guide sits, the larger the flexion gap becomes. Alternatively it may be that the AP guide chosen is too small and consideration can be given to up sizing but remember the femur should never be larger than the tibia. The most common reason is the former i.e. the AP guide is sitting too anteriorly in this situation the AP guide can be pinned, the femoral guide positioner can be removed and an initial anterior femoral cut only can be performed as shown in Fig. 114. At this stage the flexion gap is 15 mm but there is room anteriorly too remove a further 2.5 mm and provided there is enough room posteriorly the AP block is moved posteriorly by 2.5 mm and the definitive AP cuts are performed. This reduces the flexion gap from 15 to 12.5 mm as shown in Fig. 115.

The flexion gap is now checked with the spacer block to confirm that it is 12.5 mm as shown in Fig. 115. The extension gap should also be checked once more and if it is still 7.5 mm then a further 5 mm has to be removed from the distal femur to make it 12.5 mm also.

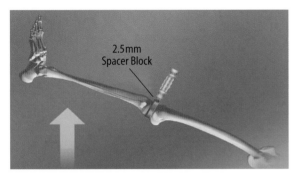

Fig. 109. Full extension

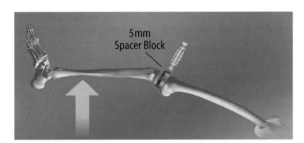

Fig. 110. Fixed flexion

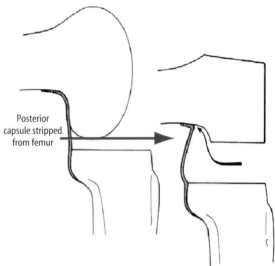

Fig. 111. Stripping posterior capsule from distal femur

Fig. 112. Balanced conservative extension gap

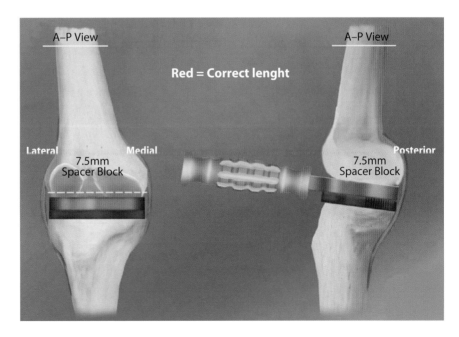

Fig. 113. Initial flexion gap 7.5 mm bigger than conservative extension gap

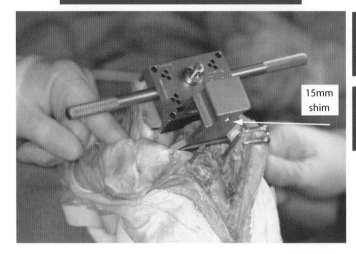

Conservative Extension Gap = 7.5mm

Difference = 7.5mm

15mm shim

Flexion Gap = 7.5mm

Fig. 114. a Initial anterior femoral cut too conservative. **b** AP resection block moved posteriorly by 2.5 mm thus reducing the flexion gap from 15 mm to 12.5 mm

Flexion Gap 15mm

AP jig moved 2.5mm posteriorly
Flexion gap goes from 15 to 12.5mm

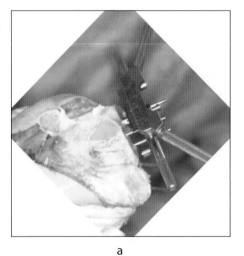

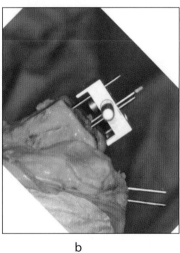

a

b

Fig. 115. Difference between the definitive flexion gap and the conservative extension gap is now 5 mm

Difference now 5mm

Second anterior cut

Flexion Gap = 12.5mm

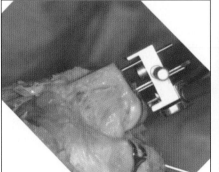

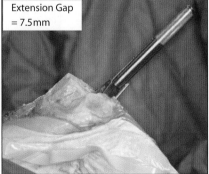

Extension Gap = 7.5mm

a

b

6 Definitive Distal Femoral Cut with the CDFCF Technique

The distal femoral resection jig is reassembled and is placed back into the femoral canal. The distal femoral cutting block can now be placed flush on the anterior femoral cut. The locking wing nut should now be loose. The distal face of the distal femoral resection block is made flush with the conservative distal femoral cut (Fig. 116). The wing nut is then locked and the block is now held firmly and flush on the anterior cut. It is then pinned using the two zero holes. The jig is removed and the distal femoral cutting block is moved back 5 mm (Fig. 117). The definitive femoral cut is now performed. The distal cutting block is removed the extension gaps and flexion gaps are checked once more to ensure that they are 12.5 mm (Fig. 118). The components can then be requested and the operation proceeds in the usual fashion.

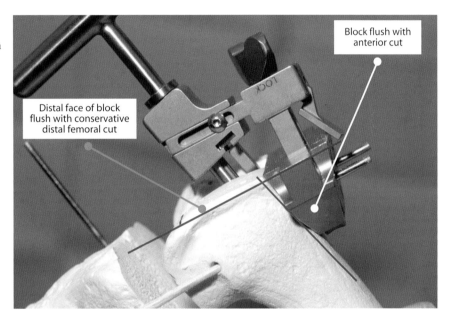

Fig. 116. Distal femoral resection jig reapplied flush with anterior femoral cut and flush with conservative distal femoral cut

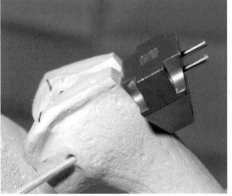 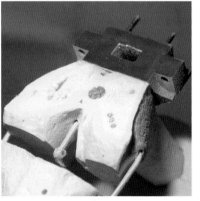

Fig. 117. Distal cutting block moved proximally 5 mm before performing definitive distal femoral cut

a

b

Fig. 118. Equal and balanced flexion and extension gaps

Balanced and Equal Flexion and Extension Gaps

Extension Gap 12.5 mm   Flexion Gap 12.5 mm

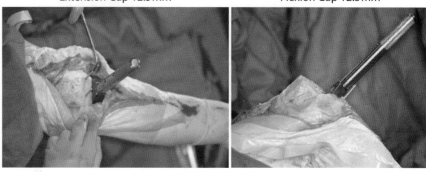

a   b

10.9 Approaching the Asian Knee

P. K. Chiu

1 Introduction

Asian patients in general have smaller body build. In 40% of Indian adults, the anteroposterior dimension of the distal femur was smaller than 55 mm [19]. This figure was the lower limit of the available sizes of femoral prostheses for Western patients. In an on-going multicenter, open study on Low-Contact-Stress (LCS) rotating platform knee prostheses in Asian patients (The "Dragon Knee Study") a small or small plus femoral component was implanted in 28 percent of knees and a large femoral component was rarely implanted (less than 3 percent). This is in contrast to sales figures from Western countries, where a small or small plus femoral component is rarely implanted (less than 3 percent), and a large or large plus femoral component is implanted in 25 percent of knees.

The native patella was also found to be relatively thin in Asian patients, with an average pre-cut thickness of 22.5 mm in male and 20.9 mm in female subjects. This means that it is more difficult to resurface the patella in Asian patients – the resurfaced patella may be too thick which can block flexion, or the post-cut thickness may be too thin which can increase fracture risk.

Apart from the size of the prosthesis, there are two other important issues. The shapes of Asian knees are also different and this may have some bearing on surgical technique when performing total knee arthroplasty (TKA). Secondly, in some Asian countries, the patients may need a higher degree of knee flexion after TKA because of cultural and religious requirements. These issues will be discussed in the following sections.

2 Asian Knees are not Only Smaller, but Different

While the prostheses available in the market can be used without any problem in most Asian patients, component miss-match does exist. On the femoral side, it is not uncommon to see sub-optimal coverage of the resected surface, despite the component being appropriately sized anteroposteriorly. This could perhaps be attributed to a wide variation of medio-lateral dimension for a given anteroposterior dimension in Asian knees. The need for a knee prosthesis specially designed and manufactured for the Asian population is being discussed, but the heterogeneity within Asian ethic groups makes it difficult, and further studies are awaited.

The rotational alignment of the distal femur in Chinese patients has been shown to be different to that reported in the Western literature. With the LCS knee, femoral rotation is set by using the "horse shoe" spacer (femoral guide positioner). At the same time this instrument creates the flexion gap by separating the femur and tibia. Provided the collateral ligaments have been balanced and the proximal tibia has been cut perpendicular to the tibial axis, then the proximal tibia and the trans-epicondylar axis will be parallel. Normally this results in slightly more bone being removed from the medial posterior femoral condyle than the lateral. However in our Chinese population we found that the amount resected from the posterior medial condyle was relatively much bigger than the lateral. This discrepancy led us to hypothesize that the usual relationship between the posterior condylar line and the trans-epicondylar axis was not 3 degrees as reported in Western patients, but was more in Asian knees. This is in line with what we found in a study that looked at the axial alignment of the lower extremity. Using anteroposterior weight-bearing radiographs of the entire lower limb in 50 young, normal Chinese subjects, the knee joint line was found to be more oblique, averaging 5 degrees [18], compared with 3 degrees in Western studies. Similar findings were reported in a group of Japanese patients with medial osteoarthritis [13]. With the joint line in 5 degrees of varus, the posterior condylar line should also form a 5 degrees angle with the trans-epicondylar axis that is perpendicular to the tibial axis. This postulation correlated very well with what we found in another study using 25 pairs of Chinese cadaveric femora. The rotational alignment

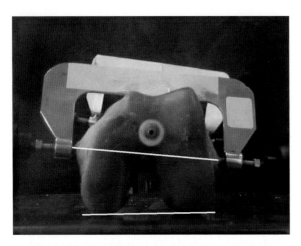

Fig. 119. In Asian femora, the angle formed between the transepicondylar axis and the posterior condylar line was not 3 degrees as reported in Western literature, but averaged over 5 degrees. In this particular specimen, the angle was 6 degrees

was such that the trans-epicondylar axis was externally rotated by more than 5 degrees relative to the posterior condylar line (Fig. 119). In other words, one may not get the necessary external rotation if the jig that usually produces only 3 degrees of external rotation relative to the posterior condylar line is used in the Asian knee. This could result in a trapezoidal flexion gap and a problem with patellofemoral tracking. This does not happen with the LCS knee because of the femoral guide positioner.

We also had the impression that the posterior tibial slope in Chinese subjects was more than the 5 to 10 degrees being reported in Western literature. We evaluated this in 25 pairs of Chinese cadaveric tibia; the fibula was left intact to ensure proper orientation. Using the intra-medullary axis as the reference, the posterior slope averaged 11.5 degrees [2]. It is important to point out that the anterior tibial crest, which is used by some surgeons as the reference to indicate tibial slope, is not parallel to the intra-medullary axis. Using the same jig, the extra-medullary alignment method will result in 3 degrees less posterior slope if its rod is placed parallel to the anterior tibial crest rather than the intra-medullary axis. If posterior slope is desired, one must put the rod parallel to the intra-medullary axis by pulling it away from the ankle distally. The problem of cutting the proximal tibia without slope in a knee with significant posterior slope is that more bone will be resected in the front thus exposing weak bone. Since the LCS prosthesis is designed to have 7 to 10 degrees of posterior slope, it suits the Asian knees better when compared with other prostheses that do not have much posterior slope especially if the posterior cruciate ligament is not retained.

Anatomic variations are perhaps more common in Asian knees. In Chinese patients, over 20 percent of varus knees showed tibial bowing to the degree that the intra-medullary alignment guide could result in an unacceptable cut of the proximal tibia [9]. In Japanese patients, it was shown that the femoral medullary canal was often not straight, and the central line of the proximal femoral diaphysis formed an angle of 2 degrees with the central line of the distal diaphysis [13]. The lateral femoral bowing could result in erroneous distal femoral cut with the intra-medullary alignment system. Such deformities may be pre-existing and could contribute to the development of osteoarthritis in Asian knees. Also Asian patients are often stoical and if reluctant to have surgery may continue to ambulate despite advanced knee deformities. It is possible that in this situation the bone may remodel in the presence of abnormal stress to produce such bone deformities. In any case, the Asian knee is technically more difficult to replace and careful pre-operative planning is a must.

3   How to Maximize Range of Motion After TKA

It has been demonstrated that 67 degrees of knee flexion is needed for the swing phase of gait, 83 degrees are needed to climb stairs, 90 degrees are needed to descend stairs, and 93 degrees are needed to rise from a chair [8]. Most recent published series reported that final flexion was between 100 degrees and 115 degrees after TKA. While this may be enough according to the criteria above, some Asian patients may need knee flexion from 120 to 150 degrees. For example, full squatting with the knees to the floor is commonly practiced every day because of the sitting environment in Japan. Similar positions are required for prayers in many religions, such as Buddhism and Islam. If knee flexion from 120 to 150 degrees is wanted, one must pay attention to every detail. The factors that affect the knee flexion range after TKA can be grouped into 4 parts, and will be discussed below.

3.1   Patient selection

It is much easier to get good flexion after TKA if the patient is thin, has good pre-operative flexion range, has a knee that was not operated before, and is co-operative and highly motivated.

Obesity has been associated with poor flexion range after TKA. Shoji et al. [16] studied 192 patients who underwent primary TKA. In patients who had more than 120 degrees of flexion, only 7 percent were obese. Of those with a range from 101 to 119, 28 percent were obese and for those who could flex for 100 degrees or less, a total of 78 percent were obese. Such findings can be attributed to the soft tissue impingement between the thigh and the leg? (between the thigh and the calf?).

Pre-operative range of motion has also been found to be an important factor influencing the range of motion after TKA. Many studies have shown that knees with good pre-operative flexion would lose flexion, and those with poor pre-operative flexion would gain flexion afterwards. However, the knees that had good pre-operative flexion would still have better flexion at the end of the day, and those with poor pre-operative flexion would not attain a very good range of flexion. It is thus important to know the pre-operative flexion range when comparing the flexion range after TKA in different series.

Whether history of prior knee surgery could affect the flexion range is controversial. While previous studies have reported reduced range of motion after TKA for failed high tibial osteotomy compared with primary TKA for OA, a recent study did not show a significant difference in knee flexion between the side with and the side without previous high tibial osteotomy in 39 patients who had bilateral TKA [12].

Motivation of patients, and their ability to withstand the pain and discomfort of rehabilitation were considered to be important. It is interesting to know that repeated manipulation without anesthesia to maximize the flexion range is being practiced in some centers in Japan. Also prior education of the patient may enable them to cope better afterwards. Another possibility is cultural difference – perhaps the Japanese patients are more tolerant and tend to obey the instructions of their surgeons.

3.2   Prosthetic Design

The early total condylar designs had limited flexion range because the posterior femoral flange engaged the posterior aspect of the tibial component at about 95 degrees of flexion. By saving the posterior cruciate ligament (PCL) and carefully balancing ligaments, motion is preserved. The latter, together with modification of the prosthetic geometry, provides greater posterior clearance and permits more flexion. Greater motion can also be achieved by substituting the PCL with the posterior-stabilized design, which has a tibial post – femoral cam mechanism. Most recent series on a single prosthesis reported that final flexion was between 100 degrees and 115 degrees after TKA, and no obvious difference existed between PCL-retaining and PCL-substituting TKA.

Several studies have compared knee flexion after PCL-retaining and PCL-substituting TKA. Becker et al. [1] reported on 30 patients who had bilateral TKA. A PCL-retaining prosthesis was implanted in one side, and a PCL-substituting knee was implanted in the other. The pre-operative flexion was 101 degrees in the PCL-retaining side and 98 degrees in the PCL-substituting side. The post-operative flexion was 111 degrees in the PCL-retaining side and 113 degrees in the PCL-substituting side. Hirsch et al. [6] studied 242 TKAs that were divided into three groups. The PCL was sacrificed in 77 knees in group I and was retained in 80 knees in group II. In group III, the PCL was substituted in 85 knees. The post-operative flexion range of group III was 112 degrees, which was significantly better than the 103 degrees achieved in Group I and 104 degrees in Group II. Dennis et al. [4] compared 20 patients who had PCL-retaining knees with 20 patients who had PCL-substituting knees. The knees were from the same system. Before surgery, knee flexion was 118 degrees for the PCL-retaining knees and 108 degrees for the PCL-substituting knees. After surgery, the maximum knee flexion was determined using video-fluoroscopy. In active weight-bearing mode, the post-operative knee flexion was 113 degrees for the PCL-substituting knees, which was significantly more than 103 degrees for the PCL-retaining knees. From these studies, it appeared that the PCL-substituting TKA gave better flexion than the PCL-retaining TKA.

Mobile-bearing TKA was not originally designed to have better flexion. However, the flexion was at least as good as the fixed-bearing TKA. Stiehl et al. [17] studied 261 rotating-platform (PCL-sacrificing) and 521 meniscal-bearing (PCL-retaining) LCS knees. The PCL-sacrificing rotating-platform prostheses were used in the difficult cases with pre-operative flexion of 95 degrees, when compared with 105 degrees for the PCL-retaining meniscal-bearing knees. One year after surgery, the flexion range was 115 degrees for the cruciate-retaining knees and 105 degrees for the cruciate-sacrificing knees. These did not differ much from the fixed-bearing outcomes in the literature.

What is important to the surgeon is therefore whether the knee prosthesis is compatible with good flexion. Modifications in prosthetic design may perhaps bring along some benefits. However, the most important part is still whether the surgeon can implant the prosthesis properly and permit the replaced knee to function as planned.

3.3   Surgical techniques

The important points are soft tissue balancing, avoiding an increase in patellar thickness and elevation of the joint line, and meticulous clearance of the posterior femoral condylar remnants.

The need to appropriately balance the ligaments cannot be over-emphasized. If any of the ligaments are tight, the range will be limited. Ritter et al. [14] reported on the balancing of the excessively tight PCL by sub-periosteally recessing the tibial attachment. The knee flexion achieved was 114 degrees for the PCL-balanced knee and 107 degrees for the standard knees. Laskin [10] studied the effect of a trapezoidal flexion gap. In the first group (92 knees), equal resection of the posterior femoral condyles combined with 90 degrees tibial

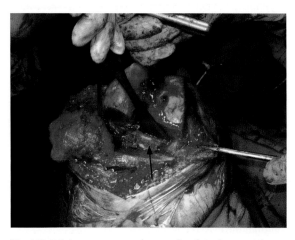

Fig. 120. It is important to make sure that there is no overhanging bone above the posterior part of the femoral prosthesis. Such remnants block knee flexion by impinging against the posterior lip of the tibial polyethylene liner. This figure shows the use of a broad chisel in removing a big piece of bone remnant (arrow) from the posterior medial condyle

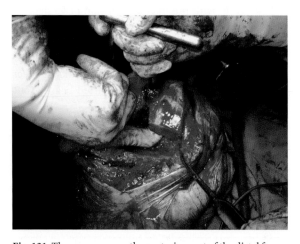

Fig. 121. The recesses over the posterior part of the distal femur are palpated for remaining bone ledge or loose bone chips that may impede knee flexion. The surgeon must be meticulous, and time spent here is often well paid back by the improved knee flexion after TKA

resection resulted in a trapezoidal flexion gap – the average pre-operative flexion was 120 degrees, and it was 100 degrees after surgery. In the second group (96 knees), the femoral resections were externally rotated by an average of three degrees to give a rectangular flexion gap – the average pre-operative flexion was 115 degrees, and it was 112 degrees after surgery.

Excessive elevation of joint line has also been shown to lead to poor knee flexion. Shoji et al. [16] studied 231 primary TKAs. If the joint line was elevated by 10 mm or less, 32 percent of knees could flex beyond 120 degrees. Only 7 percent of knees could do so if the joint line was elevated by more than 10 mm. Ryu et al. [15] reviewed 90 TKAs in 60 patients. They reported that the joint line was elevated by an average of only 2.1 mm in the good flexion group. In the poor flexion group, the joint line elevation averaged 5.7 mm.

It is important to avoid increasing the patellar thickness after resurfacing. Shoji et al. [16] found that if the patellar thickness was increased by 20 percent after TKA, 74 percent of knees could not flex more than 100 degrees; if the increase in patellar thickness was less than 20 percent, only 3 percent could not do so. Ryu et al. [15] found that the patellar thickness decreased from 19.5 mm pre-operatively to 18.7 mm after TKA in the good flexion group, and increased from 18.8 mm pre-operatively to 21.4 mm after TKA in the poor flexion group. This issue is particularly important in Asian knees, since our patellae are in general thinner.

In order to achieve 120 to 150 degrees of knee flexion, one needs to pay a lot of attention to the clearance of the posterior femoral condylar remnants. If not cleared, they may obstruct knee flexion by causing impingement against the tibial liner posteriorly (Fig. 120). One must be able to palpate the recesses at the posterior aspect of the distal femur to ensure that there is no mechanical obstruction to knee flexion (Fig. 121).

A few other points related to surgical technique remain controversial. Wakankar et al. [20] reported that the initial knee flexion after TKA was significantly better if a thigh tourniquet was not used. Perhaps there was less soft tissue swelling and discomfort without the pressure being applied. Emerson Jr et al. [5] recommended wound closure with the knee in 90 to 110 degrees of flexion. They hypothesized that loss of flexion would occur due to the relative shortening of the extensor mechanism, together with the skin tightness if the wound was closed with the knee extended. While these were not supported by similar studies, it could be that the difference was subtle if the final range aimed for was less than 120 degrees. They may be of value, if combined with other factors, in achieving range of motion well beyond 120 degrees of knee flexion. We currently perform our TKA without thigh tourniquet and close our knees in flexion.

3.4 Rehabilitation

Whether continuous passive motion (CPM) is beneficial to the range of motion after TKA has been a controversial question. Coutts et al. [3] reported that none of the 137 patients who were subjected to CPM after TKA required manipulation for poor initial flexion, while 21 % of 129 patients who did not have CPM required manipulation of the knee. However, several authors subsequently reported no long-term difference in the range of motion with CPM after total knee arthroplasty. Other series showed that there was a difference in the range of motion only in the early postoperative period but not after three months. We stopped using CPM after we found that at 3 weeks after TKA, the CPM knees had the same range of motion as knees that were immobilized in the initial period [11].

Jordan et al. [7] reported on the use of an "early flexion routine" with CPM to achieve maximum early knee flexion. The CPM was begun in the recovery room with the range set to 70 degrees to 120 degrees of flexion. Extension was advanced by 20 degrees on the first post-operative day and to full extension in the second post-operative day. They compared 50 knees subjected to this method with 50 knees subjected to a control group with conventional CPM regime. The range of motion at one year was 120 degrees in the early flexion group and 111 degrees in the control group. However, such benefit was not found in any other study. In some Asian countries orthopedic surgeons immobilize the knees in 90 degrees of flexion after TKA. There is little evidence to support such practice.

Most surgeons will agree that good post-operative pain control is very important, so as to permit the patients to do early mobilization of the replaced knee. Post-operative inflammation is occasionally a problem, and the use of cold compressive dressings may be advantageous. The patient must be fully informed about the rehabilitation program and be prepared to co-operate with the therapist. Obtaining flexion beyond 120 degrees is usually achievable with such an approach. In order to reach 140 and 150 degrees of flexion, more vigorous forms of physical therapy, such as repeated manipulations or stretching exercises under close supervision, are commonly required.

Finally, very good flexion is only necessary and can only be maintained if the patients really need it. The "unintentional" passive knee flexion imparted by the Japanese sitting-style may provide very effective functional training. Yoshino et al. [21] evaluated those patients who could squat fully after TKA and found that more than half of them were not able to do it any more after eight years. One of the main reasons was the loss of the reason to squat because of change to a Western life style.

4 Summary

Asian knees are different to their Western counterparts both in size and shape. These differences may call for prostheses specially designed and manufactured for these patients. This may also affect what Asian surgeons do during TKA. One must pay particular attention to the patellar thickness when resurfacing the patella and carefully evaluate the femoral rotational alignment. One must also be aware of the possible anatomic variations that may misguide the bone cuts.

Some Asian patients need knee flexion beyond 120 degrees, and even up to 150 degrees after TKA. This is not always achievable, and many surgeons discourage their patients from doing so in view of the potential conflict with prosthetic survivorship. If very good flexion is wanted, the patient has to be thin and have good pre-operative flexion. The prosthesis used has to be compatible with good flexion. The surgeon must balance the soft tissues and pay attention to every detail of the technique. Post-operatively early pain-free mobilization followed by a vigorous rehabilitation pro gram is important.

References

1. Becker MW, Insall JN, Faris PM (1991) Bilateral total knee arthroplasty. One cruciate retaining and one cruciate substituting. Clin Orthop 271: 122–124
2. Chiu KY, Zhang SD, Zhang GH (2000) Posterior slope of tibial plateau in Chinese J Arthroplasty 15: 224–227
3. Coutts RD, Borden LS, Bryan RS (1983) The effect of continuous passive motion on total knee rehabilitation. Orthop Trans 7: 535–536
4. Dennis DA, Komistek RD, Stiehl JB, Walker SA, Dennis KN (1998) Range of motion after total knee arthroplasty. The effect of implant design and weight-bearing conditions. J Arthroplasty 13: 748–752
5. Emerson Jr RH, Ayers C, Head WC, Higgins LL (1996) Surgical closing in primary total knee arthroplasties. Flexion versus extension. Clin Orthop 331: 74–80
6. Hirsch HS, Lotke PA, Morrison LD (1994) The posterior cruciate ligament in total knee surgery. Save, sacrifice, or substitute? Clin Orthop 309: 64–68
7. Jordan LR, Siegel JL, Olivio JL (1995) Early flexion routine. An alternative method of continuous passive motion. Clin Orthop 315: 231–133
8. Kettelkamp DB, Johnson RJ, Smidt GL, Chao EYS, Walter M (1970) An electrogoniometric study of knee motion in normal gait. J Bone Joint Surg 52-A: 775–790
9. Ko PS, Tio MK, Ban CM, Mak YK, Ip FK, Lam JJ (2001) Radiologic analysis of the tibial intramedullary canal in Chinese varus knees. Implications in total knee arthroplasty. J Arthroplasty 16: 212–215

10. Laskin RS (1995) Flexion space configuration in total knee arthroplasty. J Arthroplasty 10: 657–660

11. Lau SK, Chiu KY (2001) Use of continuous passive motion after total knee replacements. J Arthroplasty 16: 336–339

12. Meding JB, Keating M, Ritter MA, Faris PM (2000) Total knee arthroplasty after high tibial osteotomy. A comparison study in patients who had bilateral total knee replacement. J Bone Joint Surg 82-A: 1252–1259

13. Nagamine R, Miura H, Bravo CV, Urabe K, Matsuda S, Miyanishi K, Hirata G, Iwamoto Y (2000) Anatomic variations should be considered in total knee arthroplasty. J Orthop Sci 5: 232–237

14. Ritter MA, Faris PM, Keating EM (1988) Posterior cruciate ligament balancing during total knee arthroplasty. J Arthroplasty 3: 323–326

15. Ryu J, Saito S, Yamamoto K, Sano S (1993) Factors influencing the postoperative range of motion in total knee arthroplasty. Bull Hosp Joint Dis 53: 35–40

16. Shoji H, Solomonow M, Yoshino S, D'Ambrosia R, Dabezies E (1990) Factors affecting post-operative flexion in total knee arthroplasty. Orthopedics 13: 643–546

17. Stiehl JB, Voorhorst PE, Keblish P, Sorrells (1997) Comparison of range of motion after posterior ligament retention or sacrifice with a mobile bearing total knee arthroplasty. Am J Knee Surg 10: 216–220

18. Tang WM, Chiu KY, Zhu YH (2000) Lower limb alignment in Chinese adults. J Bone Joint Surg 82-A: 1603–1608

19. Vaidya SV, Ranawat CS, Aroojis A, Laud NS (2000) Anthropometric measurements to design total knee prostheses for the Indian population. J Arthroplasty 15: 79–85.

20. Wakankar HM, Nicholl JE, Koka R, D'Arcy JC (1999) The tourniquet in total knee arthroplasty. A prospective, randomized study. J Bone Joint Surg 81-B: 30–33

21. Yoshino S, Nakamura H, Shiga H, Ishiuchi N (1997) Recovery of full flexion after total knee replacement in rheumatoid arthritis – a follow-up study. Int Orthop 21: 98–100

10.10 The Rheumatoid Knee

K.J. HAMELYNCK

1   Introduction

Total knee arthroplasty (TKA) in patients with rheumatoid arthritis (RA) is challenging for the orthopedic surgeon and requires a profound knowledge of the general and local aspects of the disease as RA-patients generally may differ a lot from the well known patient with osteo arthritis (OA). Patients with RA differ from these with OA as they are sick, their physical condition is diminished because of the disease and influenced by the use of medication such as immunosuppressive drugs and corticosteroids. Their immune system is compromised by the disease and the use of these drugs, which makes these patients more susceptible to infection. Osteoporosis is a general feature of RA especially in female patients and patients with juvenile chronic arthritis. Moreover RA-patients usually have more than one joint affected by the rheumatoid disease. When joints of the upper limb are involved this may have serious consequences for the rehabilitation after TKA. When joints of the lower limb are involved a careful evaluation is needed to plan the best sequence of surgeries: total hip replacement first and sometimes operations on the forefoot as well. Sometimes operations may better be combined, like ipsilateral total hip and knee replacement or bilateral TKA. In this chapter on the surgical technique of TKA emphasis will be given to the local aspects of RA, but the surgeon must realize that successful TKA in RA-patients is simply impossible without considering the general aspects of the disease and a careful planning [2].

2   The Rheumatoid Knee

2.1   The Clinical Picture

RA of the knee is characterized in the early stage by a painful hypertrophic synovitis. A radiograph may show gradually narrowing of the joint space and juxta-artic-ular osteopenia. Erosions may be seen, but osteophytes are usually not seen. Though the radiograph may give an impression of cartilage being of normal thickness, this impression may very well be false: during arthroscopic or open synovectomy often considerable local cartilage damage (erosions) may be seen which on a radiograph of a weight bearing knee is not visible. In those knees the effect of synovectomy will be marginal and TKA is already justified.

In the more advanced stage of the disease the joint narrowing is obvious, juxta-articular deossification is evident, but the presence of osteophytes is not dominant as it is in OA. More important is the presence of bone cysts in the subchondral bone, which can be very large and very often are barely visible on routine antero-posterior and lateral radiographs (Fig. 122)! When the bone collapses due to the weakening effect of the bone cyst, the knee will show considerable deformity. Fortunately the presence of bone cysts may be shown very well on MRI.

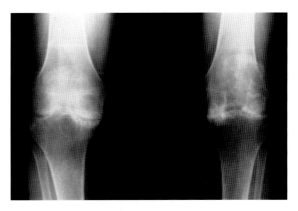

Fig. 122. Rheumatoid arthritis of the knee with marked joint space narrowing and a huge subchondral cyst barely visible in the femur

2.2   The Bone Abnormalities

Most RA-patients demonstrate minor or major bone abnormalities. The abnormality is a focal and generalized disorder affecting both cortical and cancellous bone, characterized by a loss of bone volume and strength, which results from a major increase in the rate of bone remodeling. Bone formation and resorption are increased [1]. The use of corticosteroids may exacerbate bone loss, but serious bone loss can be present in RA-patients who have never received corticosteroids, so the use of corticosteroids is not the main causing factor.

The loss of mechanical strength of bone about the knee joint has important consequences: fractures may easily occur and the fixation of components is compromised.

Fractures, like a fracture of a femoral condyle or a supracondylar fracture, may easily occur during preparation of the knee for knee replacement or during impaction of a femoral component. It has been seen that simply lifting the lower limb by the heel in an anesthetized patient has resulted in a supracondylar fracture! And fractures may occur during manipulation of the replaced knee in the postoperative period. Fortunately the healing of fractures in RA-patients is rapid provided the fractures are sufficiently stabilized.

Apart from this considerable risk of fractures, the bone loss and the loss of mechanical strength of the remaining bone offers an even more important problem, the fixation of prosthetic components becomes extremely difficult. Fixation of the prosthetic components is mostly achieved in the subchondral bone and this bone is most affected by the formation of bone cysts and osteoporosis. The stiffness of the cancellous bone of the proximal tibia of RA-patients was shown to be 675 N/mm, compared with 1287 N/mm for normal bone and 1116 N/mm for osteoarthritic bone [3, 11]. The subchondral bone may be soft enough to be compressed with finger tip pressure [5]! This abnormal quality of bone needs to be improved and the best way to achieve this improvement is bone transplantation. Resected pieces of bone, other autologous grafts or homologous grafts may be impacted in the defects. The fixation may also be improved by the use of acrylic bone cement.

2.3   The Soft Tissues

Most knees affected by RA have an almost normal range of motion, but some patients may present a serious flexion contracture, probably the result of staying in a sedentary position for to long. The position has become structural due to shortening of the posterior soft tissues, not only of the capsule but sometimes of the dorsal superficial fascia as well. Sometimes RA-patients may present an almost ankylosed knee. An other deformity not rarely seen is the fixed valgus deformity. In this deformity most often a combination of a lateral bone defect and soft tissue contracture is found.

It is hard to assess the quality of the ligaments in RA. Physical examination of patients is too painful and bone loss is often present. There is a general belief that ligaments in the majority of RA-patients are lax [4, 7, 8]. The cruciate ligaments and the popliteus tendon within the joint are covered by synovial tissue and are likely to be affected by the inflammatory arthritis, but the peripheral ligaments are extra-articular and not covered by synovium. Maybe the collateral ligaments are not weak at all, because ruptures of collateral ligaments seldom occur in RA, not even a rupture of the medial collateral ligament in a knee with a fixed flexion-valgus deformity.

3   Traditional total knee arthroplasty in RA

Insecure about the quality of the ligaments, especially the cruciate ligaments, most surgeons preferred not to rely on them and to sacrifice them during TKA. To stabilize the knee, prostheses with intrinsic constraint were used. These prostheses require long intramedullary stems and the use of acrylic bone cement for fixation. In the light of later developments the use of cementless fixation came up, but most experts nowadays still prefer the use of cement. In the Swedish Knee Arthroplasty Register [10] it is shown that non-cemented arthroplasties fail earlier and more often than cemented arthroplasties, but the impression is that the use of cement may just delay the failure of cement and design specific differences have been demonstrated.

The important question is whether fixation with cement or without cement, or the type of prosthesis and its design for fixation, is the more important factor determining lifelong fixation and/or mechanical loosening. In the light of more recent knowledge of the kinematics of the replaced knee and the forces that are being transmitted to the bone-prosthesis interface during activities of daily life it seems probable that design details of prostheses play an important role in achieving a permanent fixation or in causing mechanical loosening.

Looking at long term results of TKAs it has become evident that intrinsic constraint of a prosthesis or the inability of components to move anatomically is detrimental for lifelong fixation of components, the tibial and patellar component in particular. Free anatomical motion is a condition for the long-lasting maintenance of fixation, but stability of the replaced knee is an important condition for normal knee function.

In this conflict between the need for stability of the replaced knee and free anatomical motion between components to secure their fixation to bone a compromise seems necessary: some anatomical motion and some intrinsic stability. The relatively low activity level of RA-patients seems to be a justification of this compromise. Because of this low activity level less rotational and shear stresses than normal in more active patients will be conducted to the bone-prosthesis interface and mechanical loosening is less likely to occur. But the surgeon needs to realize that the quality of bone for the fixation of an implant in RA-patients is inferior to the quality of bone in OA-patients, which may be of greater importance for lifelong fixation than the activity level. Moreover it should be realized that RA-patients needing knee replacement are on average 10–15 years younger than OA-patients, while their life expectancy is almost the same. So the need for duration of fixation is higher. Maybe freedom of anatomical motion of a replaced knee is, for the same reason even more important in RA-patients than in OA-patients. At least this hypothesis is justified.

Additionally in RA-patients, stability of the replaced knee is important for their daily activities. In this respect it is of interest to look again at the function of the ligaments, the natural stabilizers of the knee. As written before it is hard to judge the quality of the collateral and cruciate ligaments of the rheumatoid knee. In RA the bony attachment of the ligaments may be under-

mined by proliferation of inflamed synovial tissue. The real mechanical strength of the ligaments is insecure. The thought is justified that the mechanical strength of these ligaments is not as bad as was generally believed as ligament ruptures seldom occur while tendon ruptures present very often. The tendons are usually surrounded by inflamed synovial tissue. Inflammation of the synovium may cause a local anoxemia. The ruptures occur at places of friction on an anatomical structure. The situation of the ligaments of the knee is anatomically very different. A rupture may not very probably occur. On an MRI, it is not uncommon that an intact anterior cruciate ligament can be seen (Fig. 123a,b). Preservation of cruciate ligaments in RA may be considered!

The necessity of the use of acrylic bone cement for fixation of prosthetic components is not clear. Though it is obvious that the use of cement may result in an optimal primary fixation, it is questionable whether the advantages will last. Bone cement may deteriorate with time, which has negative consequences for patients requiring lifelong fixation. Primary stability is of great importance for lasting implant fixation. When primary fixation is good the increased turnover of bone, characteristic for RA, may promote early bone ingrowth and enhance fixation of cementless implants [2]. So cementless fixation may be successful as well. The addition of hydroxyapatite to a porous surface of tibial components has shown on roentgen stereophotogrammetric analysis to give fixation not different from cemented fixation [9].

The strength of bone itself may be improved by bone transplantation. During TKA bone resected from the femoral condyles, the articular surface of the tibia and maybe the patella, can be impacted into defects in the tibial and femoral surfaces. The amount of bone is limited but usually enough to fill most cavities. If more

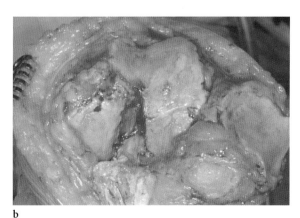

a
b

Fig. 123. a An intact anterior cruciate ligament on a MRI of a rheumatoid knee. b The same knee during surgery showing the intact anterior cruciate ligament

bone is required autograft or morselized allografts can be used. All grafts must be compacted carefully. At the tibial surface these grafts may be shaped in a dental form to reinforce the loading capacity of the subchondral bone [6].

4 The Use of the LCS Mobile Bearing Total Knee System in RA-Patients

In the LCS total knee system mobile bearings provide stability and motion of the knee. There is the possibility to retain cruciate ligaments if desirable and possible, because there is a choice between three different tibial components : one for the retention of both cruciate ligaments (BCR, Fig. 124a,b), one for retention of the posterior cruciate ligament (PCR, Fig. 125a,b) and a rotating tibial component (RP) to be used when the cruciate ligaments are absent or need to be sacrificed. Retaining cruciate ligaments should be considered only if these ligaments are healthy and sufficient and not causing a

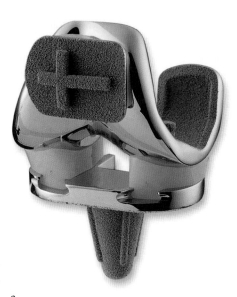

a

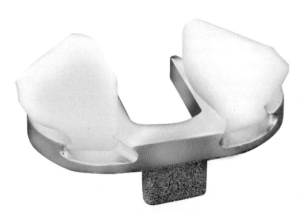

a

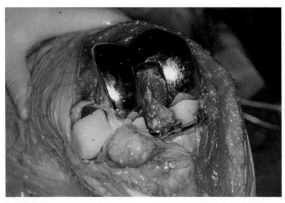

b

Fig. 124. a The bi-cruciate ligament retaining BCR tibial component. **b** the BCR tibial component implanted in the rheumatoid knee of a 25-year old patient

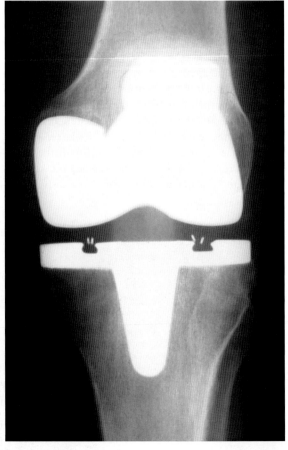

b

Fig. 125. a The posterior cruciate ligament retaining PCR tibial component. **b** The PCR tibial component implanted in the rheumatoid knee of a 36 year old patient

deformity. In most knee replacement systems retaining the anterior cruciate ligament (acl), is simply not possible because the fixation of the tibial component requires the total tibial surface and the tibial insertion of the acl is sacrificed. The question is whether mobile bearing knee arthroplasty can be done in knees of RA-patients as the ligaments play an important role in stabilizing these knees.

The components of the LCS knee may be implanted using cementless or cemented fixation. The components for cementless fixation are porous coated. Secondary fixation is meant to occur by bony ingrowth into this porous surface. The question is whether cementless fixation is possible in the soft bone of RA-patients. In RA-patients with their above mentioned increased bone turnover, this bony ingrowth is likely to occur provided a good primary fixation is achieved during implantation

The primary fixation of the BCR tibial components is limited to three short fins. The primary fixation of the PCR and RP tibial components is relying on a central cone

4.1   Clinical Experience

The Amsterdam Slotervaart Ziekenhuis is a center for the treatment of RA-patients in The Netherlands. Since 1984 the LCS mobile bearing knee system was used in all patients requiring TKA under the age of seventy. After 1990 the system was used with patients of all ages. It was the aim of the surgeons to retain the cruciate ligaments whenever these ligaments seemed sufficient during surgery. Before making bone cuts the alignment of the knees was corrected by performing subperiosteal releases. Flexion deformities were corrected by posterior capsule release, sacrifice of the posterior cruciate ligament (if the pcl was part of the deformity), and occasionally release of the external popliteal fascia. The fixation of components was mostly cementless with patients below seventy years of age and cemented above seventy and after extensive bone transplantation.. Bone grafting was considered to be of great importance to improve the quality of bone. The size of the tibial component was

chosen in such a manner as to achieve full coverage of the tibial cortices, which was not always the case, as in the early years of use of the LCS system bridging of standard and large components was not possible. Some tibial components were undersized relative to the size of the femoral component, so they did not match the surface of the resected tibia.

4.2   Materials

From November 1984 till January 1995, 783 TKAs were performed using the LCS system in 138 men and 645 women. The average age before 1990 was 59, and 65 after 1990 (Table 1).

In this chapter special attention is given to the questions whether, using the LCS mobile bearing knee system in RA-patients, fixation was reliable and ligaments remained sufficient.

4.3   Ligamentous Stability

Of 466 RA-knees, in 95 (20.4 %) both cruciate ligaments were retained and in 345 (74 %) only the posterior cruciate ligament. During a 7–17 years follow up period ligamentous instability was a reason for revision in one BCR case (1.3 %) and in four PCR cases (1.1 %). In OA cases, revision for ligamentous instability occurred in one BCR case (2.1 %) and five PCR knee replacements (2.3 %). Replaced knees of both diagnoses RA and OA completely stable after surgery and scoring 8–10 points for anterior-posterior stability according to the Knee Society score, remained stable throughout the years of follow up 7–17, average 12 years (Fig. 126). Progressive ligamentous instability mainly occurred in knees already somewhat unstable after surgery.

4.4   Fixation

In RA-patients the cementless fixation of the PCR and RP tibial components with central cone fixation was very successful: no mechanical loosening in 238 cases.

Table 1. Type of tibial component

	All		OA		RA		Other	
	n	%	n	%	n	%	n	%
BCR	149	19	48	17	95	20.4	6	18.7
PCR	578	73.8	214	75.3	345	74	19	59.4
RP	56	7.2	23	7.6	26	5.6	7	21.9
Total	783		285		466		32	

Crudibte Ligbment Tetention inaKA

Averbge AR-stbcility in Psteo Arthritis

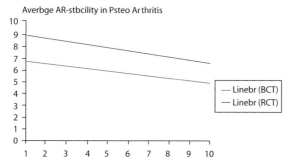

Cruciate Ligament Retention in TKA

Average AP-stability in Rheumatoid Arthritis

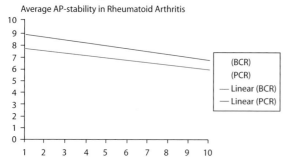

Fig. 126. The anterior-posterior stability of rheumatoid knees after retention of both cruciate ligaments (BCR) or retention of the posterior cruciate ligament only. 10 points = completely stable, 0 points = more than 1 cm translation (according to the Knee Society Score)

In 133 cases with cemented fixation one case of loosening was seen. In OA cases two loosenings were seen in 80 cases with non cemented central cone fixation and two loosenings in 157 cases with cemented cone fixation.

The BCR component with three short fins for fixation showed in the RA group four loosenings (4.2%) of cementless fixation and no loosening of two cases of cemented fixation. The three fin fixation of the BCR components in OA-patients failed in 6 of 64 cases with cementless fixation and 0 in 2 cemented cases. The 6 mechanical loosenings were associated with high tibial osteotomy. Using high tibial osteotomy as an exclusion criterion for bi-cruciate ligament retention in OA the loosening rate in OA would have been 0.

Mechanical loosening of a femoral or patellar component was never seen.

5   Discussion

The fixation of the prosthetic components of the LCS system has proven to be very reliable in RA-patients regardless of the fact whether this fixation was achieved with or without the use of bone cement. The stability of fixation was even better in RA than in OA! This may be explained by the lower activity level of most RA-patients but remains remarkable taking into account the lower stiffness of the cancellous bone of the proximal tibia of RA-patients as mentioned above. Even cementless fixation proved to be excellent demonstrating that bony ingrowth does in fact occur in the porous surfaces. The success of fixation certainly has been influenced a lot by surgical technique. The preparation of the bone bed is of great importance. After removing the articular surfaces the surgeon needs to carefully look for any soft spots and especially for the presence of subchondral bone cysts, which may not easily be detected. Any soft spot needs to be grafted preferably with autologous bone taken from the removed articular surfaces. The bone in the central part of the tibia that often needs to be removed to enable placement of the central cone of the tibial component, should not be removed but impacted. Only after reinforcing the subchondral bone will cementless fixation be successful. If allograft bone is needed to fill larger defects of subchondral bone, the subchondral bone must be carefully impacted with morselized grafts and the prosthetic component fixed to the bone with a superficial layer of bone cement.

Almost certainly the free anatomical movement of the LCS knee system relieving the bone-prosthesis interface from high rotational and shear stresses has been of great importance in enhancing permanent fixation. The biomechanics of the prosthetic design are just as important for lifelong fixation as fixation itself.

Ligamentous instability did not occur even after more than 10 years of follow up. The suggestion is that ligaments in knees of RA-patients, when found sufficient during surgery, remain sufficient for many years. This may probably not be true in elderly patients in whom degeneration of the mechanical properties of the ligaments may occur. The mere fact that ligaments function well during a considerable period of time is of great importance for RA-patients. It gives the surgeon the opportunity to perform a knee arthroplasty in a conservative manner which may be of great benefit later when revision TKA needs to be performed. The surgeon dealing with TKA in RA-patients, who are usually relatively young, must realize while performing the first knee replacement, that one day a surgeon may have to revise that knee prosthesis. Therefore a conservative attitude during primary surgery is necessary. Knowing the results mentioned above of retaining the cruciate ligaments, this may indicate the way to remain conservative during TKA in RA-patients.

6 Conclusion

- Total knee arthroplasty in RA-patients using the LCS mobile bearing total knee system has proven to be successful in a 7–17, average 12 year, follow-up study.
- Cementless fixation of components was reliable.
- Cruciate ligament retention, including retention of the anterior cruciate ligament, was reliable.

7 Total Knee Arthoplasty in the Rheumatoid Knee: Recommendations

- Soft tissue contractures must be corrected by subperiosteal releases. These releases should be done before making bone cuts.
- It is important to avoid extra stresses on bone and soft tissues as fractures may easily occur. To facilitate exposure and to provide optimal protection to bone and soft tissues an osteotomy of the tibial crest is advised.
- In ankylosed stiff knees a superficial osteotomy of the tibial articular surface may be done to facilitate the opening of the knee
- Conservative knee replacement inclusive of cruciate ligament retention is recommended in young and active patients. However cruciate ligaments being part of a deformity need to be sacrificed.
- The quality of bone must be improved by bone transplantation. During surgery the surgeon is recommended to carefully look for any weak spot in the bone. These spots must be grafted.
- Cemented fixation of implants is reliable but cementless fixation may be just as reliable when a prosthesis with free anatomical motion is used. Remember : any constraining element in the design of the prosthesis increases the stresses on the fixation to the bone, that is relatively weak in RA!

- For cementless fixation the surface of the prosthesis must be designed for bony ingrowth, e.g. with an enlarged contact surface and pores wide enough to allow bone ingrowth. Cementless implants possibly may be coated with tri-calcium-phosphate, hydroxylapatite or other material to improve the ingrowth of bone.
- The LCS has proven to be a very reliable implant in the knees of rheumatoid patients. So this implant may be safely used.

References

1. Bogoch ER, Moran EL (1999) Bone abnormalities in the surgical treatment of patients with rheumatoid arthritis. Clin Orthop 366: 8–11
2. Chmell MJ, Scott RD (1999) Total knee arthroplasty in patients with rheumatoid arthritis. Clin Orthop 336: 54–60
3. Finlay JB, Bourne RB, Kraemer WJ, Moroz TK, Rorabeck CH (1989) Stiffness of bone underlying the tibial plateaus of osteoarthritic and normal knees. Clin Orthop 247: 193–201
4. Hagena FW, Hofmann GO, Mittlmeier T, Wasmer G, Bergmann M (1989) The cruciate ligaments in knee replacement. Int Orthopaedics (SICOT) 13: 13–16
5. Hamelynck KJ. Joint replacement and osteoporosis.
6. Keblish P. Stonehedge technique of reinforcing the tibial surface. Personal communication
7. Laskin RS (1990) Total condylar knee replacement in patients who have rheumatoid arthritis. A ten-year follow-up study. J Bone Joint Surg 72 A: 529–535
8. Laskin RS, O'Flynn HM (1997) Total knee replacement with posterior cruciate retention in rheumatoid arthritis. Problems and complications. Clin Orthop 345: 24–28
9. Nelissen RGHH, Valstar ER, Rozing PM (1998) The effect of hydroxy-apatite on the micromotion of total knee prostheses. J Bone Joint Surg 80 A: 1665–1672
10. Robertson O, Knutson K, Lewold S, Goodman S, Lidgren L (1997) Knee arthroplasty in rheumatoid arthritis. A report from the Swedish Knee Arthroplasty Register on 4,381 primary operations 1985–1995. Acta Orthop Scand 68: 545–553
11. Yang JP, Woodside TD, Bogoch ER, Hearn TC (1997) Stiffness of the tibial trabecular bone in rheumatoid arthritis of the knee. J Arthroplasty 12: 798–803

Chapter 11
LCS® Multicenter Worldwide Outcome Study

11.1 The LCS Clinical Experience – An Overview of the Literature

J.B. Stiehl

1 Introduction

Mobile bearings were originally introduced with the Oxford knee in 1977 which sought to improve articular congruity for improved wear characteristics using a spherical, congruous articulation while diminishing implant constraint with a floating surface [6]. The Low Contact Stress (LCS) knee prosthesis (Depuy, Warsaw), the subject of this outcome study was a mobile bearing design with modifications of the tibial component to allow for posterior cruciate retention (meniscal bearing) or sacrifice (rotating platform). From the outset, it was recognized that a long term experience would be needed to prove the experiment that mobile bearings would solve the issues of fixation and wear through a favorable, high area of contact, wear surface and nonconstrained moveable bearings [2].

An interesting point of comparison with other fixed bearing prosthetic designs is the fact that over the years, the LCS components have remained identical in geometry from the outset of original implantation in 1977. In contrast, most implant systems have undergone substantial design changes over a period of time, thus adding complexity to any conclusions about potential long term durability. With keen interest of current prosthetic designers in the mobile bearing concept, it is important to evaluate these implants over the long term to determine which factors may predispose to late clinical failure.

This chapter will present the existing knowledge on the clinical efficacy of the LCS total knee system. We will evaluate peer reviewed publications regarding the LCS prosthesis analyzing the long term outcome and clinical performance of the femorotibial articulation, patellar resurfacing, and various issues of surgical technique such as cruciate retention or sacrifice, tibial axis alignment method of bone resection, cement versus cementless, and the lateral approach in valgus deformed knees. These results will be compared with outcome studies of total knee arthroplasty in general. We will then present the results of a multicenter outcome study evaluating the survivorship results from surgeons around the world who have extensive experience with the LCS knee.

2 LCS Clinical Experience (Literature Review)

Buechel and Pappas presented their 10 year experience with the LCS knee replacement of the first 357 total knee arthroplasties in 1989 [3]. There were 72 bicruciate retaining meniscal bearing implants, 49 posterior cruciate retaining meniscal bearing implants, and 137 posterior cruciate sacrificing rotating platform implants, with 80 revision arthroplasties. Of the entire group, there were 231 excellent results and 87 good results with 89% of the total in these categories and the remaining in fair or poor categories. In regards to complications specific to mobile bearings, there were 7 rotating platform dislocations (3.2%) and 1 traumatic meniscal bearing dislocation (0.7%). Most of the revision arthroplasties were re-revision of difficult revision cases where there was flexion instability. Factors predisposing to mobile bearing complications such as dislocation were stated to be malrotation of the tibial component allowing a meniscal bearing to sublux, late rupture of the posterior cruciate ligament, flexion/extension gap instability, and traumatic twisting of the knee joint. Three tibial components loosened (2.0%) in very heavy patients where the component poorly covered the proximal tibia. There were no femoral implant loosenings.

Buechel et al. reported their 11 year experience with the LCS metal-backed, rotating-bearing patellar prosthesis in 515 total knees of which 331 had greater than 24 month follow-up [4]. The overall postoperative fracture rate was 0.58% with avacular necrosis seen in 0.38%. There was one patellar dislocation of the entire group and no polyethylene dissociations, no polyethylene wear through and no implant loosenings. It was postulated that the deep femoral groove engagement prevented dislocation and allowed high contact, even with subluxation.

Buechel et al. studied 373 LCS total knee replacements of their initial series surviving a minimum of 10 years [1]. Of this group, 97.9% had good or excellent results with the posterior cruciate retaining meniscal bearing implant, 100% with the cemented rotating platform, and 97.9% with the cementless rotating platform. Meniscal bearing dislocation occurred in 2.5% while 5% required meniscal bearing exchange for wear at an average of 10.1 years. Rotating bearing dislocation was seen in 1.2% and there were three rotating platforms revised for wear of the overall group. Kaplan-Meier survivorship for non-infected LCS total knee replacements and mechanical loosening for any reason was 83% at 16 years for the cementless meniscal bearing group, 97.7% for the cemented rotating platform group, and 98.3% at 18 years for the cementless rotating platform group.

Stiehl et al. reported the results of the American FDA clinical trial in 147 meniscal bearing and 44 rotating platform total knees done with a cementless technique at an average of 68 months follow-up [10]. Pain was absent in 94% of meniscal bearing and 93.2% of the rotating platform knees. Range of motion averaged 120° for the meniscal bearing and 180° for the rotating platform knees (p<.001). The overall New Jersey Orthopedic Score was 93.2 for the meniscal bearing knees and 87.6 for the rotating platform knees (p<.001). The overall survivorship was 98.1% at 7 years. The overall meniscal bearing complication rate was 0.6% with one fracture and one extrusion. No rotating platform problems bearing spinouts were noted. The patellar complication rate was 1%.

Jordan et al. evaluated 473 cementless cruciate retaining meniscal bearing LCS total knees with 2–10 year follow-up (average 5 years) [7]. Mechanical failure occurred in 3.6% with meniscal bearing fracture and dislocation in 2.5%. In 1%, there was tibial subluxation resulting from ligamentous instability. Kaplan-Meier survivorship for mechanical revision for any reason was 94.6% at 8 years.

Sorrels reported the results of 525 cementless rotating platform total knees with up to 13 years follow-up [11]. The revision rate of this entire group was 5%, and tibial component exchange rate for polyethylene wear or instability was 2%. The survivorship for mechanical component failure was 92.9% (95% CI: 83–100%) at 13 years. Sorrels, et al. reported a subgroup of this experience with 117 patients younger than 65 years (average 56 years). With average follow-up of 8.5 years, the average knee score was 91 points and pain score was 27 (with a possible 30). The survivorship with revision for any reason was 88% at 14 years. The revision rate was 7% with four malpositioned implants, one infection, and one case of osteolysis. Bearing dislocation or "spin out" occurred in one case at three weeks following surgery.

Callaghan et. al. studied 114 cemented LCS rotating platform total knees with 9–12 year followup [5]. The average Knee Society clinical and functional score was 90 and 75 at final follow-up. The average active range of motion was 102° at final follow-up. In this series, there were no cases of periprosthetic osteolysis, implant dislocation, or evidence of implant loosening and none of the patients available for follow-up have been revised.

Stiehl and Voorhorst evaluated factors affecting range of motion with the LCS total knee evaluating the posterior cruciate retaining or sacrificing technique in 782 total knees [12]. Postoperative motion averaged 115° for the meniscal bearing and 104° for the rotating platform (p<0.05) but the preoperative range was significantly lower for the rotating platform. The greatest gains in motion occurred in patients with less than 90° of preoperative motion and improvement in motion was greater in patients without prior surgery.

Klebish et al. compared LCS total knees with patella u-surfacing versus LCS total knees without u-surfacing.

Keblish et al. compared resurfaced LCS total knees versus non-resurfaced LCS total knees, in 52 patients with bilateral total knee arthroplasties with an average follow-up of 5.24 years [9]. Comparing the group overall, there was no significant difference with subjective preference, performance on stairs, or the incidence of anterior knee pain. However, they recommended non-resurfacing in cases with a small patella under 19 millimeters thickness or the younger active patient and resurfacing with the very large patella and in the workmen's compensation case.

Keblish et al. reviewed their experience with the lateral parapatellar approach for the valgus deformed total knee arthroplasty in 53 patients who had undergone an LCS total knee arthroplasty [8]. The results were good/excellent in 94% of cases, and there were no failures from patellar maltracking or implant instability. They stated that a lateral release, which is needed in most of these cases, is part of the approach allowing the medial blood supply to be preserved. More recently, a coronal z-plasty has been recommended where the lateral retinacular dissection is more lateral in the superficial and then dissects medially through the synovium and fat pad allowing for a significant lateral based soft tissue mass that allows for a water tight lateral closure.

The clinical performance of the LCS total knee prosthesis remains exemplary based on long term clinical outcome studies. The incidence of bearing complications remains low, particularly with the posterior cruciate sacrificing rotating platform implant. Osteolysis and patellar problems are extremely low compared to the general total knee experience and can be cited as a primary reasons for favoring the LCS implant. Surgical technique remains an important element of success with mobile bearing implants and tibial axis alignment continues to be the preferred method of implant insertion.

References

1. Buechel FF Sr, Buechel FF Jr, Pappas MJ, D'Alessio J (2001) Twenty-year evaluation of meniscal bearing and rotating platform knee replacements. Clin Orthop Rel Res 388: 41–50
2. Buechel FF, Pappas MJ (1986) New Jersey low contact stress knee replacement system: Biomechanical rationale and review of first 123 cemented cases. Arch Orthop Tramua Surg 105: 197–204
3. Buechel FF, Pappas MJ (1989) New Jersey low contact stress knee replacement system: Ten-year evaluation of meniscal bearings. Orthop Clin N Am 20: 147–177
4. Buechel FF, Rosa RA, Pappas MJ (1989) A metal-backed, rotating-bearing patellar prosthesis to lower contact stress: An 11-year clinical study. Clin Orthop Rel Res 248: 34–49
5. Dorey F, Amstutz HC (1986) Survivorship analysis in total joint arthroplasty. J Arthroplasty 1: 63–69
6. Goodfellow JW, O'Connor J (1986) Clinical results of the Oxford knee: Surface arthroplasty of the tibiofemoral joint with a meniscal bearing prosthesis. Clin Orthop 205: 21–42
7. Jordan LR, Olivo JL, Voorhorst PE (1997) Survivorship analysis of cementless meniscal bearing total knee arthroplasty. Clin Orthop Rel Res 338: 119–123
8. Keblish PA (1991) The lateral approach to the valgus knee. Surgical technique and analysis of 53 cases with over two-year follow-up examination. Clin Orthop Rel Res 271: 52–62
9. Keblish PA, Varma AK, Greenwald AS (1994) Patellar resurfacing or retention in total knee arthroplasty. A prospective study of patients with bilateral replacements. J Bone Joint Surg 76B: 930–937
10. Stiehl JB, Voorhorst PE (1999) Total knee arthroplasty with a mobile-bearing prosthesis: Comparison of retention and sacrifice of the posterior cruciate ligament in cementless implants. Am J Orthopaedics 28: 223–228
11. Sorrels RB, Voorhorst PE, Grennwald AS (1999) The long-term clinical use of a rotating platform mobile bearing TKA. Proceedings of the 66th Annual Meeting of the American Academy of Orthopaedic Surgeons, Feb 4–8, 1999, Anaheim, CA
12. Stiehl JB, Voorhorst PE, Keblish PA, Sorrells RB (1997) Comparison of range of motion after posterior cruciate-retention or sacrifice with a mobile bearing total knee arthroplasty. Am J Knee Surg 10: 216–220

11.2 Worldwide Multicenter Outcome Study

KAREL J. HAMELYNCK, JAMES B. STIEHL, PAUL E. VOORHORST

List of Participants in the Outcome Study

BELLIER, GUY
Cabinet Goethe, Chirurgie Orthopedique & Sportive
75116 Paris, France

BEVERLAND, DAVID
Musgrave Park Hospital, Stockman; Lane
Belfast, BT9 7JB, Ireland, United Kingdom

BREITRUCK, HANS MARCEL
Rotkreuz-Krankenhaus
80634 München, Germany

BRIARD, JEAN-LOUIS
Clinique du Cèdre, Bois Guillaume
76235 Rouen-Cedex, France

CHOY, WON SIK
Department of Orthopaedic Surgery
Eulji Medical University Hospital
Choog-Ku, Taejon, 301–726, South Korea

DELCOUR, JEAN-PIERRE
C.H. Du Bois de l'Abbaye
Seraing, Belgium

DOETS, KEES
Department for Orthopaedic and Rheumatoid Surgery,
Slotervaart Ziekenhuis
1066 EC Amsterdam, The Netherlands

FRIEDERICH, NIKLAUS
Klinik für Orthopädische Chirurgie und Traumatologie
des Bewegungsapparates
Kantonsspital, 4110 Bruderholz, Switzerland

GAECHTER, ANDRÉ
Klinik für Orthopädische Chirurgie
Kantonsspital, 4110 Bruderholz, Switzerland

GEBHARD, FRANK
Klinik für Orthopädische Chirurgie und Traumatologie
des Bewegungsapparates
Kantonsspital, 9007 St. Gallen, Switzerland

HAMELYNCK, KAREL J.
Department for Orthopaedic and Rheumatoid Surgery,
Slotervaart Ziekenhuis.
1066 EC, Amsterdam, The Netherlands

HIRT, THOMAS
Klinik für Orthopädische Chirurgie und Traumatologie
des Bewegungsapparates
Kantonsspital, 4110 Bruderholz, Switzerland

JORDAN, LOUIS R.
Jordan-Young Institute, P.C.
Virginia Beach, VA 23462, USA

JUNG, YOUNG BOK
Department of Orthopaedic Surgery, Chung-ang Medical University Hospital
Yongsan-Gu, Seoul, 140–877, South Korea

KEBLISH, PETER
Orthopaedic Associates of Allentown
Allentown, PA 18103, USA

KUSTER, MARKUS
Klinik für Orthopädische Chirurgie
Kantonsspital, 9007 St. Gallen, Switzerland

MÜLLER, WERNER
4125 Riehen, Switzerland

OLSTHOORN, PAUL
Department for Orthopaedic and Rheumatoid Surgery,
Slotervaart Ziekenhuis.
1066 EC, Amsterdam, The Netherlands

RADKE, JÜRGEN
Rotkreuz-Krankenhaus, Orthopädie
80634 München, Germany

ROGAN, MACK
Morningside Clinic
Morningside, Sandton 2010, South Africa

RUTHERFORD, HOWARD
Darlington Memorial Hospital
Darlington, Co Durham DL3 6HX, United Kingdom

SORRELLS, R. BARRY
The Joint Relacement Clinic
Little Rock, Arkansas 72205, USA

STIEHL, JAMES B.
Orthopaedic Hospital Wisconsin
575 West Riverwoods Parkway, #204
Milwaukee, Wisconsin, 53212, USA

WIDMER, HEINZ
Klinik für Orthopädische Chirurgie und Traumatologie
des Bewegungsapparates
Kantonsspital, 4110 Bruderholz, Switzerland

WIESMER, THOMAS
Klinik für Orthopädische Chirurgie
Kantonsspital, 9007 St. Gallen, Switzerland

WINIA, PAUL
Department for Orthopaedic and Rheumatoid Surgery,
Slotervaart Ziekenhuis.
1066 EC, Amsterdam, The Netherlands

YAGI, TAMOTO
Yagi Orthopaedics Center
Teine-ku, Sapporo/shi 006–0029, Japan

1   Introduction

The LCS mobile bearing total knee system was designed to overcome the most important problems of total knee replacement (TKR): mechanical loosening and wear of polyethylene as seen in fixed bearing total knee systems. Mechanical loosening may result from intrinsic constraint of the components and wear is the result of high contact stresses between the components as a result of limited contact areas. Wear may cause a painful synovitis or osteolysis and subsequent loosening. Mobile bearings provide the knee with optimum, physiologically unconstrained movement. Rotational and shear forces are conducted through soft tissues rather than the prosthesis. Thus mechanical loosening may be prevented. Large contact areas are responsible for low contact stresses and so wear may be reduced to the minimum.

Thus the expectations of the use of the LCS total knee system are: anatomical motion, minimal mechanical loosening and minimal wear related problems like synovitis and osteolysis.

Another interesting aspect of the system is the possibility to retain healthy well functioning ligaments: there is a BCR tibial component with meniscal bearings for retention of both cruciate ligaments, a PCR tibial component with meniscal bearings for retention of the posterior cruciate (PCL) ligament and a RP tibial component with a rotating polyethylene platform to be used in knees where the cruciate ligaments are absent or insufficient or part of the deformity (in this condition they need to be resected). So in this system a realistic choice can be made between cruciate ligament resection or sac-

rifice. In this respect it is interesting to see that the RP tibial component has a certain amount of built in anterior-posterior stability. As a result of these options the surgeon no longer has to adapt the knee to the design of the prosthesis, but may use the prosthesis that fits the pathological condition of the patient. When the cruciate ligaments are sufficient, they may be retained. This discussion is of importance in the younger and more active patient population, where retaining cruciate ligaments may play an important role in stabilizing the knees. Elderly patients with a lower activity level and cruciate ligaments that degenerated with the arthritis, may not need cruciate ligament retention and do very well with the RP tibial component. The LCS system is the only system where a real comparison of cruciate ligament retention and sacrifice may be done because unlike other systems the articular geometry remains the same in both types of tibial components (Fig. 1).

The three different tibial components do not have the same fixation principle. The BCR component has a fixation limited to three short fins. The PCR and RP tibial component have the same tapered cone design for fixation. This fixation cannot be used in BCR components because the central cruciate bridge of the tibia is the point of insertion of the anterior cruciate ligament (ACL). Because anterior subluxation of the tibia during surgery is restricted by the presence of the ACL long fixation pegs at another location cannot be used. Looking at the results of fixation it is necessary to distinguish between these types of fixation.

The question whether the use of cement is better or worse than cementless biological fixation with bony in-

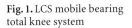

Fig. 1. LCS mobile bearing total knee system

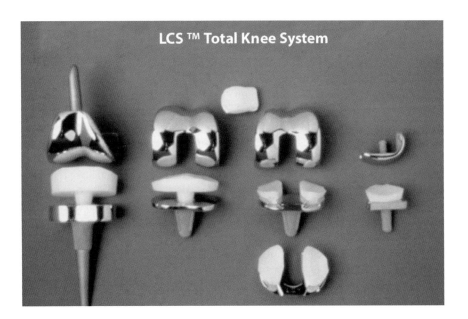

growth into a porous coated surface can only be answered by follow up studies.

The LCS total knee system comprises a well designed patellar component and a femoral component design that is nearly anatomical. In such a system the question whether the patella should be replaced or not becomes very interesting. The performance of the patellofemoral articulation in TKR does not simply depend on the design of the patellar component only. The geometry of the femoral component is equally important.

One of the intriguing questions about the use of mobile bearings is, do these bearings cause new problems that do not exist in fixed bearing knee replacement systems? This has been the fear of many orthopedic surgeons. These problems may include meniscal bearing dislocation and fracture.

For anybody studying the results of TKR it is necessary to understand that these results are dependent on more than total knee design alone. The performance of the surgeon and pathology of the patient are of great importance as well.

Correcting the overall and rotational alignment and creating balanced flexion and extension tension of the collateral and cruciate ligaments is of paramount importance when the LCS mobile bearing knee replacement system is used. Meniscal or rotating bearings are unconstrained in axial rotation, therefore subluxation or dislocation can occur when the surgeon has improperly balanced the ligaments or has not created equal flexion and extension gaps. Rotational malposition of the tibial component, especially when meniscal bearings are used, may be a reason for bearing dislocation as well. If the osteotomy of the tibial articular surface has been performed in improper anterior-posterior direction giving an inclination e.g. from anteromedial to posterolateral, this may again cause bearing dislocation. But incorrect judgement about the quality of the ligaments, may also be considered a surgical error: when the PCL is insufficient but retained by the surgeon.

It is hard to exclude the "surgical factor" in outcome studies. One way of trying to solve the problem is not to include the results of experts only, but to include as many surgeons as possible. The surgical errors will still be in the study, but the average orthopedic surgeon consulting the outcome study will be better advised, because these results may resemble more his own practice. The outcome study may also reveal that the implantation of some type of prosthesis gives a more reliable result in the hands of the average surgeon where other implantations are more difficult and probably should be restricted to specialists only.

A problem in performing outcome studies is in the fact that not every surgeon has follow up data that can be used for a study because they do not fulfill the inclusion criteria of credible studies. Best follow up is usually done in expert clinics.

The pathology of the patient certainly plays an important role in the outcome of TKR. Malalignments and deformities make high demands upon the surgeon and abnormal bone quality, bone defects and/or weakness of bone as seen in osteoporosis, requires special techniques in restoring bone quality thereby creating a better opportunity for fixation of components. In follow up studies these differences should be addressed and the question must be answered whether the use of cement is needed in conditions of poor bone quality.

The activity level of the patients is equally important. The collateral ligaments, in the absence of cruciate ligaments may be strong enough to sustain the forces of the activities of daily life, but it is questionable whether the original stability during surgery can be maintained. Progressive ligamentous instability may occur and cause serious problems in mobile bearing and fixed bearing knee replacements when ligaments stretch under the influence of excessive loads.

It is hard to find the activity level of patients in outcome studies. However there may be at least some correlation with age and disease. Generally the younger the patients the more centre they will be, and Rheumatuid patients will be less active than osteoarthritic ones. The younger the more active, and rheumatoid patients are generally less active than osteoarthritic ones.

2   Materials and methods

The purpose of the study was to document the long term survival of the LCS Knee system in a multicenter worldwide study. Centers from all over the world were asked to participate in the study. This study includes the results of surgeons from around the world with extensive experience with the LCS. The surgical technique of the LCS is standardized with a tibial cut first method utilizing instrumentation described in other chapters. Without exception, all surgeons included here utilized the recommended method. The surgeons and clinics participating in the study are listed above. Excluded were unicompartmental knee replacement and revision TKA.

Data collection was limited to those parameters required for survival analysis with the addition of patient demographic information that might impact the survival analysis results.

The only clinical parameter collected was the range of motion (ROM), since this is an objective quantifiable measure that is routinely performed by most centers. No pain, walking or other functional or clinical data were collected due to the lack of standard techniques to evaluate these parameters.

The statistical analysis was focused on survivorship using life table methods. Dorey and Amstutz suggested that survival estimates be reported only when the effective sample size is greater than 20 cases, this guideline is followed in this chapter [4]. Relationship of gender, diagnosis, previous knee surgeries, device configuration, and cement status on survival were assessed using life table methodologies.

Included were 4743 TKR's performed between February 23, 1981 and January 1, 1997. This study represents an 18 year follow-up, average 5.7 years. Over 100 cases were followed at 13 years overall.

There were 1437 males and 3306 females. The average age at surgery was 68 years. The knee was right sided in 52.2% and 47.8% left.

Diagnosis	n	%	Age
Osteoarthritis (OA)	3666	77.3	69.8.
Rheumatoid Arthritis (RA)	901	19.0	62.5
Posttraumatic Arthritis (PT)	123	2.6	62.0
Other (OTH)	53	1.1	64.1
Total	4743	100.0	68.1

In the group "other diagnoses" patients with rare diagnoses were collected. Examples are: chondrocalcinosis, haemophylia and arthritis after a previous infection e.g. tuberculosis. In this study the results of the different pathology groups will be compared.

The type of tibial component used:

	All	OA		RA		PT		OTH	
	n	n	%	n	%	n	%	n	%
BCR	324	200	61.7	114	35.2	6	1.9	4	1.2
PCR	2165	1563	72.2	541	25.0	35	1.6	26	1.2
RP	2254	1903	84.2	246	10.9	82	3.6	23	1.0
Total	4743	3666	77.3	901	19.0	123	2.6	53	1.1

The average age at surgery was:

	All	OA	RA	PT	OTH
BCR	62.8	67.6	55.6	55.5	55.8
PCR	68.1	69.8	63.9	62.2	69.1
RP	68.8	70.0	62.6	62.4	59.7
Total	68.1	69.8	62.5	62.0	64.1

Fixation: overall, 69% of all knees had cementless fixation while 31% had at least one component, either femur or tibia fixed with cement. Similarly, the patella was fixed cementless in 77% of cases. By diagnosis, for osteoarthritics, 78% of posterior cruciate retaining knees were cementless while 61% of the rotating platform knees were implanted cementless. In the rheumatoid arthritis group, 88% of the bicruciate retaining implants were cementless. Similarly, 95% of bicruciate retaining patellar implants were inserted cementless in this group. By implant type, 86% of patellas were implanted without cement in the bicruciate retaining knees; 74% were implanted without cement in posterior cruciate retaining knees; and 80% were implanted without cement in rotating platform knees.

Cementless fixation in percentages per type of tibial component and diagnosis:

	All	OA	RA	PT	OTH
BCR	75.9	67.5	88.6	100.0	100.0
PCR	74.9	77.7	66.4	82.9	76.9
RP	62.0	61.6	57.3	84.1	65.2
Total	68.8	68.8	66.7	84.6	73.6

The patella was replaced in 2838 knees (60%) and not replaced in 1905 knees (40%).

Of the replaced patellae 2198 (77.4%) were fixed without the use of bone cement and 640 (22.6%) with the use of cement.

Cementless fixation of patella components by percentage:

	All	OA	RA	PT	OTH
BCR	85.9	77.3	94.2	100.0	100.0
PCR	73.7	77.2	66.4	82.6	61.5
RP	80.1	81.9	64.4	85.1	66.7
Total	77.4	79.6	70.2	85.1	68.0

3 Results

3.1 Range of Motion

The only clinical parameter collected in this study was the range of motion, since this is an objective quantifiable measure that was routinely performed by most centers.

The overall average range of motion at last follow up examination was 110° and was similar for each type of tibial implant and barely influenced by the pathology of the patients, or whether the patients had undergone prior knee surgeries.

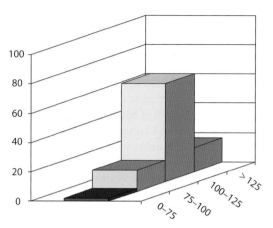

Fig. 2. Range of motion at latest follow-up: <75 degrees, between 75 and 100 degrees, between 100 and 125 degrees, and >125 degrees

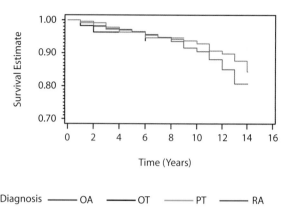

Fig. 3. Survivorship curve for all reasons of revision in the pathology groups OA, RA, PT and OT

The pre-operative results (in brackets) of all patients and pathologies are compared to those at the last follow-up.

Range of motion:

	All	OA	RA	PT	OTH
BCR	110.2 (100.6)	110.5	109.5	111.5	116.7
PCR	111.9 (94.8)	112.5	110.9	104.1	107.9
RP	108.7 (98.9)	108.9	108.4	108.1	97.6
Total	110.2	110.4	110.0	107.1	104.0

A more detailed overview of the postoperative range of motion reveals, that a considerable amount of patients acquired a range of motion of more than 125 degrees (Fig. 2).

3.2 Failure Analysis

With failure defined as revision for any reason, the survivorship was 79% (95% C.I.: 74% to 84%) at 15 years follow up this included a total of 259 (5.4%) of the entire cohort of patients.

The overall survivorship for osteoarthritic patients was 80% at 15 years while that for rheumatoid patients was 85%. By implant type, the 14 year survivorship for bicruciate retaining implants was 79%; posterior cruciate retaining implants was 82%; and rotating platform was 87%. When we look at the survivorship rates at 10 years follow-up, the comparison is 89% for bicruciate retaining, 91% for the posterior cruciate retaining, and 94% for the rotating platform implants. The overall 14 year survivorship for cementless fixation was 83% and cemented fixation, 84% (Fig. 3, 4).

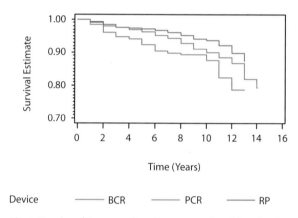

Fig. 4. Survivorship curve for all reasons of revision for the three tibial components: BCR, PCR and RP

The authors were able to distinguish four main groups of reasons for failure of TKA

- biological reasons:
  - infection,
  - other biological reasons: arthrofibrosis, ectopic bone formation;
- insufficient surgery:
  - malposition of femoral, tibial or patellar component,
  - femoral component too big,
  - knee too tight,
  - residual malalignment,
  - insufficient fixation during surgery: whenever a revision of a component was needed within one year after surgery, this was considered a mistake by the surgeon and not a failure of the prosthesis;
- failures due to trauma:
  - femur fracture,
  - tibia fracture;

- prosthesis related reasons:
  - aseptic loosening of prosthetic components,
  - bearing problems:
    meniscal bearing dislocation, fracture, polyethylene wear,
    rotating platform spinout, dislocation, polyethylene wear,   ·
  - patella problems: bearing fracture, dissociation, wear, dislocation, malposition,
  - instability: instability may be considered to be a surgical mistake as well, as will be discussed later, but may also be the result from the type of prosthesis used.

3.3   Biological Reasons for Failure

Infection. Infection was a reason for revision in 20 cases, 0.42 %. Infection was evenly distributed over the pathologies:

	n	Infection	%
OA	3666	15	0.41
RA	901	4	0.44
PT	123	0	0.0
OT	53	1	1.89
Total	4743	20	0.42

The percentage of reported infections is low and evenly distributed over the pathologies, osteoarthritis and rheumatoid arthritis especially, remarkable.

Other reasons for failure. Other biological reasons for revision were: arthrofibrosis and scar tissue in 5 cases and ectopic bone formation in 1 case, a total of 6 cases, or 0.13 % of the revisions.

3.4   Insufficient Surgery

This was as a reason for revision in 23 cases or 0.48 %. The reasons were:

- malposition femoral component   2
- malposition tibial component   5
- malposition patellar component   1
- insufficient fixation femoral component   1
- insufficient fixation tibial component   6
- insufficient fixation patellar component   1
- residual malalignment   4
- femoral component too big   2
- knee too tight   1

In 1 case only all components were revised. Other solutions were; exchange of tibial and patellar bearing in 1, revision of only the patellar component in 2, revision of only the tibial component in 12, revision of tibial and patellar component in 2, revision of femoral component and tibial bearing in 1, revision of femoral and tibial component in 1 and revision of only the femoral component in 3 cases.

3.5   Failure Due to Trauma

Revision of the prosthesis due to a trauma was needed in 6 cases or 0.13 %: There was 4 femoral fractures and 2 tibial fractures causing the need for revision.

3.6   Prosthesis Related Problems

3.6.1   Aseptic Loosening
Femoral Component. Of 4743 femoral components 2 components were revised for aseptic loosening.

Patellar Component. In this study of 4743 TKA's the patella was replaced in 2838 knees. No loosening of a patellar component was reported.

Tibial Component. The fixation of the tibial component was either with or without the use of bone cement. In cementless fixation prosthetic components with a porous coated surface for bony ingrowth were used. The survivorship for aseptic loosening was 95 % (C.I.: 91 %–98 %).
Failure of *cementless* fixation in numbers:

	All	OA	RA	PT	OTH
BCR	18	10	7	1	0
PCR	19	13	5	0	1
RP	14	13	1	0	0
Total	51	36	13	1	1

Or in percentages for the three components:

	All	OA	RA	PT	OTH
BCR	7.4	7.4	7.0	0.3	0.0
PCR	1.1	1.1	1.4	0.0	0.0
RP	1.1	1.1	0.8	0.0	0.0

The results are visualized in the survival curves:

- survival curve for aseptical loosening of cementless fixation of the three tibial components for all diagnoses (Fig. 5),

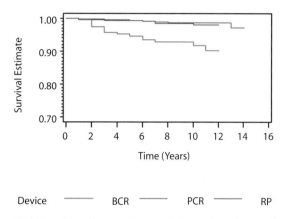

Fig. 5. Survivorship curve for aseptic loosening of cementless fixation of the tibial components BCR, PCR and RP for all diagnoses

- survival curve for aseptic loosening of cementless fixation of the three tibial components in patients with osteoarthritis (Fig. 6),
- survival curve for aseptic loosening of cementless fixation of the three tibial components for the diagnosis rheumatoid arthritis (Fig. 7).

Failure of cemented fixation in numbers:

	All	OA	RA	PT	OTH
BCR	2	2	0	0	0
PCR	4	2	2	0	0
RP	4	2	2	0	0
Total	10	6	4	0	0

Or in percentages:

	All	OA	RA	PT	OTH
BCR	2.6	3.1	0.0	0.0	0.0
PCR	0.7	0.6	1.1	0.0	0.0
RP	0.5	0.3	1.9	0.0	0.0

The results are visualized in the survival curves:

- survival curve for aseptic loosening of cemented fixation of the three tibial components for all diagnoses (Fig. 8),
- survival curve for aseptic loosening of cemented fixation of the three tibial components for the diagnosis osteoarthritis (Fig. 9),
- survival curve for aseptic loosening of cemented fixation of the three tibial components for the diagnosis rheumatoid arthritis (Fig. 10).

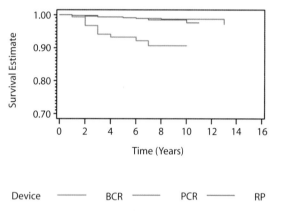

Fig. 6. Survivorship curve for aseptic loosening of cementless fixation of the tibial components BCR, PCR and RP for the diagnosis: osteoarthritis

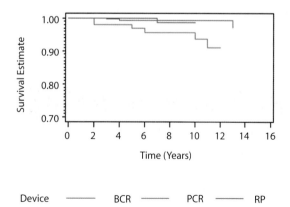

Fig. 7. Survivorship curve for aseptic loosening of cementless fixation of the tibial components BCR, PCR and RP for the diagnosis: rheumatoid arthritis

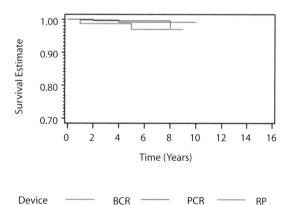

Fig. 8. Survivorship curve for aseptic loosening of cemented fixation of the tibial components BCR, PCR and RP for all diagnoses

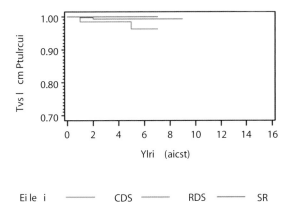

Fig. 9. Survivorship curve for aseptic loosening of cemented fixation of the tibial components BCR, PCR and RP for the diagnosis osteoarthritis

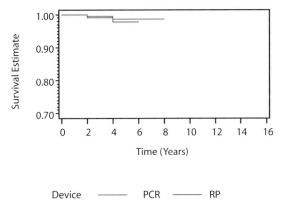

Fig. 10. Survivorship curve for aseptic loosening of cemented fixation of the tibial components BCR, PCR and RP for the diagnosis rheumatoid arthritis

3.6.2 Bearing Problems

The most common cause of revision was bearing related issues including chronic instability, bearing subluxation, bearing dislocation, or bearing failure in 1.8% of all patients

Bearing problems included meniscal bearing problems like dislocation, fracture and wear encountered in knees with BCR and PCR components and bearing subluxation or spinout and wear in rotating platform bearings as listed below.

	n	Bearing Problem n	Bearing Problem %	Bearing Exchange n	Bearing Exchange %	Revision of Tibial Component
BCR	324	7	2.2	3	0.9	4
PCR	2165	65	3.0	42	1.9	23
RP	2254	12	0.5	9	0.4	3
Total	4743	84	1.8	54	1.1	30

It is important to notice that bearing failures were not necessarily treated by revision of the tibial component. In 54 cases (64%) the treatment was bearing exchange. This treatment may be done in day treatment or require only a few days of hospital stay, is relatively inexpensive because no implants, except for a bearing, are used, and immediate weight bearing is allowed.

3.6.3 Patella Problems

The survivorship of knees that had resurfaced patellas, when considering all causes of failure was 80% at 14 years, while in the unresurfaced patellar group, survivorship was 91% at 13 years. The survivorship of the patella implants, for revision of patella related complications, was 98.5% at 15 years.

Of the 1905 non-resurfaced patellae in this study, 2 were resurfaced as a secondary procedure.

In the 2838 knee replacements with resurfaced patellae, reasons for failure were:

Surgery Related	Malposition of patellar component	4
	Subluxation and maltracking	5
	Patella baja	1
Prosthesis Related	Bearing fracture	2
	Bearing wear	13
	Bearing dissociation	5
Total		30

Not a single loosening of a patellar component was reported.

The treatment of the patellar problems: patella bearing exchange in 6, revision of patellar component in 20, removal of patellar component in 1, and a realignment procedure in 3.

3.6.4 Instability

Instability was a reason for revision in 1 BCR case (0.3%), 20 PCR cases (0.9%) and 6 RP cases (0.3%)

The treatment was revision of the tibial component in 16 cases (59%) and bearing exchange in 11 cases (41%).

	n	%	Revision of Tibial Component	Bearing Exchange
BCR	1	0.3	1	0
PCR	20	0.9	14	6
RP	6	0.3	1	5
Total	27	0.6	16	11

3.6.5   Other Reasons for Ending Follow-up

Three other prostheses were lost: 1 as result of an amputation of the femur following an infection, 1 as result of a leg amputation after fracture and 1 after revision in another hospital for an unknown reason.

4   Discussion

Total knee arthroplasties with well designed fixed-bearing prostheses have provided long-term fixation with prosthetic survival rates of 95 to 97 percent at ten to fifteen years [2]. Recent studies have failed to show substantial differences of variables such as cemented or cementless fixation; posterior cruciate retention, substitution or sacrifice; or specific prosthetic design issues such as flat on flat condylar geometry versus a more dished fixed bearing design, or the type of posterior stabilizer used in a posterior substituting design. Robertsson et al. have reported the most recent update of the Swedish Knee Arthroplasty Register in 1999 indicating that the overall revision rate for total knee arthroplasty is about 1 % per year [7]. From that study, it was difficult to isolate the performance of particular tricompartmental fixed bearing total knees as being superior or inferior due to the divergence of confidence intervals. Patellofemoral failures have been exaggerated in prior studies due to poorly designed metal backed components, patellar complications such as fracture or subluxation, and more subtle problems such as patellar "clunk". These reports have indicated an incidence of problems in 4 to 21 % of cases [6]. Polyethylene wear related osteolysis is another failure mechanism causing the need for revision with certain problematic designs noted from 16 to 30 % in certain series [5, 9].

How then can we define a prosthetic design that performs better than average and has a greater expectation of longevity and durability. In the first place, the implant must perform at least as well as the "gold standard" in terms of mechanical loosening, osteolysis, overall revision rate, and the absence of glaring issues such as patellar clunk or polyethylene failure. There must be adequate experience with a specific prosthetic design over an extended period of time. Two logical criticisms can be made of recent retrospective reports. The implants of a long-term follow-up series are commonly modified during the period of study or are no longer in vogue. Secondly, a specific problem is identified and then data analysis segregates out that data subset from the overall conclusions of the experience. The suggested implication is that the newer improved version of an implant design is better than original due to the evolutionary changes. The clinical performance of

an implant is then compared by certain favorable aspects such as mechanical loosening or absence of the need for lateral release. These conclusions may be true for the most part but realistic conclusions regarding overall outcome are called for. For example if the revision rate for a particular total knee implant is 10 % due to a poor patellar design and resulting osteolysis, the statement of favorable performance from a low mechanical femorotibial loosening rate and a survivorship of 98 % is disingenuous. A better approach would be to compare the overall revision rate or survivorship for any reason.

The LCS total knee experience is unique in several regards. Most importantly, this implant has remained successful though unmodified in nearly 25 years of continuous use. There have been some minor changes such as altering the meniscal bearing polyethylene design when it was shown that minor subluxation could cause edge fracture of the implant. The basic implant geometry continues to be considered satisfactory and evolutionary from a design standpoint. Finally, the surgical technique of the tibial axis alignment method with the tibia cut first has continued to remain the standard method of implant insertion, though several instrument improvements have been made over the years.

Outcome studies of the designer have the longest clinical follow-up and continue to show successful performance. It would be pointed out however, that the incidence of bearing failure and fracture with the meniscal bearings has proven significantly greater than that of the rotating platform after ten years though the overall revision rate continues to be about 1 % per year. Buechel et al. noted bearing dislocation in 2.5 % of meniscal bearings while only of 1.2 % of rotating platforms dislocated [1]. This was unexpected, as the meniscal bearing was projected to have greater potential for long term performance while the rotating platform was reserved for more complex and difficult cases. The contemporary view is that the rotating platform will show the greatest long term durability though some surgeons remain enthralled with the better clinical function of meniscal bearing implants. All studies compared have shown greater range of motion with the meniscal bearings and posterior cruciate retention compared to the rotating platform with posterior cruciate sacrifice.

Non-designer studies have shown similar long-term results with survivorship, revision rates, and bearing failures. It is interesting to note that the long term studies quoted in this report include primarily the initial experience of the original surgeon study group. All surgeons including Buechel, Sorrells, Keblish, and Jordan participated in the FDA Investigational Device Exemption study initiated in 1984. Sorrells has pointed out that nearly 50% of the mechanical failures in his study were related to early surgeon error due to prosthesis malalignment and ligament imbalance, mistakes that could be avoided with improved surgical technique and the availability of more implant sizes.

The current worldwide survivorship study has provided some interesting data that we believe confirm our overall opinion of the clinical durability of the LCS system.

Infection of a replaced knee remains one of the very serious complications of TKA. It is fortunate to observe this complication occurred in 0.42% of the cases of this extensive follow up study only. In the study surprisingly an even percentage of infection is seen in OA and RA patients. This does not correspond with the literature, but is the experience of the authors as well.

Arthrofibrosis may form a nasty complication. The prosthesis seems to be well implanted. Infection parameters don't show any sign of a low grade infection. The range of motion is limited and remains limited despite manipulations (not without risk) and open debridement.

In chapter 10.7 of this book a possible cause of the development of arthrofibrosis is described. There may be a strong correlation between malrotation of the femoral component and arthrofibrosis. This may be corrected surgically by revision of the femoral component. The better option is prevention. As well known by LCS surgeons, the tibial cut first technique and femoral rotation based on the use of the LCS femoral resection guide positioner will automatically result in a rotational position of the femoral component with the transepicondylar axis parallel to the cut tibial surface and perpendicular to the tibial axis.

Insufficient surgery unfortunately remains an important reason for revision. The authors wanted to distinguish the "surgeon" factor to point out clearly that perfect surgical technique still is mandatory for successful TKA.

In 0.48% of the cases insufficient surgery was a cause for revision, but the percentage is probably higher. In the part "patellar problems" of this chapter surgical errors are responsible for another 0.35% of the failures necessitating revision. In the part "instability" some of the instabilities causing revision may have been the result of insufficient surgery as well. The total percentage of surgery related causes of failure may roughly be calculated to be 1% (Fig. 11).

The capacity of the surgeon to create equal flexion-extension gaps remains the essential part of the LCS surgical technique. By creating equal flexion-extension gaps the ligaments will be in tension and stability is realized.. The question remains however whether these liga-

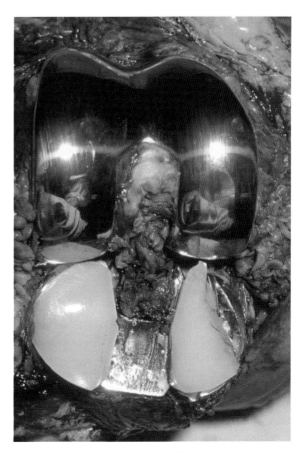

Fig. 11. Synovia blackened by metallosis due to a meniscal bearing fracture

ments will be strong enough to sustain the loads of daily life or traumatic situations. The surgeon during surgery will have to make a decision about the quality of the ligaments by eye and/or manual testing. It may be hard to judge the quality of a ligament, the PCL especially. In the chapters 4, 9.2, 9.3 and 9.4 of this book the theoretical advantages and disadvantages of cruciate ligament retention are discussed.

In the outcome study ligamentous instability was a reason for revision in 27 cases: 1 BCR component (0.3%), 20 PCR components (0.9%) and 6 RP components (0.3%). The low percentages reflect the good anterior-posterior and medial-lateral stability of the BCR and RP knee replacements.

The BCR patients were relatively younger (average 62.8 years) and probably more active. The occurrence of only 1 instability necessitating revision may be an indication that retention of cruciate ligaments is a good option in young patients as far as the condition of the ligaments is concerned.

The RP patients were on average 68.8 years. The reliability of the stability by limited intrinsic constraint of

the tibial bearing and the quality of the collateral ligaments in this category of relatively elderly people is of
great importance, because the quality of the PCL is questionable in the elderly. The result indicates that more intrinsic constraint in the absence of functioning cruciate ligaments is not necessary in these elderly patients,
which form the majority of patients needing TKA.

Retention of the PCL was not successful in 0.9% of the
cases. During revision surgery, the ligament was considered as insufficient in 14 of these cases, but sufficient in 6.
An important question is whether the PCL was sufficient
or not, at the time of surgery. And another question is;
do these ligaments become insufficient and stretch over
time. Looking at the average age of the patients, 68.1 years,
it seems obvious that at least some ligamentous insufficiency has resulted from degeneration. On the other hand
one of the authors (KH) has observed that knees stable after surgery remained stable in a ten years postop. period
(chapter 9.2). Insufficiency of the PCL probably results
from some residual instability accepted during surgery.
This may reflect the difficult choice for the surgeon to balance the PCL correctly. The surgeon may end with a PCL
that is "too loose" or "too tight", with subsequent stretching or rupture of the ligament. The authors have the opinion that during surgery the surgeon should not only think
about the present situation, but about the future (with a
possible degeneration of the PCL) as well. In the chapter
9.3 it is clearly postulated that PCL retention should be
considered in patients below 65 years. Above that age the
PCL may degenerate in future years.

Fixation does not offer a great problem in the LCS
total knee system with the exception of the BCR tibial
component.

Aseptic loosening of a femoral and patellar component virtually non-existent: of the 4743 femoral components 2 were revised. Of the 2838 resurfaced patellae not
a single was revised for loosening.

The fixation of the tibial component was cementless
in 77.4% of all cases, 85.9% of the BCR components, 73.7
of the PCR components and 80.1% of the RP components (Fig. 12).

The fixation of the BCR component relying on three
short fins only failed in 7.4% of the components with
cementless fixation and in 2.6% of the cases with cemented fixation In OA patients fixation of BCR components failed in 7.4% of non-cemented cases and in 3.1%
of cemented cases. In RA, fixation of BCR components
failed in 7.0% of cementless fixation; there were no cases
with cemented fixation. The use of bone cement considerably contributes to the fixation of the BCR tibial components with the three short fin fixation. In the extensive
experience with bi-cruciate retention TKA of one of the
authors (KH), a strong correlation was found between

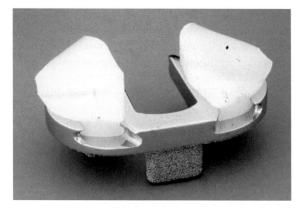

Fig. 12. Three short fin fixation of the tibial component

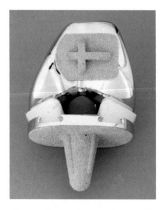

Fig. 13. Central tapered cone fixation of the PCR and RP tibial component

aseptic loosening of the BCR tibial component and previous high tibial osteotomy. This condition should be a
contra-indication against the use of the BCR component.
The PCR or RP component should be used (Fig. 13).

The central tapered cone fixation of the PCR and RP
tibial components is identical.

The percentages for aseptic loosening of these components is practically identical as well:

- Failure of non-cemented PCR components is 1.1%
  and failure of cemented fixation is 0.7%.
- Failure of non-cemented RP components is 1.1%
  and failure of cemented fixation is 0.5%.

There is a slight advantage of cemented fixation over cementless fixation at the longest follow up in OA, but not
in RA. This may be caused by the quality of bone in RA.
Cement alone is not the solution for the fixation of tibial components in RA. Before fixation the bone quality
needs improvement by the transplantation of bone.

The theoretical advantages of meniscal bearings and
rotating platform bearings, to optimize the kinematics

of total knee systems, to relieve the stresses from the interface and minimize mechanical loosening, and to reduce the contact stresses and so reduce wear, have been embraced by many orthopedic surgeons. However there has been the constant fear that these bearings might cause new problems like dislocation and fracture

In this outcome study the overall percentage of bearing problems was 1.8%: 2.2% of meniscal bearings in BCR components, 3.0% of meniscal bearings in PCR components and 0.5% in RP components. Included are all problems, not only bearing dislocations or rotating platform spinouts. It has been identified that minor subluxation could cause fracture of the flexible lip of a meniscal bearing. A minor design change of the meniscal bearing solved that problem. The basic implant geometry remained unaltered.

The original polyethylene was not always of superior quality. The implants were sterilized by gamma in air radiation, a technique which has shown to enhance subsurface oxidation and delamination of the polyethylene and was later abandoned.

Follow-up studies of the LCS system have revealed that meniscal bearing dislocations may result from surgical errors like malrotational position of the tibial component, insufficient stability in flexion and the preservation of an insufficient PCL.

Meniscal bearing problems do not necessarily need to be treated by revision of the tibial component: bearing exchange is a realistic option: 3 of 7 meniscal bearing problems were solved by bearing exchange in BCR knee replacements. 42 of 65 meniscal bearing problems in PCR knees were treated by bearing exchange as well.

As a result of these considerations it is hard to make a final judgement about meniscal bearings. It is certainly true that most of the problems are caused by surgical mistakes, early polyethylene problems and meniscal bearing design (which was changed). Using the new design meniscal bearing (1989) made of improved and well sterilized polyethylene, and implanted in a well balanced knee with equal flexion and extension gaps, may result in optimal lifelong performance of the total implant. This is of particular interest for the BCR total knee with good anterior-posterior stability. There seems to be no reason not to use this form of conservative knee replacement in the young and active patient.

The RP tibial bearing showed problems in only 0.5% of the cases. In 9 of the 12 cases the solution was bearing exchange. The performance of this implant without any doubt is excellent.

One of the reasons cited for improved mobile bearing performance has been improved polyethylene wear related to the high conformity and low surface contact stresses of the articulation. Long term clinical follow-ups certainly support this design objective as cases of overt osteolysis are virtually nonexistent. In this multi center study, like in studies reported in the overview of the literature some wear was reported, but not a single case of osteolysis. Collier evaluated the one case identified by Sorrells, et al. finding substantial polyethylene inclusions and oxidation in that particular implant. Collier has also stated that retrieval analysis of a large number of LCS implants have revealed few of the findings typical of fixed bearing retrievals such as pitting and delamination wear (see chapter 8.2). This was noted despite the prevalence of gamma in air sterilization in most of these retrievals which is known to cause surface oxidation and much higher wear rates [3].

The results of patellar resurfacing were extremely favorable with an overall complication rate of 0.5% and a 15 year survivorship of 98.5%. We attribute this to a variety of factors including the favorable anatomical shape of the femoral component with deepened intercondylar sulcus, the tibia cut first technique which optimizes femoral component external rotation, and the highly conforming mobile patellar implant that optimizes both wear issues and function.

Perhaps the most outstanding clinical performance of the LCS prosthesis has been the paucity of patellofemoral complications and satisfactory outcome with patella non-resurfacing. From all LCS clinical series noted to date including the current worldwide outcome study, the overall patellar resurfacing complication rate is about 1% despite the long-term use of a metal backed patellar component. The LCS patella is unique in several aspects, allowing high conformity for improved wear yet allowing near anatomical patellar kinematics as shown by recent kinematic fluoroscopy studies [8]. Patellar component loosening is virtually nonexistent and this may be attributed to the unconstrained mobility allowed by the implant as well as the physiological positioning allowed by the deepened intercondylar groove of the femoral component. The clinical experience with the unresurfaced patella has been equal to that of resurfacing and would be the recommended technique of many European surgeons.

The authors believe the results of this study are unique for several reasons. In the first place, this study was not performed predominantly by a small trial of surgeons from university settings but more likely in community settings by high volume practicing orthopedists. From our knowledge, neither the technique nor the implant has changed in any major way during the entire 18 year study. By including failure for any reason, we were not segregating our data to focus on some particular strength of the system at the expense of the overall experience.

5 Conclusion

This multi center worldwide outcome study has confirmed the favorable results of the LCS total knee system as reported in the literature.

The overall range of motion demonstrated in the three types of tibial components was 110 degrees, PCL retaining knees having a slightly better flexion than RP replacements. The flexion was more than 125 degrees in 16 % of the cases, indicating that this flexion is not inhibited by the prosthesis.

Infection (0.42 %), arthrofibrosis (0.13 %), surgical mistakes (0.48 %) and trauma (0.13 %) caused 1.16 % of the revisions.

Aseptic loosening of a femoral or patellar component did virtually not occur.

The fixation of the tibial components with a central tapered cone, PCR and RP, was reliable. These components are mostly used in the orthopedic world: implanted were 4743 tibial components: 2165 PCR and 2254 RP components. Failure of fixation occurred in 1.1 % of the cementless cases (PCR and RP) and in 0.7 % and 0.5 % of the cemented cases, PCR and RP respectively.

The fixation of the BCR tibial component with three short fin fixation was less reliable: the cementless fixation failed in 7.4 % and cemented fixation failed in 2.6 %.

Cemented fixation seems to give better results, but more factors are involved than the use of cement.

Bearing problems occurred in 1.8 % of all patients: 2.2 % in BCR knees, 3.0 % in PCR knees and 0.5 % in RP knees. Bearing problems like dislocation and subluxation may result from surgical mistakes (insufficient ligament balancing in flexion, malrotation position of a tibial or femoral component, retention of an insufficient PCL). Fractures and wear may also result from instability, but may also be caused by inadequate quality of the polyethylene either by production method or by sterilization. The design of the meniscal bearing was responsible as well: minor subluxations could cause a fracture of the flexible lip of the bearing. After a minor design change in 1989 this problem was not encountered anymore.

The rotating platform bearing caused problems in only 0.5 % of the cases. Bearing exchange was the simple solution for 9 of 12 problem cases out of a total of 2254 RP components.

Meniscal bearing and rotating platform bearing problems may well be solved by bearing exchange.

The survivorship of the patella implants for only revision of patella related complications was 98.5 % at 15 years. Not a single component was revised for loosening. The patella bearing may easily be exchanged. Not replacing the patella gave equally good results. Not replacing the patella is a realistic option with the LCS. This excellent performance is the result of design and surgical technique. The geometry of the femoral component with a deepened intercondylar sulcus is almost anatomical, the highly conforming mobile patellar component allows high conformity for improved wear yet allows near anatomical patellar kinematics. The surgical technique with a tibial cut first and excellent balancing of the flexion gap stability also creates perfect femoral rotation with the transepicondylar axis perpendicular to the tibial axis.

The LCS was designed in the seventies. The prosthesis has remained new and futuristic among many other designs of total knee prostheses, coming and going. Today we may show that the expectations have been realised true: implantation of this prosthesis in the vast majority of cases results in an excellent clinical performance with a low percentage of failures, which may easily be treated.

References

1. Buechel FF Sr, Buechel FF Jr, Pappas MJ, D'Alessio J (2001) Twenty-year evaluation of meniscal bearing and rotating platform knee replacements. Clin Orthop Rel Res 388: 41–50
2. Callaghan JJ, Squire MW, Goetz DD et al. (2000) Cemented rotating platform total knee replacement. J Bone Joint Surg 82A: 705–711
3. Collier JP, Mayor MB, McNamara JL et al. (1991) Analysis of the failure of 122 polyethylene inserts from uncemented tibial knee components. Clin Orthop 273: 232–242
4. Dorey F, Amstutz HC (1986) Survivorship analysis in total joint arthroplasty. J Arthroplasty 1: 63–69
5. Ezzet KA, Garcia R, Barrack RL (1995) Effect of component fixation method on osteolysis in total knee arthroplasty. Clin Orthop 321: 86–91
6. Malkani AL, Rand JA, Bryan RS, Wallrichs SL (1995) Total knee arthroplasty with kinematic condylar prosthesis. J Bone Joint Surg 77A: 423–431
7. Robertsson O, Knutson K, Lewold S, Lidgren L (1999) Knee arthroplasty for osteoarthritis and rheumatoid arthritis 1986–1995. Proceedings Annual Meeting of the American Academy of Orthopaedic Surgeons, Feb 1–4, 1999, Anaheim, CA
8. Stiehl JB, Dennis DA, Komistek RD, Keblish PA (2001) In vivo kinematics of the patellofemoral joint in total knee arthroplasty. J Arthroplasty 16: 706–714
9. Whiteside LA (1994) Four screws for fixation of the tibial component in cementless total knee arthroplasty. Clin Orthop 299: 72–76

11.3 Biological Fixation in Uncemented Mobile Bearing TKA

T. Y. Kashiwagi, J. G. Boldt, P. A. Keblish

1 Introduction

Prosthetic fixation in TKA is multi-factorial and depends on biomechanical alignment, bone quality, surgical technique, and prosthetic design of the articulating and fixation interfaces. Failures of original fixed-bearing TKA stimulated design changes to address issues of patella tracking, bearing overload, and fixation. Cementless fixation was introduced in the early 1980s to address cement-related failures in an attempt to allow for potential lifetime fixation. However, some design changes increased constraint at the articulating interface with increased fixation stress and resulted in aseptic loosening. Tibial fixation concerns without cement resulted in the addition of screws, fins, etc., to provide for initial stable fixation. Changes, such as addition of tibial platform screws, have added other problems, including easier access of backside polyethylene wear and osteolysis [14].

Mobile bearing designs address the dilemma of high constraint and fixation interface stress in TKA. Rotation and/or translation at the tibial – bearing interface, decreases the stress at the cemented prosthesis-bone or cementless (surface-coated) prosthesis bone interfaces. One of the primary goals of the LCS system is to decrease fixation interface stress by improving femorotibial congruity whilst increasing rotational/transitional mobility at the polished backside articulating surfaces. Early results with cement fixation utilizing the LCS mobile-bearing TKA were encouraging. Meniscal and rotating platforms with fully porous-coated, metallic tibial surfaces, which underwent a successful Food and Drug Administration Investigational Device Exemption (FDA IDE) protocol, have been available for general use since the early 1990s (query date). Many mobile bearing TKA designs are now available.

This study focuses on radiographic evaluation of cementless fixation in TKA in LCS meniscal bearing and rotating platform cases performed by a single surgeon, with independent clinical evaluation (TK) utilizing the Knee Society guidelines for radiographic analysis. Results will focus on radiographic zonal analysis and tibial fixation outcomes.

2 Materials and Methods

Of 709 consecutive primary cementless TKA, 567 cases with complete radiographic and clinical review entered the study. All cases were performed by one senior author or under his direct supervision between May 1984 and December 1996. Mean follow-up was 5.7 years (2.0 to 14.9). There were 369 (65.1%) females and 198 (34.9%) males with a mean age of 68.6 years (32 to 94). Primary diagnosis was osteoarthritis (OA) in 502 (88.5%) cases, rheumatoid arthritis (RA) in 47 (8.3%) cases, and other non-inflammatory diagnoses in 18 cases (3.2%).

Prosthetic components utilized were the LCS anatomic femoral and metal-backed rotating patella designs (Fig. 14).

The patella was resurfaced in 29%, and not resurfaced in 71%. Two different tibial designs were utilized, rotating platform and meniscal bearing. The tapered cone design (n=523) was utilized in both the PCL-sacrificing rotating bearing (n=168) and the PCL-retaining meniscal polyethylene bearing inserts (n=445). Both tibial designs are identical at the bone interface side (Fig. 15),

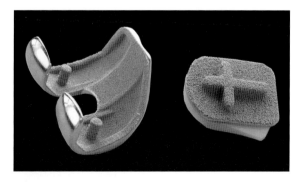

Fig. 14. Femoral and patellar design – porous-coated fixation surfaces

but different on the bearing subsurface side. The cruciate ligament sacrificing design is open centrally to accommodate for the rotating platform; the PCL-retaining design has a posterior cut-out for the PCL-retaining meniscal bearings with the same outer cone. The 3-fin design (n=44) allows for the ACL/PCL meniscal bearing polyethylene inserts, which requires retention of the

cruciate bridge and, therefore, a different fixation interface surface (Fig. 16).

The surface areas of the 3-fin design, the tapered cone configuration, and the femoral and metal-backed patel-

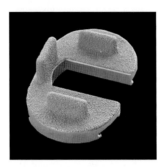

Fig. 16. 3-fin design – porous-coated fixation surface of tibial platform

Fig. 15. Tapered cone design – porous-coated fixation surface of the tibial platform

Fig. 17a–d. Autologous bone graft technique. **a** Preparation of bone graft material; **b** impaction of morcellized bone chips into the instrumented tibial anchoring zone; **c** impaction of either morcellized graft, slurry, and/or bone paste on the tibial surface with the permanent component; **d** impaction of cortico-cancellous strut grafts in the softer central tibia metaphysis

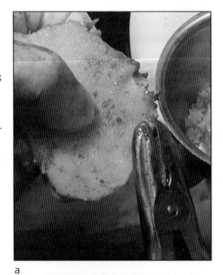

a

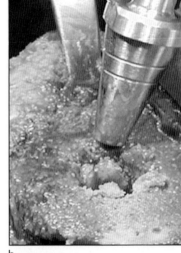

b

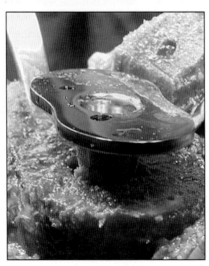

c

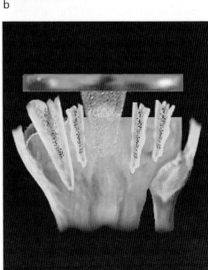

d

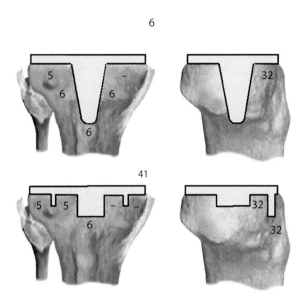

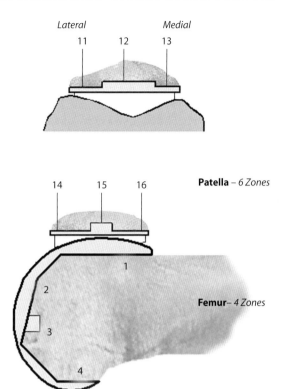

Fig. 18. Tibial interface zones of the tapered cone and 3-fin design

lar components are fully porous-coated with Porocoat (DePuy, Inc., Warsaw, Indiana, USA). The porous-coated implants described by Pilliar and Bratina [26] consisted of a sintered porous bead coating with a volume porosity of 35–45% and an average pore size of 200–250 μm.

Interference fit of the tibial interface and outer cortical coverage are most important. Proper prosthetic sizing and autograft enhancement were achieved utilizing:

- corticocancellous strut grafts for varus slope-off deformities, plateau defects, and soft rheumatoid bone support,
- cancellous graft augmentation of the central tibial metaphysis to achieve a "compaction-impaction" interference fit,
- drilling of hard sclerotic zones,
- autograft slurry for smaller surface defects, and
- prosthetic coverage = 70% of the cortical rim (Fig. 17).

The tapered cone design has the advantage of compressing the soft metaphysial bone, avoiding diaphysial fixation, allows for ease of autograft impaction. Optimum fit and fill of the upper tibia was the goal and felt to be achieved in all cases.

The scoring system utilized was a modified HSS (100 points) scale [7, 16] (pain 30, function 25, range of motion 15, deformity 12, stability 10, and strength 8). Alignment and fixation interfaces of all 567 cases were evaluated radiographically following Knee Society guidelines. Tibial zones 5 to 7 were analyzed from an anteroposte-

Fig. 19. Femoral and patellar interface zones

rior weight-bearing view and zones 8 to10 from the lateral view (Fig. 18).

Femoral zones 1 to 4, and patellar zones 14 to 16 were analyzed on a lateral radiograph. Patellar zones 11 to 13 were analyzed on a patella skyline view (Fig. 19).

Radiographic evaluations were performed preoperatively, 6–8 weeks, yearly to every 3 years, and latest available. Cases with inadequate radiographs were excluded from the study. Tibial/femoral interfaces were graded using the Knee Society guidelines and recorded as none, 0–2 mm, and >2 mm. Interim view analyses were carried out when radiographs were not available in symptom-free patients. Radiographs were reviewed at all intervals in cases that had fixation failures and/or failed for other prosthetic-related complications.

3 Results

Clinical results of all 567 cases were divided into non-inflammatory (OA) and inflammatory cases (RA). Of 520 OA cases, 493 (94.7%) had excellent or good results, 19 (3.7%) had fair results, and 8 (1.6%) had poor results. Mean preoperative score in the OA group was 54.7 points (27 to 85), and latest mean postoperative score was 87.3 points (51 to 99). Eleven patients had a decreased postoperative score at the latest evaluation, including those requiring revision surgery. Pre-operative pain scores improved from 14.0 to 28.1 points (latest), function from 11.8 to 19.7, deformity from 8.4 to 10.1, strength from 4.3 to 7.0, stability from 8.3 to 10.1, and range of motion improved from a mean of 94 to 109 degrees. Of the 47 RA cases, 40 (85.1%) had excellent or good results, 6 (12.8%) had fair results, and 1 (2.1%) had a poor result. Mean pre-operative score was 54.1 points (23 to 81), and latest score was 83.3 (52 to 98). No patient had a decreased postoperative score at the latest evaluation. Mean preoperative pain scores in the RA group improved (latest) from 12.9 to 28.3 points, function 11.3 to 18.1, deformity 8.4 to 11.8, strength 3.3 to 6.8, stability 7.4 to 9.0, and range of motion from 93 to 109 degrees.

3.1   Zonal Analysis

All femoral (n=567), tibial (n=567), and patellar (n=165) zone interfaces were analyzed immediately postoperatively and at latest evaluation at the intervals described. RLZ were analyzed in four femoral zones on lateral radiographs, six patellar zones (three zones on skyline and three on lateral radiographs), and six tibial zones (three zones on both anteroposterior and lateral radiographs). The RLZ analyses are summarized in Fig. 20 to 23.

On the femoral side, lucencies of 1–2 mm were observed in 0.2% of zone 1, 0.7% of zone 2, and no lucencies in zone 3 and 0.7% in zone 4. No lucencies >1 mm were seen in any patellar interfaces. Tibial interface lu-

cencies of 1–2 mm were detected at zone 5 (1.9%), zone 6 (3.7%), zone 7 (2.1%), zone 8 (1.4%), zone 9 (4.4%), and zone 10 (3.4%). These RLZ occurred in random fashion and were often noted at the peripheral interfaces, frequently in the areas of dense osteoarthritic bone that was incompletely removed in slope-off deformities. These areas are considered to be fibrous osseous stable [14] and represent arrested biologic remodeling if noted after 2 years. None of these cases represented clinical fixation failures. Lucencies of more than 2 mm in two or more zones were seen in four (0.7%) cases, all of which represented clinical and radiographic tibial com-

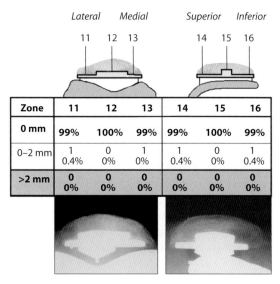

| | Lateral | Medial | | Superior | Inferior | |
	11	12	13	14	15	16
Zone	**11**	**12**	**13**	**14**	**15**	**16**
0 mm	99%	100%	99%	99%	100%	99%
0–2 mm	1 0.4%	0 0%	1 0%	1 0.4%	0 0%	1 0.4%
>2 mm	0 0%	0 0%	0 0%	0 0%	0 0%	0 0%

Fig. 21. Presence and distribution of RLL in patellar zones 11 to 16

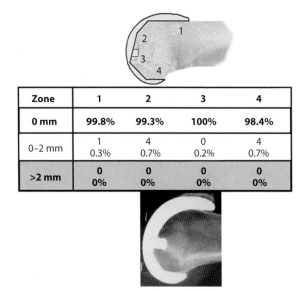

Zone	**1**	**2**	**3**	**4**
0 mm	99.8%	99.3%	100%	98.4%
0–2 mm	1 0.3%	4 0.7%	0 0.2%	4 0.7%
>2 mm	0 0%	0 0%	0 0%	0 0%

Fig. 20. Presence and distribution of RLL in femoral zones 1 to 4

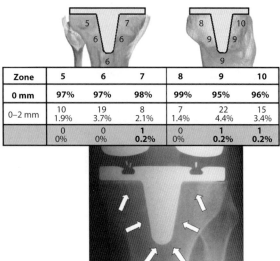

Zone	**5**	**6**	**7**	**8**	**9**	**10**
0 mm	97%	97%	98%	99%	95%	96%
0–2 mm	10 1.9%	19 3.7%	8 2.1%	7 1.4%	22 4.4%	15 3.4%
	0 0%	0 0%	1 0.2%	0 0%	1 0.2%	1 0.2%

Fig. 22. Presence and distribution of RLL in tibial zones 5 to 7 evaluating tibial cone design

ponent fixation failure. All required revision surgery. Three of these failures were ACL/PCL-retaining 3-fin designs, and one case was a PCL-substituting (rotating platform) device with a tapered cone design configuration. No prosthetic component showed bead disengagement (shedding).

3.2 Complications

Thirty-two cases (5.6%) required revision surgery related to a combination of technical and/or polyethylene failures. Four cases (0.7%) were tibial fixation failures, as noted above; one (0.2%) septic loosening, and three (0.5%) aseptic loosenings. Three of the four aseptic loosening cases were bi-cruciate (ACL/PCL) retaining meniscal bearing devices with a 3-fin design (Fig. 24), and one PCL-substituting rotating platform device (ta-

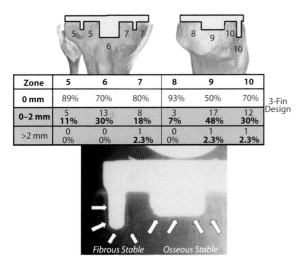

Zone	5	6	7	8	9	10	
0 mm	89%	70%	80%	93%	50%	70%	3-Fin Design
0–2 mm	5 11%	13 30%	8 18%	3 7%	17 48%	12 30%	
>2 mm	0 0%	0 0%	1 2.3%	0 0%	1 2.3%	1 2.3%	

Fig. 23. Presence and distribution of RLL in tibial zones 5 to 10 evaluating tibial cone design

pered cone) complicated by delayed sepsis. Three of the four cases that showed aseptic tibial loosening had a varus mal-position of the tibial component of >6 degrees on immediate postoperative radiographs. One case of rheumatoid arthritis (0.3%) represented a late (metastatic) septic loosening of a tibial rotating platform device which was superimposed on progressive varus subsidence at 12 years after surgery. This case is considered to be a fixation failure prior to the infection.

Of the non-fixation related failures, three other cases of tibial component failure were due to kinematic problems or progressive ligamentous instability, two of which were ACL/PCL-retaining 3-fin designs. One early tibial component revision was performed due to rotational mal-position of the PCL-retaining tibial tray, requiring conversion to a rotating platform. In five cases, polyethylene rotating platform bearings were exchanged due to wear. In nine cases, the meniscal bearings of a PCL-retaining device were exchanged. In eight cases, the meniscal bearings of an ACL/PCL-retaining device were exchanged. No femoral component and no resurfaced patellar component required revision surgery at mean follow-up of 5.7 years.

4 Discussion

Uncemented fixation remains a more controversial issue in TKA than in total hip replacements, especially at the tibial side [4, 6, 14, 18, 21, 24, 33–35, 37, 41]. Occurrences of RLZ in uncemented TKA are multifactorial and highly dependent on the type of implant, the surgical technique, and mechanical alignment. Interpretation of radiographic RLZ can be difficult and must be correlated to clinical findings. Interface (RLZ) analysis in uncemented and cemented total joint arthroplasties, and their interpretation have been of major interest since the very beginning of total joint arthroplasty

Fig. 24. Radiographs showing a fixation failure secondary to an aseptic loosening with subsidence and varus deformity

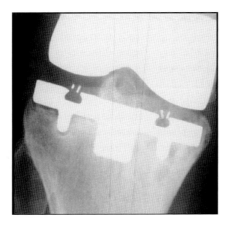

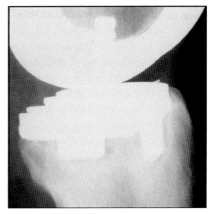

[13, 25, 42–44]. Fixation failures in cemented implants are identified radiographically at both the cement-prosthetic and cement-bone interfaces. Cementless fixation eliminates one of the variables (cement) and requires a biologic bonding at the prosthetic bone interface. Variations in type of surface treatment (porous coating, grit blast, hydroxyapatite, fiber mesh, etc.), areas of surface treatment (partial, complete), and the time relationship after implantation must be understood to properly evaluate radiographs postoperatively.

The appearance of RLZ differs in cemented and uncemented TKA components. Whereas cemented prostheses show fewer RLZ early (first year of implantation) with a tendency to increase with time, uncemented prostheses have shown the opposite tendency. The biology of the bone/implant fixation is multifactorial and has been widely studied and reported in the literature [5, 6, 8, 19, 15, 28, 32, 36, 40, 42]. Histological, radiographic, and clinical correlation of femoral stem retrievals have shown a combination of osseous and fibrous integration with radiolucent lines between 1 and 2 mm [15]. This study has established guidelines commonly used in radiographic evaluation of cementless implants, namely osseous stable, fibrous or fibro-osseous stable, or fibrous unstable. This classification has been validated by Ecker et al. [13] who reported fixation failures in TKA where RLZ occurred in a higher number of areas, or when RLZ exceeded 2 mm in size. Cook et al. [10] reported histological evidence of 50% of ingrowths into the porous coated tibial components in areas of radiographic sclerotic lines. With uncemented implants, RLZ are commonly seen within the first few months postoperatively and show radiographic improvement over time in successful cases [21].

Osseointegration is the goal of fixation at cementless interface to ensure clinical success. Osseointegration is required to eliminate the gasket effect (potential pumping of fluid and debris into the interface), that can lead to loosening and/or osteolysis. Whiteside [44] showed that circumferential porous coating was more resistant to the development of RLZ at the tibial interface. Micromotion at the interface is a major contributing factor in the success or failure of osseointegration. Micromotion of up to 0.6 mm is considered acceptable and may positively influence fibrous-osseous integration [32, 35], whereas micromotion >1.9 mm has shown a higher incidence of RLZ and clinical failure. Bone fixation dynamics of porous-coated tibial implants has been studied by Ryd et al. [33, 34] using roentgen stereophotogrammetric analysis (RSA), which demonstrated subsidence of 0.2 to 1.0 mm in successful cases, supporting the theory of bone healing under limited micromotion [17].

Major factors influencing fixation in uncemented TKA are:

- exacting interference fit [30],
- proper alignment of the knee joint,
- prosthetic design, which allows for optimum surface area articulation (low contact stress) and low constraint (tension) forces at the bone implant interface, and
- host bone quality to support the implant loads.

Since mechanical fixation sets the stage for ultimate biologic osseointegration, cortical coverage and bone surface treatment are also important in achieving immediate mechanical fixation. Any deviation of technical accuracy can unfavorably influence outcomes.

The use of autologous bone grafting has shown improvement in graft-host continuity in the investigations of Bloebaum et al. [5], who demonstrated improved bony ingrowths in retrieved tibial components 3–48 months after implantation. Bone surface treatment in our study included the generous use of morcellized cancellous autograft fill of the central tibia, corticocancellous strut grafts for slope-off deformities or soft zones (i.e., rheumatoid/osteopenic bone) of the distal femoral condyles or tibial plateaus, and bone paste for surface defects (see Fig. 17). Bone graft material is readily available and can be harvested as needed. Bone paste is best collected from saw cuts and drillings.

Prosthetic design and metal "fixation surface" treatment are important considerations in both cemented and cementless TKA. Currently, the most common uncemented TKA designs are fixed bearings with various articulating geometries, often with screw fixation for "immediate fixation" on the tibial side [43]. Porous coated (full or partial) Co-Cr is the most commonly used metal and has been used successfully in uncemented total joint arthroplasties of different types [3, 8, 9]. Porous size, coating, operative technique, and prosthetic interface design are very variable; therefore, results must be measured for the specific prosthesis utilized.

When variations of extent or number of zone lucencies exist, interpretation becomes more difficult. Individual cases must be examined in more detail if clinically warranted. Lucencies in the 1–2 mm range are more difficult to interpret if they appear in multiple zones. An example case in this study demonstrates a radiographic sclerotic zone around the tibial cone with an appearance of cancellous bony trabeculae (of different density) between the sclerotic line and the porous-coated surface in the lateral view (Fig. 25).

These areas may represent technique and/or graft-related remodeling and not fibrous fixation. The interface can remain biologically active for several months to years. Clinical correlation for a given case, especially if true radiolucent lines >2 mm are present in two or more zones, requires more specialized studies such as bone scans, fluoroscopy, etc.

Vyskocil et al. [42] recommended that only fluoroscopic investigations of the interface provide adequate and reliable information and has been recommended to be performed in every patient. Routine fluoroscopic studies of the interface are time consuming, impractical, and not cost-effective, but should be considered in the problem case. The identification and interpretation of RLZ on plain radiographs in TKA is limiting if looked at in a "single snapshot". Experience of the reviewer may vary and quality of radiographs at a given time may be

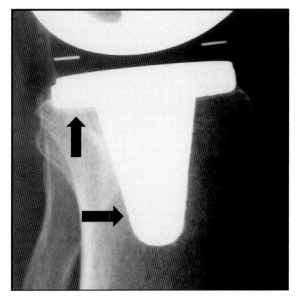

Fig. 25. Example of stable osseous and fibro-osseous fixation in tibial zones 8 to 10

less than ideal. An algorithm which outlines the course of RLZ in uncemented total joint components from immediate postoperative, to latest follow-up is proposed based on our observation using plane radiograph analysis over time (Fig. 26).

Any suggested treatment plan should correlate X-ray interpretation with the clinical status.

Reports of RLZ in uncemented TKA varies considerably in the literature and occurs most commonly at the tibial interface and more commonly in rheumatoid patients [2, 31, 39]. Most references are focused on the presence of RLZ at the uncemented metal-backed tibial interface with both fixed and mobile bearings. Results from centers using fixed tibial bearing devices showed presence of RLZ varying from 20–86 % [1, 11, 12, 22, 23, 27, 29, 45] at the tibial interface. Tibial survivorship of 99 % and 97 % were reported by Sorrells [38] and Jordan et al. [19] utilizing the LCS tapered cone meniscal and rotating platform designs. Other results with LCS cementless knee implantation have also been reported [20]. However, neither of these studies addressed specific radiolucent zonal analysis, which this study evaluates in detail.

RLZ analysis of bone-prosthetic interface is a practical method of evaluating cementless fixation and correlates with TKA clinical outcomes. Results in this study show fewer RLZ compared with reports in the literature to date, with less than 1 % tibial fixation failures, the majority of which occurred in a non-stemmed tibial device. Our results suggest that the 3-fin design should not be used for cementless implantation. The LCS tapered cone design is highly predictable (99 % fixation survivorship) in both osteoarthritic and rheumatoid patients, and can be recommended for clinical implantation.

Fig. 26. Proposed algorithm for evaluation of treatment of cementless TKA utilizing RLL radiographic analysis

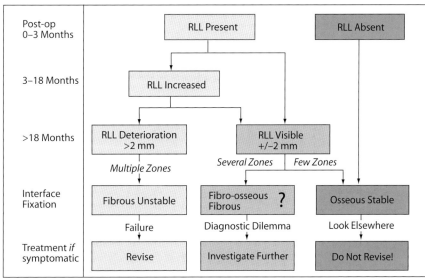

References

1. Aglietti P, Buzzi R (1988) Posterior stabilised total-condylar knee replacement. Three to eight years follow-up of 85 knees. J Bone Joint Surg [Br] 70-B: 211–216
2. Armstrong RA, Whiteside LA (1991) Results of cementless total knee arthroplasty in an older rheumatoid arthritis population. J Arthroplasty 6:357–362
3. Baldwin JL, El-Saied MR, Rubinstein RA Jr (1996) Uncemented total knee arthroplasty: report of 109 titanium knees with cancellous-structured porous coating. Orthopedics 19:123–130
4. Bloebaum RD, Rhodes DM, Rubman MH, Hofmann AA (1991) Bilateral tibial components of different cementless designs and materials. Microradiographic, backscattered imaging, and histological analysis. Clin Orthop 268: 179–187
5. Bloebaum RD, Rubman MH, Hofmann AA (1992) Bone ingrowth into porous-coated tibial components implanted with autograft bone chips. Analysis of ten consecutively retrieved implants. J Arthroplasty 7: 483–493
6. Bloebaum RD, Bachus KN, Jensen JW, Hofmann AA (1997) Postmortem analysis of consecutively retrieved asymmetric porous-coated tibial components. J Arthroplasty 12: 920–929
7. Buechel FF (1982) A simplified evaluation system for the rating of the knee function. Orthop Rev 11: 9
8. Cheng CL, Gross AE (1988) Loosening of the porous coating in total knee replacement. J Bone Joint Surg [Br] 70-B: 377–381
9. Collins, DN, Heim, SA, Nelson, CL, Smith P III (1991) Porous-coated anatomic total knee arthroplasty. A prospective analysis comparing cemented and cementless fixation. Clin Orthop 267: 128–136
10. Cook SD, Barrack RL, Thomas KA, Haddad RJ Jr (1989) Quantitative histological analysis of tissue growth into porous total knee components. J Arthroplasty 4 (Suppl): S33–43
11. Donaldson WF III, Sculco TP, Insall JN, Ranawat CS (1988) Total condylar III knee prosthesis. Long-term follow-up study. Clin Orthop 226: 21–28
12. Duffy GP, Berry DJ, Rand JA (1998) Cement versus cementless fixation in total knee arthroplasty. Clin Orthop 356: 66–72
13. Ecker ML, Lotke PA, Windsor RE, Cella JP (1987) Long-term results after total condylar knee arthroplasty. Significance of radiolucent lines. Clin Orthop 216: 151–158
14. Engh GA, Bobyn JD, Petersen TL (1988) Radiographic and histologic study of porous coated tibial component fixation in cementless total knee arthroplasty. Orthopedics 11: 725–731
15. Engh CA, Zettl-Schaffer KF, Kukita Y et al. (1993) Histological and radiographic assessment of well functioning porous-coated acetabular components. A human postmortem retrieval study. J Bone Joint Surg [Am] 75-A: 814–824
16. Ewald FC (1989) The Knee Society total knee arthroplasty roentgenographic evaluation and scoring system. Clin Orthop 248: 9–12
17. Farron A, Rakotomanana RL, Zambelli PY, Leyvraz PF (1995) Total knee prosthesis. Clinical and numerical study of micromovements of the tibial implant. Rev Chir Orthop Reparatrice Appar Mot 80: 28–35
18. Fukuoka S, Yoshida K, Yamano Y (2000) Estimation of the migration of tibial components in total knee arthroplasty. A roentgen stereophotogrammetric analysis. J Bone Joint Surg [Br] 82-B: 222–227
19. Jordan LR, Olivo JL, Voorhorst PE (1997) Survivorship analysis of cementless meniscal bearing total knee arthroplasty. Clin Orthop 338: 119–123
20. Keblish PA. Schrei C, Ward M (1993) Evaluation of 275 low contact stress (LCS) total knee replacements with 2- to 8-year follow up. Orthopaedics International Edition (Jan., Feb., March) 1: 168–174
21. Kim YH (1990) Knee arthroplasty using a cementless PCA prosthesis with porous-coated central tibial stem. Clinical and radiographic review at five years. J Bone Joint Surg [Br] 72-B: 412–417
22. Kobs JK, Lachiewicz PF (1993) Hybrid total knee arthroplasty. Two- to five-year results using the Miller-Galante prosthesis. Clin Orthop 286: 78–87
23. Konig A, Kirschner S, Walther M, Eisert M, Eulert J (1998) Hybrid total knee arthroplasty. Arch Orthop Trauma Surg 118: 66–69
24. Matsuda S, Tanner MG, White SE, Whiteside LA (1999) Evaluation of tibial component fixation in specimens retrieved at autopsy. Clin Orthop 363: 249–257
25. Matthews LS, Goldstein SA (1992) The prosthesis-bone interface in total knee arthroplasty. Clin Orthop 276: 50–55
26. Pilliar RM, Bratina WJ (1980) Micromechanical bonding at a porous surface structured implant interface–the effect on implant stressing. J Biomed Eng 2: 49–53
27. Ranawat CS, Insall J, Shine J (1976) Duo-condylar knee arthroplasty: hospital for special surgery design. Clin Orthop 120: 76–82
28. Ranawat CS, Johanson NA, Rimnac CM, Wright TM, Schwartz RE (1986) Retrieval analysis of porous-coated components for total knee arthroplasty. A report of two cases. Clin Orthop 209: 244–248
29. Ranawat CS, Flynn WF Jr, Saddler S, Hansraj KK, Maynard MJ (1993) Long-term results of the total condylar knee arthroplasty. A 15-year survivorship study. Clin Orthop 286: 94–102
30. Ranawat CS, Flynn WF Jr, Deshmukh RG (1994) Impact of modern technique on long-term results of total condylar knee arthroplasty. Clin Orthop 309: 131–135
31. Rosenqvist R, Bylander B, Knutson K et al. (1986) Loosening of the porous coating in patients with rheumatoid arthritis. J Bone Joint Surg [Am] 68-A: 538–542
32. Ryd L, Linder L (1989) On the correlation between micromotion and histology of the bone-cement interface. Report of three cases of knee arthroplasty followed by roentgen stereophotogrammetric analysis. J Arthroplasty 4: 303–309
33. Ryd L, Egund N (1995) Subsidence of tibial components in knee arthroplasty. A comparison between conventional radiography and roentgen stereophotogrammetry. Invest Radiol 30: 396–400
34. Ryd L, Lindstrand A, Rosenquist R, Selvik G (1986) Tibial component fixation in knee arthroplasty. Clin Orthop 213: 141–149
35. Ryd L, Carlsson L, Herberts P (1993) Micromotion of a noncemented tibial component with screw fixation. An in vivo roentgen stereophotogrammetric study of the Miller-Galante prosthesis. Clin Orthop 295: 218–225
36. Shaw JA (1995) Hybrid fixation modular tibial prosthesis. Early clinical and radiographic results and retrieval analysis. J Arthroplasty 10: 438–447
37. Smith S, Naima VS, Freeman MA (1999) The natural history of tibial radiolucent lines in a proximally cemented stemmed total knee arthroplasty. J Arthroplasty 14: 3–8
38. Sorrells RB (1996) The rotating platform mobile bearing TKA. Orthopedics 19: 793–796

39. Stuchin, SA, Ruoff, M, Matarese W (1991) Cementless total knee arthroplasty in patients with inflammatory arthritis and compromised bone. Clin Orthop 273: 42–51

40. Vigorita VJ, Minkowitz B, Dichiara JF, Higham PA (1993) A histomorphometric and histologic analysis of the implant interface in five successful, autopsy-retrieved, noncemented porous-coated knee arthroplasties. Clin Orthop 293: 211–218

41. Volz RG, Nisbet JK, Lee RW, McMurtry MG (1988) The mechanical stability of various noncemented tibial components. Clin Orthop 226: 38–42

42. Vyskocil P, Gerber C, Bamert P (1999) Radiolucent lines and component stability in knee arthroplasty. Standard versus fluoroscopically assisted radiographs. J Bone Joint Surg [Br] 81-B: 24–26

43. Whiteside LA (1994) Four screws for fixation of the tibial component in cementless total knee arthroplasty. Clin Orthop 299: 72–76

44. Whiteside LA (1995) Effect of porous-coating configuration on tibial osteolysis after total knee arthroplasty. Clin Orthop 321: 92–97

45. Wright J, Ewald FC, Walker PS et al. (1990) Total knee arthroplasty with the kinematic prosthesis. Results after five to nine years: a follow-up note. J Bone Joint Surg [Am] 72-A: 1003–1009

Chapter 12
Complications and Management

12.1 LCS Rotating Platform Dislocation and Spinout – Etiology, Diagnosis and Management

D. E. BEVERLAND, L. R. JORDAN

1 Introduction

Mobile bearing total knee prostheses have a potential for bearing dislocation or spinout. Surgeons must understand the etiology and management of this unusual complication if they are going to use mobile bearings. Prior reports have identified bearing dislocations as an important complication with surgical technique and surgeons' experience being important factors.

Mobile bearing total knee replacement was developed to address the problems of loosening of the tibial component and polyethylene wear. Highly congruent surfaces provide low contact stresses, thus reducing wear, whereas motion between the tibial insert polyethylene and metal tray reduces constraint, lowering shear at the tibial component-bone interface. However, despite satisfactory long-term results, some surgeons remain apprehensive about using mobile bearings because of the risk of bearing dislocation or spinout. The device permits unconstrained axial rotation but has the potential for bearing dislocation or "spinout" if laxity allows femorotibial disengagement. Correct ligament tension and balance, particularly in flexion, is a key factor in eliminating the risk of bearing spinout. The purpose of this chapter is to propose a mechanism, to discuss the etiology, to clarify the diagnosis and to discuss management.

2 Mechanism of Dislocation/Spinout

Dislocation or spinout occurs as a result of excessive rotation of the polyethylene bearing accompanied by translation of the femur on the tibia. Either the medial or lateral femoral condyle remains engaged with one side of the bearing and therefore, "spinout" is a more accurate description than dislocation as illustrated in Fig. 1.

If a fixed bearing knee dislocates, both femoral condyles become disengaged and this can occur with a rotating platform but is very rare. We feel that when discussing the rotating platform, the term spinout should be used in preference to dislocation unless both condyles disengage. The rest of this chapter relates to our experience with spinout of the rotating platform.

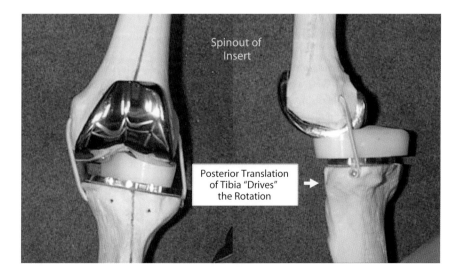

Fig. 1. Saw bone model demonstrating spinout of a rotating platform

Spinout of Insert

Posterior Translation of Tibia "Drives" the Rotation

Normally axial rotation of the bearing is dictated by femoral rotation particularly in extension where the femur and insert are fully congruent. With flexion of the LCS beyond 30 degrees the congruence between the femoral component and the rotating platform decreases thus permitting more independent axial rotation of the rotating platform relative to the femur. At the point at which the dislocation takes place the flexion gap is tighter on one side and excessive rotation of the insert is driven by the femoral condyle on this tighter side, turning the bearing around the central peg. The direction of spinout is determined by the direction of the shear force acting at the time. If an anterior shear force exists of the femur relative to the tibia, the femoral condyle on the slack side will tend to climb the anterior lip of the bearing as the tight side condyle is driven forward rotating the insert around the central peg. If sufficient shear force and/or laxity exists, then the lax condyle will jump over the anterior lip of the bearing producing a spinout as illustrated in Fig. 1. As can be seen from the lateral view of the figure the tibia translates posteriorly relative to the femur and the side of the bearing that spins out extrudes posteriorly in same direction as the tibia. This is the most common mechanism if however the tibia translates anteriorly the femur will climb the posterior lip of the bearing and thus the latter will extrude anteriorly.

3   Etiology of Bearing Spinout

The literature reports a varying incidence of bearing dislocation with rotating platforms as compared to meniscal bearing prostheses depending on the composition of the patient groups studied. For example Buechel and Pappas (1989) in a 10 year follow-up reported a 3.2% (7 out of 217) dislocation rate with the rotating platforms as compared to 0.7% (1 out of 140) in a meniscal bearing group. However of the 7 dislocations in the rotating platform group 6 were in revision knees and in fact the dislocation rate for primary rotating platforms was also 0.7% (1 out 137). In the 6 revision cases Buechel and Pappas [1] blamed the dislocations on "insufficient flexion stability". There were no revision cases in the meniscal-bearing group. When using rotating platforms the common rate of dislocation has been reported to be approximately 1% for primary surgery and almost 7% for revision arthroplasty [3]. Other authors have reported an incidence of 0.5 to 1% [4]. Since mobile bearing elements depend on the contact pressure exerted and the engagement depth of the femur in the bearing, in order to prevent extrusion, correct soft tissue balancing prior to bony resection is a critical step during the procedure.

If the flexion and extension gaps are balanced, equal and correctly tensioned, the risk of dislocation of the rotating platform should be virtually eliminated.

In primary surgery, what factors predispose to spinout of the rotating platform? From our experience, the most common cause of spinout is flexion gap instability. In the varus knee, this may result if an inadequate medial release is done before the anteroposterior (AP) femoral cuts are performed. In this situation the AP cuts will be performed in excessive external rotation as illustrated in Fig. 2.

This is because the under released medial collateral ligament (MCL) holds the femur in excessive internal rotation. At this stage the flexion gap is rectangular but not balanced. Subsequently when the surgeon realizes that the knee is tight medially in extension the MCL is then released. This release of the MCL after the AP femoral bone cuts have been done can create a trapezoidal flexion gap, which is wider, and more slack medially (Fig. 3).

As a result the knee is slack medially in flexion. It is therefore important in a varus knee to ensure that the soft tissues are balanced before the AP femoral cuts are made.

In the valgus knee, over release of the lateral collateral ligament (LCL) and popliteus from the lateral condyle prior to performing the AP femoral cuts can result in AP cuts being made in marked external rotation Fig. 4).

Even with this the flexion gap is still slack laterally in flexion. If the soft tissues are released from the lateral condyle in a valgus knee after the AP cuts then the lateral laxity and instability in flexion can be even more marked. To avoid bearing spinout in a valgus knee the lateral femoral condyle must not be stripped of all its soft tissue attachments. As can be seen from figure 4 there are three significant structures attached to the lateral condyle; the popliteus, the LCL and the lateral head of gastrocnemius. In a valgus knee, release of the iliotibial tract and the posterolateral capsule will usually create a neutral femorotibial alignment in extension. As the posterior capsule is normally lax in flexion, the AP bone cuts can safely be made at this point. If the knee remains tight in extension release of the structures attached to the lateral femoral condyle must be done carefully. The popliteus tendon does not contribute to the valgus deformity and therefore should not be released because it is an important lateral stabilizer in flexion. An alternative solution is to advance the lateral collateral epicondylar attachment by performing an osteotomy of the lateral femoral condyle. The osteotomized fragment includes the attachments of popliteus and gastrocnemius. The fragment is moved distally and slightly anteriorly, which has the effect of lengthening the tight lat-

Fig. 2. Performing the AP femoral cuts before the MCL has been released. Femur held down in internal rotation and AP cuts in excessive external rotation

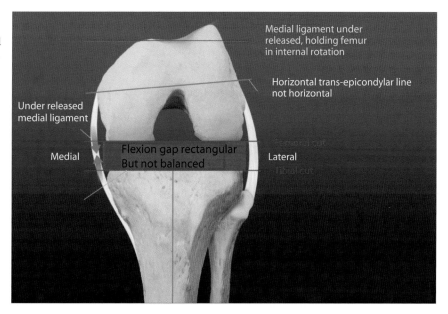

Fig. 3. Release of MCL after AP cuts have been done creates a trapezoidal flexion gap

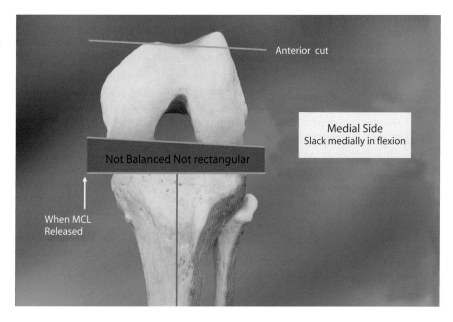

eral structures in extension while enhancing the stability of the flexion gap. This technique has been developed by Dr Jean Louis Briard of Rouen France.

In the neutral knee, where no specific releases are required to ensure equal compartment tension, rotating platform dislocation may result from inappropriate soft tissue releases or ligament balancing, therefore creating either of the scenario's as described above. In our experience patients with a prior patellectomy are particularly at risk. This is because in a normal knee the extensor mechanism plays a central role in maintaining AP stability and this is compromised by patellectomy.

In this setting, the surgeon must very carefully balance the gaps and even consider the use of a deep dish prosthesis.

4   Diagnosis of Bearing Spinout

The patient may present with sudden pain but often the patient can be totally asymptomatic. At times the clinical deformity is not gross, despite the x-ray appearances and because spin out is more common in valgus knees, from the patient's perspective the recurrence of their

Fig. 4. Release of soft tissues from lateral condyle in a valgus knee creates flexion instability. Inset shows the points of attachment of popliteus, the lateral collateral ligament and the lateral head of gastrocnemius

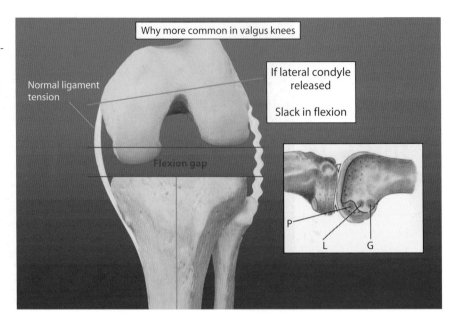

pre-operative valgus deformity does not seem abnormal. Often on inspection, it is posterior subluxation of the tibia in the sagittal plane (lateral view) that is more obvious than the deformity in the frontal plane, as can be seen in Fig. 1 and 5, shows the x-ray appearances in a typical case. At first sight these can be difficult to interpret.

Figure 6 shows the x-ray appearance of the normal LCS rotating platform. The insert contains two wire markers that run in an AP direction as can be appreciated from the lateral x-ray. In a perfect AP x-ray the wire markers are superimposed and therefore appear as a spot. Figure 1 demonstrated the pathology in a saw

bone model. As can be seen the insert spins through approximately 90 degrees. Thus in the AP x-ray of a patient with spinout the appearances of the insert are similar to those seen in a lateral x-ray of the normal post-operative knee and vice versa for the lateral x-ray. Also note the posterior subluxation of the tibia on the femur in Fig. 1 and 5. The direction in which the insert becomes extruded is always dictated by the direction in which the tibia moves. In the majority the tibia subluxes posteriorly and therefore the insert spins out and extrudes posteriorly. If the tibia subluxes anteriorly the insert will dislocate or spin out anteriorly. Thus with spinout, the bearing extrusion occurs in the same direction as the

Fig. 5. X-ray appearance in a typical case of spinout with a rotating platform

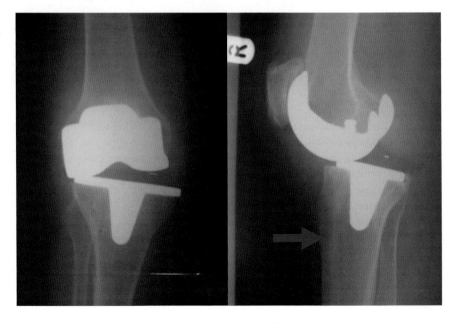

Fig. 6. X-ray appearance with a normal rotating platform

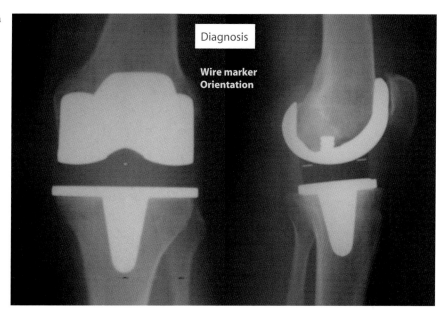

tibial translation and in the opposite direction to the femoral translation.

5   Treatment of Bearing Spinout

The majority of mobile bearing spinouts occur in the first few weeks and months following surgery. Most require open reduction but on occasion a closed reduction is possible. Before attempting a closed reduction it is important to have understood the mechanism in that particular case and to know the direction and side of extrusion. The knee is then flexed to 90 degrees and direct pressure is applied over the side of the insert that has extruded. Normally the extrusion is posterior so the pressure is applied on the appropriate side in the popliteal fossa. If the insert reduces then the knee should be flexed and extended for a number of cycles to ensure that the bearing remains reduced. If it re-dislocates it is worth reducing it again, as often stability will improve after several flexion/extension cycles. Provided the insert is reasonably stable the knee is placed in full extension, reduction is confirmed with a check x-ray and the knee is immobilized in a long leg cylinder cast. It should remain in cast for 8 weeks.

If the insert is unstable or cannot be reduced, as is often the case, then open reduction is required. This may be attempted through a small incision as often when reduced the insert is acceptably stable. A 5 cm incision is made through the original scar centered just below the level of the joint line. The insert is then exposed. In order to reduce the insert through this small incision a 3.2 mm drill is used to make a hole in the anterior face of

the insert parallel to the surface of the tibial tray. A long 4.5 mm cortical AO screw is then inserted into the insert as illustrated in Fig. 7.

A pair of vice grips is then applied to the screw and the insert is then manipulated back into place. Again the knee is put through a number of cycles and if stable the screw is removed and the wound is closed. After wound closure the knee is again immobilized in cast in full extension for 8 weeks.

If the knee remains unstable then consideration can be given to changing the insert and or correcting any soft tissue imbalance. It is important that before doing that the surgeon knows the type of insert that was used previously but it is also important to have understood the etiology of the problem. As discussed above the most common cause of bearing spinout is release of the soft tissues from the lateral condyle in a valgus knee resulting in lateral flexion instability. In this situation if a thicker insert is used, for example going from a 12.5 mm to a 15 mm insert the instability may be made worse. This is because in this situation the knee is often tight medially in flexion and if a thicker insert is used the medial tightness will be increased and may "jack out" the space laterally. This can produce "lift off" or "gapping" between the lateral femoral condyle and the bearing in flexion, which will increase the instability. On the other hand if the original procedure was performed with a classic bearing then changing to a deep dish of the same thickness will increase the stability. This is because the deep-dish component has an extra 3.5 mm of engagement height on the anterior wall. The newer universal bearing has the same configuration as the deep dish and is therefore inherently more stable than the

Fig. 7. Using an AO screw to reduce a rotating platform spinout

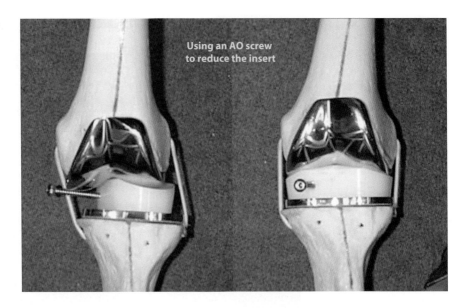

classic bearing. In cases with marked instability or situations were instability has recurred following a period in cast then other options have to be considered. These include revision to a fixed bearing knee and perhaps using a more constrained design.

One of the authors (Beverland DE) has had 10 patients with spinout out of a series of 2,300 primary LCS rotating platforms (0.43%). Of the ten six had a preoperative valgus deformity, two had a preoperative varus deformity and two were in neutral alignment. Two of the cases (one valgus, one neutral) had had a previous patellectomy several years earlier for symptomatic patellofemoral osteoarthritis. Of the ten, four cases were treated by exchange of the polyethylene insert to a deep-dish bearing. Five cases had open reduction of the original insert without bearing exchange (3 using the AO screw technique). The remaining case was managed by closed reduction. All cases were immobilized in a cylinder cast for a total of 8 weeks.

The above treatment was successful in eight cases. Two cases however had recurrent episodes of platform spinout despite considerable periods of protection in cast. One of the patients, following discussion, opted for arthrodesis. Three years following arthrodesis she is pain-free with a solid arthrodesis but obviously her mobility is significantly compromised. The other patient, due to multiple medical problems was deemed unfit for any major surgical intervention and therefore a decision was taken to cement the insert in place. To do this the knee was opened, the insert was temporarily removed, the tibial tray was scored using a diamond

tipped high-speed burr and the under surface of the insert was also roughened. The two surfaces were then cemented together. One year from surgery she is mobile with the use of a walking stick although she does now have recurvatum. Radiographs do not show any deterioration in the implant position. Despite initial success in this case, we do not advocate this technique as a means of managing rotating platform spin out but rather as a salvage procedure in medically unfit patients.

In summary, spinout of the LCS rotating platform is considered a recognized complication in primary as well as revision total knee arthroplasty. Surgical error in soft tissue balancing is the cause in the majority of cases with failure to correctly balance particularly the flexion gap. In the author's series discussed above previous patellectomy significantly increased the risk of rotating platform dislocation, as did pre-operative valgus deformity particularly in the older patient.

References

1. Buechel FF, Pappas MJ (1984) New Jersey integrated total knee replacement system: biomechanical analysis and clinical evaluation of 918 cases. FDA panel presentation Silver Spring, Maryland July 11, 1984
2. Buechel FF, Pappas MJ (1989) New Jersey Low Contact Stress knee replacement system: ten year evaluation of meniscal bearings. Orthop Clin North Am 20: 147
3. Sanchez-Sotelo J, Ordonez JM, Prats SB (1999) Results and complications of the low contact stress knee prosthesis. J Arthroplasty 14: 815
4. Sorrels RB, Stiehl JB, Voorhorst PE (2001) Midterm results of mobile-bearing total knee arthroplasty in patients younger than 65 years. Clin Orthop 390: 182–189

12.2 Complications and Management: Bearing Exchange

F. F. BUECHEL

1 Wear of LCS Mobile Bearings

Twenty-year evaluation of LCS meniscal bearing and rotating platform knee replacements [1] revealed a meniscal bearing wear rate leading to revision in 5% at an average of 10.1 years after the index operation for the cementless posterior cruciate retaining meniscal bearing device. Rotating platform bearing wear necessitating revision surgery was seen in 1.2% at an average of 9.9 years after the index operation [1]. Rotating bearing patella failures were not seen in either cemented or cementless primary knee replacements. One rotating-bearing patella (0.6%) wore through the inferior marker wire after 10.8 years in a patient who had multiple operations, causing metallosis and osteolysis. All components were revised.

The most important factors influencing wear in these bearings included poor quality polyethylene with unconsolidated fusion defects that was sterilized by a gamma irradiation in air process. Studies by Collier at Dartmouth University demonstrated a "white band" of oxidation in the subsurface layer of the polyethylene sterilized by this method [2]. This subsurface layer of oxidized ultra-high molecular weight polyethylene (UHMWPe) became more brittle over time, especially if left on an inventory shelf. Despite having lowered contact stresses, these bearing developed premature fatigue related fractures and delamination type wear patterns rather than a predicted abrasive wear pattern. It is now known that the longer these bearings are aged on the shelf, the more rapid the wear rate. As such, ethylene oxide and gas plasma sterilization methods have replaced gamma radiation in air sterilization to minimize fatigue related wear problems for these bearings in the future.

2 Etiology of meniscal bearing dislocation and breakage

Dislocation of meniscal bearings in total knee replacement was a major design concern in 1977 after considering the documented Oxford unconstrained meniscal bearing dislocation problems [3]. The use of radial tracks and biologic anterior patella tendon and posterior cruciate bone bridge stops seemed worthwhile and even necessary to prevent such problems. Excess anterior or posterior motion could allow a meniscal bearing to exit the track and be inexorably trapped out of position leading to a sudden varus or valgus instability, depending upon whether the dislocated bearing is medial or lateral.

Excessive internal or external rotation of the tibial component in full extension, to the extent that each meniscal bearing was not contained in the track, could also lead to subsequent subluxation or dislocation during flexion. This technical malposition is seen in Fig. 8.

An additional problem associated with rotary malposition of the meniscal bearing tibial component occurs in flexion when the bearing moves posteriorly over the track and begins to cantilever bend repetitively (Fig. 9). This repetitively cyclic bending can create tensile fatigue

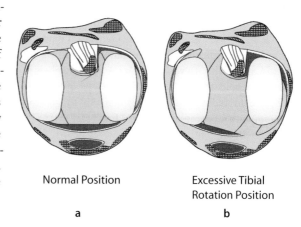

Normal Position   Excessive Tibial Rotation Position

a   b

Fig. 8. a Correct rotational positioning of the tibial component. **b** Excessive external rotation of the tibial component in full extension, showing the bearings in neutral positioning. Any rotation of the bearings due to femoral component will results in overhang of the meniscal bearings

of the polyethylene bearing at the point of bending until a fracture occurs, as described by Weaver et al. [4].

These problems have been identified as technical malposition problems occurring at surgery. They should be carefully avoided to enjoy optimal performance and longevity of meniscal bearing function.

3   Clinical manifestation of meniscal bearing dislocation and breakage

When meniscal bearings dislocate or fracture, the same clinical picture is demonstrated. If a medial meniscal bearing has dislocated, fractured or developed severe wear, the knee will produce a sudden varus deformity associated with medial instability (Fig. 10b).

If a lateral meniscal bearing has dislocated, fractured or developed severe wear, the knee will produce a sudden valgus deformity associated with lateral instability (Fig. 10c).

These developmental varus or valgus instabilities demonstrate mechanical failure of meniscal bearings and warrant emergency exploration of the knee to replace the bearing elements in the case of wear or fracture. In cases where the bearing has dislocated because of rotational malposition of the tibial component, revision of the tibial component into proper orientation or salvage to a rotating platform component would be acceptable procedure choices.

4   Meniscal Bearing Exchange, the Concept

The concept of exchanging worn meniscal bearings was part of the original design philosophy in 1977. Sliding the bearings into or out of metallic radial tracks requires exposure of the front edge of each track to provide complete clearance for the dove-tailed section of each meniscal bearing. Development of a meniscal bearing clamp to hold the bearing and allow enough seating pressure to reduce the bearing beneath the femoral component was completed in 1998 Fig. 11). Prior to this instrument, digital pressure was used to seat the bearings, a technique that is more difficult and somewhat awkward, but also effective.

4.1   Surgical Technique

Extensive exposure through the median parapatellar approach, everting the patella laterally gives the surgeon the best view of the knee components and soft tissue. Through this approach a synovectomy can be

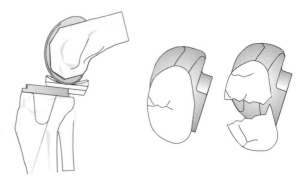

Cantilever bending due to overhang from malposition

Repetivie loading results in fatigue faliure fracture of bearing

Fig. 9. Rotary malposition of the meniscal bearing tibial component can cause the bearings to cantilever bend repetitively in flexion when the bearing moves posteriorly over the track

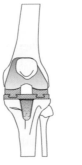 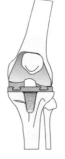 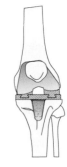

Neutral Alignment	Valgus Alignment Lateral Bearing Wear	Valgus Alignment Medial Bearing Wear
a	b	c

Fig. 10. a Correct frontal plane positioning of components. **b** Varus deformity associated with medial instability, due to a bearing that has dislocated, fractured or developed severe wear. **c** Valgus deformity associated with lateral instability, due to a bearing that has dislocated, fractured or developed severe wear

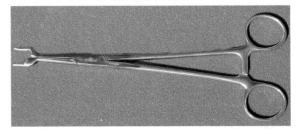

Fig. 11. Clamp developed to grasp the meniscal bearing dovetail track to aid in insertion during bearing exchange

Fig. 12. a 1/4" osteotome is used to separate a rotating patellar bearing from a well fixed back plate.
b The rotating bearing being removed from the wound, **c** a new patellar bearing being installed with the patellar clamp

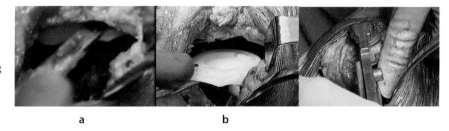

a
b

Fig. 13. Towel clips can be used to firmly grasp the meniscal bearing and aid in removal

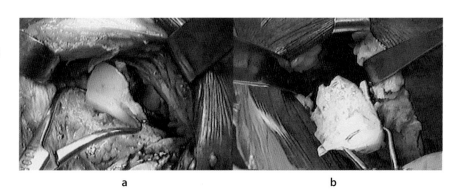

a
b

easily performed if needed and the patella bearing can be exchanged under direct vision by unsnapping the worn bearing with a 1/4 inch osteotome (Fig. 12a) and re-snapping a new bearing onto the patella anchoring plate with digital pressure or using the patella clamp (Fig. 12b). Meniscal bearings that are worn but not broken can be grasped with a towel clip and pulled forward out of their tracks (Fig. 13). Broken meniscal bearing fragments can be removed from the posterior capsular region with a pituitary rongeur (Fig. 14).

Insertion of new gas plasma sterilized meniscal bearings should restore collateral ligament stability (Fig. 15). Over time, it has been observed that minor collateral ligament instability can develop either during or as a consequence of the wear process. The instability is usually symmetrical in both compartments and perhaps represents stable but minor component subsidence. Thus, it may be useful to insert 12.5 mm bearings into the space occupied by worn out 10 mm bearings to improve collateral ligament stability in flexion and extension.

A limited exposure technique has been developed for use in situations where excessive bearing wear is accompanied by minimal synovitis in the knee. In these cases, where a synovectomy is not needed, a mid-patella to tibial tubercle skin incision is made through a portion of the previously healed incision (Fig. 16). The medial and lateral retinacula are opened up to the mid patella level proximally. All soft tissue and bony osteophytes are removed from the front of the meniscal tracks on the tibial component and soft tissues are elevated medial and laterally on the proximal tibia to give access to both

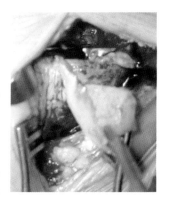

Fig. 14. Smaller fragments can be removed from the wound with a pituitary rongeur

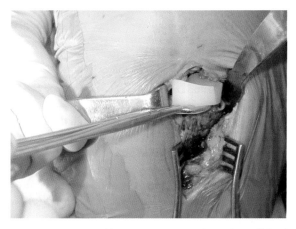

Fig. 15. New meniscal bearings are inserted into the well fixed tibial tray

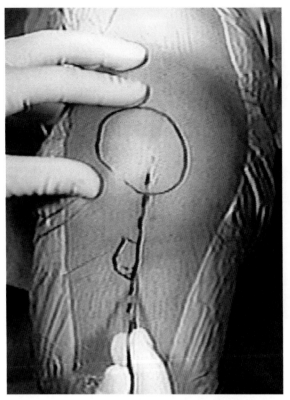

Fig. 16. A straight, midline incision is used from the mid patella to the tibial tubercle

with either digital pressure or use of the patella clamp, see figure 5. If the patella clamp is used, protect the skin over the patella with a moist sponge under the clamp. Closure is routine with careful attention to providing central patellar tracking.

5 Rotating Platform Bearing Exchange

Rotating platform bearing insertion without removing the femoral component requires an extensive exposure to sublux the medial and lateral polyethylene surfaces forward from the flexed femoral component. Once disengaged, the bearing is easily removed from its central, conical seat by digital pressure. Significant wear of the older rotating platform bearings is usually accompanied by significant synovitis and medial-lateral instability. It is important at revision, to consider a complete synovectomy to remove the bioburden of excess polyethylene-laden synovial tissue. As in meniscal bearing exchange, it is often helpful to increase the rotating platform bearing thickness to re-stabilize the collateral ligaments in flexion and extension.

5.1 Surgical Technique

Extensive exposure through the medial parapatellar approach, everting the patella laterally gives the surgeon the best view of the knee components and soft tissue. Through this approach a synovectomy can be easily performed and the patella bearing can be exchanged under direct vision by unsnapping the worn bearing with a 1/4 inch osteotome and re-snapping a new bearing onto the patella anchoring plate with digital pressure or using the patella clamp (see Fig. 12). Perform an extensive medial sleeve release on the proximal tibia to include the posterior medial corner. Elevate the lateral soft tissues to free up the lateral compartment without detaching the lateral collateral ligament. The popliteus tendon should be preserved unless there is significant scarring and posterior lateral impingement that restricts bearing motion, in which case, the popliteus may be released to facilitate exposure and collateral ligament balance.

compartments. The meniscal bearings are removed by grasping their front edge with a towel clip and pulling them forward from their respective radial tracks (see Fig. 13). Posterior bearing fragments can be removed with a pituitary rongeur. Removal and reinsertion of meniscal bearings usually requires knee flexion of about 45° combined with axial rotation of the leg. External rotation and flexion allows easier insertion of the lateral meniscal bearing, which is usually replaced first. Internal rotation and flexion allows insertion of the medial meniscal bearing, which is replaced last.

4.2 Patella Bearing Exchange

The patella bearing can be palpated through this limited incision and can be removed by inserting a 1/4 inch osteotome between the bearing and the metallic anchoring plate, then twisting the osteotome to unsnap the patella bearing. The edges of the anchoring plate must be cleared of any soft tissue or bony overgrowth to allow the new bearing to be snapped onto the trunion cone. The new gas plasma sterilized rotating patella bearing is placed into position and compressed onto its seat

Once the proximal tibia has been extensively exposed, the knee is flexed to approximately 100° and drawn forward to dislocate the rotating platform bearing from under the femoral component. A new gas plasma sterilized bearing of increased thickness is then placed into the central conical seat of the metallic tibial component and forcefully reduced beneath the femoral component at approximately 100° flexion. Once reduced, this thicker rotating platform bearing is very difficult to re-dislocate.

So, it is recommended that only the final bearings be used for this maneuver rather than any trial bearings. Closure is routine with careful attention to providing central patellar tracking.

6   Post-Operative Course

Patients tend to recover quickly from either meniscal bearing or rotating platform bearing exchange. Limited exposures cause minimal discomfort and patients are usually assymptomatic within 2 to 4 weeks. Patients can be discharged on the same day of surgery or after only an overnight observation in most cases of limited exposure bearing exchange.

Extensive exposures cause more discomfort than limited exposures, but patients report less pain than they experienced with their initial knee replacement surgery. Recovery time is similar to primary knee replacement recovery. This is in stark contrast to patients undergoing full revision of all components. The pain after full revision is generally much worse than their initial knee replacement surgery and recovery is far slower after full revision of all components.

7   Overall Appeal of Bearing Exchange Revision Surgery

After years of experience, there is no question that simple bearing exchange revision surgery is far more appealing to the patient, the surgeon and the hospital. The patient has less discomfort, less blood loss and minimal recovery time. The surgeon can perform a much simpler total knee revision operation than full component revision and perform the surgery more quickly and efficiently as well. The hospital uses less costly resources by being charged only for bearings rather than the expensive revision implants, as well as enjoying a much decreased length of hospital stay for the patient.

References

1. Buechel Sr FF, Buechel Jr FF, Pappas MJ, D'Alessio J (2001) Twenty-year evaluation of meniscal bearing and rotating platform knee replacements. Clin Orth 388: 41–50
2. Collier JP (1996) The effects of sterilization on Polyethylene. Orthop Special Edition 33–34
3. Goodfellow JW, O'Connor J (1986) Clinical results of the Oxford knee. Surface arthroplasty of the tibiofemoral joint with a meniscal bearing prosthesis. Clin Orth 205: 21–42
4. Weaver JK, Derkash RS, Greenwald AS (1993) Difficulties with bearing dislocation and breakage using a movable bearing total knee replacement system. Clin Orth 290: 244–252

12.3 The Unstable Knee

J.B. Stiehl, K.J. Hamelynck, J.L. Briard

1   Definition

Ligamentous stability in total knee arthroplasty can be defined by accurate balancing of the ligaments in relation to the intrinsic stability offered by the mechanical constraint of the prosthetic implant. The extrinsic ligamentous stability may be essential with an unconstrained bicruciate preserving LCS implant or only moderately essential in a VVC type of constrained insert device, as compared to the low requirement in the hinge total knee implant. The other important element of stability is the function of muscles about the knee. Function of the extensor mechanism is critical to total knee performance, while the hamstrings are moderately important in stability but must be present for function of gait. Instability in total knee arthroplasty can be defined as ligamentous or soft tissue laxity resulting in symptomatic discomfort and the feeling of buckling along with clinical findings of swelling and detectable gap opening on stress. It is possible for knee dislocation to occur from extensor mechanism insufficiency where the femur may dislocate anteriorly on the tibia. This problem has resulted from femoral nerve palsy or patellar tendon disruption. However, we will confine our discussion only to instability resulting from imbalance of the femorotibial ligaments. With the LCS system, a typical clinical finding has been bearing dislocation or spinout, which will be discussed in other chapters. With fixed bearing prostheses, such dislocation is not likely, and the patient more likely experiences a problematic poor result. Recent studies have shown that the percentage of revisions done for ligament instability can be as high a 39%. This is disturbing as the complication is virtually preventable in every case, and only in the most extenuating circumstances should the outcome be purely attributed to surgeon's error.

2   Etiology

The primary cause of ligamentous instability in total knee arthroplasty is extension/flexion imbalance (Fig. 17, 18). Typically, the problem is found very early after primary surgery and reflects poor balancing of ligaments such as the posterolateral capsule in a valgus knee, and will be compounded by abnormal bone cuts that do not balance the knee prosthesis in extension and flexion. Experts have mistakenly recommended that mild laxity is tolerated or even beneficial to improving postoperative range of motion. The facts would indicate that moderate postoperative laxity will only worsen with time as opposed to excellent well-balanced ligament tensioning. LCS surgeons have learned that the toleration of the unconstrained and dislocatable bearings for ligament imbalance is relatively low. The advantage of the tibia-cut-first flexion space balancing is discussed well elsewhere in this book, but we will only reiterate this inviolate concept. Surgeons who choose an anatomical fixed bone resection, given the disparate anatomy of the human knee in normal and diseased cases, will only learn the hard way.

Early instability with the LCS will generally lead to a bearing dislocation or spinout problem. With fixed bearing total knees, the patients typically experiences an early "poor" result. Late instability is a more insidious problem and is something more likely to be seen with the LCS. As we have stated, from the work of Hamelynck, if ligaments are closely balanced at the outset, late ligament stretching is unlikely. On the other hand, if the ligaments are poorly balanced, the condition is progressive and will gradually worsen over time. The other important consideration is the instability that results over the long term from implant subsidence and rarely wear, which in effect makes the knee more unstable.

Late rupture of the posterior cruciate ligament may occur if tibial resection exceeds 8 millimeters, weakening the cruciate insertion [6, 7]. We have witnessed this

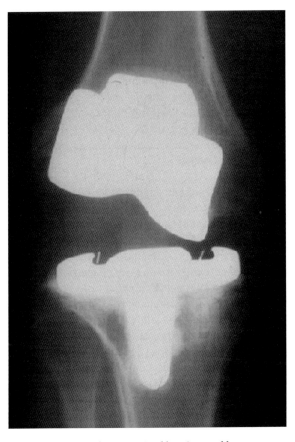

Fig. 17. Instability of LCS meniscal bearing total knee

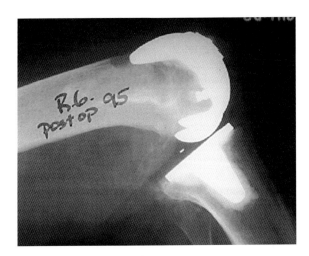

Fig. 18. Spinout or dislocation of an LCS rotating platform tibial insert. Note posterior tibial sag

imal tibia as a means of creating balance of the knee in flexion. With the mobile bearing devices, this is inviting disaster. Surgeon experience with the AP Glide would suggest that loss of the posterior cruciate ligament is tantamount to a revision for chronic instability.

Another concern is excessive joint line elevation as this may reflect a large flexion gap and difficulty gaining full extension [8, 9]. The surgeon may leave the knee lax in flexion to avoid overresecting distally. Conversely, if the distal femur is overresected, the surgeon will then insert a larger insert to balance in extension. If a smaller insert is used, it may allow adequate knee flexion, but leave the knee unstable in extension and midflexion. To avoid raising the joint line, we would advise trying to create the smallest flexion space possible, and later in this chapter such ideas are proposed. For the LCS primary technique, this usually means moving the anterior/posterior cutting block a notch or two dorsally, or even upsizing the prosthesis whenever possible. The end result is that the flexion space is reduced, the extension space becomes less, and ultimately the joint line is raised less.

With the LCS system, surgeons have learned that careful balancing of the gaps is critical to the performance of the total knee and for the avoidance of clinical instability. Our kinematic studies have shown that good clinical function demonstrates small amounts of joint space opening, on the order of three to four millimeters throughout the range of motion in both the medial and lateral compartments, with or without posterior cruciate preservation. In general, greater than 15 millimeters of anterior/posterior laxity, 10 to 15 millimeters of varus/valgus laxity in extension, and 15 to 20 millimeters of laxity in 90° flexion can be called clinical instability.

3   Ligament Balancing Problem

Most standard posterior cruciate retaining surgical techniques use anatomical bone resections based on predetermined landmarks. Examples include the Whiteside intercondylar line, the posterior condyle reference with a 3° to 5° external femoral rotation or transepicondylar line. Stiehl et al. have shown that the transepicondylar axis clearly matches the knee flexion axis and is nearly perpendicular to the mechanical axis [10]. However the transepicondylar axis may be difficult to define in primary knee arthroplasty. If the anterior/posterior distal femoral cuts are inaccurate in terms of ligamentous balance, it is difficult to perform subsequent releases to achieve matching flexion/extension balance. Krakow, et.al. has shown that the majority of ligaments

problem with the cruciate retaining meniscal bearing knees and more recently the AP Glide prosthesis which will fail if the posterior cruciate gives way. There is an American contingent, who actually believes in partially resecting or releasing the posterior cruciate from prox-

released can have indepent affects on the flexion and extension gaps [1–5]. Release of the medial and lateral capsular ligaments, lateral collateral, popliteus, and superficial medial collateral ligaments will affect both the flexion and extension gaps. Release of the pes tendons, iliotibial tract, medial and lateral gastrocnemius, semitendinosus, and biceps tendons affect balance in extension. Release of the anterior and posterior cruciate ligaments increase the flexion gap roughly 50% more than the extension gap. The problem is more difficult if the posterior cruciate ligament is spared as the options for achieving perfect flexion/gap balance become very limited indeed.

Another issue is the effect of extraarticular deformities. Should the surgeon attempt to balance the deformity through the joint, over resection of ligaments may occur with the potential of instability. Similarly if severe deformity, either in the coronal plane or with flexion contracture be addressed incorrectly, the surgeon can easily leave the knee unbalanced. With the multitude of complexities balancing ligaments, the LCS approach simplifies the problems by using the bone cuts to balance the ligaments instead of vice versa.

4 Clinical Findings

4.1 History

Flexion instability is frequently seen in poorly balanced posterior cruciate retaining fixed bearing total knee arthroplasty. Insidious pain and swelling are the hallmarks of the problem and reflect both instability and polyethylene wear. Typically, there is pain and tenderness anteriorly. Instability can be gross to the extent that the knee is described as "slopy". Patients are particularly uncomfortable walking down stairs. Symptoms can be disabling with a strong sense that the knee will buckle or give way. Some patients are so afflicted that they are uncomfortable placing weight in near extension using crutches or a walker for balance.

Patients will become aware of chronic effusion and swelling. Anterior knee pain is noted and this reflects strain on the anterior tissues due to flexion instability and abnormal anterior femoral sliding in flexion. There may be a visible posterior sag, typical of posterior cruciate ligament laxity or absence. Wasliewski et al. has described the quadriceps active test, where contraction of the quadriceps muscle with the knee in flexion causes the proximal tibia to visibly be thrust forward or anterior [11]. In full extension, there may be anterior tibial translation to the extent that the tibia appears to be more forward than normal.

The patient may relate that there was no symptom free interval following surgery. Physical therapy and bracing are usually of little benefit. The surgeon may have attempted a tibial insert exchange but this may be of little value if there is gross imbalance. Finally, the history of a postoperative knee dislocation is the hallmark of an unstable total knee arthroplasty.

4.2 Physical Findings

The patient will exhibit significant tenderness over the hamstring tendons and insertions, such as the pes, biceps, and semitendinosus tendons. The reason for this is the muscle overactivity that is naturally occuring to deal with the inherent instability (Fig. 16–21). As noted above, greater than 15 millimeters of anterior/posterior laxity, 10 to 15 millimeters of varus/valgus laxity in extension, and 15 to 20 millimeters of laxity in 90° flexion can be called clinical instability. The authors have found an easy test is to place the patient in the sitting position with the leg hanging off the edge of the table. When completely relaxed, the surgeon grabs the distal femoral condyles and then attempts to rock the tibia back and forth. With some practice, this will show amazingly well the amount of laxity in flexion. Standard radiographic studies are usually "normal" but traction radiographs centered over the joint line with 7° flexion may be illustrative. Aspiration is usually negative for bacterial growth as these cases are typically not infected, but there may be polyethylene wear debris on microscopic evaluation.

4.3 Detailed Analysis of Balancing Error

For the surgeon to understand the problems, he must go back and review the potential issues that were encountered at the time of surgery. The possibilities include good overall alignment and good ligaments, malalignment and good ligaments, and good alignment with poor ligaments. In the first case, radiographs are usually unrevealing and the surgeon must rely on the above clinical findings. In the second case, component malposition can be seen on radiographs, either from insertional error or late subsidence. In the last case, the clinical condition such as rheumatoid arthritis or polio is the culprit resulting in markedly weakened or atrophic ligaments.

Perhaps the easiest problem to understand is when technique was generally correct with good alignment and reasonable ligament balancing but postoperative instability results. With the LCS system, the most logical explanation is an error in the bone cuts or implant sizing. As the tibia must be cut in the perfect coronal posi-

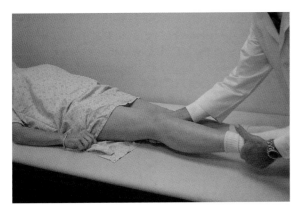

Fig. 19. Clinical examination with varus/valgus testing

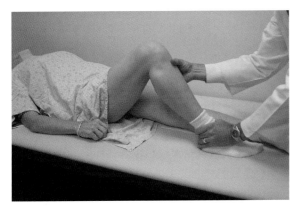

Fig. 20. Clinical examination with anterior posterior drawer

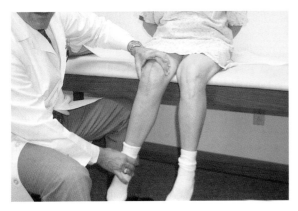

Fig. 21. Clinical examination with flexion stability testing, rocking the tibia with the knee flexion 90° and the knee totally relaxed

tion with the knee in extension, if the tibial cut is internally rotated, imbalance results with tibial varum. The reason for this is that the normal LCS tibial cut is in 7° of posterior tibial slope, and internal rotation of this cut will result in varus tibial component positioning. If the anterior/posterior flexion cut is internally or externally rotated abnormally from exact tension, imbalance results. If the patient is obese and the leg falls into ab-

duction, the heavy weight of the leg may cause the cutting block to externally rotate on the distal femur. Another common cause is overresection of ligaments in severe varus or valgus knees. As the medial or lateral collateral ligaments are released, the gaps increase but as there are more components stabilizing the extension gap, a relative over-release results in flexion. Surgeons anticipate this in the severe valgus knee but not always in the varus knee. Some of the most difficult instabilities we have seen resulted with over resection on the medial side. The knee is not as tolerant of this instability because of the natural knee valgus alignment, and conversely, a minor lateral joint laxity may be better tolerated. We would advise the surgeon to go very cautiously with these releases, titrating and testing the release, but always trying to preserve some inherent stability in the flexion space.

With posterior cruciate balancing the ultimate outcome of the case rests with the balance of the ligaments in flexion. If tensioning is "too tight", the tibia will sublux forward and stay forward throughout the range of motion. These are the knees that develop chronic stiffness and often poor flexion. If the tensioning is "too loose", the femur will slide forward on the tibia with increasing flexion, leading to the above findings of clinical instability. We believe that most total knees, especially mobile bearings like the LCS, must have adequate balance in flexion, while a bit of laxity in extension on the lateral side of the joint is more tolerated.

5   Treatment

5.1   General Considerations

For the LCS system, ligamentous instability is usually heralded by bearing dislocation or spinout. These issues are covered in above chapters. In general, the surgeon may have been close with balancing the gaps, but through trauma, late instability, or other issues, a problem has arisen. As has been shown by many surgeons, these problems can be resolved by simple bearing exchange. For example, if wear has caused late failure of a meniscal bearing implant, new and thicker bearings usually suffice. In the case of the AP Glide, if there is late posterior cruciate instability causing increased laxity, this can be resolved by a thicker, and more constrained rotating platform implant in most instances.

In an elderly patient who may be high risk for complex surgery, one may consider a period of immobilization of six to eight weeks with the knee held in extension. This may provide enough scarring to prevent gross dislocation, especially if the laxity is on the lateral side of the joint in extension.

In fixed bearing total knee implants, it establishing the correct flexion/extension gap balance has not been done correctly the problem is more difficult. A simple tibial modular insert exchange will not suffice and a revision is generally required. If the tibial base plate fixation and position is satisfactory, the surgeon may consider revising only the tibial insert and the femoral component. As a posterior stabilized femoral implant is typically needed, the surgeon must be comfortable with the type of implant utilized and the ability to use the conversion revision implant of that particular manufacturer.

In general, at the time of surgery, careful flexion/ extension gap balance is the focus of the technique. Tight balancing of 2 to 3 millimeters in both flexion and extension is the desired goal. A minor flexion contracture of up to 10° is a good idea as most of these will stretch out over the first 12 months after surgery. Finally, modular revision options as will be shown, are critical to this exercise.

5.2   Surgical Tactics

5.2.1   Extension Rebalancing

For the experienced LCS surgeon, the recommended technique of revision for flexion instability follows identical to the LCS technique in terms of the steps with posterior cruciate resection and the addition of modular solutions for the encountered problems. The first step is to gain correct balance in full extension. If instability is on the lateral side of the joint, the mistake may have been inadequate medial release in the case of severe varus deformity. This should focus on ligaments that affect primarily extension such as the superficial medial collateral ligament. If the superficial medial collateral ligament is released, it must be as a continuous subperiosteal sleeve not to loose any continuity. Then the secondary medial stabilizers in extension should be addressed including the posterior medial corner, the posterior capsule and rarely the semitendinosus insertions and even more rarely the pes insertions. One must preserve something on the medial side to prevent gross medial laxity, and this would be a careful titration of release leaving some of the posterior medial capsular ligament which will provide some stability in flexion. Similarly, on the lateral side of the joint with tight valgus deformity, the tendency is to release the iliotibial tract, the lateral capsular structures, and finally release the lateral collateral ligament from the lateral epicondyle. Something must be left on the lateral side to prevent gross opening in flexion, and this should be either the popliteus tendon or the posterior lateral capsular structures. Another option the authors have used is to release the

lateral collateral origin and popliteus as a single flake of bone from the lateral epicondyle and then advance these structures distally and anteriorly, thusly giving both release in extension and providing some stability of the knee in flexion. The extension gap must be established before one goes on to the next step, because most LCS users know, once you cut the posterior condyles, you can't rebalance the knee easily in extension.

5.2.2   Tibia Cut First

As described by Insall, the most logical method for obtaining correct balancing is to use the tibia cut first method. This preferentializes establishing the flexion gap which is the primary problem with the unstable total knee. As Stiehl has shown with the tibial axis rotation method of determining the distal bone cuts, a perpendicular tibial cut will anatomically align with the transepicondylar axis in the normal knee [10]. External alignment jigs may be used, but many revision systems utilize an intramedullary alignment for the tibia in the revision setting and there is no preference. A definite problem with intramedullary rods on the tibial side is the eccentricity both in position and alignment that they may find to the mechanical axis. Systems that allow offset of the tibial base plate may be desireable in this regard.

5.2.3   Flexion Block Method

For the LCS user, the horseshoe spacer is the "brilliant" instrument that allows tension of the flexion gap for routine anterior/posterior condylar resection. Depending on availability modular revision options either with the LCS Revision system or a fixed bearing revision system, a full complement of wedges, builds, modular stems, etc is needed. Two problems are encountered in placing the flexion block. First, the intramedullary canal may be a big "hole" not allowing placement of a firm intramedullary rod. Some systems allow placing graduated larger stem trials into the canal for stabilizing the distal femoral cutting and anterior/posterior cutting blocks. The second problem here is that this stem will tend to drift anteriorly as the stem wants to follow the natural bow of the distal femur. The PFC Sigma Modular Revision system solves this by providing a two millimeter offset of the distal stem in the dorsal direction. If all else fails, an option is to pin the anterior/posterior cutting block on one side in what you think is correct and then place tension on the opposite side of the block and then pin that in place. The final goal is assessment of the flexion space and one must have a rectangular flexion space in terms of ligament balance using the flexion spacing blocks (Fig. 22, 23).

Once the flexion space and femoral rotation is established, two additional problems arise. The first is what

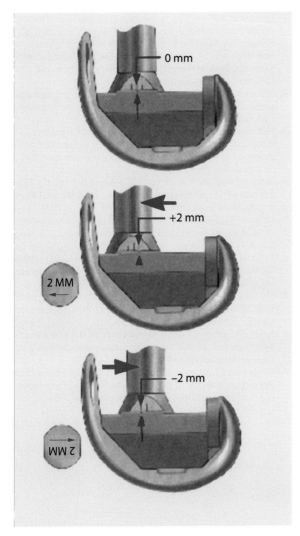

Fig. 22. Femoral component options: dorsal movement of femoral stem, posterior and distal condylar builds

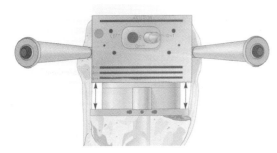

Fig. 23. Flexion spacing block method, note spacing of anterior/posterior condylar cutting block based off intramedullary rod with anterior cortical reference

to do with a poorly placed prior cut, for example if the surgeon cut the distal femur in internal rotation. In that case, the surgeon will obviously need a build on the lateral posterior femoral condyle. Contemporary flexion block jigs will allow you to cut to the defect of the con-

dyle which allows you to identify the bone loss and simply supplement with a posterior condylar build. The second problem and perhaps the most significant one of this whole discussion is what to do with an "extra large" flexion space. One of the authors, JBS has experienced a flexion gap that required 54 millimeters of material to fill the flexion space in unusual case. The following ways have been used to deal with a big flexion space. First is to try to position the axis of the femoral stem axis as far posterior as possible. As noted with the PFC Sigma, this can be done by using a 2 millimeter offset bolt. The second thing to do is to upsize the femoral component giving a greater anterior posterior diameter. This can add several millimeters, especially if the device is placed more dorsally. The final approach is to add posterior condylar builds which not only will provide stability for better fixation, but will push the implant dorsally. Correction of the space orientation can be differentially determined by adding different thickness of builds to the medial or lateral side.

5.2.4   Extension Space Determination

The last step is to take the knee into extension to determine the extension balance and create the extension gap. If done correctly, this should already be perfectly balanced and now only requires tensioning. Depending on the dimension of the flexion space, the extension space will be determined by either resecting more bone or by adding builds to the distal femoral condyle to push the joint line down. In general the joint line should be low enough to avoid patellar impingement of the tibial insert in deep flexion. This is why efforts to close the flexion gap are so important. At this point of the procedure, if there is a minor amount of extension laxity of 5 to 7 millimeters on the lateral side of the joint, the surgeon may choose a more constrained tibial post option (TC3) to prevent dislocation but any laxity should be avoided if possible. The authors have virtually no experience with collateral ligament advancement techniques for ligament instability and would not recommend them at this time. As noted above, a minor flexion contracture up to 100 limiting full extension may be a good idea, especially in the patient with hyperlax soft tissues. With posterior cruciate resection, this usually stretches out in 12 months.

6   Postoperative Management

If adequate ligament balancing has been done , these revisions may be treated like any postoperative total knee with early range of motion and gait training. For this reason, ligament advancement methods that require special bracing seem impractical. There may be certain restrictions required if a tibial tubercle osteotomy or quads snip are done.

7   Conclusion

In the authors' experience, instability is a common cause of postoperative knee problems and should be high on the differential of the painful total knee. The best solution is preventative and not to allow it to occur in the first place. With the LCS, the early problem is obvious as implant dislocation or spinout will usually occur. The treatment is excellent revision surgical technique to correctly balance the flexion/extension gaps and offers gratifying surgical results with pain-free well functioning total knees.

References

1. Krackow KA, Mihalko WM (1999a) Flexion-extension joint gap changes after lateral structure release for valgus deformity correction in total knee arthroplasty: a cadaveric study. J Arthroplasty 14: 994–1004
2. Krackow KA, Mihalko WM (1999b) The effect of medial release on flexion and extension gaps in cadaveric knees: implications for soft-tissue balancing in total knee arthroplasty. Am J Knee Surgery 12: 222–228
3. Krakow KA, Mihalko WM (2001) The effects of severe femoral bone loss on the flexion extension joint space in revision total knee arthroplasty: a cadaveric analysis and clinical consequences. Orthopaedics 24: 121–126
4. Mihalko WM, Krackow KA (1999) Posterior cruciate ligament effects on the flexion space in total knee arthroplasty. Clin Orthop 360: 243–250
5. Mihalko WM, Miller C, Krackow KA (2000) Total knee arthroplasty ligament balancing and gap kinematics with posterior cruciate ligament retention and sacrifice. Am J Orthopaedics 29: 610–616
6. Montgomery RL, Goodman SB, Congradi J (1993) Late rupture of the posterior cruciate ligament after total knee arthroplasty. Iowa Orthop 13: 167–170
7. Ochsner JL, Kostman WC, Dodson M (1993) Posterior cruciate ligament avulsion in total knee arthroplasty. Orthop Rev 22: 1121–1124
8. Pagnano MW, Hanssen AD, Lewallen DG, Stuart MJ (1998) Flexion instability after primary posterior cruciate retaining total knee arthroplasty. Clin Orthop 356: 39–46
9. Sharkey PF, Hozack WJ, Booth RE, Baldsteron RA, Rothman RH (1992) Posterior dislocation of total knee arthroplasty. Clin Orthop 278: 128–133
10. Stiehl JB, Abbot B (1995) Morphology of the transepicondylar axis and its application in primary and revision total knee arthroplasty. J Arthroplasty 10: 785–792
11. Waslewski GL, Marson BM, Benjamin JB (1998) Early, incapacitating instability of posterior cruciate ligament-retaining total knee arthroplasty. J Arthroplasty 13: 763–767

12.4 Aseptic Loosening in the LCS Total Knee Arthroplasty

L. R. Jordan, J. L. Olivio

1 Introduction

Although total knee arthroplasty has proven to be a successful surgical procedure, aseptic loosening has been and is still a perplexing complication [5, 22, 29, 46, 47, 51]. Aseptic loosening as a reason for revision has varied from 58 % to 73 % [22]. The results of these revisions in turn are less predictable and are not as successful as the primary total knee arthroplasty [26]. Thus, it is imperative to obtain initial and long-lasting fixation of the total knee components to avoid aseptic loosening and the inherent difficult technical problems and complications involved in revision total knee arthroplasty.

Total knee component designs have been evolutionary. Early cemented, fixed hinge designs such as the Guepar placed significant stress on the bone-cement interface, leading to early loosening and failure [14, 31]. Subsequently, non-hinged but highly constrained and congruent cemented designs failed because of the high shear stress placed on the bone-cement interface of the femur or tibia (Fig. 24).

Likewise, polycentric and spherocentric designs also failed because of the high stresses placed on the fixation [25, 37].

Initial tibial designs were all polyethylene components. Problems arose with polyethylene deformation, cold flow and loosening, especially with the thin polyethylene components. Metal backing was added to tibial trays to increase the support of the polyethylene, decrease cold flow, and to more evenly distribute shear forces to the component fixation interface [2, 3].

In an effort to decrease the incidence of loosening occurring with highly constrained total knee designs, there was a shift to less congruent, less constrained cemented and cementless components [28, 45, 55]. This was in anticipation that the less constrained designs would lead to decreased shear stress, improved stress distribution, and subsequently less loosening complications.

This concept, however, introduced and created a new set of problems, namely potential aseptic loosen-

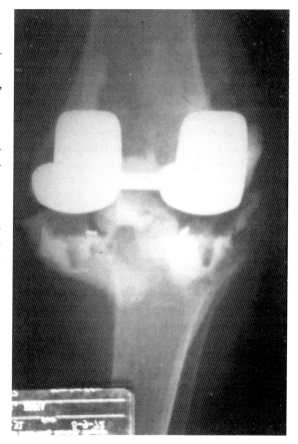

Fig. 24. Loosening of congruent but constrained total knee arthroplasty

ing secondary to osteolysis from polyethylene particulate debris [12, 17, 18, 41, 43]. By decreasing the congruity of the femoral tibial articulation in an attempt to decrease shear forces on the fixation, conformity was sacrificed. Detrimental kinematics were created, increased contact stresses occurred, resulting in higher rates of wear, polyethylene delamination, and debris formation [12, 19, 52, 60]. This particulate debris elicited a significant host response, resulting in bone osteolysis with or without loosening of the total knee components, and

whether or not the components were cemented or uncemented. When modularity was added to fixed bearing total knee designs, backside wear added to the problems of osteolysis secondary to polyethylene debris, especially when the locking mechanism was not adequate
[17, 18, 41, 43, 51].

Initial total knee designs did not include patellar
components. Because of a high incidence of patellofemoral pain, the patella articulating surface began to be replaced with an all polyethylene component. These early
designs were noted to show high levels of polyethylene
wear, and deformation secondary to large patellofemoral reactive forces. Efforts to lower the polyethylene wear
by making the patellofemoral joint more congruent resulted in increased constraint and shear forces at the
implant-bone interface and subsequent loosening [63].
Metal backing was added in the mid-1980's to reduce
polyethylene strain and improve load transfer, as well
as to allow for cementless fixation. Unfortunately, high
contact stresses and polyethylene wear of these metal-
backed components lead to an additional set of complications, including polyethylene metal dissociation, polyethylene wear and fracture, fixation peg-plate breakage,
patellar fracture, and patellofemoral joint instability
[4, 52, 53, 61]. Today, aseptic patellofemoral complications are among the most common cause of total knee
revision surgery. Complications related to the patellofemoral joint have been as high as 50 % of total knee
complications [7].

2   The LCS Mobile Bearing Total Knee Prosthesis

In an attempt to balance the high contact stresses of the
tibial femoral articulation, as well as those of the patellofemoral joint and still allow minimal constraint and
shear forces to reduce loosening problems, the LCS Total Knee system was developed [8]. The LCS Patella was
designed with a congruent, anatomic polyethylene articulating surface, free to rotate on a thin metal fixation
plate. The tibial femoral articulation consisted of a mobile, congruent polyethylene component free to articulate on a polished metal tibial tray. Both the metal fixation plate of the patella or the tibial tray could be used
with cementless or cement fixation. This construct resulted in a highly congruent polyethylene articulation to
reduce polyethylene wear with rotation to decrease constraint and shear forces resulting in minimal problems
with aseptic loosening.

Aseptic loosening remains one of the most frequent
complications of current total knee arthroplasties.
When these complications require revision, the quality
of the revision is frequently less than that of the primary

total knee arthroplasty. Thus, it is imperative to develop
a total knee component that will provide long term durability with good polyethylene wear and a low probability of loosening. This is especially true as these components are used in younger, high demand patients with
life expectancy increases.

Aseptic loosening most frequently involves the patella or tibial component and occurs in both cementless
as well as cemented arthroplasties. Fixed bearing tibial
or patellar components that are highly congruent and
conforming, to keep contact stresses and subsequently
polyethylene wear at a minimum, create excessive shear
forces at the component-fixation interface leading to
potential loosening of the components. Fixed bearing designs that have decreased the congruity to lower
shear stresses on the fixation develop increased contact
stresses and potential accelerated polyethylene wear resulting in mechanical failure of the component and potential loosening secondary to osteolysis.

Early patella and tibial components were all polyethylene designs. With the all polyethylene patella, large reactive forces at the patellofemoral joint resulted in significant polyethylene wear and deformation. In an effort to decrease the high contact stresses, more congruent patellofemoral articulations were developed. While
the congruency reduced contact stresses, constraint
forces and shear stresses increased at the implant fixation interface, resulting in fixation complications [8]. In
an effort to improve load transfer and reduce polyethylene wear, as well as facilitate fixation in cementless designs, metal backing was added to the polyethylene patellar component [28]. Discouragingly, metal-backed
fixed bearing patellar components developed additional complications, including polyethylene wear and
fracture, metallosis, polyethylene-metal disassociation,
fixation peg-plate fracture and disassociation, and metal
plate fracture [21, 53, 61]. As a result, some have advocated caution in the use of fixed bearing metal-backed
components [4, 5, 13, 61].

All metal-backed patellar components are not equal,
and the combination of a highly congruent mobile, anatomic metal-backed patella has proven to be extremely
successful [9, 32, 33, 58]. The congruent polyethylene ensures low polyethylene wear and excellent stability while
the mobility compensates for misalignment and reduces
shear stresses at the fixation interface, resulting in an extremely low incidence of polyethylene failure or component loosening.

Early all polyethylene tibial components were associated with loosening and polyethylene deformation,
especially when eccentric loads were applied to one
or the other tibial plateaus [3, 59]. In an effort to more
evenly distribute loads, decrease loosening, decrease

creep, protect the underlying, sometimes weak cancellous bone and decrease polyethylene complications, metal backing was added to the tibial polyethylene component [3, 11, 38].

Even with the metal-backed tibial components, however, aseptic loosening remains one of the most frequent causes for revisions of total knee arthroplasties. The mechanism of loosening is multifactorial and related to surgical technique, patient selection and component design [5, 13, 15–17, 19, 24, 42, 46, 51, 54].

3 Surgical Technique

Micromotion between the component and bone can result in loosening [6]. Inadequate initial fixation, whether the components are cemented or uncemented, will result in loosening. Cement must be well interdigitated into the prosthetic component and bone. Optimal fit and apposition of the porous coating to the cancellous bone must be accomplished in uncemented components. Irrespective of the type of fixation, an initial, poorly fixed

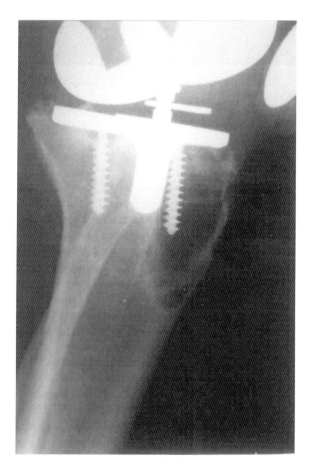

Fig. 25. Malalignment

component does not tighten or become well-fixed with time.

Malalignment must be avoided [15, 20, 69, 59, 50]. Total knee arthroplasties that are malaligned are vulnerable to eventual loosening (Fig. 25).

Excessive postoperative varus or valgus can result in off center weight bearing forces, resulting in lift off on one side and excessive loading and subsidence on the other side [30, 40]. Malalignment secondary to incorrect ligamentous balancing can cause excessive stress on the tighter side, leading to off center loading and potential increase in polyethylene wear or loosening. Equal ligamentous balancing and stability should be present throughout the entire range of motion. If ligament balancing is unequal, lift off can occur, resulting in excess compression of the polyethylene as the femoral condyles recontact the polyethylene.

Loosening can be related to the quality of bone stock that is available, and surgical techniques must be adjusted and modified to accommodate this sometimes unforeseen situation. Sclerotic bone can make cement or cementless fixation difficult to achieve. Likewise, soft, cancellous bone can lead to problems with initial fixation or later support, subsidence, and loosening. Bone loss or deficiency requiring bone grafts, augments, cement with or without additional screw fixation, must be addressed at the time of surgery.

4 Patient Selection

Excessive obesity can affect loosening, as well as anesthesia-related problems, infections, and postoperative incision complications [30, 40, 44, 46]. Patients who are 30% above their ideal weight have a 30% incidence of anterior knee pain [59]. Obese patients can also be at risk for polyethylene wear and loosening secondary to the excessively high loads across the knee joint [46].

Patients who engage in impact loading activities, the young vigorous active patient, the unrealistic, noncompliant patient who becomes overactive after total knee arthroplasty is vulnerable to loosening of the components [46]. Patients with neuropathic joints or those with sclerotic bone or deformity of Paget's disease are at risk for failure of the arthroplasty because of loosening [23, 47].

5 Component Design

Prosthetic design is related to loosening. The more constraint built into the prosthesis, the more likely loosening will occur. To decrease constraint and shear forces

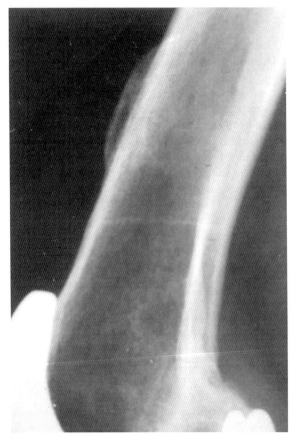

Fig. 26. Osteolysis of distal femur secondary to polyethylene debris

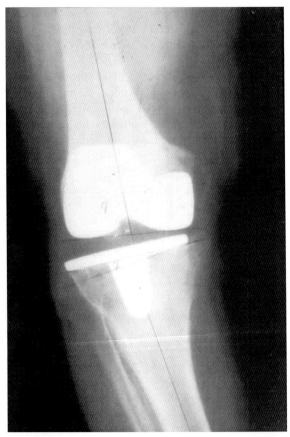

Fig. 27. Osteolysis of anterior proximal tibia secondary to polyethylene debris

in a fixed bearing design, congruity must be sacrificed. This can lead to increased contact stresses resulting in increased polyethylene wear.

Polyethylene wear can be associated with osteolysis (Fig. 26, 27).

Osteolysis can lead to component loosening in both cemented and cementless fixation [51, 17, 18, 41, 43, 54].

The LCS (DePuy) mobile, anatomic, congruent patella and mobile meniscal bearing or rotating platform total knee arthroplasty addresses the concerns of polyethylene wear and loosening. Congruity assures low contact stress and excellent polyethylene wear resistance . Mobility assures minimal shear stresses and adjusts for minor malalignment of the patella and tibial components. Proper coronal design which allows for some varus/valgus tilting and still allows for congruity and low contact stress is extremely important to keeping polyethylene wear to a minimum [3]. This concept is true not only for the femoral-tibial joint, but also for the femoral patella articulation [36] (Fig. 28a,b).

The overall survivorship at 12 years of the mobile patella is 99% with no cases of loosening [58]. Similar findings were noted in a multicenter review of 1939 knees where the patellofemoral complications were 0.9% with a 0.1% loosening complication [34]. Others have noted no cases of patellar loosening at 14 years and 20 years [9, 58].

Loosening of the femoral and tibial components of the LCS (DePuy) mobile bearing designs has been extremely low [9, 34, 36, 57, 58]. In recently reported series at 14 years and 20 years, loosening was less than 1% [9, 58]. In the author's study of 232 consecutive LCS (DePuy) mobile bearing total knee arthroplasties, there were no revisions of the tibial, femoral or patellar components for loosening and survivorship for loosening at 12 years was 100% [34, 35].

Radiolucent lines have generated interest in the LCS (DePuy) mobile bearing total knee arthroplasty. In one series, radiolucent lines occurring infrequently, were small and non-progressive [58]. Others in following the natural history and significance of radiolucent lines in the LCS (DePuy) mobile bearing knee noted that although radiolucent lines may increase during the first 12 months postoperatively, they may stabilize or even decrease thereafter [62].

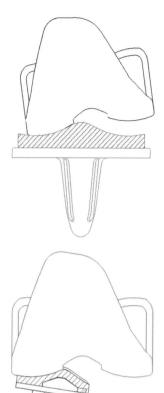

Fig. 28a,b. A common generating curve of all articulating surfaces allows fully congruent contact between lateral femoral condyle and lateral patella facet, even with mild lateral subluxation or patella tilt (From Patellofemoral success in total knee arthroplasty, DePuy Orthopaedics Inc, Warsaw, IN 1995)

6   Overview

If total knee arthroplasties are to be performed especially in anticipation that they are to last for longer periods of time, it is imperative certain principles be followed. A well-designed total knee prosthesis does not substitute or compensate for less than optimal surgical technique. Malalignment should be avoided, flexion and extension gaps should be equal and ligamentous balancing should be precise. As total knee arthroplasties are performed in younger, higher demand patients, and as life expectancy increases, emphasis should be placed on designs in which polyethylene wear will be minimal, and fixation will be long-lasting. The kinematic conflict of congruity to decrease contact stresses and polyethylene wear versus the resulting increased shear stresses resulting in component loosening can be theoretically solved with a mobile bearing total knee design. With mobility, a highly congruent polyethylene surface can co-exist with rotation, resulting in low shear forces.

Increasing number of mobile bearing total knee designs are beginning to enter the market [27]. All mobile bearing knees, however, are not the same, and all do not have long term clinical follow-up results. The LCS (DePuy) mobile bearing knee with a highly congruent femoral-tibial articulation, as well as a highly con-

gruent, anatomic patellofemoral articulation, has been in use for 25 years. The survivorship for aseptic loosening in our series of cementless meniscal bearing total knee arthroplasties for the mobile patella at 12 years has been 100%, and for the femoral-tibial components, 100%. This is similar to other series where the survivorship for loosening of the cementless meniscal bearing total knee is 100% at 16 years, and of the cemented and uncemented rotating platform is 100% at 14 years and 20 years [9, 58].

Acknowledgement: The authors sincerely thank Karen O'Brien, B.S., for her assistance and tireless effort in preparing this manuscript.

References

1. Bartel D, Burstein AH, Santavicca E, Insall JN (1982) Performance of the tibial component in total knee conventional and revision designs. J Bone Joint Surg 64 A: 1026–1031
2. Bartel DL, Burstein AH, Toda MD, Edwards DL (1985) The effect of conformity and plastic thickness on contact stresses in metal-backed plastic implants. J Biomech Eng 107: 193–199
3. Bartel DL, Bicknell MS, Wright TM (1986) The effect of conformity, thickness and material on stresses in ultrahigh molecular weight components for total joint replacement. J Bone Joint Surg 68 A: 1041–1051
4. Bayley JC, Scott RD (1988) Further observations on metal-backed patellar component failure. Clin Orthop 236: 82–87
5. Berger RA, Lyon JH, Jacobs JJ, Barden RM, Berkson EM, Sheinkop MB, Rosenberg AG, Galante JO (2001) Problems with cementless arthroplasty at 11 years follow-up. Clin Orthop 392: 196–207
6. Branson PJ, Steege SW, Wixson RI, Lewis J, Stulberg SD (1989) Rigidity of initial fixation with uncemented tibial implants. J Arthroplasty 4: 21–26
7. Brick GW, Scott RD (1988) The patellofemoral component of total knee arthroplasty. Clin Orthop 231: 163–178
8. Buechel FF (1996) Low contact stress meniscal bearing knee replacement: Design concepts, failure mechanisms and long term survivorship. In: Insall JN, Scott WN, Scuderi GR (eds) Current concepts in primary and revision total knee arthroplasty. Lippincott-Raven, Philadelphia, p 47
9. Buechel FF, Buechel Jr FF, Pappas MJ, D'Alessio J (2001) Twenty-year evaluation of meniscal bearing and rotating platform knee replacements. Clin Orthop 388: 41–50
10. Callaghan JJ, Squire MW, Goetz DD, Sullivan PM, Johnston RC (2000) Cemented rotating-platform total knee replacement. A nine to twelve year follow-up study. J Bone Joint Surg 82 A: 705–711
11. Colizza WA, Insall JN, Scuderi GR (1995) The posterior stabilized total knee prosthesis: Assessment of polyethylene damage and osteolysis after ten-year minimum follow-up. J Bone Joint Surg 77 A: 1713–1718
12. Collier JB, Mayor MB, Surprenant VA (1990) The biomechanical problems of polyethylene as a bearing surface. Clin Orthop 261: 107–113
13. Crites MB, Berend ME (2001) Metal-backed patellar components: A brief report on 10 year survival. Clin Orthop 388: 103–104

14. Deburge A (1976) A Guepar hinged prosthesis: Complications and results with two year follow-up. Clin Orthop 147: 47–53

15. Dorr LD, Boiardo RA (1986) Technical considerations in total knee arthroplasty. Clin Orthop 205: 5–11

16. Duffy GP, Berry DJ, Rand JA (1998) Cement versus cementless fixation in total knee arthroplasty. Clin Orthop 356: 66–72

17. Engh GA, Dwyer KA, Hanes CK (1992) Polyethylene wear of metal-backed tibial components in total and unicompartmental knee prosthesis. J Bone Joint Surg 74B: 9–17

18. Ezzet KA, Garcia R, Barrack RL (1995) Effect of component fixation method on osteolysis in total knee arthroplasty. Clin Orthop 321: 86–91

19. Fengel EL, Stulberg SD, Wixson RL (1994) Progressive subluxation and polyethylene wear in total knee replacements with flat articular surfaces. Clin Orthop 299: 60–71

20. Figgie HE, Goldberg VM, Figgie MP, Inglis AE, Kelly M, Sobel M (1989) The effect of alignment of the implant on fractures of the patella after condylar arthroplasty. J Bone Joint Surg 71 A: 1031–1039

21. Firestone TP, Teeny SM, Krackow KA, Hungerford DS (1991) The clinical and roentgenographic results of cementless porous coated patellar fixation. Clin Orthop 273: 184–189

22. Friedman RJ, Hirst H, Poss R, Kelley K, Sledge CR (1990) Results of revision total knee arthroplasty performed for aseptic loosening. Clin Orthop 255: 235–241

23. Gabel GT, Rand JA, Sim FN (1991) Total knee arthroplasty for osteoarthritis in patients who have Paget's disease of bone at the knee. J Bone Joint Surg 73 A: 739–744

24. Gill CS, Joshi AB, Mills DM (1999) Total condylar arthroplasty: 16–21 year results. Clin Orthop 367: 210–215

25. Gunston FH, Mackenzie RI (1976) Complications of polycentric knee arthroplasty. Clin Orthop 120: 11–17

26. Hass SB, Insall JN, Montgomery III W, Windsor RE (1995) Revision total knee arthroplasty with use of modular components with stems inserted without cement. J Bone Joint Surg 77 A: 1700–1707

27. Heim CS, Postak PD, Plaxton NA, Greenwald AS (2001) Classification of mobile-bearing knee designs: Mobility and constraint. J Bone Joint Surg 83 A (Suppl 2) : 32–37

28. Hungerford Ds, Krackow KA, Kenna RV (1989) Cementless total knee replacements in patients 50 years old and under. Orthop Clin North Am 20: 131–145

29. Insall J, Scott WN, Ranawat CS (1979) The total condylar prosthesis. A report of two hundred and twenty cases. J Bone Joint Surg 61 A: 173–180

30. Insall JN, Binazzi R, Soudry M, Mestriner LA (1985) Total knee arthroplasty. Clin Orthop 192: 13–22

31. Jones EC, Insall JN, Inglis AE, Ranawat CS (1979) Guepar knee arthroplasty results and late complications. Clin Orthop 140: 145–152

32. Jordan LR, Keblish PA, Collier DE, Greenwald A, Davenport JM (1993) Successful use of a metal-backed anatomic patella in TKA: Biomechanical rationale and clinical experience. Presented at the American Academy of Orthopedic Surgeons, San Francisco

33. Jordan LR, Olivo JL, Voorhorst PE (1997) Survivorship analysis of cementless meniscal bearing total knee arthroplasty. Clin Orthop 338: 119–123

34. Jordan LR, Olivo JL, Voorhorst PE (2000a) Survivorship analysis of a metal-backed rotating anatomic patella in total knee arthroplasty: A 14 year follow-up. Presented at the American Academy of Orthopaedic Surgeons, Orlando

35. Jordan LR, Olivo JL, Voorhorst PE (2000b) Survivorship analysis of cementless meniscal bearing total knee arthroplasty: A 14 year follow-up. Presented at the American Academy of Orthopaedic Surgeons, Orlando

36. Jordan LR, Dowd JE, Olivo JL, Voorhorst PE (2002) The clinical history of mobile bearing patella components in total knee arthroplasty. Orthopedics 25: S247-S250

37. Kaufer H, Matthews LS (1981) Spherocentric arthroplasty of the knee. J Bone Joint Surg 63 A: 545–559

38. L'Insalata J, Sterns S, Insall JN (1992) Total knee arthroplasty in elderly patients: Comparison of tibial designs. J Arthroplasty 7: 261–266

39. Lotke PA, Ecker ML (1977) Influence of positioning of prosthesis in total knee replacement. J Bone Joint Surg 59 A: 77–79

40. Moreland JR (1988) Mechanisms of failure in total knee arthroplasty. Clin Orthop 226: 49–64

41. Pagnano MW, Scuderi GR, Insall JN (2001) Tibial osteolysis associated with the modular tibial tray of a cemented posterior stabilized total knee replacement. J Bone Joint Surg 83 A: 1545

42. Parker DA, Rorabeck CH, Bourne RB (2001) Long term follow-up of cementless versus hybrid fixation for total knee arthroplasty. Clin Orthop 388: 68–76

43. Peters PC, Engh GH, Dwyer KA, Vinh T (1992) Osteolysis after total knee arthroplasty without cement. J Bone Joint Surg 74 A: 864–876

44. Ranawat CS, Boachie-Adjei O (1988) Survivorship analysis and results of total condylar knee arthroplasty. Clin Orthop 226: 6–13

45. Ranawat CS, Hansra J, Kenneth K (1989) Effect of posterior cruciate sacrifice on durability of the cement-bone interface. Orthop Clin North Am 20: 68–69

46. Rand JA (1995) Revision total knee arthroplasty for aseptic loosening. In: Lotke PA (ed) Master techniques in orthopedic surgery, knee arthroplasty. Raven Press Ltd, Philadelphia, pp 195–217

47. Rand JA (1999) Preoperative planning and prosthetic choices for revision total knee arthroplasty. In: Lotke PA, Garino JP (eds) Revision total knee arthroplasty. Lippincott-Raven Publishers, Philadelphia-New York, pp 137–156

48. Rand JA, Peterson LFA, Bryan RS, Ilstrup DM (1986) Inst Course Lect 35: 305–318

49. Rhodes DD, Noble PC, Reuben JD, Tullos HS (1993) The effect of femoral component position on the kinematics of total knee arthroplasty. Clin Orthop 286: 122–129

50. Ritter MA, Faris PM, Keating EM, Meding JB (1999) Postoperative alignment of total knee replacement. Clin Orthop 299: 153–156

51. Robinson EJ, Mulliken BD, Bourne RB, Rorabeck CH, Alvarez C (1995) Catastrophic osteolysis in total knee replacement. Clin Orthop 321: 98–105

52. Rorabeck CH, Bourne RB, Lewis PL, Nott L (1993) The Miller-Galante knee prosthesis for the treatment of osteoarthritis. J Bone Joint Surg 75 A: 402–407

53. Rosenberg AG, Andriacchi TP, Barden R, Galante JO (1988) Patellar component failure in cementless total knee arthroplasty. Clin Orthop 236: 100–114

54. Sanchez-Sotelo J, Ordonez JM, Prats SB (1999) Results and complications of the low contact stress knee prosthesis. J Arthroplasty 14: 815–821

55. Scuderi GR, Insall JN (1989) The posterior stabilized knee prosthesis. Orthop Clin North Am 20: 71–78

56. Smith BE, Askew MJ, Gradisar IA, Gradisar JS, Lew MM (1992) The effect of patient weight on the functional outcome of total knee arthroplasty. Clin Orthop 276: 237–244

57. Sorrells RB (1996) Primary knee arthroplasty: Long term outcomes: The rotating platform mobile bearing TKA. Orthopedics 19: 793–796
58. Sorrells RB, Stiehl JB, Voorhorst PE (2001) Midterm results in mobile bearing total knee arthroplasty in patients younger than 65 years. Clin Orthop 390: 182–189
59. Stern SH, Insall JN (1990) Total knee arthroplasty in obese patients. J Bone Joint Surg 72 A: 1400–1404
60. Stiehl JB, Komistek RD, Dennis DA (1999) Detrimental kinematics of a flat on flat total condylar knee arthroplasty. Clin Orthop 365: 139–148
61. Stulberg SD, Stulberg BN, Hamati Y, Tsao A (1988) Failure mechanism of metal-backed patellar components. Clin Orthop 236: 88–105
62. Varma AK, Buechel FF, Reed J, Keblish PA (1994) The natural history and significance of radiolucent zone at the bone-prosthesis interface following porous-coated total knee arthroplasty (TKA). Presented as Scientific Exhibit #41, American Academy of Orthopaedic Surgeons, New Orleans
63. Wright J, Ewald FC, Walker PS, Thomas WH, Poss R, Sledge CB (1990) Total knee arthroplasty with the kinematic prosthesis: Results after five to nine years. A follow-up note. J Bone Joint Surg 72 A: 1003–1009

12.5 Patella Complications

G. HOOPER

1 Introduction

Early total knee arthroplasty (TKA) was essentially resurfacing of either the medial or the lateral compartment with little thought paid to the patellofemoral articulation. However, a high instance of anterior knee pain [8] prompted the development of a femoral trochlea and patella component, for instance the duo condylar knee became the duopatellar knee. Cemented polyethylene dome components were used but the earlier results revealed an alarming incidence of complications with maltracking and wear being the primary problems [5].

Metal backed patellar components were developed to accommodate uncemented fixation and to support the polyethylene, decrease deforming forces on the polyethylene, and to allow a more even distribution of patellofemoral force. This however, had the disadvantage of reducing the thickness of polyethylene, and, with continuous point loading of the polyethylene, these early metal backed patellae often failed [1]. Up to 50 percent of all early total knee arthroplasty revision procedures were due to patellofemoral complications [1, 5]. Although recent design modifications and improved surgical techniques have improved the outcome of TKA, the incidence of patellofemoral complications continues to be reported between 2–10 percent.

The LCS total knee arthroplasty has a unique approach to the patellofemoral joint with a mobile polyethylene component which moves during knee flexion to maintain congruity with the femoral trochlea. This polyethylene mobile bearing is "saddle shaped" and maintains high congruity throughout 90 degrees of knee flexion. As the patella tracks in its normal serpentine path through flexion the mobile bearing is able to rotate and maintain maximal contact of the polyethylene with the trochleal groove. This produces normal tracking with minimal stress to the polyethylene.

2 Patellofemoral Instability

Patellofemoral instability following the LCS TKA is a rare but disabling complication. The first observation often made by surgeons changing from a fixed bearing knee system to the LCS system is the low requirement for a lateral release. This is due to the high congruity of the patellar polyethylene and the mobility of the tibial polyethylene which helps to self center the patellar. This accommodates any small malrotation of the tibial or femoral components. Revision of the femoral or tibial component because of malrotation has not been common with the LCS knee. This is probably due to the emphasis on maintaining ligament balance as an important aspect of the surgical technique. Once ligament balance has been achieved with equal flexion and extension gaps and a well aligned leg, then the extensor mechanism will also be well aligned and biomechanically advantaged.

The most common error in balancing flexion and extension gaps occurs in the valgus or post high tibial osteotomy knee. In this situation, an insufficient lateral release leaves a relatively tight lateral compartment which can result in malrotation of the femoral component. It is important for the surgeon to create equal flexion and extension gaps, and in flexion for the lateral compartment to be slightly lax compared with the medial compartment as in the normal knee. Problems with patellofemoral instability may arise if in flexion the medial compartment is lax compared to the lateral.

Patella instability with or without pain may be difficult to diagnose following TKA unless active or passive subluxation is observed clinically. A single skyline view of the patella is not diagnostic for active subluxation and often a detailed clinical examination is required to support this diagnosis (Fig. 29).

A CT scan may help show subluxation but must be performed with the quadriceps contracted to show the "active" position of the patella. Femoral or tibial malrotation can be assessed by CT scan. Dynamic fluoroscopy

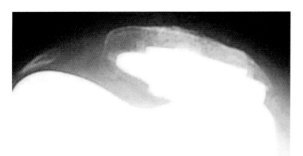

Fig. 29. Skyline view (30 degree flexion) showing marked lateral suluxation of the patellar component. The patient was asymptomatic with a knee that was rated excellent

may have a role in diagnosing patellar instability but is difficult to perform and is operator dependent.

As symptomatic subluxation with this prosthesis is rare any anterior knee pain must be thoroughly investigated before proceeding with surgical correction. The use of a stabilizing patellofemoral brace may help to support the diagnosis of patella instability. A diagnostic manipulation under anesthesia and occasionally an arthroscopy may be required to demonstrate instability. A thorough assessment of the limb alignment as well as ligament balance should be made prior to any lateral release. Technical errors resulting in medial collateral ligament laxity, excessive valgus or femoral internal rotation are the commonest cause of patella dislocation with this prosthesis and should be addressed prior to any extensor mechanism realignment procedures. It is important that the appropriate cause of patellofemoral instability is found prior to any surgical treatment.

In the absence of other causes of patella instability a lateral release can be performed and the patella tracking assessed intra operatively. If the patella is still unstable then a proximal vastus medialis advancement can be performed. Finally a distal tibial tubercle realignment may be required. The osteotomy should be a relatively long fragment, as reported by Whiteside, secured with screws, or wire if the bone is osteoporotic. Immobilization with protected weight bearing is advised for 4 to 6 weeks.

3   Fracture

Although patella fracture has been seen in other series of TKA [2, 7], mostly in rheumatoid arthritis, we have not encountered this problem in over 6,000 procedures. Initially, the patella base plate was secured to the patella with a cruciform post which did require significant bone resection and potentially could have created a significant stress riser in the patella. This component has now been changed to a more conventional three peg design.

Undisplaced or minimally displaced fractures with stable implants and an intact extensor mechanism should be treated with immobilization for 4 to 8 weeks. Open reduction and wire fixation should be restricted to displaced fractures with a compromised extensor mechanism, where the patella implant is stable. For unstable implants we would recommend implant removal and reconstruction of the patella remnants to produce a bony patellar «button» which can articulate within the trochleal groove. Patellectomy may be required as a last resort but will result in inferior function particularly in the meniscal bearing LCS implant which has increased AP excursion. If a patellectomy is contemplated in the presence of a meniscal bearing LCS implant then consideration should be given to increasing the stability of the implant by converting it to a rotating platform.

4   Polyethylene Dissociation

This complication is specific to the LCS rotating patella. The rotating polyethylene bearing can only rotate 45 degrees (30 degrees for the 3 peg device) and any force beyond this causes dissociation of the polyethylene from the base plate (Fig. 30).

At the time of implantation of the patella component the surgeon must be aware that on everting the patella the transverse axis of the patella extends an angle of approximately 20 degrees with the joint line. It is important when placing and positioning the patellar cutting instruments that this is appreciated. This can simply be checked by placing the patella in the normal position with the patella jig in place to confirm that the transverse axis of the patella base plate is parallel to the joint line. Early experience from the LCS clinical trials noted implant dissociation if the patella base plate was angled with respect to the joint line.

We have seen this complication on five occasions, each has been subsequent to a significant traumatic incident often involving falling on the flexed knee with a rotational force. Patients will immediately notice that their TKA is not normal and often complain of crepitus. Swelling may not be a significant clinical finding initially. If this complication is recognized early it is a relatively simple manoeuvre to exchange the polyethylene bearing with no long term sequelae related to the TKA. However, if this complication is diagnosed late then significant burnishing of the femoral component and patella base plate can occur which may necessitate revision of these well fixed components.

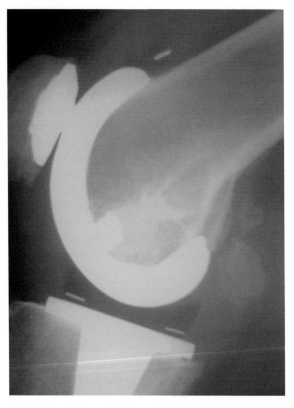

Fig. 30. Lateral view of the knee of a patient who had just fallen down a flight of stairs, twisted the knee. The metal marker of the patellar polyethylene is visible in the suprapatellar bursa. This was simply replaced with no long term effect on the TKA

5   Loosening and Wear

This complication is also rare with the LCS rotating patella. When we have encountered significant loosening of the patella, it has always been in the revision situation where the patella component was cemented. In these revision situations, the patella is often sclerotic and thin resulting in compromised fixation with cement. The patella component coming loose in the presence of this sclerotic bone often makes re-implantation of a further patella prosthesis impossible. It has been our practice to either leave the patella unresurfaced in these situations or to perform a patelloplasty where a deliberate longitudinal fracture is made within the patella so that the patella adopts a V shape allowing some stability within the trochleal groove of the femoral component. An alternative is the grafting procedure of Hansen, where the patella remnant is packed with allograft to a conforming surface and then covered with a piece of fibrous tissue.

Thin polyethylene in other metal backed patella components have been the source of excessive wear and subsequent osteolysis with patella failure [4]. The thin poly-

ethylene on the lateral side of the patella component has been a source of concern with regard to potential wear. However, we have not seen any significant wear and resultant osteolysis associated with this component. Nonetheless, if the tibial polyethylene insert is being exchanged after several years for wear, we would opt for patella implant exchange as well as this is usually a simple and innocuous procedure.

6   Patella Infera

It is common to see a degree of patella infera in most TKA's and this is no different with the LCS knee system. Patella infera can be difficult to measure on a lateral x-ray because of the difficulty of visualizing the patellar tendon. Often the patellar tendon appears to be attached to the anterior aspect of the tibia directly below the joint line rather than being attached to the tibial tubercle alone. This is a reflection of scarring in this region secondary to the knee replacement. Although it is commonly accepted that patella infera is associated with decreased knee function and increased knee pain following TKA we have not been able to demonstrate any increase in pain scores or decrease in function scores secondary to this complication with our results (Knee Society Score, WOMAC) [6]. Even in the presence of marked patella infera there has been no resultant patella impingement or patella dysfunction.

If at the time of the index procedure there is significant patellar infera the surgeon may take the option of not resurfacing the patella to avoid subsequent impingement. Excision of osteophytes around the proximal pole of the patella may also improve the patellar tracking in this situation.

7   Clinical Results

Keblish et al. [7] reported on 52 patients who underwent bilateral TKA where one knee was resurfaced and the other was not. At a minimum of 5.24 years there were no reoperations to address patellofemoral problems.

Buechel et al. [2] reported on the 11 year follow up of 515 knees. There were 3 patellar fractures, one was an undisplaced intraoperative fracture and the other two were in revision TKA's. There was only one dislocation and no polyethylene disassociation or wear problems. They were criticized because of the lack of radiological follow-up.

The Christchurch Orthopaedic Group has been using the LCS total knee system exclusively since 1989 and has now performed over 6000 arthroplasties. Our initial

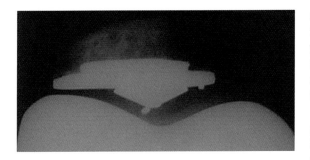

Fig. 31. Measurement of lateral subluxation in a single skyline view. The position of the patella cone is compared to the through of the femoral trochlea from a fixed point on the lateral aspect of the femoral component

study group of 568 patients has been assessed for patella complications. Within this group there have been 6 (1 %) reoperations for patellofemoral problems. Four subluxations and 1 dislocation have been treated with soft tissue realignment procedures with a satisfactory outcome. One patient disassociated the polyethylene from the patella base plate when falling while jumping a creek. The polyethylene was replaced with no further problems.

Patellofemoral subluxation was measured (Fig. 31).

Those knees with more than 5 mms of lateral subluxation of the patella were compared to the rest of the study group. There was no difference in the overall function or pain scores (Knee Society Score, WOMAC) between the two groups. These findings support the view that a congruent patellofemoral joint during active quadriceps contraction will evenly distribute forces across the polyethylene and result in minimal wear, even in the presence of relatively thin polyethylene.

The radiological assessment showed an overall incidence of radiolucent lines of 0.9 % and there were no progressive radiolucent lines up to a minimum of 7 years following surgery. There was no patella osteolysis. This study addressed the perceived deficiencies in Buechel's study by showing minimal radiological wear and osteolysis, adding support to the concept of low contact stress producing decreased polyethylene wear [3].

In conclusion the LCS rotating patella has given good to excellent results in the median term (minimum 7 years) when compared to other studies. The incidence of complications was rare and the results of this metal backed patella component were at least as good as all polyethylene components.

References

1. Barrack RL, Wolfe MW (2000) Patellar resurfacing in total knee arthroplasty. J Am Acad Orthop Surg 8: 75–82
2. Buechel FF, Rosa RA, Pappas MJ (1989) A metal backed, rotating-bearing patellar prosthesis to lower contact stress. A 11 year clinical study. Clin Orthop 248: 34–49
3. Buechel FF, Pappas MJ, Makris G (1991) Evaluation of contact stress in metal-backed patellar replacements. A predictor of survivorship. Clin Orthop 273: 190–197
4. Castro FPJ, Chimento G, Munn BG, Levy RS, Timon S, Barrack RL (1997) An analysis of food and drug administration medical device reports relating to total joint components. J Arthroplasty 12: 765–771
5. Dennis DA (1992) Patellofemoral complications in total knee arthroplasty: A literature review. Am J Knee Surgery 5: 156–166
6. Hooper GJ (1996) Not all metal-backed patellae are bad. Presented Combined English Speaking Meeting, Auckland
7. Keblish PA, Varma AK, Greenwald AS (1994) Patellar resurfacing or retention in total knee arthroplasty: A prospective study of patients with bilateral replacements. JBJS (B) 6: 930–937
8. Rand JA (1990) Patellar resurfacing in total knee arthroplasty. Clin Orthop 260: 110–117

12.6 The Evaluation and Treatment of the Painful Replaced Knee

B. Thomas, J.B. Stiehl

The results of the LCS mobile bearing knee arthroplasty meet or exceed the best results reported for fixed bearing total knee replacement. However, while most patients have enjoyed clinical success with these implants, an occasional patient will be referred with pain, swelling and stiffness, which may be severe enough to consider revision surgery. A thorough evaluation will help to determine a specific diagnosis in most cases. However, if a specific diagnosis cannot be determined, the results of revision surgery are likely to be unsatisfactory.

1   History

Evaluation of the painful total knee should always start with a complete history. Does the patient have a history of diabetes mellitus or underlying neurovascular disease or any potential sources for infection? Ask the patient to characterize his pain in terms of its' location as well as what activities exacerbate the pain and what maneuvers relieve it. It is important to differentiate rest pain from activity related pain. Establish the exact onset of the patient's symptoms, has he had pain ever since the surgery or was there a period when the knee pain was relieved and then some event after which the symptoms began. Have these symptoms been progressively worsening or are they stable? What specific activities make the pain worse, what relieves the pain and are any medications helpful?

A history of swelling requires having the patient distinguish between the sensation of tightness around the joint and true swelling. Localizing the swelling as well as timing its' appearance and disappearance is helpful as well as documenting its' presence and degree by an independent observer.

Any previous problems with the knee should be documented beginning with the index diagnosis, as well as the symptoms in the knee before the most recent surgery. What surgeries preceded the knee arthroplasty, were there any perioperative complications, any history of problems with the wound or with rehabilitation.

Family history should be reviewed in particular regarding history of gout, systemic lupus erythematosis or ankylosing spondylitis. In addition the patient should be questioned about his ability to lead a normal life, his ability to ambulate with crutches, cane or walker as well as the distance or time he is able to walk. Can he ascend or descend stairs, and is this performed normally or one step at a time. Is there any sensation of instability on either ascending or descending stairs? Difficulty arising from a chair should be noted. The patient's specific complaints before surgery should be reviewed along with his expectations before and after surgery. Employment history is often helpful in placing the patient's function in perspective as is any history of underlying psychiatric disease or treatment with antidepressants or other psychiatric medications.

Medications including corticosteroids and immunosuppressive agents may have serious side effects and any recent change in the dose of corticosteroids should be noted since a flare of disease activity may take place when these drugs are suddenly discontinued or reduced. Patients with cardiovascular disease who complain of joint pains should be asked whether they are taking Hydralazine or Procainamide since these may induce a Lupus-like syndrome.

Finally determine who the patient feels is responsible for his knee condition. Is this a workman's comp related case, a personal injury case or medical malpractice and is any medical-legal action pending? A discussion of what physical therapy and rehabilitation measures have been performed post-operatively and over what time course is useful as well.

2   Physical Examination

Physical examination can be exceedingly useful in assessing the painful total knee arthroplasty. Pain about the knee may result in muscle atrophy and weakness. The patient's gait should be evaluated and over all alignment of the limb in varus or valgus noted. The patient's ability to arise from a chair should be observed as well as his ability to ascend and descend a step without assistance. The character of the wound should be noted. In particular, observing any evidence of erythema, induration and abnormal warmth. Swelling should be graded and intra-articular effusion differentiated from generalized soft tissue edema by balloting the patella. When evaluating swelling about the knee, swelling in the prepatellar bursa or popliteal bursa must be distinguished from that in the knee joint proper. Palpation of the areas medial and lateral to the patella can provide information about synovial hypertrophy. Large intra-articular effusions are easily detected by balloting the patella after compressing the suprapatellar bursa to displace the fluid that it contains. Small amounts of fluid in the knee joint can be elicited by stroking the lateral aspect of the joint, thus moving the fluid back into the medial aspect of the knee. The "bulge sign" may then be observed on the medial aspect of the knee. Limitation of motion should be documented and specific range of motion noted in the patient's chart. Next the knee should be palpated for specific areas of tenderness. Tenderness should be elicited from all three compartments, the patellofemoral, medial and lateral compartments as well as areas overlying the medial and lateral femur and medial and lateral tibia. The function of the extensor mechanism should be assessed and any crepitance or grinding in the patellofemoral joint noted. Strength for extension and flexion of the knee should be documented on a 0–5 scale. Patellar tracking should be checked for subluxation or dislocation. Extensor lag or fixed contractures should be measured and documented. Knee stability should be evaluated both in the AP and medial lateral plane. Varus and valgus stability to stress should be assessed in full extension as well as 30° of flexion and 90° of flexion.

In addition to thorough examination of the knee, examination of the back and abdomen are also important to rule out the possibility of referred pain. The back should be evaluated for tenderness or deformity. The abdomen should also be evaluated for areas of irritability or tenderness. Full examination of the hip is required to document range of motion as well as assessing the hip as a source of referred pain to the knee. Flexion contracture of the hip can be demonstrated using the Thomas test by having the patient flex the contralateral thigh to the chest while lying supine. Examination of the hip has been particularly helpful in my experience since several patients have presented complaining of dissatisfaction and pain with a knee replacement only to be found to have severe arthritis in the ipsilateral hip. In these cases addressing the hip problem relieved the knee complaints as well. Evaluation of the foot for malalignment

is also useful since significant deformities can cause abnormal stress and pain at the knee.

3   Radiographic Assessment

Plain radiographs can determine the type of implant used, the alignment and positioning of the components, and malrotation of the components, as well as gross evidence of polyethylene wear. Anteroposterior, lateral and sunrise views should be taken tangential to the joint. The position of the joint line should be compared to the unoperated opposite knee. Elevation of the joint line of more than 1 cm is associated with patellofemoral problems. Metal backed components may show evidence of metal debris if there has been wear through of the polyethylene. Complete or progressively widening radiolucent lines at the cement prosthesis interface or cement bone interface suggest loosening. Similarly a shift in the position of the implants confirms loosening.

Cementless implants are more difficult to assess and tangential views are critical in this regard since 5° of flexion or rotation can obscure a 1 mm radiolucency as can 6° or greater angulation of the x-ray beam or more than 2.5 cm offset of the beam. Metal backed components obscure the interface with as little as 4° of flexion. Fluoroscopic positioning is useful to obtain true tangential views for the AP and lateral radiographs.

The relative position of the patella to the joint line may be assessed on a lateral view. In addition, the thickness of the patellar reconstruction should approximate the pre-operative thickness of the patella. Tracking may be assessed radiographically by obtaining merchant or sunrise views at 15°, 30°, 45° and 60° of flexion. Stress radiographs can also document medial or lateral instability as well as anterior posterior instability.

When a knee arthroplasty develops pain postoperatively, infection should always be suspected. A complete blood count, erythrocyte sedimentation rate and C reactive protein level are recommended. Aspiration of the joint gives the most direct evidence of infection. Cultures should be sent for routine aerobic and anaerobic cultures as well as fungal and TB. We have occasionally encountered fungal infections as the source of pain after joint reconstruction since the vast majority of patients are treated with prophylactic antibiotics at the time of surgery. We have occasionally repeated aspirations on two or three occasions when the initial aspiration is no growth or if the culture is positive for a suspected skin contaminant.

Technetium diphosphonate bone scans have been particularly useful in assessing the painful knee in our practice because of the difficulty in clearly demonstrating loosening on plain radiographs (Fig. 32). While bone scans have been noted to remain positive for one year after surgery, bone remodeling and local synovitis as well as early osteolysis may contribute to increased activity

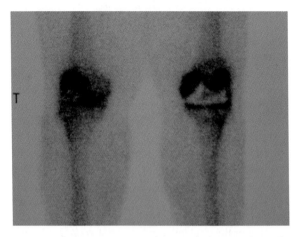

Fig. 32. Technetium scintography reveals increased uptake about the implant of the left knee consistent with implant loosening or infection

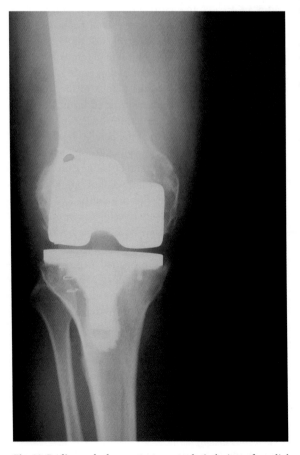

Fig. 33. Radiograph demonstrates osteolytic lesion of medial femoral condyle

in a significant number of asymptomatic patients even after one year. If, however, a patient with a symptomatic knee replacement presents with a normal bone scan, the probability of loosening or infection is low. Indium 111 labeled white cell scans are useful in evaluating for infection. If diphosphonate and Indium 111 scans are negative the likelihood of infection is low, as is the likelihood of component loosening. CT scans are helpful in assessing the degree of bone loss behind the femoral component (Fig. 33, 34).

Aspiration of the joint is critical in ruling out infection. Arthrogram has not been particularly helpful in assessing for component loosening in our experience. A technetium diphosphonate bone scan may also be useful in suggesting other possible locations for referred pain. For instance a patient with a negative scan of the knee may have increased uptake in the ipsilateral hip or low back suggesting that investigation into these areas might be illuminating. For instance, a patient with increased uptake in the low back might be evaluated with an MRI or CT scan to rule out the presence of involvement of the lumbosacral nerves. Doppler studies may also assess for possible occlusive vascular disease.

4 Causes of Pain After Total Knee Arthroplasty

There are many specific factors which can cause pain after total knee arthroplasty.

4.1 Polyethylene Wear

Currently, the most common type of prosthetic failure is caused by polyethylene wear (Fig. 35). Polyethylene damage can occur without pain. With significant polyethylene wear, synovitis may develop along with an effusion. The synovitis can cause pain and chronic synovitis can cause weakening of the ligaments and instability. Polyethylene wear should therefore be treated aggressively with polyethylene exchange. When malalignment is the cause of premature polyethylene wear, revision of the metal components may be required as well.

4.2 Soft Tissue Impingement

Soft tissue impingement may cause pain if the femoral or tibial implants overhang the edge of the bone. This problem is diagnosed by palpating directly over the area of involvement. This problem may also be diagnosed radiographically, and bone scan will often localize the in-

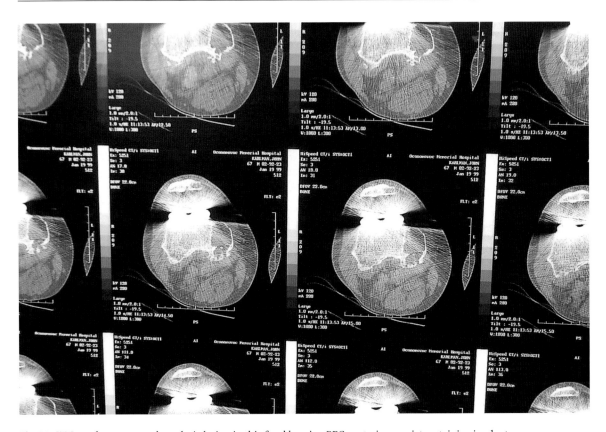

Fig. 34. CT Scan demonstrates large lytic lesion in this fixed bearing PFC posterior cruciate retaining implant

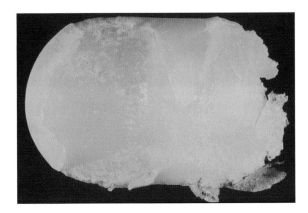

Fig. 35. Polyethylene failure of this oxidized rotating platform insert

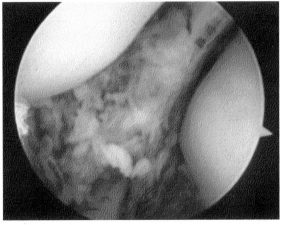

Fig. 36. Polyethylene impingement from the sharp lip of this custom posterior stabilized rotating platform tibial insert

volved area. Treatment usually requires exchange for smaller components (Fig. 36).

4.3 Component Loosening

Loosening may be caused by malalignment, prosthetic wear or instability (Fig. 37, see Fig. 18). Infection may also cause loosening. If there is any question, an aspi-

ration should be performed. Radiographic evidence of component loosening includes migration of the implants, complete radiolucent lines greater than 2 mm in width, and a change in alignment of the extremity with subsidence of the implant. Loose cementless implants may shed the beads used as an ingrowth surface. Loose components should be revised promptly to avoid further bone loss or ligament damage.

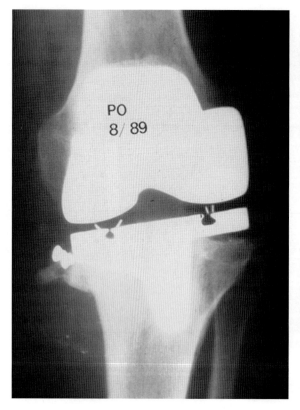

Fig. 37. a Anterior/posterior radiograph will demonstrate implant loosening; b Rotating platform "spinout"

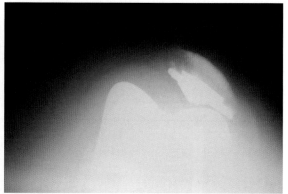

Fig. 38. Lateral patellar subluxation with this LCS rotating platform TKA

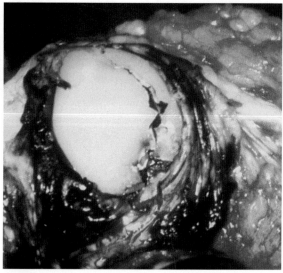

Fig. 39. Patellar metal backed failure of polyethylene

4.4 Patellar Complications

Lateral subluxation of the patella is common after total knee arthroplasty (Fig. 38). This may lead to dissociation from the metal backed patellar component (Fig. 39). A significant effusion may develop if there is polyethylene wear. On physical examination, a grating sensation is noted and often a click on ballotment of the metal backed patella. Radiographically, the polyethylene component may be displaced. In metal backed patellar components, metallic debris may be present. Aspiration may show polyethylene fragments on centrifugation or the fluid may be discolored secondary to metallosis. Patellar loosening or dissociation usually requires patellar realignment including lateral retinacular release and may require revision of the femoral and tibial components to improve external rotation of these components.

4.5 Infection

Infection is characterized by pain that is constant, rather than only with activity. The knee may present with an effusion, as well as erythema and drainage from the knee wound. Often, however, the onset is more insidious with no obvious drainage or erythema. Physical exam may show tenderness to palpation and irritability on bending the knee. Radiographs may show loosening and lysis of the bone or more often no obvious changes. Erythrocyte sedimentation rate, complete blood count with differential, and C-reactive protein may or may not be altered. Technetium[99] diphosphonate bone scan and Indium[111] labeled WBC scans may also be positive. Diagnosis is made most reliably with aspiration for culture and sensitivity. Treatment is surgical irrigation and debridement, usually including component removal, with staged reimplantation after parenteral antibiotics.

4.6 Reflex Sympathetic Dystrophy

Reflex sympathetic dystrophy should be considered when pain is out of proportion to the objective findings on examination. The pain is present from the immediate postoperative period, and is associated with a very slow postoperative recovery. Flexion is usually limited and the skin may be hypersensitive and may be warmer than the unoperated knee. Reflex sympathetic dystrophy may be diagnosed with lumbar sympathetic blockade, which relieves the pain confirming the diagnosis. Treatment is multidisciplinary and needs to be early and aggressive to improve the prognosis. Occupational and physical therapy help decrease pain and prevent stiffness. Antiedema measures include elevation and massage. Contrast baths improve blood flow and desensitize the patients. The leg should be placed in warm water for one minute, then alternate with cold water for ten minutes.

Phenoxybenzamine may inhibit the adrenergic effects seen in patients suffering from complex regional pain syndrome (the modern term for RSD). The usual starting dose is 10 mg./day orally. This may be increased by 10 mg./day every two days until pain is relieved. The initial dose should be maintained for at least five days before increase. Treatment usually lasts six weeks. Side effects include postural hypotension and phenoxybenzamine is contraindicated in several cardiac and asthmatic conditions.

Guanethidine may be used in a single oral dose for eight weeks. Side effects include mental depression, loss of appetite, impotence, and orthostatic hypotension.

Propranolol has been used to treat complex regional pain syndrome (CRPS), with less orthostatic hypotension but is contraindicated in patients with cardiac arrythmias or asthma.

Clonidine used as a transdermal patch may diminish hyperesthesia in patients who have had a positive response to sympathetic blockade.

Nifedapine, a calcium channel blocker relaxes peripheral smooth muscle and improves circulation. The starting dose is 10 mg. TID and may be increased weekly to a maximum of 30 mg. TID. Side effects include headache.

While non-steroidal anti-inflammatories are often ineffective, high dose prednisone may decrease edema and pain. Because of the risks of complications the dose should be quickly tapered.

If symptoms are not relieved promptly by oral medications combined with physical and occupational therapy, a trial of lumbar sympathetic blocks in the lower extremity may provide pain relief. If pain relief is achieved blocks may be repeated to a maximum of twelve blocks. Patients with legal, psychiatric, or disability issues frequently fail to maintain improvement.

When only temporary pain relief occurs after sympathetic blockade, surgical sympathectomy may be considered. Alternative treatments include calcitonin which alters osteoclast activity and decreases pain. Side effects include nausea, stomach upset and headaches. Electrical stimulation has had varying levels of success in treating RSD. Acupuncture may release endorphins in the central nervous system to relieve pain refractory to other treatments. Amputation may ultimately be required to control persistent infection and painful physical contact but has been unreliable in providing pain relief.

In summary a multidisciplinary approach with early aggressive management offers the best prognosis in management of complex regional pain syndrome (CPRS) or RSD.

4.7 Flexion Contracture

A fixed flexion deformity can result from posterior osteophytes being incompletely removed at the time of initial surgery. Failure to resect sufficient distal femur at the time of the surgery thus shifting of the joint line distally can result in a fixed flexion deformity. Flexion contracture preoperatively is frequently associated with postoperative fixed flexion deformity. All patients should be treated with aggressive physical therapy postoperatively and recalcitrant cases may benefit from bracing or even casting in the postoperative period.

4.8 Inadequate Flexion

Normal walking requires 67 degrees of flexion, Stair climbing requires 83 degrees, descending stairs requires 90 degrees. Sitting comfortably requires 93 degrees of flexion, bending to tie shoes 106 degrees, and lifting an object from the floor 117 degrees of flexion. If the flexion gap is left too tight, this may interfere with flexion of the knee. A femoral component that it is too large will limit flexion as will cutting the tibia with an anterior tilt. Contracture of the posterior cruciate ligament will also cause the knee to be tight in flexion. If the joint line is moved proximally, the posterior cruciate ligament may be too tight in flexion. If the patella is left too thick, flexion may be impaired. These technical errors may require surgical correction if physical therapy fails to achieve adequate flexion. Unfortunately, results after surgery have been less than ideal in our experience.

4.9   Instability

Patients may complain that the knee gives way when they walk on uneven ground. Ascending or descending stairs may also cause a sensation of instability. Physical examination will confirm laxity on varus, valgus, anterior, or posterior stress. The overall limb alignment should also be assessed, and the diagnosis may be confirmed objectively with stress radiographs. Bracing for six weeks may allow adequate soft tissue healing to stabilize the knee. If this is ineffective revision to more stable implants is indicated with rebalancing of the ligaments (see chapter 12.3).

5   Conclusion

We have learned that a thorough and systematic approach to evaluating the painful total knee reveals a proper diagnosis and treatment in most cases. For the most part, implant loosening, prosthetic infection, and chronic ligamentous instability require operative intervention. However, we can also recommend that if a conclusive diagnosis is not apparent, these conditions are not static and will worsen with time. On the other hand, if these serious conditions are not the problem, then waiting a period of time may be curative as the patient will get better. All reconstructive knee surgeons must deal on occasion with the stiff painful knee. Though reflex sympathetic dystrophy and other rare causes may be at fault, often it is simply the patient and the surgeon's misfortune. This is the time when the surgeon must follow his Hippocratic teachings. Firstly he must not resort to ill-conceived operations that may make the patient worse. Secondly, he must not resort to surgery because this what he knows how to do and he wants to get paid for it. But most importantly, he must stay at his patient's side and offer support and benefit even if it is no better than counseling and refilling chronic pain medication. Telling the patient, "there is nothing more that I can offer, you must go somewhere else", is an abrogation of the physician's ethical obligation!

References

1. Archibeck MJ, White RE Jr (2001) What's new in adult reconstructive knee surgery. [Journal Article] Journal of Bone & Joint Surgery – American Volume. 83-A(9): 1444–1450
2. Lonner JH (2001) Identifying ongoing infection after resection arthroplasty and before second-stage reimplantation. Am J Knee Surg 14(1): 68–71
3. Lucas TS, DeLuca PF, Nazarian DG, Bartolozzi AR, Booth RE Jr (1999) Arthroscopic treatment of patellar clunk. Clin Orthop Rel Res 367: 226–229
4. Mason JB, Fehring TK, Odum S, Griffin W, Nadaud M (2000) The value of white blood cell counts to revision total knee arthroplasty. Annual Meeting of the American Association of Hip and Knee Surgeons; 2000 Nov 3; Dallas, Tx
5. Mont MA, Waldman BJ, Hungerford DS (2000) Evaluation of preoperative cultures before second-stage reimplantation of a total knee prosthesis complicated by infection. A comparison-group study. J Bone Joint Surg Am 82: 1552–1557
6. Scott WN, Clarke HD (2000) The stiff knee: causes and cures. Orthopedics 23(9): 987–988
7. Shaw JA, Chung R (1999) Febrile response after knee and hip arthroplasty. Clin Orthop Rel Res 367: 181–189
8. Smith SL, Wastie ML, Forster I (2001) Radionuclide bone scintigraphy in the detection of significant complications after total knee joint replacement. Clin Radiol 56(3): 221–224
9. Waslewski GL, Marson BM, Benjamin JB (1998) Early, incapacitating instability of posterior cruciate ligament-retaining total knee arthroplasty. J Arthroplasty 13(7): 763–767

Chapter 13
Revision

13.1 Mobile Bearings in Revision TKA

F. F. Buechel

1 Revision TKR Concepts

Revision knee replacement surgery requires a thorough knowledge of normal and pathologic anatomy, especially when mechanical implant failure is accompanied by bone and soft tissue loss. The bone defect classification of Engh [8] is useful to quantitate the extent of bony and soft tissue pathology in the tibia and femur (Fig. 1).

In contained defects, such as Engh type I femoral or tibial defects, primary cemented or cementless components may be used with either morselized bone grafts in the case of cementless fixation or Rebar type screws to stabilize and reinforce fixation in the case of cemented fixation [4].

Structural defects, such as Engh type II or III femoral or tibial defects, require the use of intramedullary stems to gain stable fixation for articulating knee replacement

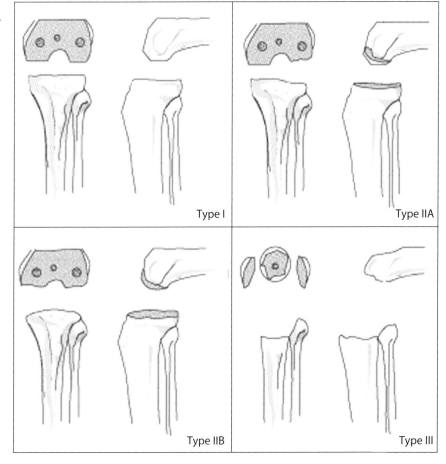

Fig. 1. Engh bone classifications for bone defects in revision knees

Type I

Type IIA

Type IIB

Type III

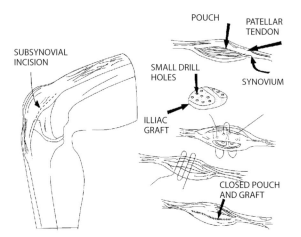

Fig. 2. Patellar tendon bone grafting technique for the patellectomized patient

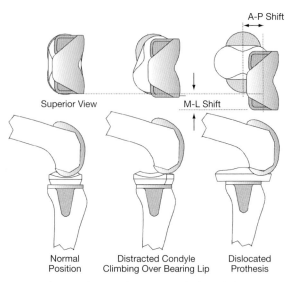

Fig. 3. Failure mechanism for rotating platform dislocations

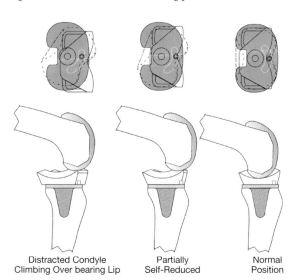

Fig. 4. Rotational stop tibial design prohibits bearing spinouts from occurring

surfaces. These stems should be canal filling and of sufficient length to prevent varus-valgus or anteroposterior "toggle" loosening; usually two medullary canal diameters beyond the defects in the femur or tibia. Allografts or Rebar screws and cement may be used to stabilize these modular components once the proper sizes have been determined.

Management of the patella during revision surgery depends upon the available bone stock remaining. In simple bearing exchange of a failed rotating-bearing, no treatment other than snapping on a new bearing to a well-fixed anchoring plate is needed, proving the original placement of the anchoring plate is correct. In cases where the failed patella replacement must be removed from the bone, the patella bony remnant needs to be evaluated for sufficient integrity to anchor a new patella component. In situations where the patella bony remnant is too thin or severely deficient, it is best to trim the bony borders to allow central tracking of the "resection arthroplasty", which is well tolerated by the anatomic femoral groove of the LCS prosthesis [5]. In patellectomy conditions, it is useful to consider bone grafting the patella tendon to restore a lever arm to the extensor mechanism [3] (Fig. 2).

2 Use of Mobile Bearings for TKA Revision

Mobile bearings, usually rotating platforms are particularly useful in revision TKA since wear resistance is improved and axial rotation of the tibial component is self-adjusted by the tibial bearing. Flexion and extension gap balance, however, is extremely important to prevent bearing dislocation which has been the major mechanical complication seen in 5% of cemented and 6.7% of cementless revision rotating platform cases [2]. An in-

sufficient or loose flexion gap allows the bearing to pivot under the femoral component, which usually maintains good contact with one side of the femoral component (Fig. 3). Revision with a thicker bearing or deep dish component usually solves this problem, but occasionally recurrent deep-dish rotating platform instability has required improved component stability, such as the use of a rotational stop pin on the tibial component which has been effective in stabilizing such recurrent dislocations [6] (Fig. 4). Prior to the availability of this improved tibial component, additional surgery was required at least once more in 17.5% of cemented and 20% of cementless cases to achieve a satisfactory overall outcome in 95% of cemented and 89.1% of cementless revision arthroplasties [2].

Importantly, the rotating platform with rotational stop has reduced primary and multiply-operated TKA dislocations form 1.6 % [7] to 0 % in the most recent review of the fist 170 cases followed over a ten year period [6]. This significant improvement in dislocation resistance has not compromised implant performance in primary or revision situations, while continuing to avoid the major intercondylar femoral resection required when using posterior-stabilized-type femoral components.

3 Revision TKA Surgical Technique

3.1 Preparation and Draping

The patient is placed in the supine position on the operating table. Prep and drape the knee in a sterile fashion. A sterile non-permeable stockinet is applied to allow for palpitation of the anterior tibial and malleolar contours. The leg is elevated for one minute to allow for venous run-off and then the previously applied tourniquet is inflated.

3.2 Skin Incision

The previous midline skin incision or the most recently healed incision that will provide an extensile exposure to the knee without creating a compromised skin flap is used (Fig. 5a).

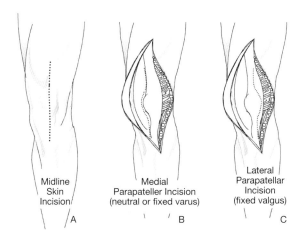

Fig. 5. a Previous midline or healed incision is used. **b** A median parapatellar deep incision for neutral or fixed varus deformities. **c** For fixed valgus knees, a lateral parapatellar deep incision

3.3 Deep Incision

A median parapatellar deep incision for neutral or fixed varus deformities combined with a proximal quadriceps snip or V-Y quadriceps turn down to allow lateral eversion of the patella is utilized to gain exposure to the knee (Fig. 5b).

For fixed valgus knees, a lateral parapatellar deep incision and a reverse quadriceps snip or tibial tubercle osteotomy is used to evert the patella medially and gain access (Fig. 5c).

3.4 Soft Tissue Balancing

Fixed varus deformities require a proximal subperiosteal medial sleeve release of the MCL and pes tendons from the tibia to allow correction to neutral mechanical axis alignment [9]. Fixed valgus deformities require a sequential, lateral, subperiosteal soft tissue sleeve release of the ITT, popliteus and LCL to allow a similar correction to neutral alignment [1].

3.5 Evaluation of Failed Components

All knee replacement components are inspected for deformation, malalignment, wear and/or loosening. It is imperative to attain neutral alignment by necessary soft tissue releases before removing any failed components. These components provide leverage for applying varus or valgus stress to the knee in extension during the soft tissue balancing part of the procedure. Thereafter any loose, worn or malaligned components are removed and any component that remains stable, properly aligned and without signs of wear or infection may be retained.

3.6 Technique of Removal

3.6.1 Femoral Component
An osteotome or Gigli saw is used under the anterior flange and the other surfaces of the femoral component to loosen the bone-cement interface, or in the case of cementless fixation, the bone-prosthesis interface. The lateral margins of the femoral component are impacted alternately until the component becomes dislodged.

3.6.2 Tibial Component
Two osteotomes are driven under the flat fixation plate of the tibial component to assess its stability in the cement mantle or the bone if a cementless device was used.

If the component surface lifts free from the tibia and the central fixation stem (if available) becomes grossly loose, then the osteotomes are gradually increased in thickness under the fixation plate until complete loosening is achieved.

If the tibial component remains well-fixed, a small 2×3 cm cortical window in the proximal medial tibia can be made, under the medial soft tissue sleeve, to allow access to the short metaphyseal stem. A curved osteotome can be used to remove cement or interrupt the bone prosthesis interface, so that the tibial component can be driven upward with an impactor until completely removed. The cortical window is replaced after a new tibial stem is inserted. The medial soft tissue sleeve will maintain stability over the bony window. In lateral approaches, the cortical window can be centered on Gerdy's tubercle and the closure of the anterior compartment fascia will maintain lateral stability of the bony window.

3.6.3   Patella Component

A small osteotome can be driven under the edges of the patellar component until it breaks free from its central fixation. Malaligned patellar replacements sometimes require a corrected bony cut at the level of the quadriceps tendon, which will facilitate removal of a solidly fixed component.

If this is a New Jersey knee revision and if the Rotating-Bearing Anchoring Plate is well-aligned and well-fixed but the Patella Bearing shows signs of wear, a 1/4" osteotome can be inserted between the bearing and the anchoring plate followed by a twist of the osteotome to dislodge the bearing from the trunion cone. A new bearing is snapped on by digital pressure or use of the Patella Clamp.

3.7   Tibial Preparation

The tibial resection guide is positioned perpendicular to the tibial shaft axis in the frontal plane placing the Distal Alignment Rod on the anterior tibialis tendon, which represents the position of the ankle joint center (Fig. 6a). The Guide is inclined posteriorly 10 degrees with respect to the anterior tibial shaft and pinned into place at the level which resects the minimal amount of bone to create a flat surface on at least one side. The Guide is adjusted by moving it upward or downward on the previously placed fixation pins. After the proper level is set, the proximal tibia is resected with a power saw (Fig. 6b).

If significant bone loss is encountered, 2 or more Rebar Screws may be inserted medially or laterally in

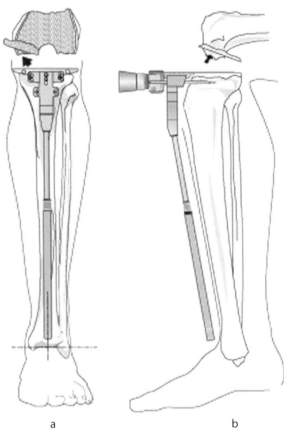

a   b

Fig. 6. a The tibial resection guide is positioned perpendicular to the tibial shaft axis in the frontal plane placing the Distal Alignment Rod on the anterior tibialis tendon which represents the position of the ankle joint center. **b** Lateral view showing proper tibial guide placement and resection

the best bony bed (Fig. 7). The screws are placed into 1/8" pre-drilled holes and are adjusted with a hexagonal screw driver until the Tibial Template-Reamer Guide makes light contact. This assures that the tibial component cement mantle or bone graft will have additional structural support in the region of bony deficiency.

A Reamer Sleeve of appropriate internal diameter is inserted into the Reamer Guide Tube (Fig. 8a). The intramedully canal is reamed through the hole in the Reamer Guide, which is pinned into place after it is centered in the A-P and M-L plane to obtain the best coverage without overhang. Sequential, blunt-tipped, straight reamers are passed through the cylinder portion of the Reamer Guide using sequential centering sleeves (Fig. 8b). The depth of reaming should engage the endosteal cortex and bypass any proximal cortical defects by at least 2 tibial shaft diameters. Minor A-P or M-L adjustment of the Tibial Template position may be necessary to remain centered on the tibial canal in cases of severe bony deficiency or malalignment. During this process the Tem-

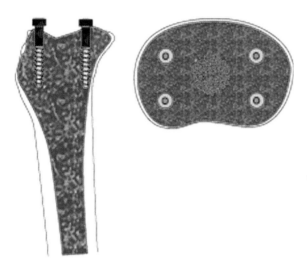

Fig. 7. Rebar screw placement in defects of tibial component

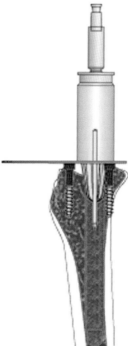

Fig. 9. Conical reamer used to fashion the proximal tibia

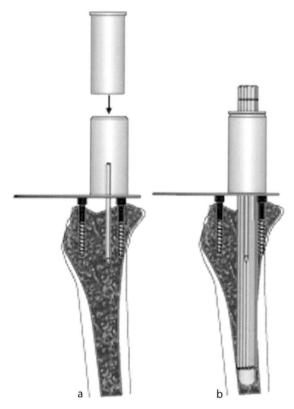

Fig. 8. a Reamer sleeve placed in the reaming guide to provide for central reaming. **b** Straight, blunt tipped reamer used to fashion the intramedullary canal

plate may be moved, or even decreased in size to obtain the best combination of canal centering and tibial plate fit.

The Sleeve and Reamer are removed and the depth of the reamed hole is noted from the inferior surface of the

Tibial Template. From this dimension the overall length of the modular stem and unconnected tibial component can be determined. Be sure that the overall length is less than the depth of the reamed hole. The conical Reamer is then passed through the Reamer Guide to fashion the hole for the proximal tapered cone of the Revision Tibial Platform (Fig. 9). Often the Reamer will not touch any bone in severe proximal deficiencies.

The revision Tibial Trial is assembled by first screwing a Trial Extension Adapter to the distal end of the Trial Tibial Component. If a +10 mm Thick Revision Tibial Component is to be used, the Trial Tibial Thickness Adapter is added (Fig. 10). The appropriate length and diameter Modular Trial Stem is selected from the reaming. This length must be added to 55 mm, which represents the length of the unconnected Tibial Component. The Modular Tibial Trial is then pressed into position in the prepared tibia. Further femoral preparation is preformed with the Tibial Trial in place. This protects the proximal tibial preparation and provides a stable platform to adjust flexion and extension gaps.

3.8 Femoral Preparation

The 9 mm Drill Guide is removed from the appropriate size A/P Femoral Resection Guide by unscrewing it from its bayonet mount. This guide is positioned in the same fashion as for primary LCS knee surgery (see chapter 10.1). The Reamer Sleeve is placed onto the bayonet mount, and the desired diameter Reamer Bushing placed into the Sleeve (Fig. 11).

The Femoral Guide Yoke is assembled onto the A/P Femoral Resection Guide. Place and align the assembled guide on the distal femur in the usual manner, such that the Yoke is centered on the femoral shaft and the Femoral Resection Guide is centered between the epicondyles (Fig. 12). Bone pins are used to stabilize the Guide aligned with the femoral epicondylar axis. The desired size reamer is then used to ream the hole in the femur sufficiently deep to allow implantation of a stem of desired length. Holes of increasing size using sequentially larger Reaming Bushings and Reamers while maintain-

ing a constant position for the Guide without migrating anteriorly (Fig. 13). Use the straight, blunt-tipped reamers to engage the endosteal cortex and prepare a length of at least 2 femoral shaft diameters above the most proximal femoral defect. Once completed remove this Guide and Pins. If necessary the anterior and posterior femoral resections can be made after setting up the Guide in the usual manner.

3.9   Femoral Trial Component Placement

The appropriate length and diameter Modular Trial Stem is selected to be used. For the femur the Modular Stem length must be added to 36 mm which represents the length of the unconnected Femoral Component (Fig. 14). It is important to note the overall length

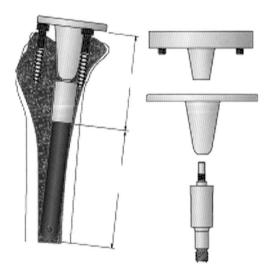

Fig. 10. Assembly of the tibial trial first by screwing the extension adaptor to the tibial trial, and then by screwing the trial extension to the tibial trial

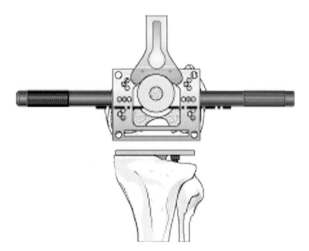

Fig. 12. Alignment of the AP resection block and reaming guide

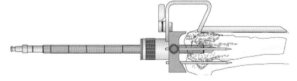

Fig. 13. Blunt tipped reamers used to create the intramedullary canal in the femur

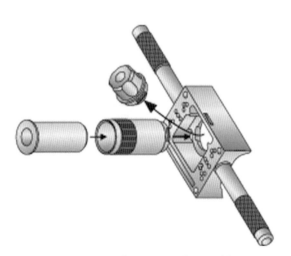

Fig. 11. AP resection and reaming guide assembly

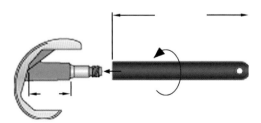

Fig. 14. Femoral trial assembly

of the assembled Femoral Component is less than the depth of the reamed hole.

When bone stock deficiency in the distal femur is excessive the Femoral Trial is used to establish extension tension. The appropriate size and thickness Trial Tibial Bearing is assembled onto the Tibial Trial and then the Trial Femoral Component with its Modular Stem into the distal femur and a check is performed for proper ligamentous tension. Different thickness Trial Tibial Bearing are inserted as needed to obtain proper flexion tension (Fig. 15a).

Superior-inferior position is adjusted by placing the Trial Femoral Component while at 90 degrees flexion, into the position that allows an equal anterior and pos-

terior drawer test. This places the collateral ligaments into a vertical or neutral position, which balances the extension gap to the flexion gap. The balance of the medial and lateral collateral ligaments also provides the correct axial orientation of the Femoral Trial relative to the femur. The position of the Anterior Femoral Flange is marked on the distal femur, and then removed to place 1 or 2 Rebar screws into the distal femoral condyles, if needed, to adjust the Trial Femoral Component into the correct distal position.

The leg is then placed in full extension and ligamentous extension tension is checked (Fig. 15b). Additional Rebar Screws may be inserted into the distal femur to help provide a stable position of the Femoral Trial. If tension is not proper, the position of the Femoral Trial may be adjusted by adjustment of the Rebar Screws until proper ligamentous and Femoral Trial stability are achieved.

3.10 Patella Preparation

If a New Jersey Rotating-Bearing Patellar Anchoring Plate or another type of patella device has been removed, the remaining bone stock is examined for quality and alignment of cut, making sure that the bony cut is parallel to and at the level of the quadriceps tendon insertion to give equal amounts of bone medially-laterally and superiorly-inferiorly (Fig. 16a). If ample bone stock exists after the facing cut has been completed, the appropriate Patellar Template is placed onto the resected bony surface of the patella with the patella reduced into its normal anatomical position (Fig. 16b). The Template should be oriented perpendicular to the patellar tendon and the tibial shaft in this position. The patella is then everted and the patellar template orientation maintained which is usually downward by approximately 30 degrees (Fig. 16c). It is important to center the template on the patella at this angle and mark the channel position with a marking pen. The patellar burr is used to create the fixation channels for the patellar component.

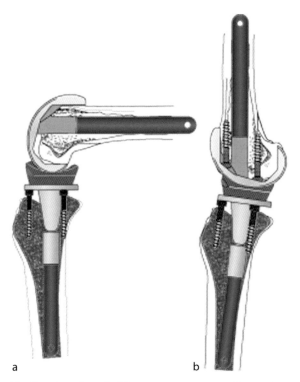

Fig. 15. a Insertion of trial components to assess ligamentous stability. b Placement of Rebar screws to provide for proper femoral positioning

Fig. 16. a The patellar remnant is resected to provide a horizontal platform for the patella to rest on. b The Patellar template is placed perpendicular to the patellar tendon. c The patellar is everted and position of the template noted

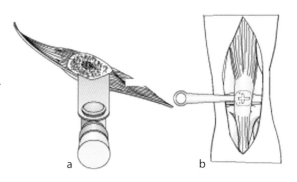
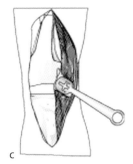

3.11 Final Implant Placement

3.11.1 Tibial Component

The proper size Tibial Component and Modular Stem are assembled by inserting the conical end of the Modular Stem into the distal recess of the Tibial Component and then insert the Clamping Screw into the other recess (Fig. 17a). Tighten the Clamping Screw using the Torque Screwdriver until a click indicating proper torque is heard (Fig. 17b). The bony surfaces are cleared of all loose soft tissue debris, and the Rebar screws are maintained in their properly aligned positions. Bone cement is applied to the proximal region of the tibia and Rebar screws, leaving an opening for the entrance of the modular stem. The modular stem is placed into the tibial canal, and the component is allowed to seat on the Rebar screws for proper positioning. Excess cement is removed from the edges of the prosthesis and allowed the to fully set.

3.11.2 Femoral Component

Assemble the proper size Femoral Component and Modular Stem in the same manner as the tibial component (Fig. 18). Again, the bony surfaces are cleared of all loose soft tissue debris and the Rebar screws are maintained in their properly aligned positions. Bone cement is applied to the distal region of the femur and Rebar screws, leaving an opening for the entrance of the modular stem. The knee is flexed to 110 degrees and the modular stem is inserted into the femoral canal. The knee is brought into 80 degrees of flexion and allowed to seat on the Rebar screws for proper positioning. Excess cement is removed from the edges of the prosthesis and the knee is extended fully to allow the cement to completely set.

3.11.3 Patellar Component

Bone cement is placed onto the resected patellar surface and with finger pressure the cruciate fixturing channels outlined. The cruciate fixturing fins or the three fixation pegs are pressed into the cement mantle and final seating is secured with the patellar clamp. Excess cement is removed from the edges of the prosthesis.

3.12 Rotating Hinge Component

There are three optional techniques for the implantation of the New Jersey Rotating Hinge Knee. The appropriate choice depends upon the soft tissue and bone availability.

The first technique may be used when the joint has sufficient laxity and flexibility. This technique is the same as that of the modular components except that after the Hinge Tibial Component is implanted the knee is placed in hyperflexion and the stem of the Femoral Component-Hinge Assembly is inserted slowly into the

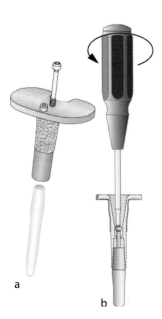

Fig. 17 a The modular extension is inserted into the tibial component. **b** The torque screwdriver is used to tighten the clamping screw

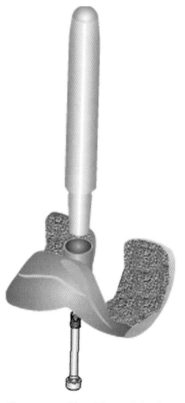

Fig. 18. Assembly of the modular femoral component

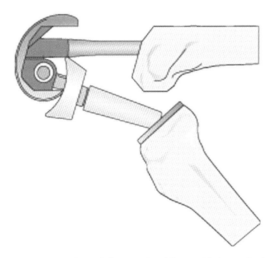

Fig. 19. Insertion of the rotating hinge with hyperflexion of the knee

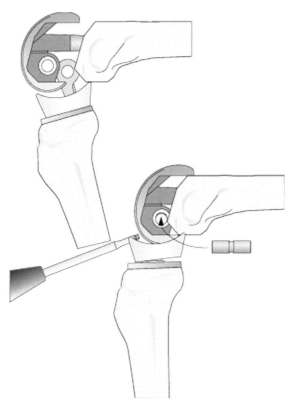

Fig. 20. Insertion of the rotating hinge by disconnecting the carriage from the hinge femoral component prior to installation, and reconnecting once seated

femur until the end of the Carriage Bearing is adjacent to the conical cavity in the Tibial Component. The yoke end is then inserted into this conical cavity and the Femoral Assembly fully seated on the distal femur (Fig. 19).

The second technique is used where the use of the first is impractical due to insufficient laxity or flexibil-

ity of the joint. In this technique loosening the Hinge Set Screw holding the Hinge Pin, about four turns, and removing the Hinge Pin disassemble the Hinge. The Hinge may now be uncoupled.

The Hinge Tibial Component is implanted using the same method as used for the Modular Tibial Component. The Hinge Carriage and Bearing Assembly are then inserted into the conical cavity in the Tibial Component. The Hinge Femoral Component, with the desired Modular Stem attached, is partially inserted onto the prepared distal femur.

The holes in the Femoral Component and Carriage are now aligned and the Hinge pin inserted into the holes and centered in the Femoral Component. The Set Screw is then inserted into the Femoral Component and tightened using the Torque Screw Driver to complete the Hinge assembly. The Femoral Component is now fully seated onto the Femur (Fig. 20).

The third option is a variation of the second used where there is a substantial distal femoral bone deficiency. Here, the final preparation of the distal femur is carried out by inserting the Femoral Component and removing bone needed to allow coupling of the components that are fully seated.

3.13 Cementless Option

The previous technique may be modified for use with bone graft augmentation. Each case should be individualized for specific bone graft requirements. Rebar screws should be recessed into bone grafts by 2 mm prior to final impaction of tibial and femoral components. The same principles of stable flexion and extension gaps as well as central tracking of the patella must be maintained.

3.14 Closure and Post-operative care

The tourniquet is released and the wound is copiously irrigated with antibiotic saline solution. Motion is checked with the tourniquet down. The deep retinacular tissues are closed using #1 absorbable suture, and the subcutaneus tissue with a 2–0 absorbable suture and the skin using staples or a vertical mattress suture. A suction drain may or may not be used (Fig. 21). A Robert Jones compression dressing is applied to the extremity followed by a long leg knee immobilizer. If pressure is needed to gain full extension, apply a long leg cast to hold full extension for two days.

The patient may be out of bed on the first post-operative day and may begin isometric quad setting exer-

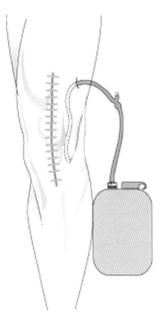

Fig. 21. Routine closure

cises of at least ten per hour. Suction drains are removed, if used, after 48 hours. The patient may transfer with weight-bearing to tolerance on the first post operative day and may begin gravity-assist and active-assistive range of motion. Should wound healing be a problem, flexion is deferred until the wound quality appears satisfactory. An anticoagulation program is administered beginning on the first post-operative day [10].

Physical therapy is performed, consisting of progressive ambulation with weight bearing to tolerance, daily for the first two weeks and then three times weekly over the next four weeks. Knee swelling may persist consistent with the rehabilitation status of the quadriceps

mechanism. Post operative swelling with a well-functioning quadriceps generally subsides within 6–12 weeks following knee replacement. Isometric quad setting exercises are continued until knee effusion (swelling) has subsided. Once this effusion has subsided, progressive resistive quadriceps exercises begin to improve strength and endurance necessary for normal gait.

References

1. Buechel FF (1990) A sequential three step lateral release for correcting fixed valgus knee deformities during total knee arthroplasty. Clin Orthop 260: 170–175
2. Buechel FF (1991) Cemented and cementless revision arthroplasty using rotating-platform total knee implants: A 12-year experience. Orthop Review 71–75
3. Buechel FF (1991) Patellar tendon bone grafting for patellectomized patients having total knee arthroplasty. Clin Orthop 271: 72–78
4. Buechel FF (1997) Rebar screws: an inexpensive alternative in revision TKA. Presented at the 13 Annual Current Concepts in Joint Replacement Meeting. Orlando, Florida
5. Buechel FF (1998) Mobile-bearing joint replacement options in post-traumatic arthritis of the knee. Orthopedics 21(9): 1027–1031
6. Buechel FF (2001) Recurrent LCS rotating platform dislocation in revision TKR: mechanism, management and report of two cases. Orthopaedics (In Press)
7. Buechel Sr FF, Buechel Jr FF, Pappas MJ, D'Alessio J (2001) Twenty-year evaluation of meniscal bearing and rotating platform knee replacements. Clin Orthop 388: 41–50
8. Engh GA (1997) Bone defect classification. In: Engh GA, Rorabeck CH (eds) Revision total knee arthroplasty. Williams and Wilkins, Md, pp 63–120
9. Insall JW (1984) Surgical approaches to the knee. In: Insall JN (ed). Surgery of the knee. Churchill Livingston, New York, pp 4–54
10. Zimlich RN, Fulbright BM, Freidman RJ (1996) Current status of anticoagulation therapy after total hip and total knee arthroplasty. J Am Acad Orthop Surgeons. 4:54–61

13.2 Revision of Hinge to Rotating Platform – Techniques and Results

J. G. Fitzek

According to a widely used algorithm, failed knee arthroplasties are replaced by components with enlarged surface available for anchorage and with increased intrinsic stability [9, 14]. This technique has limitations, such as, if the failed implant is a cemented hinged prosthesis. Here, the question is, whether reliable function of the knee joint can be restored with techniques of biological reconstruction of bone defects and with smaller implant volume and components with reduced constraint.

1 Deficiencies after failed hinged prostheses

1.1 Extent of bone defects

Primarily the intercondylar bone resection during insertion of the hinged prosthesis reduces the stability of the femoral condyles. Additionally, implant axes that are transepicondylarly fixed, increase the primary bone loss. After implant failure and removal of the components with débridement, frequently only the egg-shell-cortical wall of the femoral condyles remains. Often there are concomitant structural defects of the posterior

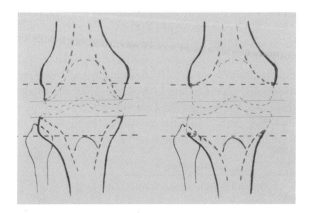

Fig. 22. Bone defect classification in revision knee arthroplasty [8]: type 3

and distal femur. In loosened cemented implants with former diaphyseal fixation, there is regularly sclerotic diaphyseal bone at the interface and enlargement of the medullary channel of the distal femur and the proximal tibia. Bone quality is also mostly compromised by metaphyseal osteoporosis resulting from stress shielding caused by changed bone loading in implants designed for diaphyseal fixation [15, 16]. These defects are not especially referred to in the AORI – (Anderson Orthopaedic Research Institute) classification [6]. Therefore, in the authors' bone defect classification, these defects are referred to as type 3 with subcategory A (contain) or B (uncontain) according to the remaining supportive cortical wall in the area between the primary line of resection and the epicondylar line [8] (Fig. 22).

1.2 Extent of Ligamentous Deficiencies

For primary implantation of a hinged prosthesis the insertions of the collateral ligaments are only tangentially dissected. Consequently, the ligaments can reattach under conditions of changed tension. Therefore, at revision of such implants, there is regularly a stable soft tissue envelope.

2 Reconstruction of Bone Defects

In analogy to revision hip arthroplasty, extensive contained defects can be reconstructed with the impaction grafting technique [3, 4, 24]. Small and moderate defects can be treated with metal wedges. For more extensive defects allogeneous femoral heads can be applied [5, 18, 20]. Excessive metaphyseal defects as in type 3 of the AORI classification can only be treated with bulk allografts (distal femur or proximal tibia grafts) [5, 20]. The aims are supportive femoral and tibial condyles to prevent diaphyseal loading.

3   Choice of Implant in Revisions of Failed Hinged Prostheses

If a cemented hinged prosthesis is chosen for revision knee arthroplasty of the same type of implant, this necessitates even longer stems and more cement. The reduced bone quality, especially the sclerotic surface of the intramedullary canal, makes reliable interdigitation of the cement questionable [10, 13]. Modular systems provide defect reconstruction with metal wedges. The length of the stems can be individually chosen according to the extent of constraint guaranteed by the revision implant. Additionally either cementless or cemented stems can be chosen. Despite the obvious advantages of the rotationally stable press-fit stem that avoid diaphyseal cementing, there are some inherent disadvantages: The position of the press-fit stems is influenced by the intramedullary canal and this can lead to an offset position of the prosthesis plateau in relation to the bony condylar surface. Special offset stems can minimize this problem but not eliminate it. Further disadvantages of the press-fit stems are: the occurrence of pain at the end of the stem and the inferior stability in the presence of constraint forces [1, 21].

In complex revisions with severe ligamentous insufficiency, an increased intrinsic stability of the implant is necessary. Therefore either varus-valgus-constraint mechanisms or hinged prostheses with rotational mechanism are used. Especially these later implant systems are increasingly applied, as they reduce the rotational constraint forces and provide reconstruction of the joint line without complicated bone reconstructions [2, 12, 23].

4   From Constraint to Rotating Platform – Personal Experience

In the present series 19 hinged prostheses were revised from 1/90 to 4/99 (Fig. 23).

In 17 patients, revision was performed with the non-modular LCS Classic revision system. In two cases the modular LCS Universal was used. In contrast to the primary LCS components, the non-modular system is characterized by a longer conical stem with a short porous-coated area near to the joint surfaces. The articulation is provided by a rotating platform with a standard or a deep dish version. As a result of the different congruencies of the liners, the jump factor for the standard version is 6.1 mm and for the deep dish version 9.1 mm. A residual laxity of the collateral ligaments or the posterior capsule must be below this critical limit in order to avoid spin-out of the platform or dislocation.

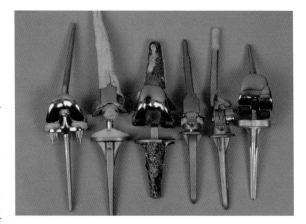

Fig. 23. Types of explanted hinged prostheses

The revisions were performed in 18 patients (4 male, 14 female) with a mean age of 71.3 years (range, 35–82 years). According to the Knee Society Score [11] four patients belonged to category A, seven to category B and seven to category C. The original diagnosis leading to the implantation of the primary implant was osteoarthritis in all cases, for three patients it resulted from trauma. In five knees the failed hinged prosthesis was implanted as a revision arthroplasty (four revisions of unicondylar arthroplasties, one revision of a bicondylar implant). In 14 knees the hinged prosthesis was the primary implant. Eight of these 14 knee arthroplasties had mean 5.6 preceding operations (range, 2–14 operations). The mean time between implantation and revision of the hinged prosthesis was relatively low: mean 5.6 years (range, 0.5–12 years). The reasons for failure were multiple: aseptic loosening: 8, periprosthetic infection: 4, fracture of the implant: 4, untreatable patella pain: 3, chronic painful effusion as result of polyethylene and metal wear: 1. The explanted hinges were: 11 rotating prostheses (8 Dadurian, Orthoplant; 3 Endo-Rotation, Link), five fully constraint hinges (1 Endo, Link; 2 Blauth, Aesculap; 1 GUEPAR, Benoist Girard) and four so-called gliding hinged prostheses (3 GSB, AlloPro; 1 S&G, S&G-Implants). After removal of the failed hinged prostheses the bony defects were categorized according to authors´ classification: At the femoral side there were three type 3 A, twelve type 3 B and four type 4 (= type 3 according to the AORI classification). The tibial defects were 16 type 3 A and three type 3 B.

5   Operative Technique – Surgical Approach

In all cases the lateral-parapatellar approach with osteotomy of the tibial tubercle was used [17]. This provides an excellent approach to all parts of the joint. It allows for medial and lateral release techniques exclusively at the tibial condyle. Additionally there is the option of transferring the tibial tubercule after insertion of the components in order to adjust the patella height to the joint line.

6 Reconstruction of the Bone Defects – Tibial Side

Reconstruction of the central defects was performed with impaction grafting in fourteen revisions, in the remaining four cases the before mentioned sandwich technique was applied. For the impaction-grafting-technique, the conical stem of the LCS-Classic-revision-system has several advantages: If it is necessary, the stem can be inserted excentrically to the tibial longitudinal axis, while the tibial tray still completely covers the cortical rim. At the same time, a slight tibial slope (–7°) is still possible. As the length and the diameter of the stem proportionally increase with the implant size, the cancellous bone can gradually be impacted in axial and radial direction by the use of successive trial components. Alternatively the sandwich technique (Fig. 24) can be used especially in presence of uncontained defects of the tibial wall. Here the intramedullary canal is filled with solid cancellous slices of 10 to 15 mm height. After contouring with a high speed burr, these slices are hammered into the intramedullary canal to achieve tight press-fit fixation. The trabecula of the grafts are positioned parallel to the tibial longitudinal axis. When the defect has been filled up in this way, the central hole for the conical stem is created by a reamer or a high speed burr.

7 Reconstruction of the Bone Defects – Femoral Side

The complexity of the defect situation required 15 structural reconstruction of the condyles. In 11 cases, femo-

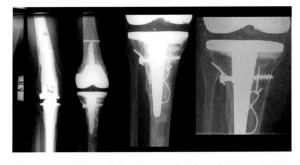

Fig. 24. Remodeling following sandwich-technique: 3/1997, left: failed hinged prosthesis, right: revision with LCS system, femoral side with distal femoral allograft, tibial side with sandwich-technique. 6/1997, tibial cancellous bone slices are clearly shown. 10/2001, 4.5 years after surgery, longitudinal formation of the trabecula

ral heads were fixed with osteosynthesis. In two cases, a proximal femoral allograft and in another two cases a distal femoral allograft (see Fig. 24) were applied. These four bulk allograft were inserted in inlay technique into the metaphyseal ice cone like defect. The bulk allografts were fresh frozen and were received from a commercial American or European tissue bank. All femoral heads were fresh frozen and were provided by the authors´ bone bank. In an average 2.8 femoral heads were used per patient (range, 1–5). In three patients additional autologous cancellous bone and tricortical iliac crest grafts were used.

8 Dimension, Fixation and Position of Implants

As result of the relatively short and conical stem of the LCS revision system, all implants could be exactly placed on the bony surface without overlapping. In five cases the femoral component was intentionally positioned more posteriorly in order to compensate for a relatively large flexion gap. This was simultaneously treated by bone augmentation of the posterior condyles. The tibial volume of the implants (tibial tray and liner) influences extension and flexion gap at the same time and determines the position of the joint line. For all 19 revisions, the tibial implant volume was mean 17.5 mm (range, 10–25 mm). In three patients patella infera could not be avoided. Fourteen revisions had an abnomal patella position. In one patient revision could not influence patella position. A severe metallosis following implant fracture led to excessive granuloma in one patient which necessitated patellaectomy. Patella replacement was done in only 6 cases, in the remaining patients moderate shaping of the patella surface was done. Component fixation was cementless in eight revisions both at the femoral and the tibial side. In five cases there was femoral cemented fixation and tibial cementless fixation. Six patients had cemented both implants. If cement was used, the application was restricted to the bone cut surface. There were 15 deep-dish and four regular polyethylene platforms. Adequate soft tissue release technique led to a sufficient ligamentous stability in all cases. After operation none of the patients required braces.

9 Aftertreatment

After operation, all patients started with assistive physiotherapy and active motion. If it was necessary, continuous passive motion was also applied. The patients started walking three days after surgery with two crutches or a rolator. Weight bearing was reduced to 15 kg for 10 to 12 weeks.

10   Follow-up

At the most recent follow-up, 17 patients with 18 revisions were available. One patient was lost to follow-up. The mean follow-up was 5.3 years (range, 0.7–10.5 years). The Knee Society score [11] was mean 74.9 points (range, 0–94 points). The functional score was mean 68.1 points (range, 0–100 points). The range of motion was mean 93.3° (range, 0–120°). At the time of the most recent follow-up examination three patients with three revised knee arthroplasties had died because of diseases that were unrelated to the revision arthroplasties. Two of these patients had a five-year follow-up with a Knee Society score of 93 and 85 points, the functional score was 100 and 80 points. The clinical results did not change until death. Eight months after knee revision with a distal femoral allograft the third patient died from pulmonary embolism during a contralateral primary knee arthroplasty. At the time of this operation, the Knee Society score was 85, the functional score was 45. Another patient, who had a two-staged knee revision arthroplasty after septic loosening, had a successful eradication of the infection. But one and a half years after the index surgery a haematogenous infection with totally different bacteria occurred during treatment of a tooth infection. One year after the index operation the Knee Society score was 83, the functional score was 80. In the following two-staged revision, the S-ROM mobile hinged bearing implant was used. In another patient, two years after surgery, a fibrous unstable tibial component had to be revised, the Knee Society score before re-revision was 48, the functional score was 45. After a successful re-revision, a haematoma was released half a year later with resulting periprosthetic infection and arthrodesis performed in another hospital. Two patients were wheel chair bound at the time of the most recent follow-up. One patient had a severe Alzheimer disease, the Knee Society score of 84, the functional score was 0 points (follow-up 10.5 years). The second patient was excessively overweight and had a contralateral amputation of the mid-femur because of untreatable periprosthetic infection. After the index operation a dislocation of the liner occurred, this is documented by radiographs since 11/99. The patient reported several adequate traumata as the reason for the luxation. Until now she has refused re-revision. The Knee Society score is 0, the functional score is also 0 (follow-up 7.5 years). Another patient has a severe lumbar stenosis with a Knee Society score of 94 and a functional score of 45 at a follow-up of eight years. Apart from the aseptic loosening of the tibial component in this series there is only one poor outcome as a direct result of the index operation. This patient had a two-staged revision following infection. The implants are stable. There is an anterior knee pain in the presence of patella baja without patella replacement. The Knee Society score is 59, the functional score is 50 (follow-up 2.5 years). If those four patients are excluded, whose functional score is merely reduced by the comorbidity, for the remaining patients there is a mean functional score of 81.1 (range, 50–100). The mean Knee Society score is 81.2 (range, 59–94), if those patients are excluded, whose index operation was influenced by implant loosening, secondary infection or trauma (n=3).

11   Ligamentous Stability

The analysis of ligamentous stability generally favors constrained implants when compared to un-constrained systems. A recent analysis of ligamentous stability was only possible in 13 patients of the altogether 19 knee revisions because of the circumstances mentioned above. In 20° flexion six knees had a physiological mediolateral stability, four had a slight medial instability, two a slight mediolateral instability. None of the patients reported giving away phenomena.

12   Radiographic Evaluation

For eighteen knee revisions standard a.p., sagittal and patella sky views were available. The radiographs were taken either at the last follow-up before death (3 cases) or before re-revision (2 cases) or at the most recent follow-up. Only the above mentioned revised cementless tibial component showed criteria for loosening. In the second patient with re-revision as a result of infection, both components were stable. Re-sorption or collapse of the structural graft was not visible and isolation of the components was not detectable. In all cases the extensive central cancellous bone graft revealed remodeling with trabecula growing according to the direction of loading (Fig. 25, 26).

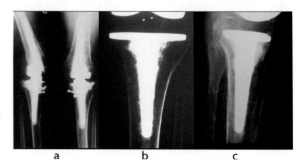

a   b   c

Fig. 25. a Remodelling following impaction grafting; **b** failed hinged prosthesis and **c** distinct trabecula formation in both planes, stable cementless tibial component

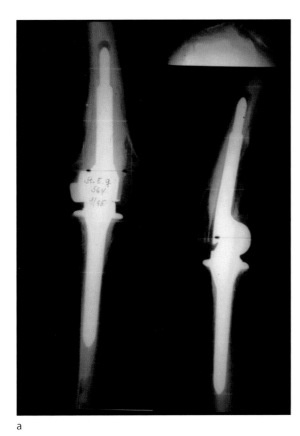

a

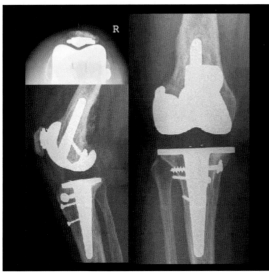

b

Fig. 26a,b. Patient B.S. **a** Loosened malaligned femoral component with posterior supracondylar fracture, dislocated patella. **b** Stable cementless components, remodeling of the impacted morselised bone, well aligned patella, follow-up 6 years

This was especially seen in the sandwich-technique, where the remodeling occurred even sooner. Radiolucent lines with a width of less than 1 mm were seen in a few cases in the zones 1 and 4 at the femoral and tibial side [7]. The lines never occurred in combination. In 25 % of all cases a dense sclerotic halo was found at the peripheral stem. There was no progression of this halo. The femorotibial angle was mean 5.1° (range 1°–11°). The patella was aligned and did not show tilting. In all cases the six cementless patella replacements had bone ingrowth.

13 Perioperative complications

The overall rate of perioperative complications was 47.4 %, but this did not influence the outcome. The most frequent complication was a longitudinal fissure at the tibial condyle during surgery (6 cases). The fissure healed primarily following intra-operative screw fixation. Two postoperative haematoma were treated with irrigation. In one patient the tibial tubercle dislocated postoperatively as a result of adequate trauma. After fixation with cerclage wires the tubercle healed.

14 Critical Résumé

The present series of revision knee arthroplasties is characterized by a great homogeneity of parameter: The failed implants are all hinged prosthesis, there are only severe bone defects and the LCS-revision-system is systematically used. At midterm follow-up mechanical loosening only occurred in one component. The satisfying results are due to several factors. Special attention was given to the press-fit fixation of the components at the femoral condyles and to the fixation of the structural grafts. This was particularly important, as the stem of the non modular LCS revision components is rather short. Impaction grafting as well as the sandwich technique provide a high primary stability and lead to a reliable secondary stability of the implants concomitant with an evident bone remodeling. Additionally, it is particularly important that the constraint forces are essentially reduced by the mobile bearing revision system used in this series. Thus long cemented or uncemented stems could be avoided. Slight ligamentous instability, as found in the present series, can be tolerated, as long as the critical limit for spin out of the polyethylene liners is not surpassed.

Finally, downgrading of the bone defects by the presented methods is an essential aspect: In case of a re-revision, the bone defects are less extensive as at the time of the index operation. So prognosis for the patient after re-revision can definitively be improved. In conclusion the present series shows the special advantages of the mobile bearing revision system combined with massive bone grafts as a treatment option in demanding cases of revision knee arthroplasty.

References

1. Barrack RL, Rorabeck C, Burt M, Sawhney J (1999) Pain at the end of the stem after revision total knee arthroplasty. CORR 367: 216–225
2. Barrack LR, Lyons TR, Ingraham RQ, Johnson JC (2000) The use of a modular rotating-hinge component in salvage revision total knee arthroplasty. J Arthropl 7: 858–866
3. Bradley GW (2000) Revision total knee arthroplasty by impaction bone grafting. CORR 371: 113–118
4. Channer MA, Glisson RR, Seaber AV, Vail TP (1996) Use of bone compaction in total knee arthroplasty. J Arthropl 6: 743–749
5. Clatworthy MG, Ballance J, Brick GW, Chandler HP, Gross AE (2001) The use of structural allograft for uncontaint defects in revision total knee arthroplasty. JBJS 83-A 3: 404–411
6. Engh GA (1997) Bone defect classification, In: Engh GA, Rorabeck CH (eds) Revison total knee arthroplasty. Williams & Wilkins, †, pp 63–120
7. Ewald F (1989) The knee society total knee arthroplasty roentgenographic evaluation and scoring system. CORR 248: 9–12
8. Fitzek JG, Barden B (2000) Rekonstruktionsmöglichkeiten nach Fehlschlägen in der Knieendoprothetik. In: Imhoff AB (Hrsg) Fortbildung Orthopädie, Bd 3. Steinkopff, Darmstadt, S 157–172
9. Hoeffel DP, Rubash HE (2000) Revision total knee arthroplasty. CORR 380: 116–132
10. Inglis AE, Walker PS (1991) Revision of failed knee replacements using fixed-axis hinges. JBJS 73 B: 757–761
11. Insall J, Dorr L, Scott R, Scott N (1989) Rationale of the knee society clinical rating system. CORR 248: 13–14
12. Jones RE, Skedros JG, Chan AJ, Beauchamp DH, Harkins PC (2001) Total knee arthroplasty using the s-rom mobile-bearing hinge prosthesis. J Arthropl 3: 279–287
13. Kim YH (1967) Salvage of failed hinge knee arthroplasty with a total condylar iii type prosthesis, CORR 221: 272–277
14. Kirk PG (1997) Selecting an implant: a comparison of revision implant systems. In: Engh GA, Rorabeck CH (eds) Revision total knee arthroplasty. Williams & Wilkins, S 137–165
15. v. Lenthe GH, De Waal Malefijt MC, Huiskes R (1997) Stress shielding after total knee replacement may cause bone resorption in the distal femur. JBJS 79 B 1: 117–122
16. Lonner JH, Klotz M, Levitz C, Lotke PA (2001) Changes in bone density after cemented total knee arthroplasty. Influence of stem design. J Arthropl 1: 107–111
17. Markus PA, Friederich NF, Widmer H, Müller W (1999) Lateral approach to the knee combined with an osteotomy of the tibial tuberosity. Op Orthop Traum 3: 224–232
18. McAuley JP, Engh GA (1997) Allografts in revision total knee arthroplasty. In: Engh GA, Rorabeck CH (eds) Revision total knee arthroplasty. Williams & Wilkins, S 252–274
19. Scuderi GR (2001) Revision total knee arthroplasty. How much constraint is enough? CORR 392: 300–305
20. Tsahakis PJ, Beaver WB, Brick GW (1994) Technique and results of allograft reconstruction in revision total knee arthroplasty. CORR 303: 86–94
21. Vince KG, Long W (1995) Revision knee arthroplasty. The limits of press fit medullary fixation. CORR 317: 172–177
22. Wang JS, Tägil M, Aspenberg P (2000) Load-bearing increases new bone formation in impacted and morselized allografts. CORR 378: 272–281
23. Westrich GH, Mollano AV, Sculco TP, Buly RL, Laskin RS, Windsor R (2000) Rotating hinge total knee arthroplasty in severely affected knees. CORR 379: 195–208
24. Whiteside LA, Bicalho PS (1998) Radiologic and histologic analysis of morselized allograft in revision total knee replacement. CORR 357: 149–156

13.3 Hinge Total Knee Arthroplasty

R. D. Jones

1 Introduction

Walldius first reported use of a hinge knee prosthesis for primary total knee arthroplasty [24]. This chapter will outline the development of hinged knee arthroplasty from that early report to the present day, third generation mobile hinge knee system. The hinge total knee mechanically links the femoral component with the tibial component to provide enhanced stability to the prosthesis. Early designs of hinged knee systems were characterized by sagittal motion only in an attempt to reproduce the "hinge" action of the human knee. These early designs were found to have high rates of complications and failures [3, 8, 10, 25, 28]. Poor results were attributed to the highly constrained articulation, and other design flaws. Hinged knee systems have progressed from those early, first generation implants to an intermediate stage of second generation prostheses, and to the currently used third generation, mobile-bearing, rotating hinged knee systems.

2 Evolution of the Hinge Total Knee Arthroplasty

2.1 First Generation

Over 4 decades ago, Walldius reported on his design of a hinge total knee. The Walldius prosthesis was a fixed device allowing motion only in the sagittal plane with flexion limited to 90 degrees [24]. Other first generation hinge prostheses followed and reports appeared in the 1950's through the 1970's and included the Shiers, Guepar, and Stanmore prostheses [3, 8, 10, 15, 25]. These early hinge components were designed to be used as primary knee replacements. They were characterized by high levels of constraint, unidirectional motion, metal-on-metal load transmission at the articulation, minimal selection of implant size, and a flattened trochlea region.

2.2 Second Generation

To correct the problems associated with the detrimental stresses seen in the early systems, new designs were created to decrease the constraint but maintain the stability of the knee systems. Systems which incorporated axial freedom and decreased direct transmission of torsional forces across the joint included the Herbert knee, the Spherocentric knee, the Kinematic rotating hinge knee prosthesis, the Rotaflex knee, and the Noiles rotating hinge prosthesis.

The Noiles hinge total knee was a second generation system that had an uncemented tibial stem set within a cemented sleeve, allowing a 20° arc of both medial and lateral rotation in flexion, as well as allowing axial rotation [22]. While the early results of the Noiles hinge total knee arthroplasty were promising [1, 7], long-term follow up studies revealed flaws in the design of the implant that led to high rates of complications [16, 22]. Shindell et al. found a 56 % failure rate at an average of 32 months postoperatively [22]. Kester et al. reported extensive wear of the polyethylene tibial components [16].

2.3 Third Generation

The problems associated with the initial Noiles hinge total knee arthroplasty engendered extensive changes in the design of the implant creating the S-ROM Noiles Rotating Hinge Knee System. A review of those changes is instructive in understanding the process of design changes leading to better clinical results. The modifications of the Noiles system have achieved inherent stability, load-sharing through broad articulating surfaces to decrease the context stresses, and the accommodation of gait kinematics with a mobile-bearing. In fact, Noiles, an engineer with U.S. Surgical Corporation, patented the first mobile-bearing in the mid-70's. The S-ROM, Noiles rotating bearing allows stresses to be distributed more evenly thereby protecting the bone-cement-implant interfaces. It is suggested that these modifications and the incorporation of metaphyseal loading sleeves have accounted for the low incidence of radiolucencies around the implant and the very positive results reported in recent studies [4, 12, 13].

3 Principles and Design

The single axis movement of early hinges led to significant torque under axial load that caused deleterious stresses on the bone-cement-implant interface which led to higher wear rates and implant loosening [14]. Thusly, all evolutionary designs of hinge knees featured some increase in degrees of freedom at the knee joint usually by a mobile, rotating type bearing. This change better accommodated the gait-related flexural and rotational stresses at the knee and diminished the excess sheer stresses applied at the implant interfaces. The use of polyethylene at the axle yoke mechanism and on the femoral and tibial condylar bearing surfaces also diminished the particulate metal debris. A broader range of sizes for selection of an implant that would match patient anatomy also proved useful. In the Noiles system the addition of specialized intramedullary stems designed for press-fit and metaphyseal filling and loading sleeves further distributed the stresses throughout the hard and soft tissue anatomy.

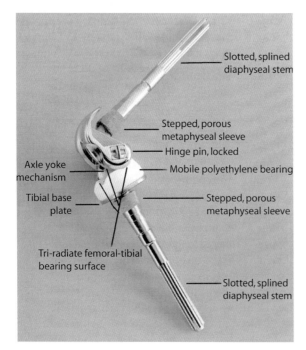

Slotted, splined diaphyseal stem

Stepped, porous metaphyseal sleeve

Hinge pin, locked

Mobile polyethylene bearing

Axle yoke mechanism

Tibial base plate

Stepped, porous metaphyseal sleeve

Tri-radiate femoral-tibial bearing surface

Slotted, splined diaphyseal stem

Fig. 27. The S-ROM Noiles mobile-bearing hinge knee prosthesis

The modern design of the S-ROM Noiles Rotating Hinge has a mobile-bearing that allows axial rotation between the inner tibial bearing and outer tibial sleeve. The system has highly polished cobalt chrome alloy bearing surfaces which broadly articulate both on the condylar surfaces and the axle yoke mechanism with good stress distribution throughout the tri-radiate bearing. The distinguishing feature of this rotating hinge system from other hinge implants is the ability to use modular sleeves and stems in a range of sizes to provide optimal fit and fill to manage a wide range of possible metaphyseal deficiencies. This also allows for fill which promotes intramedullary load sharing, fixation into intact bone, a decreased need for fixation with intramedullary bone cement, and the ability to bypass stress risers in situations of bone deficiencies [12].

The sleeves of the S-ROM Noiles hinged knee system are stepped and textured with beads having interbead pore diameters of approximately 200 microns, creating the possibility of bony ingrowth. The femoral and tibial stems are slotted and fluted to increase the diaphyseal fit and rotational stability, and more closely match the stiffness of bone. The implant has metallic augmentation blocks that are available for cases with distal femur or proximal tibial bone loss (Fig. 27).

The S-ROM Noiles hinged knee arthroplasty has a deepened femoral trochlear groove. The articulating surface on the top of the tibial tray and the inside of the stem receptor area are highly polished in order to create a broad mobile surface for the ultra-high molecular weight polyethylene tibial bearing. There is now a congruent articulation between the polyethylene bearing and the medial and lateral femoral bearing surfaces, as well as with the axle-yoke assembly. Physiologic valgus has been fixed into the femoral component at 7°. The modifications of the system have achieved inherent stability, load sharing through broad articulating surfaces to decrease contact stresses, and the accommodations of gait kinematics [12].

4 Indications and Surgical Technique

Most revision total knee arthroplasties that are performed in patients with significant deformity and instability can be done with the increased constraint provided by a posterior stabilized system or constrained condylar type of total knee system. However, there is a group of patients with severe anatomic loss of bone, supporting soft tissue structures, or both that require a linked knee prosthesis. While such hinged knee systems are usually used in revision circumstances, there are primary indications such as knee arthrodesis take down, paralytic knee deformities with minimal muscular support, or severe post-traumatic arthrosis. The senior author's preferred surgical technique when a linked knee system is required is to use the S-ROM Noiles rotating hinge total knee system. This selection is based on extensive personal experience with the prosthesis and the excellent mid-term results that have been reported using the system [4, 12, 13].

Revision knee is approached using and excising previous skin incisions. The prosthesis is removed with preservation of as much bone as possible. Complete debridement of hard and soft tissues is performed, and a final assessment of bone loss and soft tissue support is accomplished. The S-ROM Noiles intramedullary mounted instrument system provides for reaming the canal to the appropriate size and cortical feel/medullary fill, metaphyseal broaching with intramedullary pilots to rotational stability, and bone cuts made off the stem-sleeve aligned intramedullary guides. Appropriate augments are used to obtain the correct joint line. Assembly of the trial component is then performed. The modular components are then assembled on the back table. The medullary stems and metaphyseal sleeves are designed to be press-fit. Patch grafting with local bone or more extensive grafting with allograft bone usually particulate, can be used to augment any major defects and hard tissue that may be encountered [11] (Fig. 28).

Since the S-ROM Noiles Modular Knee System provides sleeves that fit and fill the large bony defects often seen in salvage knee replacement, these patients usually do not require bulk allograft reconstruction. Therefore, operating time efficiency is greatly enhanced. Jones and Barrack reported a mean operative time of 135 minutes in their series of 30 knees using the S-ROM Noiles Hinge Knee System[12]. Westrich [27] reported mean operating times of 198 minutes using the Finn hinge knee system for the same type of salvage knee arthroplasty patient. In comparing the two series, it is apparent that the intramedullary-mounted instrument system and availability of modular sleeves in the S-ROM system was advantageous.

5 Clinical Results

Jones et al. [13], Barrack et al[4], and Jones, Barrack and Skedros [12] have all reported outstanding mid-term results using the S-ROM Noiles Hinge Knee System. The

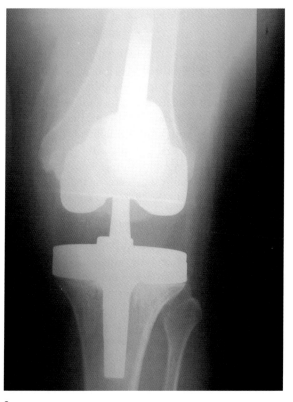
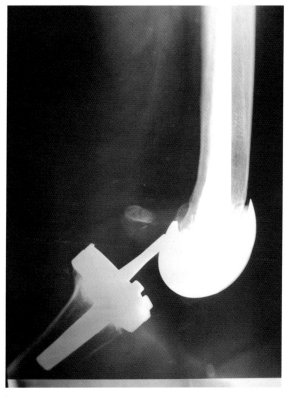

a   b

Fig. 28. a,b A.p. and lateral radiographs of a 49 year old female post fourth revision total knee with coronal and sagittal plane instability and huge flexion-extension gaps

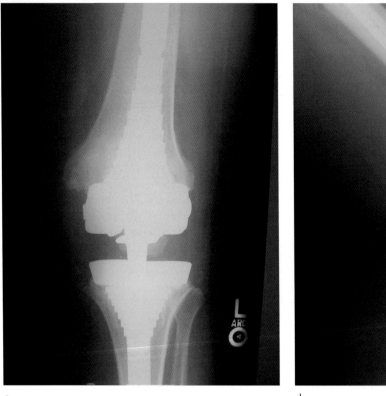
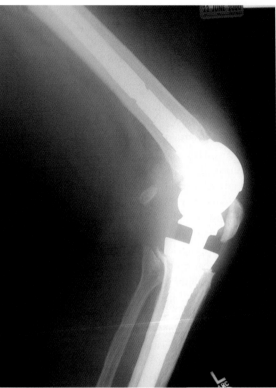

c   d

Fig. 28. c, d a.p. and lateral radiographs 2 years pot conversion to S-ROM Noiles modular mobile-bearing hinge

combined series from Dallas (Jones et al), and from New Orleans (Barrack et al), documented 30 knees that underwent revision using the S-ROM Knee System. The patients were followed up at a mean time of 49 months and ranged in age from 33 to 83 years. There were dramatic differences in the Knee Society Clinical Scores with preoperative means of 52 and post-operative mean scores of 134 points. Additionally, the mean range of flexion improved from 81° to 100° in this group of patients. There were no mechanical failures of the prosthesis. Radiographic analysis of the patients at follow up showed that all patients with press-fit femoral and tibial sleeves and stems showed bony apposition and no implant-interface radiolucencies. Three patients sustained intraoperative fractures during canal preparation and were treated by cerclage wire or cable fixation and the intramedullary rods that are part of the implant construct. No changes in post-operative treatment were necessitated because of the stable constructs achieved.

6   Conclusions

The current third generation, modular, mobile-bearing hinge knee systems can now be used with increasing

confidence. While Rand et al [20] recommended the use of a condylar type stabilized knee prosthesis in cases of revision total knee arthroplasty with medial instability and avoidance of a hinged knee prosthesis, we can make a contrasting recommendation. The excellent mid-term follow-up studies with modular mobile-bearing hinge knee system suggest that the orthopedic surgeon when confronted with catastrophic salvage knee arthroplasty can display increasing confidence in the selection of such hinge systems. In fact, Barrack (Knee Society, San Francisco 2001) stated that the current third generation hinge knee systems may be a more conservative approach than the constrained condylar systems. Specifically, the constrained condylar systems cause significant post wear because of the lack of mobile bearing capacity. Therefore, polyethylene wear may be a bigger issue in revision knees using constrained condylar systems than it has been demonstrated to be in revision knees using third generation mobile hinge knee systems. Our follow up studies which demonstrate minimal radiolucencies also suggest that third generation linked knee systems with dynamic, bipolar motion at the tibial femoral articulation are sufficient to decrease the deleterious stresses that contributed to the failures of earlier designs of hinge knee systems. Orthopedic surgeons faced with catastrophic salvage revision knees can select modular, mobile-bearing hinged knee systems with assurance of good results.

References

1. Accardo NJ, Noiles DG, Pena R, Accardo Jr NJ (1979) Noiles total knee replacement procedure. Orthopedics 2: 37–45
2. Bain AM (1973) Replacement of the knee joint with the Walldius prosthesis using cement fixation. Clin Orthop 94: 65–71
3. Bargar WL, Cracchiolo A, Amstutz HC (1980) Results with the constrained total knee prosthesis in treating severely disabled patients and patients with failed total knee replacements. J Bone Joint Surg 62 A: 504–512
4. Barrack RL, Lyons TR, Ingraham RQ, Johnson JC (2000) The use of a modular rotating hinge component in salvage revision total knee arthroplasty. J Arthroplasty 15: 858–866
5. Churchill DL, Incavo SJ, Johnson CC, Beynnon BD (1998) The transepicondylar axis approximates the optimal flexion axis of the knee. Clin Orthop 356: 111–118
6. David HG, Bishay M, James ETR (1998) Problems with the rotaflex: a 10-year review of a rotating hinge prosthesis. J Arthroplasty 13: 402–408
7. Flynn LM (1979) The Noiles hinge knee prosthesis with axial rotation. Orthopedics 2: 602–605
8. Hui FC, Fitzgerald RH (1980) Hinged total knee arthroplasty. J Bone Joint Surg 62 A: 513–519
9. Insall JN, Aglietti P, Baldini A, Easley ME (2001) Meniscal-bearing knee replacement. In: Insall JN, Scott WN (eds) Surgery of the knee, 3rd Edition. Churchill-Livingstone, New York, p 1721
10. Jones EC, Insall JN, Inglis AE, Ranawat CS (1979) GUEPAR knee arthroplasty results and late complications. Clin Orthop 140: 145–152
11. Jones RE (1996) Management of the bone deficient knee: management of complex revision problems with a modular total knee system. Orthopaedics 19:802–806
12. Jones RE, Barrack RL, Skedros JG (2001) Modular, mobile-bearing hinge total knee arthroplasty. Clin Orthop 392: 306–314
13. Jones RE, Skedros JG, Chan AJ, Beauchamp DH, Harkins PC (2001) Total knee arthroplasty using the S-ROM mobile-bearing hinge prosthesis. J Arthroplasty 16: 279–287
14. Kabo JM, Yang RS, Dorey FJ, Eckardt JJ (1997) In vivo rotational stability of the kinematic rotating hinge knee prosthesis. Clin Orthop 336: 166–176
15. Karpinski MRK, Grimer RJ (1987) Hinged knee replacement in revision arthroplasty. Clin Orthop 220: 185–191
16. Kester MA, Cook SD, Harding AF, Rodriquez RP, Pipkin CS (1988) An evaluation of the mechanical failure modalities of a rotating hinge knee prosthesis. Clin Orthop 228: 156–163
17. LaFortune MA, Cavanaugh PR, Sommer III HJ, Kalenak A (1992) Three-dimensional kinematics of the human knee during walking. J Biomechanics 25:347–357
18. Lettin AWF, Kavanagh TG, Scales JT (1984) The long-term results of Stanmore total knee replacements. J Bone Joint Surg 66B: 349–354
19. Matthews LS, Goldstein SA, Kolowich PA, Kaufer H (1986) Spherocentric arthroplasty of the knee: a long-term and final follow up evaluation. Clin Orthop 205: 58–66
20. Rand JA, Chao EYS, Stauffer RN (1987) Kinematic rotating-hinge total knee arthroplasty. J Bone Joint Surg 69 A: 489–497
21. Ritter MA (1977) The Herbert total knee replacement: a longer than three year follow-up. Clin Orthop 129: 232–235
22. Shindell R, Neumann R, Connolly JF, Jardon OM (1986) Evaluation of the Noiles hinged knee prosthesis: a five-year study of seventeen knees. J Bone Joint Surg 68 A: 579–585
23. Trent PS, Walker PS (1976) Ligament length patterns, strength, and rotational axes of the knee joint. Clin Orthop 117: 263–270
24. Walldius B (1960) Arthroplasty of the knee using an endo-prosthesis: 8 years' experience. Acta Orthop Scand 30: 137–148
25. Watson JR, Wood H, Hill RCJ (1976) The Shiers arthroplasty of the knee. J Bone Joint Surg 58B: 300–304
26. Watt NAR, Hughes SPF (1987) Early results with Rotaflex rotating hinge knee replacement. J R Coll Surg Edinb 32: 361–365
27. Westrich GH, Anthony VM, Sculco TP, Buly RL, Laskin RS, Windsor R (2000) Rotating hinge total knee arthroplasty in severely affected knees. Clin Orthop 379: 195–208
28. Wilson FC Venters GC (1976) Results of knee replacement with the Walldius prosthesis. Clin Orthop 120: 39–46

Design Worldwide Trends in Mobile Bearing TKA

IV

Chapter 14
Design Considerations of Existing Mobile Bearing TKA

J. B. STIEHL

1 Introduction

The emergence of the mobile bearing articulating poly-ethylene surfaces in total knee arthroplasty reflects the effort of designers to optimize wear while dealing with complex function. In vivo dynamic video fluoroscopy has provided extensive knowledge of the precise mechanisms of articulation in total knee arthroplasty [1, 3, 4, 8, 9, 10–12, 15]. The convergence of kinematic data with the analysis of prosthetic retrievals from failed total knees has given a clear understanding of the functional requirements for improved mobile bearing total knee devices [1]. Design issues include femoral condyle geometry, single versus polycentric radius of curvature, devices that restrict certain bearing motions and disarticulation such as stops or pegs, a medial versus more central longitudinal axis of rotation on the proximal tibia, surgical technique, implant stability, contact area, and patellofemoral design. The question of posterior cruciate retention, sacrifice, or stabilization in regards to mobile bearing designs remains an unresolved variable. Current mobile bearing designs will be reviewed with available technical information.

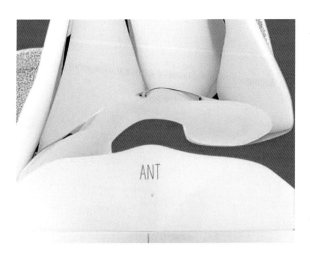

Fig. 1. Diagram of LCS Rotating Platform shows potential for both condylar liftoff and medial lateral translation while maintaining high conformity in extension

2 Mobile Bearing Design Considerations

With over twenty five years of continuous successful use with an unmodified design, the Low Contact Stress (LCS) Mobile bearing knee system has become the gold standard by which all future designs are to be compared. This design had an anatomical femoral component that allowed virtually complete area contact in extension up to 34° of flexion and decreasing radii of the posterior femoral condyles to optimize the ability for flexion. In the coronal plane geometry allowed stability with the potential for medial-lateral translation while maintaining high conformity (Fig. 1). The geometries of the tibia and patella were matched to articulate with a common area on the anterior distal femur. The femoral intercondylar groove was deepened to match the normal anatomical position. Finally, tibial trays and polyethylene inserts were developed that allowed bicruciate retention, posterior cruciate retention, or cruciate sacrifice (Fig. 2). A more recent modification was the AP-Glide rotating platform device designed for use with a rotating platform shaped insert, such that posterior cruciate retention was possible. The tibial insert is allowed to rotate and translate based on the use of a control arm that has a cone that fits into the original tibial tray (Fig. 3).

Over fifteen different mobile bearing devices have been developed in recent years following the clinical success of the LCS Knee system. With limited and unproven track record in the majority, it is unknown if they will perform satisfactorily to the level of the LCS or other fixed bearing designs with over 20 years follow-up. Therefore, analysis of general design features and surgical technique may offer important insight to the potential for long term performance and function (Table 1).

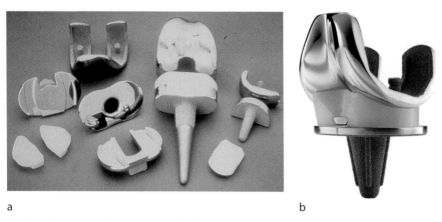

a   b

Fig. 2. a LCS System of implants including bicruciate, cruciate sacrificing, cruciate retaining, and unicondylar arthroplasty; **b** LCS universal A/P glide posterior cruciate retaining implant

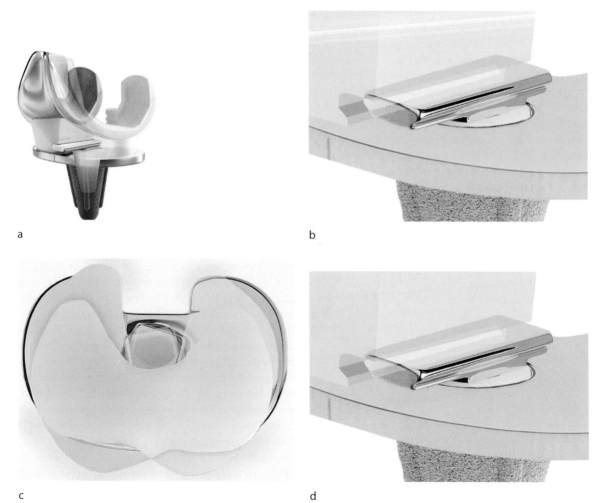

a   b

c   d

Fig. 3. a LCS AP Glide prosthesis; **b** the control arm used with the rotating platform insert to allow for posterior cruciate retention; **c** top view of tibial insert demonstrates multiplanar motion; **d** schematic view of control arm positioned in tibial tray to control tibial insert position

Table 1. Currently available Mobile Bearing total knee prostheses with general features

Prosthesis	Technique	Insert Engagement	Contact Area Extension	Radius of Curvature	Anatomical Rotating Patella	Femur, Coronal Plane Conformity	Free Rotation & Translation No "Stops"
LCS Depuy	Bicruciate, PCR, PCS	Stem in stem polyethylene	902 mm²	Multiple	Yes, Yes	Yes	Yes, (all)
Rotataglide Corin	PCR, PS	2 Pin on Slot	NA	Single	No, No	Yes	No
HLS Tornier	PS	1 Knob	NA	Multiple	No, No	Yes	No
Genesis II Smith Nephew	PCR	1 Pin on Slot	NA	Multiple	No, No	Yes	No
Natural Sulzer	PCR	Stem in stem polyethylene	566 mm²	Multiple	No, No	No	No
SAL Sulzer	PCR	1 Pin on Slot	551 mm²	Single	Yes, No	Yes	No
Trac Biomet	PS	Stem in stem polyethylene	NA	Dual Radius	No, No	Yes	No
MBK	PCR, PCS	2 Pin on Slot, Bumper	530 mm²	Single	No, No	Yes	No
AMC MKII	PCR, PS	Rim Bumper	NA	Multiple	Yes, Yes	Yes	No
Legacy	PS	1 Pin on Slot	NA	Multiple	No, No	Yes	No
Profix	PCR	1 Pin on Slot	NA	Multiple	No, No	Yes	No
PFC Sigma	PS, PCR	Stem in stem polyethylene	407 mm²	Multiple	No, No	Yes	Yes (RP)
Interax Howmedica	PCR	1 Pin on Slot	553 mm²	NA	No, No	Yes	No
Oxford Biomet	NA	NA	NA	NA	No, No	Yes	No
Innex Sulzer	PCR, PCS	Stem in stem metal	NA	Multiple	No, No	Yes	Yes

2.1 Single Versus Polycentric Radii of Curvature of the Femoral Component

With the idea of maximizing area of contact throughout the range of motion, engineers chose a single radius of curvature in certain designs. This was considered reasonable as the posterior condyle seems to define a fairly circular sagittal shape and the implant would mimic this shape. The disadvantage however is that the total radius must be significantly smaller than that of the normal distal femoral surface which may reduce area contact and cause a degree of instability in extension. High conformity in flexion may be desirable for contact area but leads to an inflexible articulation that must follow the kinematics of femoral tibial contact. Dennis has shown that some posterior cruciate retaining total knees that are tight in flexion cause the femoral tibial contact to remain far posterior on the proximal tibia [2] (Fig. 4). A lesser constrained polycentric curvature has greater accommodation for this motion while the single radius design may "slide off the back" as was shown by the original Oxford meniscal bearing design. A second related issue is "jumping distance" for disarticulation that must be lower for the single radius design (Fig. 5). For the di-

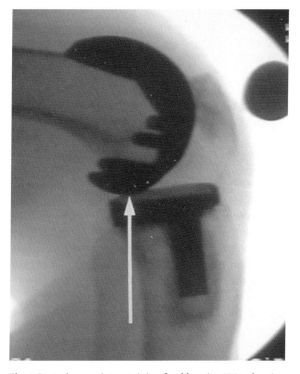

Fig. 4. Posterior cruciate retaining fixed bearing TKA showing posterior femoral tibial contact in deep flexion

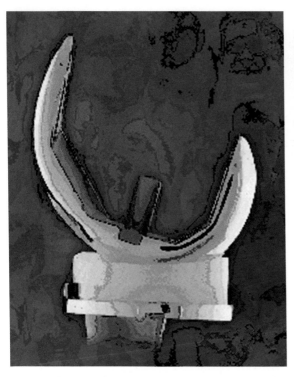

Fig. 5. Single radius of curvature increases contact area throughout range of motion at the expense of total area in extension and a lower jumping distance with greater instability in deep flexion

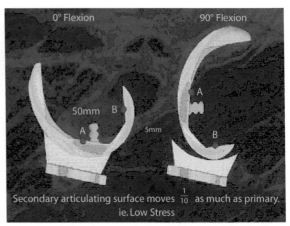

Fig. 6. Multiple radii of curvature allow for deep flexion and increase "jumping distance" in deep flexion

minished polycentric radius, the condyle must "go up the hill" and travel further to disarticulate [7] (Fig. 6).

Recently, a fixed bearing knee prosthesis was developed with a medial pivot joint that has a near fixed radius of the medial femoral condyle to minic the relatively fixed articulation of the normal medial condyle. The object of the medial pivot is to replicate the longitudinal axis of rotation of the normal knee that Freeman has shown to be medial to the center of the proximal tibia [5]. The down side of the equation is the potential for abnormal kinematics of medial condylar sliding associated with anterior cruciate deficiency that may overload the medial pivot joint.

Similiarly, certain designs have changed the center of rotation from a central position such as the LCS rotating platform to a more anterior position to accommodate the insert post into the tibial base stem that has been located more anteriorly. This creates an eccentric position for the rotation of the tibial insert offsetting the insert position for a given amount of tibial rotation. Certain abnormal kinematics which have been shown to occur, such as tibial external rotation would place the tibial insert more medial than normal, which if compounded with the normal proximal lateral translation of the femoral condyle could result in exaggerated contact on a medial tibial eminence or post.

2.2 Stops, Articulations, Mechanical Restraints

Mobile bearing tibial inserts require certain degrees of freedom that are absent with fixed bearing devices. The original Oxford and LCS clinical experience demonstrated the problem of bearing dislocation and "spinout" associated with poor surgical technique. These problems can be diminished with capture pegs, sliding control arms (LCS AP Glide is more unconstrained than the meniscal bearing LCS) and capture rims. The downside is constraint and associated polyethylene wear that could be expected with certain "pin on slot" designs (Fig. 7). Also, designs that will articulate with normal motion (such as a post cam) can be expected to wear over time. Abnormal kinematics from poor surgical technique or unaccommodated normal kinematics will likely cause exaggerated wear. An example of the later is the TRAC II total knee that is highly conforming in the coronal plane. With coronal medial-lateral translation known to occur in the normal knee, this implant will wear much like a constrained condylar revision device (Fig. 8).

2.3 Surgical Technique

The options are bicruciate retention, posterior cruciate retention, posterior cruciate sacrifice, and posterior cruciate substitution or stabilization. Experience with the Oxford unicondylar meniscal bearing device has shown that bicruciate retention is essential for success of this implant. The LCS experience has shown that posterior cruciate retention with the meniscal bearing is possible but must be implemented very carefully because of the risk of flexion instability. Too tight or too loose in flexion will lead to implant dislocation. The primary disadvan-

Fig. 7. a "Pin on slot" designs are potentially a high stress area for increased polyethylene wear especially if the articulation is a normal motion restraint; **b** Interax mobile bearing demonstrates pin on slot mechanism

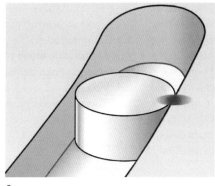
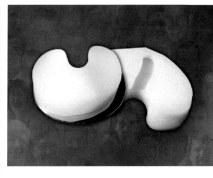

a   b

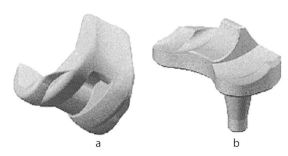

a   b

Fig. 8a, b. TRAC mobile knee demonstrates tight condylar constraints which prevent functional frontal plane translation. **a** Femoral component; **b** tibial component

tage of the "distal femoral cut first" method is the inability to accurately adjust the flexion space on final trialing. The LCS technique has evolved into a "tibial cut first", spacer block technique as pioneered by Insall. This has been an important element to the long clinical success of that implant. Posterior cruciate sacrifice with the tibial cut first technique has proven to be easy for most surgeons, reproducible, and clinically durable over the long term for the LCS.

Posterior cruciate stabilization is a common feature of the majority of new rotating platform designs. The primary advantage is the ability to enforce a degree of posterior femoral rollback that will improve flexion. In addition, an element of stability is added from the jumping distance of the post/cam mechanism that ranges from 1.1 to 1.4 cm. There are however known liabilities of the post/cam mechanism that include decreased patellofemoral articulation of the area of the box and the potential for soft tissue impingement or clunk in the box. Recent retrievals of posterior stabilized inserts have demonstrated a significant wear potential, which interestingly may involve the medial and lateral post surfaces as well as the posterior surface where spine wear would logically be seen [6].

2.4 Patellofemoral Articulation

The patellofemoral articulation has been problematic for posterior stabilized designs with a high incidence of patella fracture, subluxation, or implant loosening. Possible causes with some of these older designs include an inherent "boxy" shape of femoral components that do not anatomically restore the patellofemoral groove. The loading forces of the patellofemoral joint are poorly understood, hence question arises regarding the future performance of new posterior stabilized designs in this regard. For the LCS design, patellofemoral problems are rare in most series despite a relatively thick, mobile, metal backed patella. This could relate to the anatomical positioning of the femoral prosthetic intercondylar sulcus that relies on the unique shape of the LCS design and the 15° distal cut required for implantation.

Other issues that affect patella performance include the surgical technique and abnormal functions that may arise from abnormal kinematics. Clearly, femoral components placed in exaggerated internal rotation and tibial components with internal rotation in relation to the tibial tubercle will cause the need for lateral release, and may exaggerate problems of patellar subluxation and implant failure. Kinematic studies have shown exaggerated abnormal tibial external rotation, which when combined with abnormal lateral condylar liftoff, must strain the extensor mechanism and place a lateral thrust on the patella.

2.5 Implant Stability

Implant stability may become an issue for certain designs if there is not high conformity especially in the frontal plane. This has been a problem with early designs such as the Minn prosthesis. As noted from kinematic studies, the potential for abnormal motions is significant in total knee arthroplasty. Surgical technique is an important factor in this regard, as the design must be able to accommodate difficult problems in the hands of lesser experienced surgeons. With the LCS, and other mobile bearing implants, careful attention to flexion-extension gap spacing and ligamentous balancing are essential to eliminate this problem. Measured bone resections, typical of current fixed bearing designs have the inherent weakness of error in certain cases that fall out of the normal range of anatomy. This will likely compromise the success of surgical technique in certain cases.

2.6 Contact Stress

Wear can be related directly to the contact stress of two articulating bodies and from the engineering literature had a direct relationship to the differences of the principle radii of curvature. This obviously relates as well to the area of contact, such that two articulating surfaces with similar conforming radii with high area of contact will have lower contact surface stress than those of dissimiliar radii and much lower area contact. An interesting contradiction however is that the applied load relates only to the cube root of the material stiffness and area of contact such that increases in load or body weight in total knees does not dramatically increase the contact stress. Reducing contact stress then is the other principle benefit of a mobile bearing articulation by dramatically increasing the area of contact. In regards to current mobile bearing designs, the LCS which has very high conformity in full extension has a contact area of 902 mm^2 for the rotating platform while the MBK with a single radius of curvature has 530 mm^2 of contact area. The latter reduction is both a function of design and the fact that a single radius of curvature in total knees must be diminished with smaller contact area compared to polycentric radii. Early wear simulator studies have shown that the LCS has diminished polyethylene wear compared to typical fixed bearing designs by a factor of three. Recent wear simulation studies have shown that the wear of fixed bearings with complex out of plane motion such as sliding translation and liftoff may be four to five times that of simple linear articulation. It remains to be seen if newer mobile bearing designs with much lower contact area and conformity compared to the LCS will have the favorable long term outcome in terms of wear reduction. A comparative table and representative photos of currently available mobile bearing prostheses is shown (Table 1).

3 Conclusion

Recent advances in the understanding of kinematics and materials properties have increased the interest in mobile bearing articulations in total knee arthroplasty.

The gold standard of these implants is the Low Contact Stress mobile bearing design. Factors that may have a significant impact on the performance of newer designs, include choice of single versus multiple radius of curvature femoral component, presence of articulating stops and pegs, surgical technique, the patellofemoral articulation, implant stability, and the ability of the design to optimize contact stress and functional kinematics.

References

1. Blunn GW, Joshi AB, Minns RJ, Lidgren L, Lilley P, Ryd L, Engelbrecht E, Walker PS (1997) Wear in retrieved condylar knee arthroplasties: A comparison of wearin different designs of 280 retrieved condylar knee protheses. J Arthroplasty 12: 281–290
2. Dennis DA, Komistek RD, Hoff WA, Gabriel SM (1996) In-vivo knee kinematics derived using an inverse perspective technique. Clin Orthop 331: 107
3. Dennis DA, Komistek RD, Stiehl JB, Walker SA, Dennis KN (1998) Range of motion after total knee arthroplasty. J Arthroplasty 13: 748–752
4. Haas B, Stiehl JB, Komistek RD (2002) Kinematic comparison of posterior cruciate sacrifice versus substitution in a mobile bearing total knee arthroplasty. J Arthroplasty
5. Pinskerova V, Iwaki H, Freeman MAR (1999) The movements of the knee: A cadaveric magnetic resonance imaging and dissection study. Transactions of the Annual Meeting, American Academy of Orthopaedic Surgeons, Feb 5–8, 1999, Anaheim, CA, pp 82
6. Puloski SKT, McCalden RW, MacDonald SJ, Bourne RB. Rorabeck CH (2000) Tibial post wear in posterior stabilized TKA: A source of polyethylene debris. Proceedings 67th Annual Meeting, American Academy of Orthopaedic Surgeons, March 15–19, 2000, Orlando, FL, pp 573
7. Stiehl JB (2001) Knee kinematics and mobile bearings: new design considerations. Curr Opin Orthop 12(1): 18–25
8. Stiehl JB, Komistek R, Paxson RD, Hoff WA (1995) Fluoroscopic analysis of kinematics after posterior cruciate-retaining knee arthroplasty. J Bone Joint Surg 77B: 884–889
9. Stiehl JB, Dennis DA, Komistek RD, Keblish PA (1997) Kinematic analysis of a mobile bearing total knee arthroplasty. Clin Orthop 345: 60–65
10. Stiehl JB, Dennis DA, Komistek RD (1999a) Detrimental kinematics of a «flat on flat» total condylar knee arthroplasty. Clin Orthop 365: 139–148
11. Stiehl, J.B., Dennis, D.A., Komistek, R.D., Crane, H.S.: Invivo Determination of Condlyar Liftoff and Screw Home In a Mobile Bearing Total Knee Arthroplasty. Jl Arthroplasty 14: 293–299, 1999b.
12. Stiehl, J.B., Dennis, D.A., Komistek, R.D.: The Cruciate Ligaments in Total Knee Arthropalsty: A Kinematic Analysis. Jl Arthroplasty 15: 545–550,2000a
13. Stiehl JB, Dennis DA, Komistek RD, Keblish PA: Invivo Kinematic Comparison of a Posterior-Cruciate-Retaining and Sacrificing Mobile Bearing Total Knee Arthroplasty. American Journal of Knee Surgery, 13: 13–18, 2000b
14. Stiehl, J.B., Dennis, D.A., Komistek, R.D., Keblish, P. A. Kinematics of the Patellofemoral Joint in Total Knee Arthroplasty. Jl. Arthroplasty 16: 706–714, 2001a
15. Stiehl, J.B., Komistek, RD, Haas, B., Dennis, DA: Frontal Plane Kinematics in Mobile Bearing Total Knee Arthroplasty. CORR 392: 56–61 2001b

Chapter 15
Mobile Bearing Knee Prosthesis – Description and Classification

J.-L. Briard

1 Introduction

Mobile bearing knees were designed to address the issue of polyethylene wear, considered to be a significant potential problem, particularly where knee arthroplasty is performed in patients under 75 years of age.

The mobile bearing concept was first deployed in knees by the Oxford group. They described the principle of creating congruent contact at the femorotibial interface, whilst allowing the polyethylene tibial bearing to move relative to the tibial tray. Allowing this movement reduced the potential for stress transmission at the prosthesis/bone interfaces, thus maintaining the security of implant fixation whilst allowing normal knee motion.

The Oxford Uni-compartmental knee was first described in 1976 and has been used continuously since then. It allows the tibial "meniscal" bearing to move freely on the top of a highly polished tibial tray and therefore relies heavily upon competent collateral and cruciate ligaments to infer stability and prevent bearing dislocation.

In the mid to late 1970s, Buechel and Pappas sought to address the potential for polyethylene wear by designing knee prosthesis with highly congruent bearing surfaces. It was clear that only the mobile bearing concept allowed the potential for maximal bearing contact areas without inhibiting knee motion and threatening fixation integrity. They therefore utilized meniscal bearings like the Oxford group, adapting the concept to increase stability and usability by guiding the bearings in axially orientated dovetail grooves in the tibial tray. Shortly thereafter, they also mated a tri-compartmental femoral component with a single congruent tibial bearing which rotated around a central axis.

Buechel and Pappas developed a complete knee system which offered a uni-compartmental prosthesis as well as tri-compartmental bi-cruciate and posterior cruciate retaining and cruciate sacrificing prosthesis. This system known as the New Jersey Knee was subsequently commercialized by DePuy as the LCS Knee System.

The LCS Knee in its various forms was subjected to a rigorous US FDA Investigational Device Evaluation through much of the 1980 s. Following restricted evaluation in 25 centers, it was approved for general clinical use in the USA and it remained the only approved mobile bearing knee in that market until 2000.

Despite the restricted availability of mobile bearing knees in the USA, many other design groups adopted and adapted the concept throughout the 1980 s and 90 s. Continued recognition of the potential for wear, osteolysis and loosening and the pursuit of even better knee motion accelerated an adoption of the mobile bearing concept, encouraged by the favorable clinical results reported with the LCS Knee System.

The concept was further endorsed by Dr. John Insall, one of the great pioneers of knee arthroplasty. In lectures from 1997 onwards, he proposed that mobile bearings might provide a solution to the remaining challenges of knee replacement, particularly polyethylene wear and the restoration of a full range of motion.

There are now a growing number of mobile bearing knee prosthesis, either in evaluation or on the market. It is therefore perhaps useful to examine the major differences that exist between the various designs to allow for comparison and classification in order to aid selection.

There are a variety of ways in which one could attempt to do this, but it seems appropriate to remember the adage of what represents a successful knee replacement. It should be pain free, stable, mobile and durable. The objective of pain relief is of course common to all forms of arthroplasty and will not be addressed specific to mobile bearing knee design. The remainder of this chapter will therefore address some of the design variables of mobile bearing knees according to their means of conferring durability, mobility and stability. Classification is not straightforward as there are many independent and inter-related design variables, however some of the descriptions provided below may allow for evaluation and comparison of the key features of the various prosthesis on offer.

2   Durability

The primary motivation behind the development of
mobile bearing knees was a desire to improve the durability of polyethylene articular surfaces. It is now uni-
versally accepted that increased congruency between
the femoral component and the surfaces of the tibial and patellar bearings is likely to reduce the potential for various forms of polyethylene wear and damage.
The proponents of mobile bearing knee design have always pointed out that most fixed bearing knee prosthesis (certainly up until the mid 1990s) were designed so
as to permit contact stresses in excess of those recommended by the manufacturers of the polyethylene used
in orthopedic implants.

There has however been a divergence of opinion
among designers of mobile bearing knees as to how
large contact areas need to be and whether femorotibial area contact should be maintained throughout the
range of motion.

This divergence has existed since the beginning of
the mobile bearing knee era. The LCS prosthesis provides maximal femorotibial contact near extension
with reduced congruency in flexion, whereas the Oxford prosthesis exhibits constant congruency throughout the range of motion. This significant difference in
femorotibial loading provides one avenue for comparison and classification.

Two distinct design concepts can be described thus:

- multi-radius (polycentric) sagittal femoral geometry
  (Fig. 1):
  – extensive area contact near extension,
  – circular line contact in flexion;

- constant radius sagittal femorotibial geometry
  (Fig. 2):
  – area contact in extension,
  – area contact in flexion.

The LCS Knee tri-compartmental femoral component
was designed so as to provide a constant sagittal radius
of curvature against which the patella (or patellar prosthesis) could articulate from 5 to 105 degrees of flexion.
This allows for fully congruent prosthetic patellofemoral geometry and allows the unresurfaced patella to articulate against a constant sagittal radius. This may facilitate adaptive remodeling of the bony patella, reducing
stress and the potential for micro-trabecular fractures.

However, this fairly large radius of curvature also
mates with the tibial bearing through approximately the
first 30 degrees of flexion. The LCS knee was designed to
provide sagittal femorotibial congruency from the most
anterior to the most posterior aspects of a tibial bearing
in extension and in early flexion. It is proposed that this
is desirable as a significant majority of load bearing activity occurs within the first 30 degrees of flexion (for instance loaded phase of gait). Erosion of femoral articular cartilage is often most marked distally and this perhaps supports the idea that wear and damage occur as a
result of cyclic loading near extension. This may justify
the concept of maximizing prosthetic congruency (and
therefore minimizing stresses) near extension.

However, the radius of curvature of the LCS femoral
component has to reduce posteriorly in order to permit
flexion. This reducing radius does not match that of the
tibial polyethylene in the sagittal plane, resulting in reduced congruency and increased contact stress in flexion. Although the knee may be loaded in flexion much

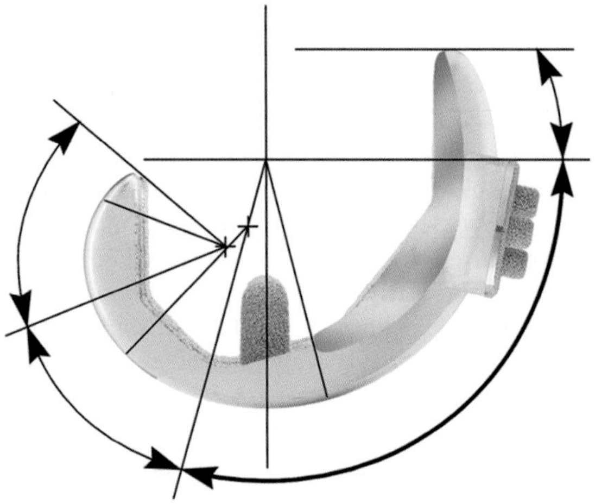

Fig. 1. LCS (DePuy), Interax ISA (Howmedica), Genesis II/
Profix (Smith & Nephew), PFC Sigma (DePuy), Innex/Natural
(Sulzer)

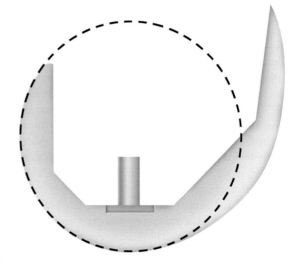

Fig. 2. Rotaglide (Corin), SAL (Sulzer), TRAC (Biomet), MBK
(Zimmer), Oxford TMK (Biomet)

less frequently than near extension, the loads encountered in flexion activities (for instance stair climbing) are notably high.

There are therefore a number of mobile bearing knee prosthesis that seek to address this by maintaining a "constant" sagittal condylar radius which interacts with the tibial bearing through much or all of the normal range of motion.

This design feature does maximize the contact area (and reduce compressive stresses) when the knee is loaded in flexion, but in order to permit the desired range of motion, the sagittal radius of curvature which loads in extension tends to be somewhat smaller than in polycentric designs such as the LCS (i.e. a radius of approximately 25 mm in the MBK design compared with 50 mm in the LCS). In extension, the polycentric designs appear to provide contact from the most anterior to the most posterior aspect of the tibial bearing. By contrast, the "constant radius" designs tend to offer less sagittal contact (and less contact area in extension), loading somewhat more posteriorly.

However, proponents of the "constant radius" designs suggest that the contact area they provide in extension is sufficient to offer contact stress levels consistent with limiting polyethylene wear and damage.

Opponents of the "constant radius" philosophy suggest that while the above is true if the knee is loaded normally through both condyles, the potential for femoral lift off in gait may result in single condyle loading and thus expose the polyethylene in the prosthesis to excessive stress.

The vast majority of knee replacements used over the last 20 years have utilized a polycentric femoral component and it is reasonable to say that this design variant is well proven, not least in the LCS mobile bearing prosthesis. However, the "constant radius" concept has produced encouraging wear results with the Oxford Uni-compartmental design and may prove valuable in well-designed tri-compartmental prosthesis.

Another design variation in sagittal femorotibial geometry is the use of a compressively loaded intercondylar spine. Where this concept is employed (i.e. in the T.R.A.C. Knee, Biomet) significant compressive load is accommodated through cylindrical contact between an intercondylar cam and spine mechanism.

Differences in the coronal femorotibial geometry of mobile bearing knees also provide a point of comparison. The majority of designs offer "curve-on-curve" coronal femorotibial conformity, usually with a radius of curvature that matches the sagittal radius, thus producing spherical contact. Some designs (e.g. T.R.A.C. and Natural) offer more "flat-on-flat" coronal contact. There are now several posterior stabilized mobile bearing knee prosthesis which offer intercondylar spine and cam mechanisms to control anterior-posterior motion. Where a prominent tibial spine exists, a coronally congruent knee should perhaps account for the potential for varus/valgus movement (condylar lift off). This may be achieved by increasing the gap between the inner edge of the condyle and the tibial spine or by reducing the coronal femorotibial radius of curvature.

Mobile bearing knee prosthesis are generally designed to provide femorotibial compressive contact stress levels of less than 10 mPA. At normally accepted levels of loading, this requires a total contact area of around 300mm². Increasing contact area from 100 to 300 mm² produces a significant diminution in contact stress, however extending congruency beyond that magnitude provides a diminishing reduction.

Designs offering 600 mm² or more in contact area over both condyles provide a minimum 300 mm² through which to dissipate stress under single condyle loading (varus/valgus "lift off") conditions. Greater contact areas are considered likely to reduce abrasive wear, but no direct functional relationship has been calculated.

Greenwald et al. have carried out extensive evaluation of the femorotibial contact areas provided by various mobile bearing knee designs. Such evaluation initially relied upon the use of a thin film technology, capable of measuring loads at the femorotibial interface (Fuji film). Subsequent evaluations have used Finite Element Analysis (F.E.A.) methods to predict the contact area and contact stress of various designs. Measuring the magnitude and distribution of compressive load and contact stress is helpful in identifying the potential for fatigue and abrasive wear.

Greenwald et al have also used three-dimensional (3D) F.E.A. techniques to predict the location and magnitude of other forms of stress. Computer models created using F.E.A. techniques provide guidance as to the potential for pitting and delamination of the polyethylene bearing (relative to the magnitude of maximum principal stresses and Von Mises stresses, respectively).

Most of the mobile bearing knee designs evaluated in this way exhibit stress levels considered compatible with extended longevity and superior to those achieved in fixed bearing design. However, publications by Greenwald et al. do allow for objective comparison of the some of the features that might affect long-term clinical outcome.

Femorotibial congruency as a means of dissipating compressive load is perhaps the most obvious factor associated with the durability of polyethylene. There are however other interfaces at which polyethylene wear and damage could occur and these should also be considered in comparing mobile bearing knee designs.

In addition to the spine and cam in posterior stabilized designs, one should consider the effects of shear and torsional stresses on the upper tibial surface, particularly where bearing movement is inhibited. Several mobile bearing knee designs employ "stops" which inhibit rotation and/or translation and these have the potential to increase stress concentration at the upper tibial surface.

The same is true of the interfaces at the lower surface of the tibial bearing. Part of the US FDA regulatory analysis of the LCS Knee involved simulator tests of the design under extreme "lateral thrust" loading conditions. These evaluated the potential for damage at the junction of the meniscal bearings and dovetail tracks and also at the interface between the polyethylene and metal cones in the rotating platform. In addition to analyzing how interfaces between the tibial tray and polyethylene bearing might perform under "lateral thrust" conditions, one should consider how other metal/polyethylene interfaces would dissipate stress (shear and torsion) under load, particularly where bearing motion is restricted or guided. Most mobile bearing knee designs pay great respect to the principles of congruency and low contact stress at the upper tibial surface and yet many utilize bearing control mechanisms that offer only very limited line contact at best under significant load (Fig. 3).

Another variation in mobile bearing design that may affect polyethylene wear is the way in which the bearing is permitted to move relative to the tibial tray. The initial LCS Knee variants (meniscal bearing and rotating platform) allow only uni-planar (in both instances axial) motion. Although this motion may create linear "wear tracks", the bearing will constantly move across these tracks in the same manner. However, where bi- or multi-planar movement is permitted (anterior/posterior

translation as well as axial rotation), there is a potential for "crossing patterns" of motion. In vivo studies indicate that this may increase the potential for wear at the under-surface of the tibial bearing. Although there is evidence that mobile bearing knees offering multi-planar movement produce less wear than fixed bearing designs, one may wish to consider uni-planar versus multi-planar bearing motion in evaluating the relative potential for polyethylene wear in mobile bearing knees.

- Designs offering uni-planar motion:
    - LCS meniscalbearing/rotating platform,
    - Natural Knee (mobile bearing),
    - Genesis II/Profix (rotating only),
    - T.R.A.C., Interax ISA,
    - PFC Sigma RP.
- Designs offering multi-planar motion:
    - SAL, Rotaglide, LCS AP Glide,
    - MBK/LPS Flex, Oxford (Uni and TMK)
    - Genesis II/Profix (rotating/translating)

One might also wish to consider the choice of materials used at articulating surfaces and the quality of manufacturing processes used to create them. Where well designed mobile bearing knees address all of the other threats to polyethylene durability, they might benefit from employing improved polyethylene materials (highly cross linked or compression moulded). Abrasive wear might also be reduced by using ceramic surfaces or coatings on femoral and tibial components. Finally, optimized manufacturing processes (e.g. tight dimensional tolerance and optimal surface finish) might yield differences in the potential for wear.

3   Stability

Stability can be provided by the soft tissue structures around the knee (extrinsic to the prosthesis), by design elements of the prosthesis (intrinsic constraint) or by a combination thereof ("load sharing"). There are theoretical advantages to retaining and utilizing natural structures (i.e. ligaments) where they exist and continue to function. In sharing load with design elements of the prosthesis, they may dissipate stress so as to reduce the potential for wear and loosening. Retained ligaments may remodel under load (Roux's Law) and become more competent.

Some of the contemporary mobile bearing knee systems provide variants to address either different disease states or variations in surgical philosophy. The LCS System offers variants which rely upon complete ligamentous competence (Uni-compartmental and bi-cruci-

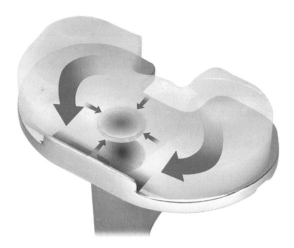

Fig. 3. Diagram – pin in slot stress problem

ate retaining tri-compartmental). It also offers variants intended for use with a competent PCL (PCR meniscal bearing and AP Glide). Where the PCL is absent (either as a result of disease or surgical choice/resection) a more stable Rotating Platform variant can be used and if required, a posterior Stabilized or even varus-valgus constrained prosthesis can be selected.

There are variations in the way in which mobile bearing knee prosthesis provide the required forms of stability:

- medial-lateral,
- varus-valgus,
- anterior-posterior,
- axial.

Almost all designs employ some form of intercondylar eminence to control medial-lateral motion. This tends to work in concert with coronal "curve-on-curve" congruency and balanced collateral ligaments to confer stability. Medial-lateral instability is not often specifically reported as a problem in total knee arthroplasty.

A few contemporary mobile bearing knee systems offer a varus-valgus constrained variant for use in instances of collateral ligament incompetence. Those that do (LCS VVC and Biomet Dual Articular) use a conventional intercondylar spine and cam mechanism with enhanced "jump height" combined with close contact between a polyethylene tibial spine and a femoral "box".

A number of mobile bearing knee prosthesis allow extensive anterior-posterior movement of the femur relative to the tibia. This is usually provided at the "secondary" interface between the polyethylene bearing and tibial tray. However, some designs used in the presence of an intact PCL use a bearing that rotates, but does not translate. Prosthesis of this type (e.g. PFC Sigma RP) rely upon reduced femorotibial congruency in flexion to permit anterior-posterior motion and therefore roll-back. Mobile bearing knee prosthesis that initially rely on an intact PCL for stability may of course become unstable as a result of progressive ligamentous incompetence or rupture.

It may therefore be valuable for a clinician to consider how a given prosthesis will function if the PCL deteriorates. Will the prosthesis confer sufficient stability? Will it predispose dislocation? How easily might a revision be performed?

There is an increasing trend (in both fixed and mobile bearing arthroplasty) towards posterior cruciate sacrifice. Where the PCL is sacrificed, the prosthesis often provides a constraint mechanism to confer appropriate anterior-posterior stability.

Such stability can be provided by a combination of well balanced collateral ligaments and a sagittally concave polyethylene insert. This configuration has been well proven in the LCS Rotating Platform knee and is available in various other designs. Additional prosthetic stability can be provided by increasing the engagement depth of the tibial bearing (vertical distance between the most inferior and superior elements of the bearing). This may be particularly useful in maintaining stability and resisting femur/bearing dislocation in cases of revision or significant pre-operative deformity. The LCS prosthesis originally offered a "deep dish" rotating bearing for such indications, but the most significant characteristics of the design (i.e. increased anterior "jump height") are now offered in standard LCS Complete inserts. The effective "jump" height over which the femur would have to lift to produce a dislocation is also affected by the inclination of the posterior resection of the tibia. The "jump" or engagement height of the tibial bearing and its control elements in combination with tibial posterior slope provides a significant point of comparison between competing designs.

There are now a number of posterior stabilized designs available for where even greater prosthetic anterior-posterior stability is required or desired. In addition to controlling the anterior-posterior excursion of the femur on the tibia, posterior stabilized designs are likely to further reduce the potential for mobile bearing dislocation or "spin out." These posterior stabilized designs tend to use a polyethylene tibial spine articulating with a femoral cam mechanism, as found in well proven fixed bearing prosthesis.

All mobile bearing knees provide axial rotation at the interface between the polyethylene bearing and tibial tray. However, some limit the extent of bearing rotation. The limit to rotation may be imposed to prevent excessive bearing "over-hang" (where the bearing protrudes beyond the tibial tray, potentially impinging soft tissues) or to prevent a form of dislocation sometimes referred to as "spin out" (this is where the rotating bearing disengages from the femoral component, potentially rotating as much as 90 degrees relative to the femur and tibial tray).

Such dislocation can occur in an imperfectly balanced knee where a femoral condyle is able to move superiorly over the anterior or posterior lip of the tibial bearing. This only happens where the extent of ligamentous laxity exceeds the effective "jump height" (engagement depth) of the femorotibial articulation.

Another potential complication, specific to mobile bearing knees may occur where excessive ligamentous laxity or inappropriate loading allows the tibial bearing to disengage superiorly from its control mechanism. This was addressed in the LCS Knee with a deep engaging cone or captured meniscal bearings. There are other designs which capture the tibial bearing to prevent lift off or disassociation. Those with a shallow, non-captured bearing control mechanism may be vulnerable to this phenomenon.

There is variation in the constraint levels provided by various prosthesis. Those that are least constrained and which rely most on natural structures to confer stability, are perhaps most sensitive to compromised surgical technique or progressive ligamentous incompetence. However, those that rely on prosthetic constraint may fail to take advantage of the ability of natural structures to "load share" and dissipate the stresses that can lead to wear and loosening.

4   Mobility

Knee prosthesis are designed to permit a useful range of motion from full extension, usually to at least 120 degrees of flexion. A growing number of specialized designs seek to accommodate a greater range of flexion (up to 155 degrees), as this is considered desirable in some populations and cultures.

Most designs accommodate the varus/valgus movement (condylar lift off) that has been observed occurring in the post-arthroplasty knee in a number of fluoroscopic studies.

The variables of movement that provide most potential for comparison and classification of mobile bearing knee designs are anterior-posterior translation and axial rotation of the femur relative to the tibia.

In some designs, anterior-posterior movement occurs only between the femoral component and polyethylene bearing. It is able to occur only in flexion, permitted by the reducing sagittal congruency of a polycentric femoral component. The LCS Rotating Platform design allows limited anterior-posterior motion in this way, but fluoroscopic evaluation has indicated that translation tends not to occur, with the femoral component remaining in the center of the tibial bearing throughout the range of motion. Other designs that do not allow anterior-posterior movement of the tibial bearing do seek to allow or even induce "roll-back" of the femur on the tibia. This occurs either as a result of retaining the PCL or using a posterior-stabilizing spine and cam mechanism that drives the femur posteriorly at a given angle of flexion (e.g. PFC Sigma P/S RP design). However, the extent of roll-back may be inhibited by the fact that the femur has to "climb" up the posterior lip of a sagittally concave bearing against soft tissue constraint.

Many mobile bearing knee prosthesis provide femoral roll-back in flexion by allowing anterior-posterior translation between the polyethylene bearing and the tibial tray. This design feature tends to be used in PCL retaining prosthesis.

PCL sacrificing knees like the LCS rotating platform have been documented as providing excellent clinical function and survivorship with an absence of induced roll-back. It is however proposed that inducing the femur to roll-back relative to the tibia may reduce the potential for impingement of posterior femoral structures on the posterior lip of the tibial bearing. Another potential advantage is that roll-back increases the lever arm and efficiency of the quadriceps mechanism, whilst reducing compressive load on the patella. These potential benefits might persuade surgeons to consider designs which use a retained PCL or P/S mechanism to induce roll-back. The classifications of PCL retaining, PCL sacrificing and PCL substituting are shared with fixed bearing knees and many of the same surgical and design principles apply.

The following table describes how bearing movement is permitted and/or controlled in various prosthesis designs (Table 1).

Although many of the designs described above seek to allow for the translation and rotation found in the normal knee, it has been observed in various fluoroscopic studies that sacrifice of the ACL predisposes abnormal ("paradoxical") motion.

In the normal knee with intact cruciate ligaments, the medial condyle translates minimally, with greater translation occurring at the lateral condyle. The greater posterior translation with flexion of the lateral condyle creates a medialized axis of rotation at the knee.

Potential for this pattern of motion is provided by many of the PCL retaining designs described above. There has been criticism of the fact that the PCL sacrificing rotating platform designs do not accommodate "normal" knee motion – that a central axis of rotation generates abnormal movement with one condyle having to move anterior if the other moves posterior.

However, the clinical function and survivorship of the LCS Rotating Platform prosthesis suggest that this is not a problem, perhaps because sacrifice of the PCL and other changes to the structures and kinematics of the knee greatly change its patterns of motion following arthroplasty. Also, the sagittal incongruency of the LCS polycentric femoral component in flexion does allow for offset rotation as each condyle can translate differentially to some extent, independent of bearing rotation.

Table 1. Bearing movement in various prosthesis designs

Bearing Movement	Brand/Design	Bearing Control Mechanism
Free anterior-posterior translation with rotation	LCS Meniscal Bearing	Axially curved dove-tail grooves
Anterior-posterior translation with rotation. Uninhibited rotation, but bearing control mechanism limits translation	SAL, Oxford TMK, Genesis II/Profix (PCL retaining)	Cylindrical metal element projecting superiorly from tibial tray, engaging elongated space in poly bearing
Anterior-posterior translation with rotation. Bearing control mechanism limits both translation and rotation	Rotaglide, MBK	2 metal elements projecting superiorly from tibial tray, engaging spaces in poly bearing
Translation linked to medial axis rotation – guided bearing motion	Interax/Duracon/Kinemax ISA	2 metal elements projecting superiorly from tibial tray, engaging curved slot in poly bearing
Rotation only (uninhibited)	LCS, PFC Sigma RP, T.R.A.C., Natural,	Poly cone or cylinder projecting inferiorly from bearing into tibial stem
	Innex PC Sacrificing Genesis II/Profix (PCL sacrificing)	Metal element projecting superiorly from tibial tray, engaging round space in poly bearing

5   Summary

The inherent benefits and potential of mobile bearing knees have attracted growing interest, particularly over the last 10 years. This has undoubtedly been encouraged by the well-documented clinical and commercial success of the LCS Knee System. Each of the major orthopedic companies now offers at least one mobile bearing brand in markets outside the USA. A number of smaller companies have also developed mobile designs.

A growing body of research data allows comparison between the design variables of these devices. As noted above, this allows comparison of the features postulated to confer durability and the stability and mobility required in various surgical situations.

Laboratory data and computer simulations can be considered alongside the observations resulting from dynamic fluoroscopic analysis and clinical follow up.

It is unlikely that all mobile bearing designs will provide acceptable clinical function and survivorship, but if they do, some will prove better than others. It is reasonable to suggest that after 25 years of evaluation, the design of the LCS Knee provides an excellent benchmark against which to compare other devices. It can be considered as a "Gold Standard" in mobile bearing total knee replacement.

However, the clinical success of even the best-designed prosthesis will continue to depend heavily on the surgical skills of those responsible for selecting and implanting them.

Future Trends with the LCS

V

Chapter 16
Introduction

J.B. STIEHL

Over the past thirty years dramatic strides have been made in the field of orthopedic surgery and total knee arthroplasty has become one of the most common and successful interventions in medicine. Worldwide, 608,000 total knees will be performed in 2002, The evolution of this operation has included development of reproducible surgical technique, durable prosthetic devices that will function over long periods of time, and a thorough understanding of the intricacies of the method such as dealing with complex diseased knees, complications, and late prosthetic failure.

Where will we go in the future? This section will explore areas of knee reconstruction that represent evolutionary changes over the next few years. Prosthetic improvements will be slight if not imperceptible. We will discuss the new LCS Complete and Revision systems. These new devices are only subtle and often cosmetic improvements on the accepted and proven LCS design. There are not departures from the original implant geometry or concepts.

What we do find intriguing and futuristic are new biomaterials in total knee arthroplasty and innovative new surgical techniques. Polyethylene improvements are eminent with newer concepts of cross linking and annealing. Metal surface improvements will result both from manufacturing innovations as well as newer ceramic surface treatments, known to enhance the finish for improved wear. For us surgeons, however, the new vista is what we do best and that is surgery and how it can be enhanced. The buzz word of the millennium is minimally invasive surgery, or surgery done through small holes with less morbidity and shorter recovery. I recently had both inguinal hernias repaired endoscopically by a master surgeon on a Monday morning and by Wednesday was on a airplane to New York city to participate as faculty on a total knee course. By the following Monday, I was back in the operating room with a full schedule.

Unicondylar hemiarthroplasty is presently on the rise as it can be done through a small incision and with much less morbidity than the classic total knee arthroplasty. For the elderly and often higher risk patient, this method will provide a quick solution with better immediate function and a very short hospital stay. Whether the unicondylar method will surpass the results of high tibial osteotomy or even total knee arthroplasty in the younger patients is unknown at this time.

Amazingly, the most common cause of revision from a recent study was surgical misadventure. Primarily this would be ligamentous instability, component malalignment, or malpositioning of implants. This means that we as surgeons are producing outcomes that reflect our errors or lack of understanding of how to get it right. Given the complexities of lower extremity limb alignment and the variations thereof, this is not too surprising. Add to that, deformity, prior surgical procedures, and the bone destruction of certain conditions, and it is understandable why we are failing. Most radiographic assessments done today reflect frontal and sagittal plane images and fails to encompass complex rotational issues and the vagaries of ligament balancing.

Will surgical navigation or other methods help us in the future? Most likely they will but is going to take a lot better understanding of our knees before the application of these technologies will be feasible. I predict that a lot of effort will be made to enhance surgical technique with better instrumentation, radiographic assessment, computer generated modeling of the extremity, and ultimately complex algorithms of biomechanical function. These efforts will be expensive and will require research initiatives beyond the usual skills of us practicing surgeons. They are achievable and offer the potential of even better overall surgical outcomes. The following section will discuss many ideas that are being evolved in knee reconstruction surgery.

Chapter 17
The A/P-Glide Knee Prosthesis – Rationales, Kinematics and Results

R.D. Oakeshott, R.D. Komistek, J.B. Stiehl

1 Introduction

The Low Contact Stress (LCS) knee prosthesis, (Depuy, Warsaw, IN) was originally designed with a tibial component that allowed for posterior cruciate retention (meniscal bearing) or sacrifice (rotating platform) [1]. The femoral component was designed with polycentric radii of curvature which approximated the condylar shape of the normal distal femur. Clinical reports have demonstrated comparable midterm clinical results with either posterior cruciate retention or sacrifice using this implant and osteolysis has been a rare event [2, 8, 11, 20]. With longer follow-up beyond ten years, investigators found increasing rates of fracture, wear and dislocation of the original meniscal bearings as compared to the rotating platform tibial insert [3]. The rotating platform was originally developed for more difficult cases and early clinical results with this implant may have been biased from that factor

[1]. However, the implant gained increasing popularity as long term results have been shown to be durable even in younger patients, and the surgical technique is generally simpler with less technical challenge [13].

The LCS anterior posterior (A/P) glide tibial insert was a later modification of the rotating platform which incorporated a control arm mechanism to articulate with the cone shaped insert tibial stem (Fig. 1).

By allowing unconstrained sagittal plane motion, this device could then be inserted with posterior cruciate retention, which continues to be a desirable technique for preservation of function while minimizing anatomical alterations such as joint line elevation. Clinical investigations with this implant have been favorable though few published reports exist at this time. This chapter

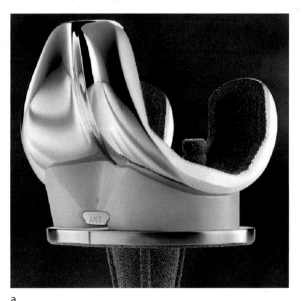

a

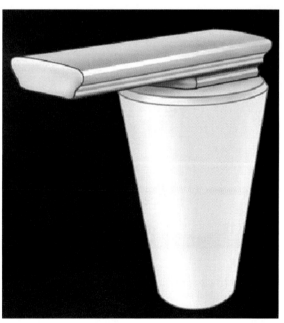

b

Fig. 1a, b. A/P glide prosthesis showing control arm and metal track for the tibial insert. **a** Diagram of A/P glide prosthesis; **b** control arm. The A/P glide components are protected by European patent 0519873 Bl. BA patent 5395401. Japanese patent 2741644 and Swiss patent 689539 which are licensed to DePoy International by Mr André R. Baehler

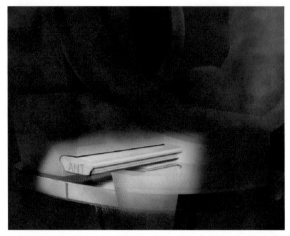

c

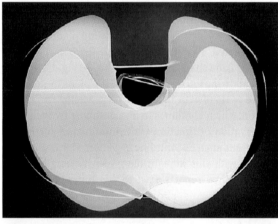

d

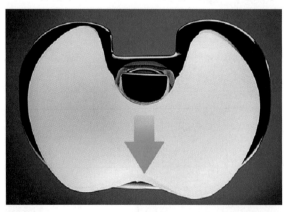

e

Fig. 1c–e. A/P glide prosthesis showing control arm and metal track for the tibial insert. **c** position of control arm within the polyethylene tibial insert; **d** unconstrained anterior/posterior motion; **e** unconstrained rotational motion

will discuss our fluoroscopic kinematic and clinical experience with the A/P glide implant.

2   Fluoroscopic Kinematic Analysis

Knee kinematics were assessed for ten subjects implanted with a Low Contact Stress anterior/posterior glide (LCS A/P Glide) mobile bearing total knee arthroplasty (Depuy International, Leads, England). All total knee arthroplasties were judged clinically successful (Hospital for Special Surgery Rating Scores >90), with no ligamentous laxity or pain. The operative procedures were performed by one surgeon (RJO) who utilized an identical technique previously described for this posterior cruciate retaining system. All surgeries were done using a posterior cruciate retaining technique with initial resection of the proximal tibia followed with ligament and soft tissue balancing in extension.

Each subject was asked to perform two activities:

- weight-bearing deep knee bends to maximum flexion, and
- a non weight-bearing bend to maximum flexion.

During the weight-bearing deep knee bend, each subject placed the foot, of their leg to be studied, on a designated marker. The subjects were initially fluoroscoped at full extension and throughout the flexion cycle (Fig. 2a).

While under non weight-bearing conditions, the leg to be analyzed was passively manipulated to maximum knee flexion (Fig. 2b). Patients were examined using a Siemens Siremobil 2000 Digital X-ray image intensifier system (Iselin, NJ). The fluoroscopic images were stored on videotape for subsequent redigitization using a frame grabber. Weight-bearing and non weight-bearing knee kinematics was analyzed for all ten subjects using the RMMRL model-fitting software package. Using a model fitting approach, the relative pose of knee implant components was determined in three dimensions from a single-perspective fluoroscopic image by manipulating a CAD model in three-dimensional space. Individual fluoroscopic frames at specified degrees of flexion were digitized. The images were projected onto the image plane, and the corresponding implant models added to the scene. The operator manipulated the models to create an accurate fit. The correct fit was achieved when the silhouettes of the femoral and tibial implant components perfectly matched the corresponding components in the fluoroscopic image (Fig. 3).

The pose of each component was then recorded and each measurement of interest was extracted using a CAD-modeling program. The process was performed at

Fig. 2a, b. Subject performing a weight-bearing deep knee bend (**a**) and a non weight-bearing knee flexion (**b**)

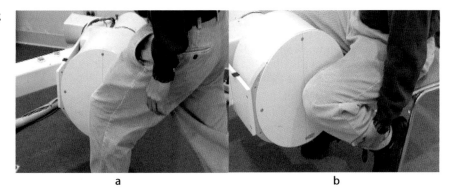

a   b

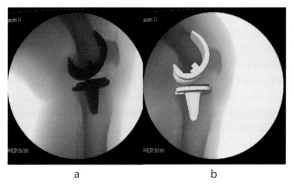

a   b

Fig. 3a, b. Example of a fluoroscopic image (**a**) and a 3D overlay (**b**)

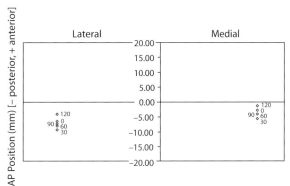

Fig. 4. Average medial and lateral condyle anterior-posterior contact while performing a weight-bearing deep knee bend

the flexion angles of 0°, 30°, 60°, 90° and 120° to determine knee kinematics (A/P contact, axial rotation and condylar lift-off. The distances from the medial and lateral condyles to the tibia plateau were measured and the difference between these two measurements was used to determine condylar lift-off.

An error analysis was conducted using a fresh cadaver. Discrete points were defined on the femoral and tibial components. Using an Optotrack system, these points were digitized and the femur was defined relative to the tibia, in the tibial reference frame. Each orientation of the femur, relative to the tibia was fluoroscoped. Using the 3D model-fitting software package, the relative orientation of the femur with respect to the tibia was predicted and compared to the known orientation determined using the Optotrack system. The relative error, derived for 75 orientations was consistently less than 0.5 degrees in rotation and 0.5 mm in translation [7].

2.1 Anteroposterior Translation

Under weight-bearing conditions, on average, the subjects experienced a posterior contact of the medial (average = –2.7 mm, range = 2.0 mm to –6.7 mm) and lateral (average = –6.3 mm, range = 0.2 mm to –12.3 mm) condyles at full extension (Fig. 4).

From full extension to 30° of knee flexion, on average, both condyles moved in the posterior direction to a medial contact position of –5.5 mm (–1.5 to –10.2) and lateral of –9.3 mm (–5.6 to –12.8). At 60° of knee flexion, both condyles moved in the anterior direction to an average medial position of –4.1 mm (1.8 to –8.3) and lateral position of –7.9 mm (–4.2 to –10.2). At 90° of knee flexion, on average, both condyles experienced minimal motion change with a medial condyle contact position of –4.5 (1.2 to –19.3) and lateral position of –7.2 mm (3.6 to –16.0). At 120° of knee flexion, on average, both condyles experienced an anterior change in contact position to a final medial position of –1.1 mm (2.6 to –3.3) and lateral position of –4.0 mm (–0.3 to –6.8). Nine of 10 subjects were able to achieve at least 120° of knee flexion under weight-bearing conditions. Only four of the subjects experienced a posterior motion of their medial condyles from full extension to 120° of knee flexion, while all subjects experienced an anterior motion of their lateral condyles.

Under non weight-bearing conditions, on average, subjects experienced a posterior contact of the medial (average = –1.8 mm, range = 1.7 mm to –4.1 mm) and lateral (average = –3.2 mm, range = 0.7 mm to –7.3 mm) condyles at full extension (Fig. 5).

From full extension to 30° of knee flexion, on average, the medial contact position moved in the anterior direction to –1.2 mm (3.5 to –4.1), while the lateral condyle contact position moved in the posterior direction to –3.4 mm (2.3 to –9.8). At 60° of knee flexion, both condyles moved in the anterior direction. Both condyles experienced an anterior contact position, where the average medial contact position was 3.4 mm (14.9 to –3.2) and lateral contact position was 0.2 mm (6.9 to –5.1). At 90° of knee flexion, on average, both condyles again experienced an anterior contact position. On average, the medial condyle contact position was 3.5 mm (15.7 to –

4.3) and lateral position was 0.5 mm (6.9 to –4.7). At 120° of knee flexion, on average, both condyles experienced a posterior change in contact position to a final medial position of –0.3 mm (12.6 to –11.2) and lateral position of –3.0 mm (4.4 to – 8.2). All of the subjects were able to achieve at least 120° of knee flexion under non weight-bearing conditions. Five of the subjects experienced a posterior motion of their medial condyles from full extension to 120° of knee flexion and six of the 10 subjects experienced posterior femoral rollback of their lateral condyles.

From full extension to 90° of knee flexion, the average A/P contact position for the subjects in this study were significantly more anterior under non weight-bearing conditions compared to weight-bearing conditions (Fig. 6, 7).

At 120° of knee flexion the average contact positions during weight-bearing and non weight-bearing conditions were similar. Using a Student-T test the A/P position data was statistically different for the lateral condyle at full extension (p=0.02), the medial (p=0.009) and lateral (p=0.003) at 30° of knee flexion, the medial (p=0.0002) and lateral (p=0.0001) at 60° of knee flexion, the medial (p=0.001) and lateral (p=0.001) condyles at 90° of knee flexion. There was no statistical difference in the position data at 120° of knee flexion. The average variance for the weight-bearing data was 14.07 compared to an average variance of 19.58 for the non weight-bearing data.

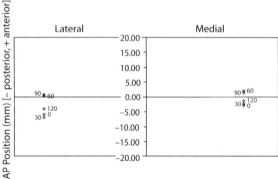

Fig. 5. Average medial and lateral condyle anterior-posterior contact while performing a non weight-bearing knee flexion

Fig. 6a–c. Example of a subject under weight-bearing conditions displaying a posterior contact position. Shown is the fluoroscopic image (**a**), the 3D overlay (**b**), sagittal view (**c**)

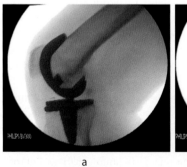 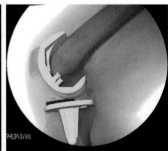 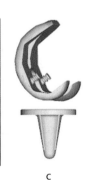

a   b   c

Fig. 7a–c. Example of a subject under non weight-bearing conditions displaying an anterior contact position. Shown is the fluoroscopic image (**a**), the 3D overlay (**b**), sagittal view (**c**)

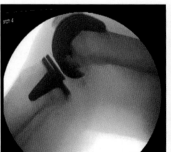 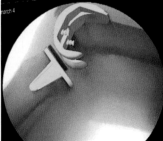 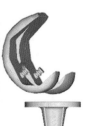

a   b   c

2.2 Axial Tibial-Femoral Rotation

On average, the subjects experienced normal axial rotation during non weight-bearing knee flexion, but opposite axial rotation during a weight-bearing deep knee bend. During non weight-bearing knee flexion, the average axial rotation from full extension to 120° of knee flexion was 1.8° (–9.1 to 10.8) (Fig. 8).

Under weight-bearing conditions, the average axial rotation was –2.0° (-11.9 to 1.6; Fig. 9). Under non weight-bearing conditions, seven of 10 subjects experienced a normal axial rotation pattern from full extension to 120° of knee flexion, while under weight-bearing conditions, only four of nine subjects (one subject did not achieve 120° of knee flexion) experienced a normal axial rotation pattern. Under non weight-bearing conditions, on average, subjects experienced a normal axial rotation pattern from full extension to 30° of knee flexion (1.1°), from 30 to 60° of knee flexion (1.4°) and from 90 to 120° of knee flexion (1.0°). From 60 to 90° of knee flexion, on average, these subjects experienced –0.4° of opposite axial rotation while performing non weight-bearing knee flexion. Under weight-bearing conditions, on average, subjects experienced a normal axial rotation pattern from full extension to 30° of knee flexion (0.3°). From 30 to 60° of knee flexion, on average, subjects experienced no axial rotation. From 60 to 90° of knee flex-

ion subjects experienced an average opposite axial rotation pattern of –1.4° and from 60 to 90° of knee flexion, on average opposite axial rotation pattern of –2.6°.

Using a Student-T test, the axial rotation was statistically different for weight-bearing vs. non weight-bearing conditions at full extension (p=0.03), but was not statistically different at the other flexion angles (p=0.31 at 30°, p=0.58 at 60°, p=0.74 at 90°, and p=0.69 at 120°).

2.3 Condylar Lift-off

Nine of 10 subjects experienced condylar lift-off during weight-bearing and non weight-bearing conditions. Under non weight-bearing conditions, the maximum amount of condylar lift-off was 2.5 mm, which was lateral condyle lift-off occurring at 60° of knee flexion. Under weight-bearing conditions, the maximum amount of condylar lift-off was 3.3 mm, which again was lateral condyle lift-off, occurring at 30° of knee flexion. Under non weight-bearing conditions four subjects experienced greater than 1.0 mm of condylar lift-off just after full extension, 3/10 at 30° of knee flexion, 3/10 at 60° of knee flexion, 2/10 at 90° of knee flexion and 5/10 at 120° of knee flexion. Under weight-bearing conditions only one subject experienced greater than 1.0 mm of condylar lift-off just after full extension, 4/10 at 30° of knee flexion, no subjects at 60° of knee flexion, only 1/10 at 90° of knee flexion and only 1/10 at 120° of knee flexion. Therefore, although one subject experienced more than 3.0 mm of condylar lift-off during weight-bearing conditions, the incidence and magnitude of condylar lift-off was greater during non weight-bearing conditions.

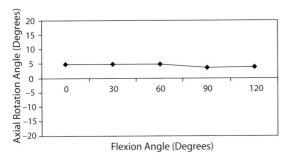

Fig. 8. Average axial rotation for the subjects during the non weight-bearing flexion activity

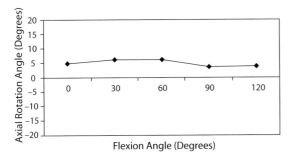

Fig. 9. Average axial rotation for the subjects during the weight-bearing flexion activity

2.4 Range-of-Motion

The average non weight-bearing range-of-motion was 129.3° (120–138). The average weight-bearing range-of-motion was 118.8° (84–135). If the one subject who only achieved 84° of weight-bearing range-of-motion was removed, the average weight-bearing range-of-motion increased to 122.7°.

3 Clinical Experience

Since August 1997, 426 hydroxapatite (HA) impregnated A/P glide tibial components were implanted by the one surgeon (RDO). The tibial implant was substantially different from the previous LCS tibial component involving a change to the area of porocoating and adding hydroxapatite. The first change was occasioned by attempting to

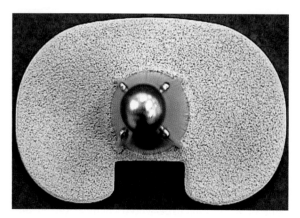

Fig. 10. Modifications of LCS tibial base plate cone with removal of porocoat from the and the addition of hydroxyappatite to the base plate

increase the ease of revisability and involved reducing the metaphyseal cone to a smooth surface except for the proximal 2 mm (allowing for a seal with the bone to prevent a 'sump pump' effect of polyethylene wear particles). The second change involved the addition of the HA to improve the bone/implant interface bonding (Fig. 10).

This is of necessity a very preliminary report of the first 368 components with a follow up minimum of 6 months and maximum of 4 years. The average age was 65.8 (30–96 years) with 167 females and 201 males. Osteoarthritis was the primary diagnosis in 89%, rheumatoid arthritis in 3%, post-traumatic in 1%, and other in 7%.

The pre-operative hospital for special surgery knee score (47.6) and American Knee Society clinical rating score (including the total knee score [24] and total function score [45.3]) are also comparable to most published series. The ultimate post-operative scores are very reflective of co-morbidities amongst the patient population (HSS – 92.1 AKSR TK score 94.6 TFS 91.7). The outstanding feature however is the range of motion, which improved from a mean of 103.1° to 124.6°.

The majority of knees (91%) as expected were varus in alignment and required release of the medial capsule from the tibia with very occasional release of the posteromedial capsule. Additional bone resection of the femur for flexion contraction was required in 36% of knees due to the severity of the deformity. Lateral retinacular division occurred in less than 1% of cases (2 knees) and there were no patella replacements. The fat pad was significantly resected in all knees and patella osteophyte resection was mandatory with particular attention being given to the inferior pole to prevent impingement problems. The latter has been resolved with a change to the anterior prominence of the tibial polyethylene insert and the requirement for significant resection of the fat pad has also been almost eliminated. In-

terestingly the anterior cruciate ligament was absent in 8.2% of knees but there were no cases where the posterior cruciate was not present as this is an absolute contradictation to the procedure. No components were cemented (excluded from the series) and minor bone grafting occurred in 7% of cases.

There have been 4 *limited* revisions in the series; none of these have involved the removal of the metal components but only changes in the tibial polyethylene. 2 occurred within the same patient who had had bilateral simultaneous TKR's and who complained of a painful posterolateral click in the knee with active extension (not reproducible under general anesthesia). Arthroscopic evaluation and popliteus release failed to give relief and conversion to a rotating platform bilaterally totally eliminated the problem. A third patient required revision following a fall down stairs, on to a flexed knee, which resulted in a rupture of the posterior cruciate ligament. Subsequently she developed chronic synovitis and anterior knee pain when negotiating stairs and with other bent knee activities. Complete resolution of symptoms occurred with exchange of the polyethylene to a rotating platform variety. The fourth revision occurred with a patient who complained of anterior knee pain also, but in whom clinical evaluation and later operative inspection revealed an intact posterior cruciate ligament. Pre-operatively she had complained of significant anterior knee pain also and a bone scan (Tc 99) subsequently revealed increased activity levels in the patella. Some reduction in her pain occurred with change of the implant to a rotating platform in combination with a patella replacement.

In the first 30 patients there was a significant incidence (60%) of synovitis and recurrent effusion, which resolved after the first year without intervention in all but 2 patients. These patients both had arthroscopic fat pad resections, when it was realized that anterior impingement was the cause of their symptoms. Following these cases routine resection of the fat pad was undertaken as part of the primary procedure eliminating the problem. Further changes to the polyethylene have subsequently been implemented obliterating the necessity for such radical fat pad resection.

Radiologically, the tibial implant has done very well within the confines of this very preliminary report. There are no instances of complete lucencies (>1.5 mm) under the plate in any zone on AP or lat fluoroscopic guided views. The metaphyseal cone is also devoid of lucencies suggesting that bone ingrowth on the compression surface has been excellent. There have been 6 cases of peripheral bone resorption at the limits of the most lateral and medial edges seen on the AP radiograph only which may have its origin in the process of HA as all cases were early in the series and the process has now been very much refined and assured. Despite the successful appraisal of the AP glide the tibial tray has been improved further with the introduction of 4 peripherally based pegs. This follows extensive stability testing conducted by Dr William Walsh of the Prince of Wales Hospital, Sydney, Australia, which convincingly shows that the Duofix tray, which has been developed from this tray, will be superior again.

4   Discussion

Posterior cruciate retention as a surgical technique in total knee arthroplasty has been advocated to improve clinical function, optimize transmission of forces across interfaces, and limit anatomical distortion such as joint line elevation. However, recent concern has grown regarding articular surface wear of certain "flat on flat" posterior cruciate retaining total knee arthroplasties [17]. Line contact in these designs can cause high contact stress known to aggravate articular surface wear particularly if increased sliding distances occur with function. Kinematic studies of femoral tibial contact using video fluoroscopy and roentgen photogrammetry have demonstrated significant aberrations from the normal condition [4, 5, 19, 20]. Stiehl et al. defined abnormal lateral condyle motion in posterior cruciate retaining total knee arthroplasties with femoral tibial sagittal plane contact found to be posterior in extension followed by abnormal anterior translation with flexion on deep knee bend [15].

Stiehl et al. evaluated the LCS meniscal bearing posterior cruciate retaining prosthesis finding posterior contact in extension compared to normal, but some degree of posterior femoral rollback up to 60° of flexion [16]. With deep knee bend, there was anterior translation of femoral tibial contacts from 60° to 90° of flexion. The early femoral rollback seen with the meniscal bearing prosthesis was attributed to the high articular conformity noted from 0° to 40° flexion. Nilsson, et al. using RSA with 15 Newton joint loads found a similar result with a posterior contact in extension followed by gradual anterior translation with flexion to 50° [12].

The LCS AP-glide prosthesis demonstrated a posterior position of both condyles at full extension followed by mild posterior translation or femoral rollback to 30° flexion followed by anterior translation up to 120° flexion. This anterior position and translation was significantly greater from 00 to 90° flexion in non weight-bearing knees. We may hypothesize that this difference reflects the posterior tibial shear force exerted with active weight-bearing. With a flexion position of 120°, the

femoral tibial contact points were similar under weight-bearing and non weight-bearing conditions.

Stiehl et al. have found significant condylar lift-off and screw home rotation with the LCS posterior cruciate sacrificing rotating platform total knee arthroplasty [18]. They found a maximal medial condyle lift-off of 2.1 mm whereas the greatest lateral lift-off was 3.5 mm. Screw home rotation was variable ranging from 9.6° of tibial internal rotation with knee flexion to 6.2° of external rotation. Nilsson et al. investigated the LCS meniscal bearing total knee prosthesis finding that initial extension started with a more externally rotated tibia than normal and had minimal internal rotation during flexion [12]. As previously suggested by Jonsson et al. and Karrholm et al. this may represent an alteration demonstrated by anterior cruciate deficient total knees [9, 10].

In the current study, the greatest amount of condylar lift-off occurred with the lateral condyle at 30° flexion, and 9 out of 10 patients experienced condylar lift-off. For screw home rotation, a similar variability was noted as compared to the prior LCS rotating platform study. Under non-weight bearing conditions, the total knees analyzed in this study had a range of 10.8° of internal tibial rotation to 9.1° of external tibial rotation, with increasing flexion. Under weight bearing conditions, only four of nine subjects experience normal axial rotation with one knee having external tibial rotation of 11.9°. The important findings of altered rotation and condylar lift-off relate to the need for contemporary total knee designs to accommodate these kinematic functions. The LCS AP-glide prosthesis is rotationally unconstrained and allows for condylar liftoff in the frontal plane without sacrificing conformity or developing edge loading.

Dennis et al. have previously evaluated non-weight bearing versus weight bearing range of motion with posterior cruciate and posterior stabilized fixed bearing TKA [6]. The average weight bearing flexion in that study was 103° for the posterior cruciate retaining fixed bearing TKA and 113° for the posterior stabilized fixed bearing TKA. The present study demonstrated substantially greater flexion compared to a fixed bearing PCR TKA with an average non-weight bearing flexion of 130° and weight bearing of 119°. We attribute this finding to at least two potential factors. The surgical technique was optimized by a highly experienced surgeon with subtle balancing of each knee. This may be confirmed by the fact that none of our knees were tight in flexion with persistent posterior femoral tibial contact and all demonstrated laxity to allow anterior translation. Secondly, patient selection for the kinematic study was optimized where patients with severe deformity and decreased postoperative motion were not considered. From our prior studies, it is likely that greater range of motion may be expected with a well-done posterior cruciate retaining technique compared with the cruciate sacrificing rotation platform prosthesis.

The final issue of the kinematic analysis is the potential safety of the A/P glide prosthesis compared with earlier devices. Anterior soft tissue impingement has been noted anecdotally by European surgeons who have used this implant, which has lead to the recommendation of fat pad excision. Our experience with this problem was significant early on and as noted above, an alteration of the tibial insert was needed to help resolve this issue. The A/P glide prosthesis is totally unconstrained in the sagittal plane and the kinematic study has shown the potential for anterior translation in the non-weight bearing condition. Flexion space balancing must be accurate and not too tight to allow adequate flexion, but if too loose may allow for abnormal anterior translation and potential fat-pad impingement. Another problem has been potential instability that may result from posterior cruciate disruption. Surgeons have preserved a bone block at the insertion of the posterior cruciate ligament to prevent late ligament failure. From the current study, such an abnormally increased flexion gap could lead to abnormal anterior-posterior motion and clinical symptoms requiring revision.

In conclusion, we have investigated the kinematics of a posterior cruciate retaining mobile bearing total prosthesis finding typical abnormal anterior-posterior translation, condylar liftoff and screw home rotation compared with other reports. Range of motion and potential instability were greater under non-weight bearing conditions, clearly demonstrating the difference that load bearing adds to these functions. As this prosthesis is unconstrained with sagittal plane translation or rotation and relies primarily on ligamentous balancing for proper articulation, surgical technique with appropriate extension and flexion spacing must be done. We have shown that goal to be achievable with this prosthesis.

The A/P glide prosthesis clinically and radiologically has proven to be as successful as its design rationale suggested. The marriage of the concepts associated with the benefits of the meniscal bearing design and the rotating platform have produced a stable kinematically correct TKR with appropriate roll back in flexion, a medial pivot and an superior range of motion. It demands however, an appreciation and embracing of the "soft tissue balance – first" philosophy and is not the universal panacea for all arthritic knees.

References

1. Buechel FF (1994) Cementless meniscal bearing knee arthroplasty: 7 to 12 year outcome analysis. Orthopedics 17: 833–836
2. Buechel FF, Pappas MJ (1986) The New Jersey Low-Contact-Stress knee replacement system: Biomechanical rationale and review of first 123 cemented cases. Arch Orthop Trauma Surg 105: 197–204
3. Buechel FF, Pappas MJ (1989) New Jersey Low Contact Stress knee replacement system. Ten-year evaluation of meniscal bearings. Orthop Clin North Am 20: 147–177
4. Dennis DA, Komistek RD, Hoff WA, Gabriel SM (1996) In vivo knee kinematics derived using an inverse perspective technique. Clin Orthop 331: 107–117
5. Dennis DA, Komistek RD, Colwell CE, Ranawat CS, Scott RD, Thornhill TS, Lapp MA (1998) In vivo anteroposterior femorotibial translation of total knee arthroplasty: a multicenter analysis. Clin Orthop 356: 47
6. Dennis DA, Komistek RD, Stiehl JB, Walker SA, Dennis KN (1998) Range of motion after total knee arthroplasty. J Arthroplasty 13: 748–752
7. Hoff WA, Komistek RD, Dennis DA, Gabriel SA, Walker SA (1998) A three dimensional determination of femorotibial contact positions under in vivo conditions using fluoroscopy. J Clin Biomech 13: 455–470
8. Jordan LR, Olivo JL, Voorhorst PE (1997) Survivorship analysis of cementless meniscal bearing total knee arthroplasty. Clin Orthop 338: 119–123
9. Jonsson H, Kärrholm J (1994) Three-dimensional knee joint movements during a step-up: evaluation after anterior cruciate ligament rupture. J Orthop Research 12: 769–779
10. Kärrholm J, Selvik G, Elmqvist L-G, Hansson LI (1988) Active knee motion after cruciate ligament rupture. Acta Orthop Scand 59: 158–164
11. Keblish PA, Schrei C, Ward M (1993) Evaluation of 275 low contact stress (LCS) total knee replacements with 2- to 8-year follow-up. Orthopaedics (International Edition) 1: 168–174
12. Nilsson KG, Kärrholm J, Gadegaard P (1991) Abnormal kinematics of the artificial knee: roentgen stereophotogrammetric analysis of 10 Miller-Galante and five New Jersey LCS knees. Acta Orthop Scand 62: 440–446
13. Sorrells RB, Stiehl JB, Voorhorst PE (2001) Midterm results of mobile-bearing total knee arthroplasty in patients younger than 65 years. Clin Orthop 390: 182–189
14. Stiehl JB, Voorhorst PE (1999) Total knee arthroplasty with a mobile-bearing prosthesis: Comparison of retention and sacrifice of the posterior cruciate ligament in cementless implants. Am J Orthop 28: 223–228
15. Stiehl JB, Komistek RD, Dennis DA et al. (1995) Fluoroscopic analysis of kinematics after posterior-cruciate-retaining total knee arthroplasty. J Bone Joint Surg 77B: 884–889
16. Stiehl JB, Dennis DA, Komistek RD, Keblish PA (1997) Kinematic analysis of a mobile bearing total knee arthroplasty. Clin Orthop 345: 60–65
17. Stiehl JB, Dennis DA, Komistek RD (1999) Detrimental kinematics of a «flat on flat» total condylar knee arthroplasty. Clin Orthop 365: 139–148
18. Stiehl JB, Dennis DA, Komistek RD, Crane HS (1999) In vivo determination of condylar lift-off and screw-home in a mobile-bearing total knee arthroplasty. J Arthroplasty 14: 293–299
19. Stiehl JB, Dennis DA, Komistek RD (2000) The cruciate ligaments in total knee arthroplasty: A kinematic analysis. J Arthroplasty 15: 545–550
20. Stiehl JB, Dennis DA, Komistek RD, Keblish PA (2000) In vivo kinematic comparison of a posterior-cruciate-retaining and sacrificing mobile bearing total knee arthroplasty. Am J Knee Surg 13:13–18

Chapter 18
LCS Complete

18.1 Primary Total Knee Replacement System

D. J. KILGUS

The LCS Total Knee System was introduced in 1977 by doctors Frederick Buechel, M.D. and Michael Pappas, Ph.D. as the New Jersey LCS (low contact stress) Knee. The original LCS knee was available in three main design variations, including the Rotating Platform Knee, which was designed to sacrifice both the anterior and posterior cruciate ligaments, the Bi-Cruciate Retaining Meniscal Bearing Knee (a design that saved both the anterior and posterior cruciate ligaments), and the Posterior Cruciate Retaining Meniscal Bearing Knee, a posterior cruciate ligament sparing design. All three variations of this knee were initially sold for use as uncemented knees. The uncemented variations of the knee gained acceptance in United States, as well as in Europe and in Australia, New Zealand, and South Africa. Approval for use as a cemented knee was granted in the United States in 1985, and the first publication that described early results of the LCS Mobile Bearing Knee was published in 1986 [4].

The LCS Rotating Platform Knee has become the most popular version of the three basic design variations of the knee in the United States and in many other countries worldwide. Outstanding long-term clinical success has been reported by a number of authors [3, 6, 7, 8]. Implant survivorship between 96 % and 100 % has been reported in these studies with follow-up time intervals of four to twenty years.

The long-term clinical success of the LCS Rotating Platform Knee has been attributed to a number of innovative design features. What are probably the most important of these design features have been:

- the rotational freedom of the polyethylene insert on the polished cobalt-chrome tibial tray, and
- the large area of contact (approximately 877 mm^2) that exists between the femoral condyles and the tibial polyethylene insert during the weight bearing portion of the walking cycle.

By having a large (spherical) area of contact between the femoral condyles and the tibial polyethylene insert, the weight bearing stresses are distributed over a very large area (approximately 877 mm^2) in comparison to alternative total knee designs. This has been accomplished as a result of the fact that the medial-lateral and the anterior-posterior radii of curvature of the femoral condyles are identical (creating a large, spherically shaped area of contact between the femoral component and the tibial polyethylene insert) during the weight bearing portion of the walking cycle (Fig. 1).

In addition, the unique, anatomic, design of the mobile bearing patellar component also allows for a large, fully congruent, area of contact to exist between the polyethylene insert of the patellar component and the femoral condyles from full knee extension to approximately 110 degrees of flexion. These unique design features are also responsible for the outstanding long-term function of the mobile bearing patellofemoral joint as well.

The shape of the patellofemoral groove of the LCS femoral component was designed to allow a congruent, large area of contact with a constant radius of curvature (throughout S2 portion of the sagittal radius of curvature of the femoral component) in order to maximize the contact area between the rotating polyethylene insert of the resurfaced patella and the femoral condyles throughout the normal arc of flexion of the knee. The sulcus groove angle of femoral component (130 degrees) was maintained from the original LCS femoral component design in order to mimic the anatomy of the normal patella. In addition, because many surgeons prefer not to resurface the articular surface of the natural patella in many cases, the shapes of the femoral condyles of the LCS femoral component were designed to allow a congruent path with a constant radius of curvature (throughout the S2 portion of the sagittal radius of curvature) in order to maximize the contact area between the natural (un-resurfaced) patella and the femoral condyles throughout the normal arc of flexion of the knee. In addition, a sulcus groove angle of 130 degrees was maintained in order to mimic the anatomy of the normal patella.

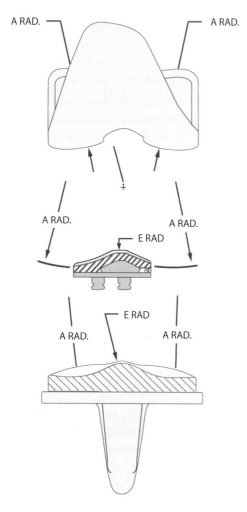

Fig. 1. The medial-lateral and anterior-posterior radii of curvature of the S-2 portion of the femoral components are identical. This allows for a large area over which the weight bearing stresses can be distributed

Despite the outstanding clinical results of the LCS Rotating Platform knee over the past 25 years, a number of refinements have been made to the system. The "LCS Complete Total Knee" system was designed in order to improve the ease of use of the system and to improve the inter-compatibility of the different sizes of the femoral, tibial, and patellar components. These refinements were the result of suggestions provided by many surgeons who have used the LCS Total Knee System for many years. The composite of these refinements have been combined as the LCS "Complete" Total Knee System. These refinements of the LCS "Complete" Total Knee System will be described below (Fig. 2).

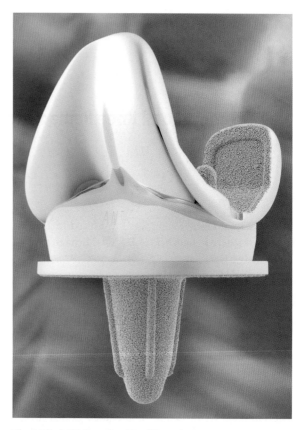

Fig. 2. The LCS Complete Total Knee System

1 Femoral Component Design of the LCS "Complete" Total Knee System

Several subtle design modifications to the femoral component have been made in order to facilitate ease of insertion of the femoral component, to expand the range of sizes of the femoral components, and to make slight refinements in the shape of the anterior flange of the femoral components to enhance component fit for a larger range of patients.

Anthropometric data was collected from a variety of surgeons, worldwide, in order to improve ease-of-use and component sizing for patients of all sizes.

The range of femoral component sizes has been increased from six to seven sizes by the addition of a "medium" size between the traditional "small plus" and "standard" sizes (Fig. 3).

In addition, two minor changes have been made to the anterior flange of the femoral components. The medial and lateral edges of the anterior flange were reduced in width by several millimeters, in order to fit a greater number of patients. In addition, the height of the anterior flange was extended proximally by several mil-

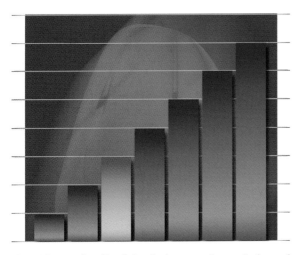

Fig. 3. The new "medium" size fits between the small plus and standard sizes

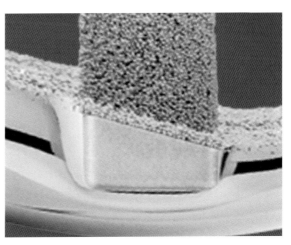

Fig. 5. Impaction slots have been added to the medial and lateral femoral condyles to aid in femoral component disimpaction

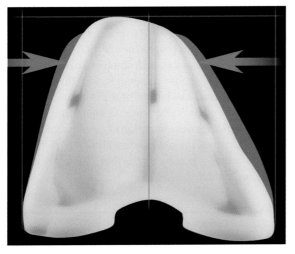

Fig. 4. The anterior flange of the femoral component has been "narrowed down" in the medial-lateral plane. It has also been made several millimeters taller to enhance tracking of the patella

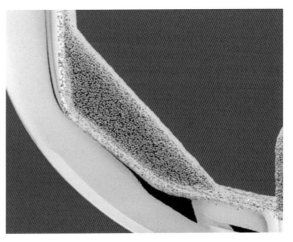

Fig. 6. The interior shape of the trochlear groove has been straightened to simplify resection of the trochlear groove

limeters in order to enhance the capture of the patella in patients who have a relative degree of "patella alta" (Fig. 4).

In order to enhance the ease of femoral component removal (should that become necessary), "impaction slots" have been added to the distal femoral condyles in order to improve the interlock of the instruments used to disimpact the medial and lateral femoral condyles (Fig. 5).

In addition, the fixation pegs of the femoral component were modified by "smoothing" the external shape of the femoral pegs. The outer diameter of the femoral fixation pegs now has a constant diameter to enhance component removal. In addition, the overall size of the

femoral fixation lugs varies with the different sizes of the femoral components.

The shape of the interior surface of the "trochlear groove" has been straightened to simplify resection of the femoral groove (Fig. 6). And, finally, the depth of the "graft pockets" of the uncemented femoral components and the "cement pockets" of the cemented femoral components have been slightly reduced in order to "optimize" the fixation interfaces (Fig. 7).

The shape of the S2 curve has been maintained from the original LCS design in order to maximize the congruency and the large contact area of the femoral condyle-tibial bearing interfaces during the weight bearing portion of the gate cycle when contact pressures are maximal (Fig. 8).

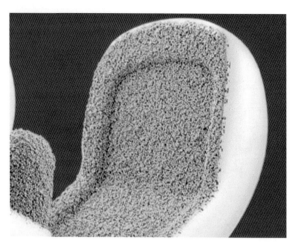

Fig. 7. The graft pockets of the uncemented femur (and the cement pockets of the cemented femur) have been made less deep. The femoral pegs now have a constant diameter

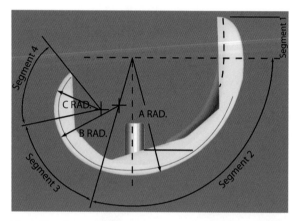

Fig. 8. The shape of the segment 2 curve has been left unchanged. Because the medial-lateral radius of curvature of the femoral condyles has the same radius of curvature as does the anterior-posterior of the S-2 portion of the femoral component, a spherical area of contact is created between the femoral condyles and the tibial poly insert during the weight bearing portion of the gait cycle

Congruency of the femoral component-polyethylene bearing geometry in the coronal and anterior-posterior planes has been maintained an order to maximize the extensive area of contact between the femoral component and the tibial polyethylene insert during the weight bearing portion of the gait cycle. Congruent femoral component/polyethylene bearing contact geometry has been maintained in the medial-lateral plane in order to maintain the large area of contact (approximately 877 square millimeters) that exists between the femoral condyles and the tibial polyethylene insert. This congruent bearing contact geometry is maintained during varus/valgus lift-off in order to prevent edge load-

ing between the femoral component and the tibial polyethylene insert (see Fig. 8). This design feature allows a very large area of contact between lateral and/or medial femoral condyle and tibial polyethylene insert (approximately 438 square millimeters) even when the knee is tilted into varus or valgus. These design features of the femoral-tibial interface permit the largest total area of contact and lowest resultant contact stresses (the smallest areas of contact stresses above 2 MPa) of any total knee design.

The internal geometry of the femoral component incorporates a 15 degree distal femoral angle in order to compensate for the femoral bow and the normal posterior slope of the proximal tibia. (This configuration was kept from the original LCS knee. It was designed to facilitate equalization of the flexion and extension gaps).

The fixation interface options of the original LCS femoral, tibial and patellar components have also been maintained. The LCS "Complete" Total Knee System is available with grit-blasted textured tibial, femoral, and patellar components for cemented fixation. It is also available with Porocoat porous coated femoral, tibial, and patellar components for uncemented fixation when indicated. An all polyethylene patellar component with three fixation pegs for cemented fixation continues to be available.

A number of clinically proven design features of the original LCS knee were intentionally kept unchanged in order to continue the outstanding clinical performance that has been observed over the past 25 years with that total knee system.

2   Tibial Component Design

The Mobile Bearing Tibial (M.B.T.) trays were designed to maintain the outstanding clinical function that has been realized by the original LCS Rotating Platform tibial tray. The M.B.T. trays are manufactured from cast cobalt chromium-molybdenum alloy, and they are gamma sterilized. The trays are available with either cemented or porous coated surface finishes. Cement pockets have been incorporated on to the bottom of the cemented tibial trays to enhance cement fixation and adhesion to the textured surface of the tray. The M.B.T. trays are designed to be inserted with a seven degree posterior slope as was the original LCS rotating platform tibial tray.

The M.B.T. trays are now manufactured in nine sizes (in place of the original seven sizes that were offered with that original LCS Rotating Platform tibial components) in order to enhance bone coverage of the proximal tibia (Fig. 9).

The proximal surface of the tibial components remains highly polished. The shape of the tibial tray has

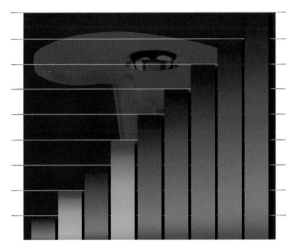

Fig. 9. Two addition sizes of tibial trays have been added to the LCS "Complete" Total Knee System

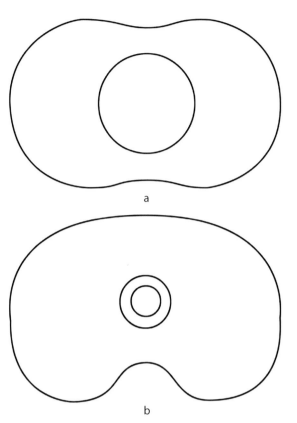

Fig. 10. a Shape of the original LCS Rotating Platform tibial component. **b** The "kidney bean" shape of the LCS Complete Tibial Tray maximizes coverage of the proximal tibia

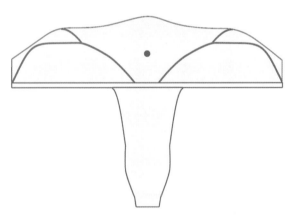

Fig. 11. New shape of the LCS Complete tibial polyethylene inserts

been modified from the traditional kidney bean-shape in order to increase the coverage of the proximal tibial bone surface (Fig. 10a,b).

The shape of the cone of the tibial polyethylene inserts has been modified from that of the original LCS Rotating Platform knee (Fig. 11).

The portion of the tibial polyethylene inserts that makes contact with the femoral condyles is no longer symmetric in the A-P plane. The height of the anterior lip of the LCS Complete tibial polyethylene inserts has been increased 2.4 mm (to 10 millimeters in order to increase subluxation resistance) and the height of the posterior lip of the tibial inserts has been reduced by 0.4 mm to 2.7 mm from the original LCS Rotating Platform tibial inserts in order to facilitate insertion of the inserts (the height of the posterior lip of the original LCS Rotating Platform inserts was 3.1 mm).

The dimensions of the conical portion of the tibial polyethylene inserts are now universal for all sizes of the LCS Complete RP tibial inserts. (The conical portion of all sizes of the LCS Complete RP tibial inserts will fit into all sizes of the LCS Complete tibial trays.) In addition, a cylindrical region has been added to the distal portion of the stems of the tibial polyethylene inserts in order to enhance subluxation resistance.

The dimensions of the conical stem of all sizes of the polyethylene inserts will now fit into all sizes of the LCS Complete tibial trays. However, *the size of the tibial polyethylene insert must be selected to match the size of the "femoral component"* in order to achieve the large area of contact that is desired between the femoral components and tibial polyethylene inserts. The number of tibial inserts sizes has been increased to seven in order to correspond with the seven sizes of femoral components that are now available in the LCS Complete Total Knee System.

The LCS Complete tibial trays are available with both standard (non-keeled) and keeled tibial stems. In addition, the LCS Complete tibial trays are available with porous coated surface finishes using Porocoat for uncemented fixation and with textured surfaces for cemented fixation.

References

1. Buechel FF, Pappas MJ (1990) Long term survivorship analysis of Cruciate-Sparing versus Cruciate-sacrificing prostheses using meniscal bearings. CORR 260: 162–169
2. Callaghan JJ, Insall JN, Greenwald AS, Dennis DA, Komistek RD, Murray DW, Bourne BB, Rorabeck CH, Dorr LD (2000) Mobile Bearing Knee Replacement: concepts and results. JBJS (A) 82(7): 1020–1041
3. Callaghan JJ, Squire MW, Goetz DD, Sullivan PM, Johnston RC (2000) Cemented Rotating Platform Total Knee Replacement. JBJS (A) 82(5): 705–711
4. Jordan LR, Keblish PA, Collier J, Greenwald AS, Davenport JM (1993) Successful use of a metal-backed rotating anatomic patella in TKA: Biomechanical rationale and clinical experience. Am Acad Orthop Surg
5. Jordan LR, Olivio JL, Voorhorst PE (1997) Survivorship analysis of cementless meniscal bearing TKA. CORR 119–123
6. Keblish PA, Schrei C, Ward M (1993) Evaluation of 275 Low Contact Stress (LCS) total knee replacements with two to eight year Follow-up. Orthopaedics (International Edition) 168–174
7. Sanchez-Sotelo J, Odonez JM, Prats SB (1999) Results and complications of the low contact stress knee prosthesis. J Arthroplasty 815–821
8. Sorrells RB (1996) Primary knee arthroplasty: Long-term outcomes using the rotating platform of mobile-bearing TKA. Orthopaedics 793–796

18.2 Knee Revision System

B. D. Haas

The designers want to bring the kinematic advantages of the LCS Complete Primary system to the revision surgeon. The previous LCS revision system lacked the advantages of modern systems. Lack of intraoperative flexibility was a deterrent to the use of the system in complex revision cases. The absence of a posterior cruciate substituting or varus-valgus constrained option limited the system to those revisions where flexion and extension balance could be obtained. Ligamentous instability could not be addressed with the current system.

The potential advantages of the LCS Complete are even more compelling in the revision situation. The congruency of the bearing gives the patient excellent stability in gait. The mobile bearing allows rotation to occur at the bearing component interface, lessening the stress at the prosthetic interface, which is compromised in the revision situation. The excellent patellar kinematics aids the postoperative tracking of the patella. The focus of the chapter will be to highlight the objectives of the design team in the quest to provide a "Complete" system to address the vast needs of the revision surgeon.

1 Implant Selection Criteria

While the principles of revision TKA are similar to those of primary arthroplasty, numerous additional difficulties are often encountered including soft tissue scarring, bone loss, flexion-extension gap imbalance, ligamentous instability and disturbance of the anatomic joint line. To deal with these difficulties, use of a revision implant system, which includes various levels of prosthetic constraint, augmentations, and diaphyseal-engaging stems, is imperative.

In designing the LCS Complete revision implant system, the designing surgeons took into account multiple variables. The coronal and sagittal geometry of the LCS implant was maintained to provide proper kinematic function in gait. Because of the complexity of each procedure, no single implant can be used for all cases. In-

creasing levels of prosthetic constraint, ranging from posterior cruciate retention, posterior cruciate substitution and a varus-valgus constrained, will be available within the system. Thus, the new LCS Complete System will have many more levels of constraint available.

Prosthetic constraint should be minimized to enhance the durability of fixation. In many cases however, posterior cruciate ligament deficiency is common and choice of a posterior cruciate substituting device is wise. In most revisions, either large bone defects or weakened condylar bone is encountered, necessitating use of either press-fit or cemented diaphyseal-engaging stems for additional fixation and load distribution. The LCS Revision System will have all these options to address all situations and surgeon preferences.

2 Posterior Cruciate Retaining Revision TKA

The use of a posterior cruciate retaining (PCR) total knee arthroplasty in revision total knee arthroplasty requires a surgeon skilled in appropriate balance of the posterior cruciate ligament. Indications for revision TKA with PCR components is uncommon in our practice and should be limited to cases with minimal deformity, instability, and bone loss. Preoperative assessment of both flexion and extension stability and the competence of the posterior cruciate ligament are essential in order to utilize this type of device.

Principles of posterior cruciate retention in revision total knee arthroplasty are the same as in primary total knee arthroplasty. If present, the posterior cruciate ligament may be retained if the operative surgeon can attain flexion and extension balance with maintenance and competence of the posterior cruciate ligament and restoration of the anatomic joint line. Advantages of the use of PCR designs in revision knee arthroplasty are the preservation of bone stock and the theoretical advantages for retention of the posterior cruciate ligament found in primary total knee arthroplasty. The majority of cases using this type of implant today are those were polyethylene failure has led to wear and the need for revision. In these cases, the original primary implant remains well fixed and posterior cruciate ligament integrity is maintained.

Disadvantages of the use of PCR designs are the difficulty of balancing the posterior cruciate ligament, restoring the joint line to its anatomical position, and obtaining adequate flexion stability in revision cases in which the competency of the existing posterior cruciate ligament may be difficult to evaluate. Collateral ligament instability may necessitate further levels of constraint, which prohibit the retention of the posterior cruciate ligament. In the author's experience, the use of these devices is limited secondary to the difficulties discussed above. However, the LCS Complete System will have available the option to use the meniscal bearing, the A/P glide, as well as the PCL sacrificing Rotating Platform in revision situations. The designers anticipate the use of PCR LCS designs to be limited secondary to those considerations listed.

3   Posterior Cruciate Substituting Revision TKA

The use of a posterior cruciate substituting (PCS) devices remains the designers implant choice for the majority of revision TKA cases. The LCS Complete will have a PS substituting option available. Advantages of use of this design include reliable substitution for an absent or incompetent posterior cruciate ligament, assistance in easier correction of deformity, increased flexion stability, and increased range of motion [5, 9] secondary to forced posterior femoral rollback. This can be beneficial in those cases where preoperative stiffness is problematic.

The LCS Posterior cruciate substituting TKA design will incorporate a cam and post mechanism to enhance flexion stability and posterior femoral rollback. The cam and post will not engage during lesser flexion activities such as gait. Polyethylene post wear in traditional PCS TKA designs has been limited. It is not yet known if post wear will become problematic in the LCS Complete design, however, previous designs have not shown this to be problematic.

Potential problems encountered with use of PCS TKA implants include posterior dislocation of the cam relative to the post [10, 14], increased bone resection resulting in condylar fracture [15] and an increased incidence of patellar clunk syndrome [2, 11, 16]. While mechanically enhancing flexion stability, the surgeon must still strictly adhere to the principle of obtaining flexion-extension gap balance to lessen the risk of dislocation. The

risk of femoral condylar fracture is typically increased in the multiply revised TKA in which excessive distal femoral bone resection has previously been performed.

While the incidence of patellar clunk syndrome has been higher in PS TKA, [2, 11, 16] the incidence is clearly design related. Designs with a more "boxy" (rectangular) sagittal geometry and those with a higher (more proximal) margin of the intercondylar box are at greater risk. The design of the LCS PS will promote less clunk by using an anatomic patellar design not allowing flexion of the patella in deep knee bend. We will attempt to lessen the chance of synovial entrapment by bringing the coverage of the box as far distal to not allow the opening to be exposed as far in the flexion cycle as possible.

Lastly, one must realize that traditional PCS TKA designs do not provide stability against varus or valgus loads and therefore do not provide stability in cases of advanced collateral ligamentous laxity or loss. Likewise, the LCS PS will not afford the surgeon collateral stability. Constrained TKA devices must be considered in these cases.

4   The LCS Constrained Revision Total Knee Arthroplasty System

Constrained TKA implants provide stability in both the frontal and sagittal planes. They are indicated in cases with severe collateral ligamentous insufficiency or loss and in those with substantial flexion-extension gap imbalance in which flexion stability cannot be obtained using traditional ligamentous balancing techniques and joint line restoration.

Constrained designs can be classified as unlinked or linked. The LCS system will initially only have an unlinked constrained design. It will have an enlarged tibial polyethylene post (height and width) which interlocks into a deepened femoral intercondylar box (Fig. 12).

It will be designed to have varus valgus constraint and enhanced subluxation resistance. Disadvantages of use of unlinked constrained designs include premature tibial polyethylene post wear [18], and premature component loosening [6, 19, 20] due to increased load transmission to the fixation interfaces and implant dislocation. It is hoped that the mobile bearing will allow rotation to occur decreasing stress at the bone prosthetic interface.

Use of linked constrained devices in our practice is very uncommon and limited to cases with medial collateral ligament loss, severe flexion instability, uncontrolled hyperextension deformities, and in patients with massive bone loss from tumor resection or comminuted supracondylar femoral fractures.

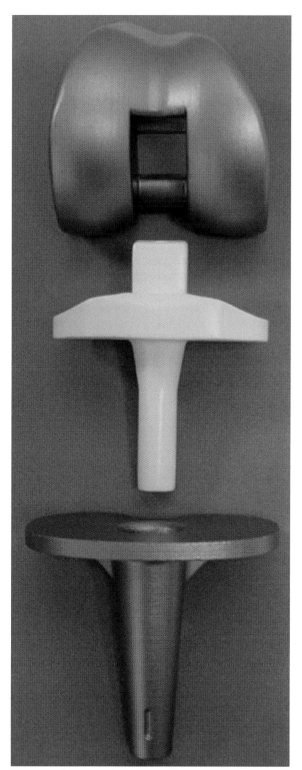

Fig. 12. Prototype of the varus-valgus constrained LCS complete revision total knee

Linked hinge designs are often excessively constrained and suffer from the same problems (premature polyethylene wear and prosthetic loosening) as unlinked constrained devices. Early linked hinges allowed no rotational laxity and failed prematurely due to component loosening [1, 4, 12].

To maximize the longevity of constrained devices, surgeons must still concentrate on restoration of normal limb alignment, balancing the remaining soft tissue envelope and not totally depend on implant constraint to provide knee stability.

5 Modular Stems and Augmentations

Use of diaphyseal-engaging femoral and tibial stems has clearly improved the results of revision TKA [7, 8, 17]. Stems enhance fixation of revision TKA components by dispersing load from weakened condylar bone.

Controversy exists whether the stem should be fully cemented or press-fit. Equivalent results have been reported using both techniques [7, 8, 17]. The LCS Complete System will offer both types to address both the type of revision as well a surgeon preference. Cementless stems will be canal filling and provide rotational stability. Cemented stems will have rounded contours decreasing stress to the cement and to facilitate removal if necessary. Modular locking mechanisms will be secure to prevent fretting or stem dissociation [13]. Due to the canal filling nature of press-fit stems, the condylar position of the femoral or tibial component is determined by the stem position within the medullary canal. The design will take this fact into account. However, this fact may preclude their use in cases with angular deformity, particularly in the metaphyseal or diaphyseal regions. Offset tibial trays or offset intramedullary stems can be helpful in these situations, and will be available. Cemented stems are favored in patients with anatomic deformity, severe osteopenia, and in those cases in which rigid fixation cannot be obtained with a press-fit design. The LCS Complete will have a full complement to choose from.

Modular femoral and tibial augmentations are useful to fill moderately sized (<2 cm) osseous defects. A common surgeon error in revision TKA is failure to recognize the amount of distal femoral bone loss. Failure to do so results in joint line elevation and possibly an unsatisfactory result. Distal femoral augmentations are quite beneficial to assist joint line restoration and will be available in multiple widths.

Modular tibial component augmentations will be available in multiple shapes (angular vs. rectangular) and sizes. Angular augmentations are often more bone

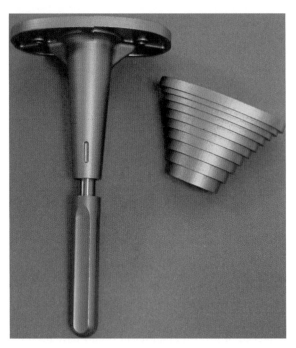

Fig. 13. Mobile bearing revision tibial component with optional metaphyseal sleeve

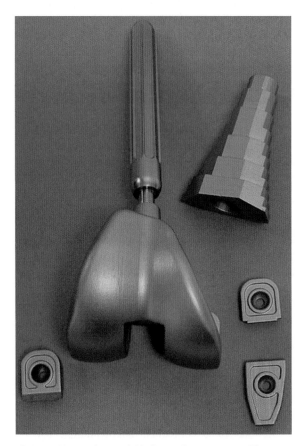

Fig. 14. LCS complete revision femoral component with posterior and distal augments with optional metaphyseal sleeve

preserving whereas rectangular augmentations have been shown to be more stable biomechanically due to reduced shear forces [3]. Both will be available. Metaphyseal augments are being considered to help when metaphyseal bone is absent. These will be porous coated and cemented. They will be available on both tibial and femoral stems (Fig. 13, 14).

---

6   Summary

To successfully manage the myriad of problems faced in revision TKA, a modular revision TKA system is favored. The LCS Complete will provide multiple levels of prosthetic constraint, femoral and tibial augmentations, and diaphyseal-engaging stems. The use of the LCS Revision implant system will allow the surgeon to assemble the desired prosthetic components based on intraoperative findings. It is the hope of the design team to offer a Revision System with the advantages of rotating bearings and the options needed in the revision situation.

References

1. Bargar WL, Cracchiolo III, A, Amstutz HC (1980) Results with the constrained total knee prosthesis in treating severely disabled patients and patients with failed total knee replacements. J Bone Joint Surg 62 A:504–512
2. Beight JL, Yao B, Hozack WJ, Hearn SL, Booth RE Jr (1994) The patellar "Clunk" syndrome after posterior stabilized total knee arthroplasty. Clin Orthop 299: 139–142
3. Chen F, Krackow KA (1994) Management of tibial defects in total knee arthroplasty. Clin Orthop 305: 249–257
4. DeBurge A, GUEPAR (1976) Guepar hinge prosthesis; complications and results with 2 years follow-up. Clin Orthop 120: 47–53
5. Dennis DA, Komistek RD, Stiehl JB, Walker SA, Dennis KN (1998) Range of motion after total knee arthroplasty. J Arthroplasty 13: 748–752
6. Donaldson WF, Sculco TP, Insall JN, Ranawat CS (1988) Total condylar III knee prosthesis. Long term follow-up study. Clin Orthop 226: 21–28
7. Engh GA, Herzwurm PJ, Parks NL (1997) Treatment of major defects of bone with bulk allografts and stemmed components during total knee arthroplasty. J Bone Joint Surg 79 A: 1030–1039
8. Haas SB, Insall JN, Montgomery W 3rd, Windsor RE (1995) Revision total knee arthroplasty with use of modular components with stems inserted without cement. J Bone Joint Surg Am 77 A(11): 1700–1707
9. Hirsh HS, Lotke PA, Morrison LD (1994) The posterior cruciate ligament in total knee surgery. Clin Orthop 309: 64
10. Hossain S, Ayeko C, Anwar M, Elsworth CF, McGee H (2001) Dislocation of Insall-Burstein II modified total knee arthroplasty. J Arthroplasty 16: 233–235
11. Hozack WJ, Rothman RH, Booth RE Jr et al. (1989) The patellar clunk syndrome: A complication of posterior stabilized total knee arthroplasty. Clin Orthop 241: 203–208
12. Hui FS, Fitzgerald RH Jr (1980) Hinged total knee arthroplasty. J Bone Joint Surg 62 A: 513–519

13. Lim LA, Trousdale RT, Berry DJ, Hanssen AD (2001) Failure of the stem-condyle junction of a modular femoral stem in revision total knee arthroplasty. J Arthroplasty 16: 128–132
14. Lombardi AV Jr, Mallory TH, Vaughn BK, Krugel R, Honkala TK, Sorscher M, Kolczun M (1993) Dislocation following primary posterior-stabilized total knee arthroplasty. J Arthroplasty 8(6): 633–639
15. Lombardi AV Jr, Mallory TH, Waterman RA, Eberle RW (1995) Intercondylar distal femoral fracture. An unreported complication of posterior-stabilized total knee arthroplasty. J Arthroplasty 10(5): 643–650
16. Lucas TS, DeLuca PF, Nazarian DG, Bartolozzi AR, Booth Jr, RE (1999) Arthroscopic treatment of patellar clunk. Clin Orthop 367: 226–229
17. Murray PB, Rand JA, Hanssen AD (1994) Cemented long-stem revision total knee arthroplasty. Clin Orthop 309: 116–123
18. Puloski SK, McCalden RW, MacDonald SJ, Rorabeck CH, Bourne RB (2001) Tibial post wear in posterior stabilized total knee arthroplasty. An inrecognized source of polyethylene debris. J Bone Joint Surg 83 A: 390–394
19. Rand JA (1991) Revision total knee arthroplasty using the total condylar III prosthesis. J Arthroplasty 6: 279
20. Rosenberg AG, Verner JJ, Galante JO (1991) Clinical results of total knee revision using the Total Condylar III prosthesis. Clin Orthop 273: 83–90

Chapter 19
Navigation and Soft-Tissue Balancing of LCS TKA

J. M. Strauss, J.-L. Briard, W. Rüther

1 Introduction

Of all orthopedic surgical procedures, endoprosthetic total joint replacement is the most frequent one today. While the frequency of total knee replacements in Europe is on a constant rise, in the US total knee replacement has already become more frequent than total hip procedures.

However, the primary success of total joint replacements is compromised by two main factors, namely unprecise intraoperative implant positioning and, as a long-term complication, aseptic loosening of implant components. Today, aseptic loosening is very rare as an early or mid term complication, rather it is observed later, due to wear, which is frequently associated with malpositioning.

In case of the knee joint, exact positioning of the prosthesis relative to the ligamentous structures of the knee is of highest importance and essential for optimal implant function. Even slight flaws in positioning the implant components will increase the mechanical stress on the implant fixation manifold. This may lead to a chronic overcharge of the interface and ultimately result in loosening of the implant.

A meta-analysis of 9879 patients [2] revealed the need for revision surgery (after only 4 years) in 4% of cases, stressing the importance of exact initial positioning as the failure rate corresponded to the radiological evidence of malpositioning. The correlation between malpositioning and premature loosening of the implant was underlined in several different studies. In a study of 421 patients, Ritter [9] (using a flat on flat design) showed that implantation in a varus position resulted in a threefold increase of the loosening rate (15%) as compared to positioning in correct alignment (5%). These results have been confirmed by other authors [1, 4].

The attempt to improve the positioning of the prosthesis by help of navigation systems or robots is not a new concept. Kienzle et al. [5] developed a computer- and robot-assisted system to plan and carry out tib-

ial and femoral cuts. Using a three-dimensional reconstruction of CT data, the surgeon can plan the placement of the tibial and femoral components. The matching of CT data and surgical object is achieved by use of fiducial markers on tibia and femur. During the operation patient and robot are tightly connected to the operating table. A different robot system [3, 6] retrieves information about the appendage and origin of the knee ligaments from the CT data source and employs them to simulate the kinematics of the prosthesis.

Another group [7] proposes a different concept., Instead of tightly connecting patient and robot, an opto-electronic navigation system follows the movements of the patient, made possible by light emitting diodes (LED) which are fixed to tibia and femur. As a basis for the component implantation, the axis of tibia and femur as well as the mechanical supporting axis of the limb are determined by various technical processes (direct digitalization of anatomical landmarks, determination of the center of rotation in the hip and ankle by "pivoting"). Without the aid of further CT data, the osseous base for the prosthesis can then be formed using an LED-equipped cutting jig and a simple navigation interface.

However, the above mentioned existing concepts have important limitations:

The postoperative outcome after total knee arthroplasty depends to a considerable degree on the soft tissue tension after implantation of the components. Today there is wide agreement among surgeons that TKR is mainly a soft tissue operation. Fadda et al. [3] carried out a kinematic analysis which is based on the length of ligaments. This method, however, is very prone to error because the ligaments are not directly visible in the CT and other essential soft tissue structures such as tendons and capsules are not taken into account. What is more, at the time of CT registration, osteophytes were still present and therefore soft tissue registration was not reliable. Algorithms published by Leitner et al. [7] for the determination of articular centers do not have sufficient reliability. In addition, the system is limited to a specific type of prosthesis because of its special cutting jigs. The user-interface does not contain individual visualization on the basis of standard x-rays.

Up to date, the use of robots requires the fixation of the patient to the robot, inadvertently leading to a larger approach and more soft tissue damage. With current techniques, the employment of robots does allow fitting of the interface with highest precision, but soft tissue balancing cannot be influenced, which, in our opinion, represents the most important aspect of total knee replacement. What is more, a CT, which is an essential requirement for robot-assisted surgery, is time-consuming and not routinely available in the OR setting.

Other authors improved the quality of 3D visualization of bony surfaces during surgery without the need of a CT scan by developing a "Bone Morphing Technique". Fleute and Praxim used anatomical data of different anatomical specimen to calculate a mathematical model of an average femur and tibia. This procedure allows morphing of the virtual average bone in relation to a cloud of points captured on the bony surface of the respective patient intra-operatively: Firstly, some reference points are captured to orientate anatomical landmarks and relate to the mathematical average model later on. A graffiti on the extremity is performed until an average of 1000 points is captured, creating a cloud of points (Fig. 1 a,b). Then transformation equations are calculated to morph the average bone to the actual bone of the patient. Missing data is interpolated and the result is a 3D visualization of the patient's bone. The average error of calculating the virtual anatomy is less than 1 mm compared to the real bony surface.

Due to the above mentioned disadvantages of the existing navigation- and robot-systems, a new freehand navigation system for the implantation of LCS prosthe-

ses was developed in cooperation with the Maurice-E.-Mueller-Institute in Bern, Switzerland (Chair L.P. Nolte) and the Department of Orthopedics, University Hospital Hamburg-Eppendorf, Germany (Chair W. Rüther). This system was designed to fulfill three requirements:

1. An exact reproduction of the relevant anatomical structures and given statics. This was to be achieved rapidly and efficiently by the digitalization of anatomical landmarks, thereby serving two purposes: exposure to additional CT radiation is not necessary and "matching", i.e. the intraoperative comparison between the real anatomy and the CT anatomy, which is difficult and prone to error, is not needed any more.

2. A high enough degree of openess and complexity. It was demanded that the surgeon should have complete visual control over each degree of freedom of the implant during any given timepoint throughout the procedure. Valgus/varus, flexion/extension and rotation of both femoral and tibial components should be controllable and the surgeon should be able to manually change them at all times, including the prospective postoperative joint line.

3. Most importantly, a computer-assisted soft-tissue balancing in flexion and extension allowing optimal functional positioning of the LCS implant. It is problematic to measure soft tissue balance with a computer without specialized sensors. In lack of such sensors, soft tissue balance can only be gauged by indirect measurement using distractors. In addition, it is difficult for the surgeon to translate the figures given by the computer to the intraoperative situation because the release in extension influences the release in flexion and vice versa. Furthermore, the tibial resection level is an important denominator of soft tis-

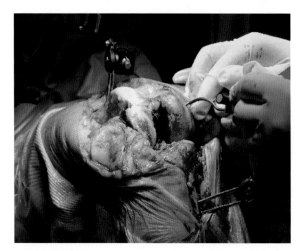
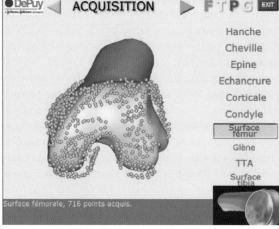

Fig. 1a, b. "Bone morphing technique": A cloud of points is captured by touching the surface of the femur with a pointer device (**a**). A 3D model of the distal femur is visualized by morphing an average femur to fit to the cloud of points (**b**)

sue tension. Additionally, the optimal position of the bone cuts needed to obtain an ideal balance between the axis of the extremity and the resulting ligamenteous tension is not known to date. Therefore, we intended to design a system that allows the integration of desirable future developments, such as sensors for pressure and tension, at a later timepoint.

2 Description of the System

A newly created software module, designed to meet the criteria outlined above, was integrated into the optoelectronic navigation system "SurgiGATE" (Medivision; Fig. 2).

The setup consists of an optoelectronic camera (Optotrack 3020, by Northern Digital) with which the motion of the instruments relative to a coordinate system of tibia and femur are monitored. To achieve this, so-called dynamic reference bases (DRBs) are attached to tibia and femur. The coordinates of these DRBs as well as all instruments (Fig. 3) connected to the so-called stroberbox (pointer, stille-hook, virtual keyboard, navigation clamp) are transferred to the computersystem (Sun Ultrasparc III). Thus anatomical data of hip, femur,

tibia and ankle can be read via the so-called pointer and visualized. Within this virtual anatomy, the motion of the instruments can then be monitored and calculated (Fig. 4).

A so-called virtual keyboard is placed on the OR table under sterile conditions. All relevant navigational options are represented on the virtual keyboard as seen on the computer screen. The virtual keyboard is used to pilot the entire navigation program intra-operatively (Fig. 5).

Except for some minor modifications, we could use the conventional "LCS Milestone-II" instruments with the current navigation system. Only the cutting jigs had to be slightly modified by drilling three scanning points into each jig to allow registration of the jigs for calibration. The navigation of the cutting jig as such is made possible by the fixation of a navigation clamp (see Fig. 3) that can be attached to any of the three cutting jigs (tibia, femur a.p., distal femur).

3 Operative Procedure and Navigation

The computer-assisted operation is performed in five steps guided by the user: *tools, anatomy, soft tissue, planning, navigation.*

3.1 Tools

First, the calibration of all instruments is checked for accuracy to rule out that potential mechanical damage leads to erroneous reading of anatomical data. In addition, the camera position as well as the presence of all instruments on the monitor is checked during this step.

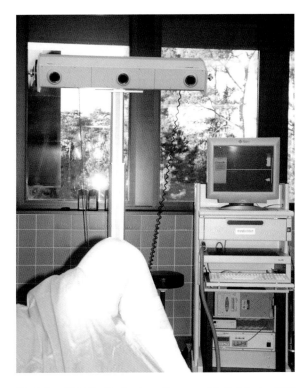

Fig. 2. SurgiGATE Navigation System (Medivision): LED equipped instruments are tracked by an optoelectronic camera (Optotrack 3020). Calculation and visualization is carried out by a SUN Ultrasparc III Computer System

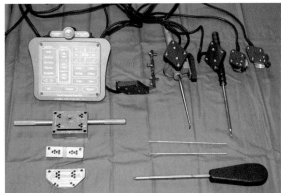

Fig. 3. LED equipped instruments for navigation (background from left to right): virtual keyboard, navigation clamp, Stille hook, Pointer, Dynamic Reference Base for femur and tibia. Front: standard cutting jigs, K-wire, Screwdriver

Fig. 4. Capture of anatomical landmarks using a Stille hook. The screenshot shows the virtual anatomy already registered (medio-lateral [left] and a.p. [right] views of the knee joint) and a 3D visualization of the instrument in real-time

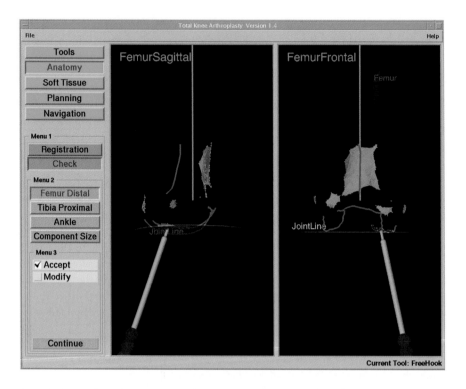

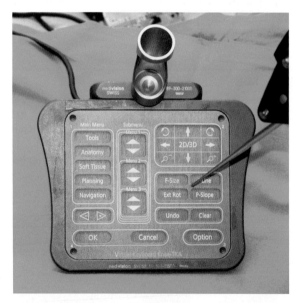

Fig. 5. Virtual keyboard: All relevant navigational options are represented on the virtual keyboard as seen on the computer screen. The virtual keyboard is used to pilot the entire navigation program intra-operatively. Action is performed by bringing the tip of the pointer close to the button on the virtual keyboard

3.2   Anatomy

In order to define the mechanical axis of the lower extremity, it is required to determine the center of the hip,

knee and ankle joints. For the knee, this determination is complex as two relevant anatomical centers account for the relative motion that exists between femur and tibia. This aspect is of importance e.g. when using an a.p.-glide inlay or in order to detect potential problems like the roll back phenomenon. Therefore it is reasonable to determine one center at the distal femur and another at the proximal tibia.

3.2.1   Hip joint
The center of the hip joint is defined by the so-called *"Pivot Algorithm"*: The pointer is attached to the anterior superior iliac spine to define a fixed reference.

The invasive fixation of an additional hip DRB, as commonly required by other systems, is not needed. Now the femur, with the attached femoral DRB, is pivoted, producing a cloud of points as a result of the relative motion of the femoral DRB to the fixed hip reference. The computer calculates the hip joint center from this cloud of points, the other joint centers (distal femur, proximal and distal tibia) are calculated from pre-read anatomical landmarks. Sequential readings of each landmark are averaged, so that by increasing redundancy of the system, the calculation of the center is again based on a cloud of points. Due to the pathological changes of the knee, the Pivot Algorithm should not be used for the joint in question which is to be replaced.

3.2.2 Knee Joint

The anatomical landmarks of the distal femur are the medial and lateral epicondyle, the anterior and posterior cortex, the contour of the femoral condyle in the horizontal and sagittal plane both anteriorly and posteriorly, bony defects and the femoral joint line. These data are used to calculate the distal center of the femur, the size of the femoral implant component and the relative position of the jointline. The landmarks of the proximal tibia are used to calculate the proximal center of the tibia and the jointline (which, in the standing position, is identical to the femoral joint line) and include the following: anterior rim of the tibia, intercondylar tibial spine, tibial tubercle, bony defects and the tibial joint line. In order to determine the degree of rotation of the lower leg, the tibia is brought into the desired post-op rotation in extension, if necessary, after a soft tissue release. In this position the femoral transepicondylar axis is projected onto the tibial plateau, thereby defining the mediolateral axis.

3.2.3 Ankle Joint

The center of the ankle is defined by digitalization of both the lateral and medial malleolus as well as the tendon of the tibialis anterior muscle. Given these centers (3.2.1–3.2.3), the anatomical axis of the extremity is determined and deviations from the mechanical axis (Mikulicz line) can be defined as varus/valgus, flexion/extension and rotation (Fig. 6).

Now the "joint play" can be visualized and quantified. Evaluation of soft tissue can only be done after exposure, excision of all osteophytes and release of adhesions. After this first registration of relevant soft tissue, tests are carried out to see if correct alignment through the whole range of motion can be achieved. If not, capsulo-ligamentous procedures may have to be performed and the soft tissues must be reevaluated for final validation. At this point, the bone cuts can be planned.

3.3 Soft Tissue

Next to the given axis deviation, the following criteria are essential for the calculation of the bone cut positioning:

- resection level 2 mm below the deepest articular defect,
- conservation of the joint line,
- small inlay size,
- balanced soft tissue in flexion and extension, and
- identical joint gap width in flexion and extension.

The first tibial resection is carried out minimally and preliminary, navigated with default 4 mm below the joint line and with 7° slope, in order to obtain a good approach to the soft tissue, in particular to the dorsal capsule and the popliteus muscle. Next, a distractor is placed into the joint gap first in extension, then

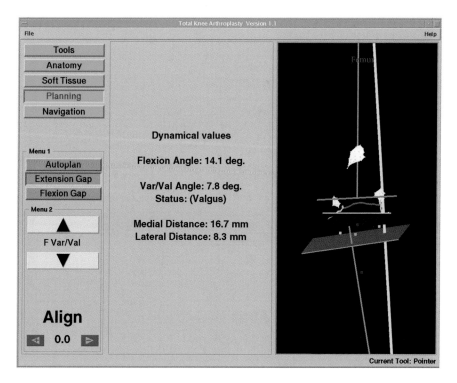

Fig. 6. A.p. view of the virtual anatomy of a left knee with a combined valgus and flexion deformity: the screenshot shows the femoral and tibial axis, the mechanical axis (Mikulicz line [yellow]), anatomical landmarks and preliminarily calculated cuts to restore the mechanical axis. Soft tissue behavior is not yet registered

in flexion. The resulting ligament tension should correspond to the desired postoperative situation. Now the computer displays the residual axis deviation in varus/valgus, flexion/extension, rotation in extension and the external rotation of the femur in flexion. A conventional soft tissue release is performed until the desired alignment is achieved in flexion and extension.

3.4 Planning

The position of femur and tibia are registered in flexion and extension with the distractor in place (Fig. 7a,b) and the corresponding bone cuts are calculated with the so-called autoplaner (Fig. 7e) according to the criteria described above. If the surgeon does not intend to correct the axis deviation completely (e.g. in cases of a consolidated dislocated femoral fracture or tibial plateau fracture), or if complete alignment cannot be achieved by soft tissue manipulation, all implantation parameters can be changed manually for each component (e.g. flexion or external rotation of the femoral component or changes of the femoral implant size in order to vary the relation of the extension to the flexion gap). Based on the changed parameters, the computer recalculates the optimal cuts for a new planning (Fig. 7c,d).

The resulting data (e.g. level of distal femoral resection, tibial re-cut, achieved correction) are processed for navigation.

3.5 Navigation

After such planning, the cuts can be performed in a quick sequence (tibial re-cut, a.p. and distal femoral resection). Each time the corresponding cutting jig is calibrated with the navigation clamp. At this point, the monitor displays the planned and actual resection plane for each jig (Fig. 8), and, when a perfect match is obtained, the block is attached to bone with pins in this position. It is not necessary to open the marrow cavity. A quality control can now be carried out with conventional spacer blocks to check the extension and flexion gaps. After implantation of the original components, the axis is checked by lifting off the leg held by the big toe. Finally, the motion of the prosthetic joint is recorded from full extension to maximal flexion with and without the application of varus/valgus stress.

4 Early Results

4.1 Analysis of Precision (Cadaver Study)

To obtain an idea of the precision of the system before clinical application, we tested the exactness of the calculation of the centers of hip, distal femur and ankle in CT-controlled intra- and interobserver cadaver studies. The matching of the CT data with the coordinates of the navigation system was made possible by the implantation of three so-called "fiducial markers" into femur and tibia before the CT was done. The intraobserver study (one

Fig. 7a–e. Soft tissue balancing: The position of femur and tibia is registered in flexion and extension with the distractor in place. Screenshot **a** (extension gap) and **b** (flexion gap) show the unbalanced situation before the soft tissue release. The release can be performed either manually-which allows correction of the orientation of tibial and femoral components – (**c** and **d**) or automatically (**e**). The screenshot shows the aligned situation after a successful soft tissue release. The bone cuts are calculated with the so-called "auto-planer" according to the criteria described in the text. Tibial and femoral resection height, joint line deviation and component size are also listed on the screen

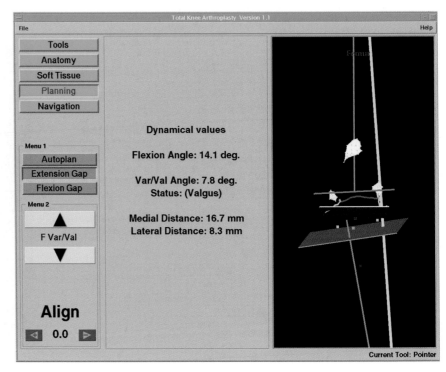

Fig. 7b

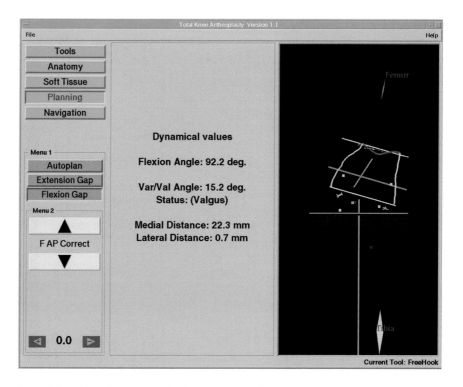

Fig. 7c

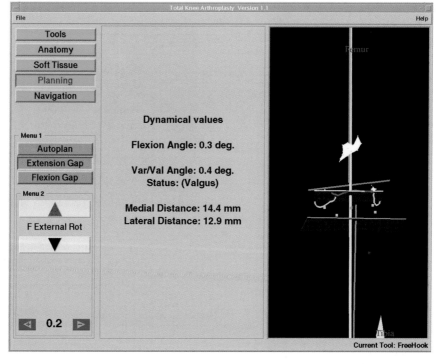

surgeon, five readings of the anatomical landmarks with the navigation system for each cadaver [n=6]) yielded a mean deviation of the center as defined by CT of 0.7 mm at the hip, 1.1 mm at the knee and 1.8 mm at the ankle. The interobserver study (five surgeons, single reading of landmarks for each cadaver [n=6]), resulted in slightly higher deviations: 1.1 mm at the hip, 1.2 mm at the knee and 2.4 mm at the ankle. To put this into perspective, it should be kept in mind that a 1° deviation of the axis of the extremity corresponds to a 7 mm dislocation of the knee center. The precision of the system was influenced more significantly by the manual skills of the sur-

Fig. 7d

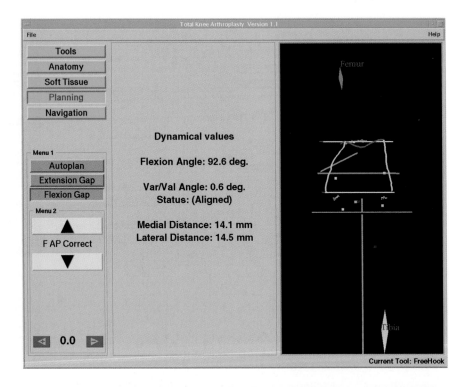

Fig. 7e

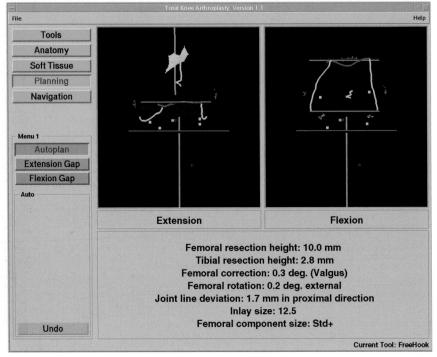

geon with respect to the resection as such. For instance, the difference between the planned and real resection planes of the distal femoral cut was 1.6° in the frontal plane and 1.9° in the sagittal plane.

4.2   First Clinical Results (Preliminary)

A first study, done with 30 gonarthritis patients, resulted in a post-op axis deviation from the ideal line (measured by x-ray a.p. and lateral of the entire extremity in stand-

Fig. 8. Navigation of the tibial cut: After calibrating the tibial cutting jig with the navigation clamp, the monitor displays the planned (yellow) and actual (red) resection plane for the tibia while the surgeon tries to fix the jig to the bone

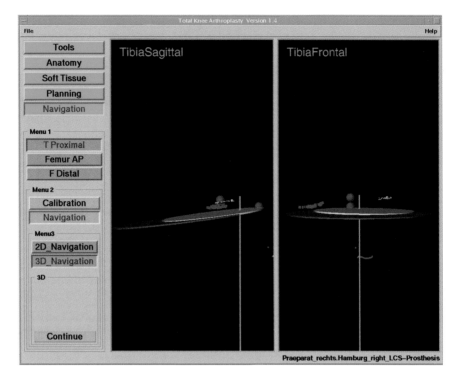

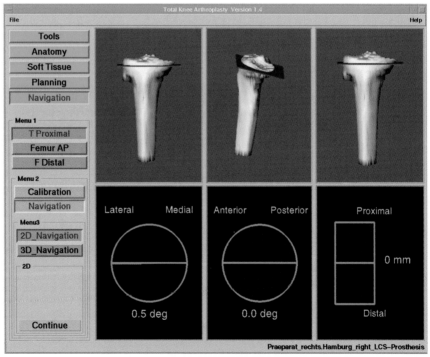

ing position) of 1.7° in the frontal plane and 3.9° in the sagittal plane for the navigated group (n=15). The control group (n=15), operated without navigation, yielded a 1.9° deviation in the frontal plane and 4.4° in the sagittal plane. The differences between the navigated and the control group were not statistically significant. However, the range in the non-navigated control group was clearly wider and it comprised the cases with the largest postoperative axis deviation of all (occurring in two cases of extreme obesity and in one valgus deformity of more than 30°). Such extreme deviations were not found among similar patients of the navigation group. The quality of the ligament stability (varus/valgus stress) was comparable in both groups, but the imbalance (difference between medial and lateral stability) was smaller in the navigated group. After analysis of all data including a power-analysis, a prospective randomized study will be performed to look for statistically significant differences in axis deviation as well as positioning of both tibial and femoral components. In particular such a study will reveal whether the quality of the component positioning achieved by this navigation system is equal for all the implantation criteria outlined above.

5   Summary and Future Perspective

The disadvantage of the current system is that it takes longer to perform the operation (19 minutes on average, range: 12 to 62 minutes) and that the setup is more complex compared to a non-navigated standard procedure. However, compared to other existing navigation systems, the advantages are apparent:

1. The system is minimally invasive thanks to the percutaneously applied reference bases.
2. While the surgeon does not have to give up his familiar handling, he receives extra information online about the optimal bone cuts, joint line displacement and the current ligament tension.
3. As all degrees of freedom of each component can be manually manipulated and the consequences of these changes for the post-op situation are displayed in the planning module, the optimal result for the patient can be found *before* the cuts are carried out.
4. The precision of the system is sufficient (cadaver study) and first clinical results are promising.
5. Last but not least the navigation system can be used by the surgeon to document the quality of his work.

The lack of statistically significant postoperative differences between the navigated and the control group in the clinical study was found with another navigation system as well [8]. This can be explained by the small number of patients in the clinical studies and the relatively small percentage of complex deformities within the cohort, because it is this particular subgroup of patients that is expected to profit from a navigated procedure. The lack of statistical power can also be accounted for by the limited precision of the post-op x-ray mea-

surement which includes up to 3° deviation due to rotational effects. In the future, a standardized and more precise way of evaluating the operative results will be needed.

The development of next generation navigation systems will be characterized by improved 3D visualization of a patient's anatomy without CT thanks to the above described "bone morphing technique". The quality of soft tissue handling will be improved by the introduction of objective measurements (pressure sensors) and the quality of the bone cuts (the major limiting factor within the present system) may be further optimized by the introduction of a minimal robot system for milling the cuts.

References

1. Bargren JH, Blaha JD, Freeman MA (1983) Alignment in total knee arthroplasty. Correlated biomechanical and clinical observations. Clin Orthop 173: 178–183
2. Callahan CM, Drake BG, Heck DA, Dittus RS (1995) Patient outcomes following unicompartimental or bicompartimental knee arthroplasty. A meta-analysis. J Arthroplasty 10: 141–150
3. Fadda M, Bertelli D, Martelli S, Marcacci M, Dario P, Paggetti C, Carmella D, Trippi D (1997) Computer assisted planning for total knee arthroplasty. In: Troccaz J, Grimson E, Moesges R (eds) CVRMed-MRCAS'97. Springer, Berlin Heidelberg New York Tokyo, pp 663–671
4. Feng EL, Stulberg SD, Wixson RL (1994) Progressive subluxation and polyethylene wear in total knee replacements with flat articular surfaces. Clin Orthop 299: 60–71
5. Kienzle TC III, Stulber SD, Peshkin M, Quaid A, Lea J, Goswami A, Wu C-H (1996) A computer assisted total knee replacement surgical system using a calibrated robot. In: Taylor RH, Lavallée S, Burdea GC, Moesges R (eds) Computer integrated surgery: technology and clinical applications. The Mit Press, London, pp 409–423
6. La Palombara PF, Fadda M, Martelli S, Marcacci M (1997) Minimally invasive 3D data registration in computer and robot assisted total knee arthroplasty. Med Biol Eng Comput 35: 600–610
7. Leitner F, Picard F, Minfelde R, Schulz H-J, Cinquin P, Saragaglia D (1997) Computer assisted surgical total knee replacement. In: Troccaz J, Grimson E, Moesges R (eds) CVRMed-MRCAS'97. Springer, Berlin Heidelberg New York Tokyo, pp 629–637
8. Mielke RK, Clemens U, Jens J.-H, Kershally S (2001) Navigation in der Knieendoprothetik – vorläufige klinische Erfahrungen und prospektiv vergleichende Studie gegenüber konventioneller Implantationstechnik. Z Orthop 139: 109–116
9. Ritter MA, Faris PM, Keating EM and Meding JB (1994) Postoperative alignment of total knee replacement. Its effect on survival. Clin Orthop 299: 153–156

Chapter 20
Cementless Fixation Options in Total Knee Arthroplasty

W.K. Walter, B. Zicat

1 Introduction

The increasing need for arthroplasty in younger patients, and encouraging results with various cementless implants in hip and knee surgery, has provided the impetus to persist with cementless fixation for all components of knee arthroplasty. Historically, cementless femoral components have always provided reliable and longlasting fixation. Patellar fixation has been plagued by high failure rates of a few specific designs. Tibial fixation has been more controversial, due to inconsistent results with a wide variety of implant designs.

2 Femoral Fixation

Femoral component fixation with cementless implants has been the most reliable of any of the components of knee arthroplasty. The design of the femoral component, with a 'captured' geometry, provides the opportunity to achieve excellent initial stability. This stability is essential to development of bone ingrowth. In this setting, surface coating of the implant is less crucial, and virtually all types of porous or hydroxyapatite coated surfaces have been successful at achieving reliable and consistent ingrowth.

There have been some long term failures of cementless femoral components, but this appears to be isolated to particular design features. One example is the development of posterior condyle stress fractures of femoral components [3]. These occasional problems underline the reliability of cementless femoral components, as mechanical failure of these implants is exceedingly rare.

Although titanium alloys have demonstrated better osseointegration than cobalt chrome alloys, they have performed poorly as bearing surfaces due to the softer mechanical characteristics of the metals, and they offer less scratch resistance. The inferior osseointegration properties of the cobalt chrome materials has not affected the reliability of ingrowth in femoral compo-

nents, likely due to the quality of initial fixation of these components, a result of the mechanical nature of the initial fit.

Stress shielding is uncommon behind femoral components of knee arthroplasty, but can occur to a limited extent in the intercondylar notch, although this has not been shown to be of clinical significance, and has been similar in severity to that seen behind cemented components [8].

3 Tibial Fixation

The development of radiolucent lines at the bone/cement interface under cemented tibial components has long been a concern after knee arthroplasty. This finding suggests the development of a fibrous membrane, and when progressive, indicates loosening of the implant. This has been of particular concern in younger, high demand patients, and limits the long term success of cemented fixation in this group. The need for improved and long lasting fixation in these groups of patients has led to the development of various cementless component designs.

There are a number of design issues that need to be addressed in tibial fixation. Initial stability must be sufficient to resist micromotion. The bone ingrowth surface must be of suitable quality to achieve consistent and reliable ingrowth in the first few weeks after implantation. Finally, the implant must resist the development of polyethylene induced osteolysis, as polyethylene debris is inevitably generated by the bearing surfaces.

We have studied some of these design features in detail, in benchtop as well as clinical studies. The initial stability of the implant is dependent on the features on the undersurface of the tibial component. Many different features have been used to achieve this initial stability, and these include stems, pegs, keels and screws, among others. We know from studies of stability that 'lift-off' of the tibial component from the underlying bone can occur with eccentric loading, the lift off oc-curring on the side not under load [4]. This lift off is well resisted by screw fixation, and this has been suc-cessfully used in a number of different designs. Unfor-tunately, screw fixation has two major drawbacks. The first is that the screw holes provide a pathway for mi-gration of polyethylene debris from the joint to the tib-ial cancellous bone, thereby increasing the effective joint space first described around hip arthroplasty [10]. The second is that the presence of irregularity of the tibial component surface, as a result of the screw holes, limits the usefulness of these implants as mobile bearing com-ponents, where there is an articulation between the un-derside of the tibial polyethylene and the surface of the tibial component.

In order to assess the effect of these various design features, we performed a cadaveric study using 6 lead-ing cementless tibial component designs [6]. These com-ponents were implanted into surgically prepared tibias, as would be performed in knee arthroplasty. The con-structs were loaded eccentrically to 700 Newtons at 3 lo-cations (anterior, middle and posterior) over the medial and lateral condyles, and lift off or subsidence was mea-sured using optical sensors. The relative displacement of the implants was measured compared to the displace-ment of the bone immediately adjacent to the implant in those locations. In addition, the implants were cycli-cally loaded (5,000 cycles) to simulate the conditions of initial weight bearing as seen in vivo during the first few weeks after surgery.

The results of this testing showed that all of the im-plants had excellent initial stability, with mean displace-ments of less than 100 microns, well within the range previously described as being required to achieve bone ingrowth fixation [1] (Fig. 1). In addition, there was no significant degradation of that stability during the cy-clical load testing, showing that this fixation was ade-quate to provide continued initial stability while allow-ing some early weight bearing (Fig. 2).

When we looked at the particular design features of the various implants, we found that the absence of stems, keels, pegs or screws in isolation did not result in any difference in the degree of initial stability in these commercially available designs. However, the geome-try of the components did have a statistically significant influence on the initial stability, with asymmetric im-plants having greater stability than symmetric implants (Fig. 3). This was felt to be due to improved cortical cov-erage of the tibia as measured using a digitized image analysis program.

Initial stability is a necessary condition for bone in-growth, but is insufficient without an appropriate in-growth surface. Many ingrowth surfaces have proven

track records, having been used in other components of arthroplasty, such as femoral stems, or acetabular cups. Porocoat is one of these proven ingrowth surfaces. It has the porosity characteristics required for successful in-growth with a long history of reliable fixation about the hip, and on the femoral component of knee arthroplasty components.

Hydroxyapatite has more recently been shown to encourage early and reliable osseointegration, but has shown a tendency to be eroded, particularly in areas of unstable fixation [5]. We have investigated the combi-nation of hydroxyapatite on Porocoat using an in vivo sheep model, to confirm the effectiveness of this com-

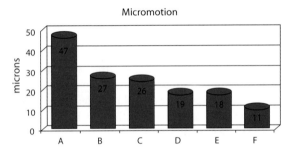

Fig. 1. Mean micromotion under cementless tibial tray

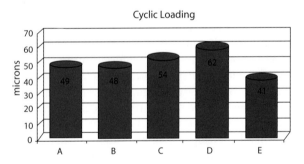

Fig. 2. Mean micromotion after cyclical loading, 5,000 cycles

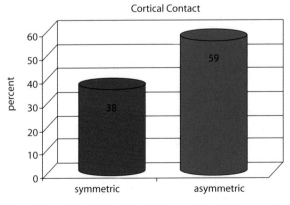

Fig. 3. Comparison of mean cortical contact between symmet-ric and asymmetric designs, p<0.05

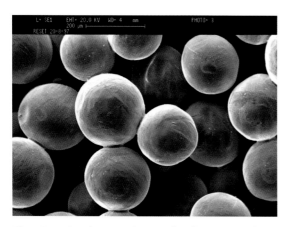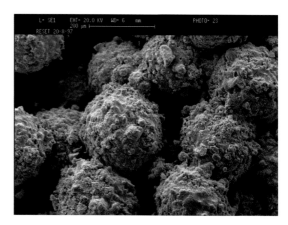

Fig. 4. Scanning electron micrographs of Porocoat and Porocoat with hydrosyapatite (Duofix) coating surfaces

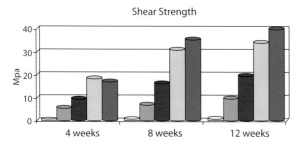

Fig. 5. Shear strength of push-out specimens

bination for providing early, reliable and potentially longlasting ingrowth.

We looked at five different surface coatings, first in a titanium alloy, and later manufactured of cobalt chrome [11]. The coatings were: highly polished, grit blasted, grit blasted with hydroxyapatite, Porocoat and Porocoat with hydroxyapatite (Fig. 4). Small dowels (15×6 mm) were implanted in a randomized location in a bilateral bicortical sheep tibia model. Specimens were harvested at 4, 8 and 12 weeks, and split for examination by histology and for mechanical testing of push out strength.

The result of this investigation was that the shear strength with the highly polished surfaces was close to zero (Fig. 5). The grit blasted and Porocoat surfaces had progressively higher push out shear strength at all time points. The addition of hydroxyapatite improved this shear strength, and the improvement was greater for the grit blasted surface than for the Porocoat, although not statistically significant for either.

In addition to the shear strength information, histological evaluation of the fracture planes revealed that the junction between the new woven bone and hydroxyapatite was very strong, and tended to remain together during fracture propogation. The fracture planes in the hydroxyapatite coated specimens was at the junction of the mature lamellar bone, and the new woven bone. The

result was the rapid development of a strong interface in the hydroxyapatite coated specimens.

This cortical model does not reproduce the exact conditions found under the tibial surface, that is predominantly cancellous bone. An ovarectomized sheep model is being developed to simulate those conditions, and may demonstrate some differences in the mechanics or histology of that clinical condition. However, the bone healing environment adjacent to the hydroxyapatite is similar to those seen in other studies, and correlates with the clinical work we have done, that also shows very reliable early fixation with this surface coating.

4   Clinical Experience

We have had a long experience with the use of cementless tibial components, including the PCA, Miller Galante and Miller Galante II implants. The MG and MGII tibial components gave excellent clinical results with high ingrowth rates, particularly using hydroxyapatite coated MG II implants. However, the development of osteolysis associated with polyethylene wear that has been described around these and other tibial components fixed with screws is of concern to us [7].

We have therefore been using a cementless component that is stabilized using a combination of pegs and a stem, with the Porocoat and hydroxyapatite coating (Duofix), and that does not require any holes on the surface of the tibial component that may permit the egress of polyethylene particles (Fig. 6). We have been very satisfied with this implant. It demonstrates excellent stability at the time of implantation, even in relatively osteoporotic bone. We use cementless fixation in virtually all of our patients, regardless of age or bone quality.

We have been using this implant since November 1995, and have now implanted 570 components. We performed 337 of these prior to January 1999. All our patients are reviewed annually or bi-annually, and clinical and radiographic information is stored on a relational database. The mean age of these first 337 cases was 71 years, with a wide range from 42 to 97 years, reflecting our preference for cementless fixation in all age groups, including the elderly and osteoporotic. Diagnosis in the majority of these cases was osteoarthritis (94%), with a smaller number of patients having inflammatory arthropathy (6%).

Tibial bone quality as assessed subjectively at the time of surgery was judged to be good in 84% of patients, and fair or poor in 8% each. Medial bone defects associated with excessive wear were documented in 2% of cases. These defects were reconstructed by minimally increased tibial resection, and occasional augmentation with cancellous grafting under the tibial component in more severe cases.

One patient required revision 12 months following her surgery, for persistent flexion contracture. She had a well fixed tibial component, and was revised to another identical implant after further resection of the proximal tibia, with good result.

Follow up radiographic evaluation of this series has demonstrated excellent ingrowth of the implants, with

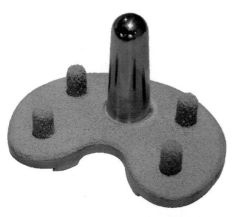

Fig. 6. Duofix Cementless Tibial Component, with Porocoat and HA

only one patient having persistent radiolucency under the tibial component. This patient was felt to have fibrous ingrowth, and was having pain.

Apart from this single case of radiolucency developing under the tibial component, we have seen the occasional radiolucent line (1%) develop under the medial aspect of the tibial component on the A/P view. This has been in cases where resection was performed through very sclerotic bone, and we feel it reflects local necrosis of the bone in the first few weeks after surgery. These lucencies have all stabilized within a few months, and have shown no evidence of progression (Fig. 7).

Other than these few instances of radiolucent line formation, there has been no indication of loss of fixation in any implant in this series. The typical appearance is of osseointegration of the undersurface of the tray, and the area around the pegs. We expected a fibrous line to develop around the highly polished stem, similar to that seen around polished stems of hip arthroplasty, the so called 'tree in the wind' sign. This has not occurred in more than a few cases, and may be related to the loading conditions on the tibial component, that are more axial compressive than bending.

Radiographic examination of our cases is done with screened fluoroscopic views, and this produces true tangential views of the undersurface of the tray. This appearance of ingrowth has been consistent out to our longest current radiographic follow up of 5 years (Fig. 8). The bone ingrowth rate for these implants was 99.5%. In addition, there has been no osteolysis in these cases to date, although follow up is somewhat short for this assessment.

We have had a further failure of fixation in an implant performed recently. A 95 year old osteoporotic patient has had anterior subsidence of the tibial component between 2 and 4 months after surgery. This was most probably due to technical error, with inadequate coverage of the anterior tibia at the index surgery.

We feel that polyethylene wear continues to be the Achilles' heel of knee arthroplasty, and are now using mobile bearing arthroplasty in an effort to reduce polyethylene stress, and hopefully, wear. The fixation tech-

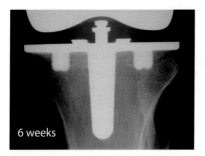
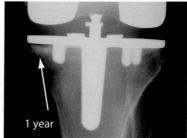
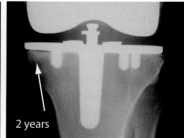

Fig. 7. Development of medial lucency under tibial component, stable

Fig. 8. Typical appearance of ingrown implant at 5 years

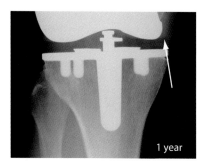
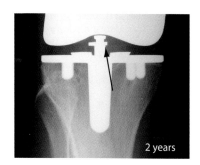

1 year

2 years

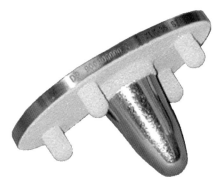

Fig. 9. Duofix MBT Cementless Tibial Component

nique that we have developed is well suited to this type of implant, as it can be performed without the need for additional screw fixation. We are currently using a similar design cementless tibial component, in conjunction with the LCS knee system, with excellent early results (Fig. 9).

5 Patellar Fixation

Cementless fixation of the patella has been plagued with spectacular failures in a small number of specific designs. Our experience with the Miller Galante cementless component, similar to others with the same implant [9], has demonstrated failure from wear through of the polyethylene, and resulting articulation of the metal backing and the femoral component. This typically produces audible squeaking, severe metallosis, and femoral component damage requiring exchange at the time of revision. Although this experience has given us cause for concern in using metal backed patellar components, many other designs have had far superior results in relation to fixation, and lack of wear through or failure [2].

One of these implants is the metal backed mobile bearing component in the LCS system, and is now our preferred component for patellar resurfacing. It has a long history of success, with very low failure rates.

6 Conclusions

Our experience with cementless fixation in knee arthroplasty has been quite favorable, but depends on proper implant selection, and attention to initial stability of tibial and femoral components. In the presence of good initial stability, implants with a reliable ingrowth surface, particularly when augmented by hydroxyapatite, provide consistent fixation, and this fixation is durable. There is no reason to believe that this fixation will not be adequate to support even the young high demand patient, in the absence of polyethylene wear and osteolysis.

References

1. Bobyn J, Cameron H, Abdulla D, Pilliar R, Weatherly G (1982) Biologic fixation and bone modeling with an unconstrained canine total knee prosthesis. Clin Orthop 166: 301–312
2. Buechel F, Rosa R, Pappas M (1989) A metal-backed, rotating-bearing patellar prosthesis to lower contact stress. An 11-year clinical study. Clin Orthop 248: 34–49
3. Campbell M, Duffy G, Trousdale R (1998) Femoral component failure in hybrid total knee arthroplasty. Clin Orthop 356: 58–65
4. Dempsey A, Finlay J, Bourne R, Rorabeck C, Scott M, Millman J (1989) Stability and anchorage considerations for cementless tibial components. J Arthroplasty 4(3): 223–230
5. Geesink R, de Groot K, Klein C (1987) Chemical implant fixation using hydroxyl-apatite coatings. The development of a human total hip prosthesis for chemical fixation to bone using hydroxyl-apatite coatings on titanium substrates. Clin Orthop 225: 147–170
6. Kershner J, Walsh W, Zicat B, Walters B (2000) Micromotion of cementless tibial components. Crit Rev Biomed Eng 28(1–2): 17–22
7. Lewis P, Rorabeck C, Bourne R (1995) Screw osteolysis after cementless total knee replacement. Clin Orthop 321: 173–177
8. Mintzer C, Robertson D, Rackemann S, Ewald F, Scott R, Spector M (1990) Bone loss in the distal anterior femur after total knee arthroplasty. Clin Orthop 260: 135–143
9. Rorabeck C, Bourne R, Lewis P, Nott L (1993) The Miller-Galante knee prosthesis for the treatment of osteoarthrosis. A comparison of the results of partial fixation with cement and fixation without any cement. J Bone Joint Surg Am 75(3): 402–408

10. Schmalzried T, Jasty M, Harris W (1992) Periprosthetic bone loss in total hip arthroplasty. Polyethylene wear debris and the concept of the effective joint space. J Bone Joint Surg Am 74(6): 849–863

11. Svehla M, Morberg P, Zicat B, Bruce W, Sonnabend D, Walsh W (2000) Morphometric and mechanical evaluation of titanium implant integration: comparison of five surface structures. J Biomed Mater Res 51(1): 15–22

Chapter 21
New Materials for Mobile Bearing Knee Prosthesis – Titanium Nitride Counterface Coatings for Reduction of Polyethylene Wear

V.C. Jones, D.D. Auger, M.H. Stone, J. Fisher

1 Introduction

Wear of polyethylene is widely recognized as a cause of osteolysis and failure in artificial hip joints [2]. Recent studies of tissues surrounding knee prosthesis [1] have shown the accumulation of micron and sub micron size polyethylene wear debris, at similar levels to that found in the hip, hence indicating the potential for longer term osteolysis. In the hip damage or scratching to the femoral counterface has been shown to accelerate polyethylene wear [6] and it is now recommended to use alumina ceramic femoral heads, which are more damage resistant and can deliver lower long term wear rates [5]. Similar damage has been found in knees [4]. The complexity of the femoral and tibial tray geometries in the knee do not readily lend themselves for replacement of the metallic bearing counterfaces with monolithic ceramic materials. An alternative approach is to modify the polished metallic bearing surface with hard smooth 'ceramic like' coatings.

A further complication in total knee replacement is that a small percentage of patients experience some degree of nickel sensitivity. This precludes them from receiving a standard Cobalt Chromium (CoCr) alloyed component. Finding an alternative bearing surface for these patients, which performs as well as CoCr in vivo was an additional goal of the study.

The main aim of this study was to investigate the application of Titanium Nitride TiN coatings to femoral and tibial counterfaces for the reduction of polyethylene wear under standard conditions and conditions that simulate the presence of third body counterface damage.

2 Materials and Methods

Arc Evaporation Physical Vapour Deposition (AEPVD) Titanium Nitride (TiN) coating were laid down on polished metallic substrates. The thickness of the titanium

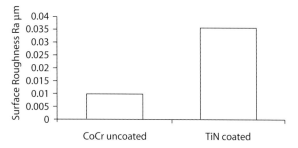

Fig. 1. Surface roughness Ra of the uncoated and TiN coated counterface

nitride coating was 8 m. After coating the surface roughness was increased considerably due to the formation of micro droplets. Post coating polishing was carried out to remove the droplets and to produce a smoother surface. Figure 1 shows the surface roughness Ra of the Cobalt Chrome uncoated counterfaces and the TiN coated counterfaces.

3 The Wear

GUR1050 ultrahigh molecular weight polyethylene sterilized with gas plasma was studied when sliding against the uncoated and coated metallic counterfaces. Polyethylene wear specimens were made in the form of 20 mm diameter pins, which were slid against the uncoated and coated metallic counterfaces. The counterfaces were tested in their smooth conditions and additionally with deliberate scratching to simulate third body damage.

A new multidirectional wear test methodology has been developed [3] to simulate wear on mobile bearing knees. It consisted of a reciprocating motion of the plate (±10 mm) and a separate rotation of ±8 degrees of the polyethylene pin. A load of 180 N was applied to each pin, which produced a contact stress of 0.6 MPa. Tests were run for 1.4 million cycles or 25 km. Measurements of wear were made every 300,000 cycles. Tests were carried out in a 25 % solution of new born calf serum, which was also changed every 300,000 cycles. Three replicates of the polymer pins were slid on each of the uncoated and coated counterfaces initially when smooth and then subsequently when deliberately scratched. Wear surfaces were analyzed at the beginning and end of tests using both non-contacting white light interferometry, contacting Talysurf and SEM. Wear was determined gravimetrically and expressed as volume wear rate mm³ per million cycles.

4   Results

The relative wear rates of the polyethylene sliding against the smooth uncoated and Titanium Nitride coated counterfaces are shown in Fig. 2.

The wear rate on the TiN coated counterface was higher than on the uncoated counterface. The difference was not statistically significant. The increase in wear found on the coated surface is explained by the surface roughness values given in Figure 1. Although the TiN coating were polished after coating the final surface roughness was not as low as the original uncoated surface. The coefficient of friction on the TiN coated surface was slightly lower than the uncoated surface (Fig. 3).

The scratches to replicate third body damage were produced with a 2 N load on a 40 m radius diamond stylus. Scratches were applied in the direction of sliding.

Figure 4 shows the height Rp of the scratches on the uncoated and coated counterfaces. The TiN was much harder than the substrate alone and the resulting scratch damage was much less with much lower values of Rp. When polyethylene pins were worn on the scratched surfaces, the wear rate on the uncoated surface increased significantly and was much higher than on the scratched coated counterface (Fig. 5).

The hard TiN coating provided resistance to third body scratching and this resulted in lower polyethylene wear rates compared to the uncoated counterface.

5   Discussion

The wear of polyethylene and the potential for wear debris induced osteolysis remains a long term potential concern for the survivorship of artificial knee joints. A low contact stress multidirectional wear model of mobile bearing knees has been developed [3]. The model which applies a load of 180 N is effectively a one fifth scale model of the mobile bearing knee. The wear rates in this model can be multiplied by a factor of five to achieve an approximate prediction of wear in a total knee replacement.

Retrieved knee prosthesis have shown evidence of scratching on both the femoral counterface and tibial tray [4]. In the hip, resistance to this scratching is achieved through the use of alumina ceamic femoral heads [5], and this is predicted to reduce long term wear

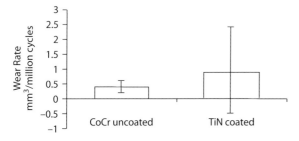

Fig. 2. Wear rate of polyethylene against the uncoated and TiN coated counterfaces

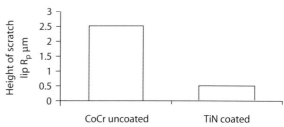

Fig. 4. Height of the scratch lips Rp for the uncoated and TiN coated counterface

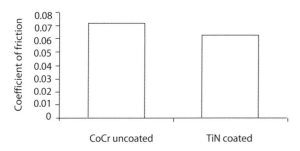

Fig. 3. Coefficient of friction for the uncoated and TiN coated counterfaces

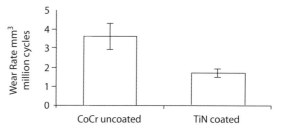

Fig. 5. Wear rate of polyethylene on the scratched uncoated and scratched TiN coated counterfaces

rates of polyethylene. In the knee monolithic ceramic components are not available and the use of ceramic surface coatings is of interest. The surface roughness of the coating is important, as the increase in roughness after coating (see Fig. 1) can lead to an increase in polyethylene wear (see Fig. 2). The benefit of the coating is shown in its resistance to scratching (see Fig. 4). Under these conditions of simulated third body scratching the wear rate of the polyethylene in the TiN coated surfaces with smaller scratch lips was significantly less than on the scratched, uncoated Cobalt Chrome counterface. Ceramic like coatings have the potential to reduce long term wear in knee prosthesis.

Acknowledgement: V.C. Jones was supported by an EPSRC Case Studentship and by DePuy International.

References

1. Howling GI, Barnett PI, Tipper JL, Stone MH, Fisher J, Ingham E (2001) Quantitative characterization of polyethylene debris isolated from periprosthetic tissue in early failure knee implants and early and late failure Charnley hip implants. J Biomed Mater Res 58: 415–420
2. Ingham E, Fisher J (1999) Biological reactions to wear debris in total joint replacement. Proc Instn Mech Engrs 214 H: 21–37
3. Jones VC, Barton DC, FitzPatrick DP, Auger DD, Stone MH, Fisher J (1999) An experimental model of tibial counterface polyethylene wear in mobile bearing knees: The influence of design and kinematics. Biomed Mater Eng 9: 189–196
4. Jones VC, Williams IR, Auger DD, Walsh W, Barton DC, Stone MH, Fisher J (2001) Quantification of third body damage to the tibial counterface in mobile bearing knees. Proc Instn Mech Engrs 215 H: 171–179
5. Minakawa H, Stone MH, Wroblewski BM, Lancaster JG, Ingham E, Fisher J (1998) Quantification of third-body damage and its effect on UHMWPE wear with different types of femoral head. J Bone Joint Surg 80-B: 894–899
6. Tipper JL, Ingham E, Hailey JL, Besong AA, Fisher J, Wroblewski BM, Stone MH (2000) Quantitative analysis of polyethylene wear debris, wear rate and head damage in retrieved Charnley hip prostheses. Materials Science, Materials in Medicine 11: 117–124

Chapter 22
Minimally Invasive Unicompartmental Knee

D. A. Fisher, G. C. Keene

1 Historical Review of Unicompartmental Knee Arthroplasty (UKA)

The treatment of gonarthrosis with unicompartmental knee resurfacing dates back to the 1950's with the McKeever and MacIntosh metallic interpositional arthroplasties [14, 16].

Satisfactory clinical results with unicompartmental replacement have been documented in numerous early publications [6, 9, 15]. Problems encountered in these early series have been attributed to poor patient selection, poor implant positioning, and disease progression in the unresurfaced compartments.

The indications for unicompartmental replacement have been controversial. General recommendations have included: Age over 60 years, weight less than 82 kg (180 pounds), low or moderate activity level, noninflammatory arthropathy, no pain at rest, less than 5 degree flexion contracture, and less than 15 degree of correctable angular deformity [13]. The reported short term benefits of UKA are not without recognition. Less bone resection leads to less blood loss and need for transfusion. Rehabilitation has been more rapid and range of motion is superior with UKA compared with TKA [4, 17]. In addition, although we are aware of no large series that confirms our suspicion, the authors have seen lower incidences of deep venous thrombosis and sepsis with UKA compared to their TKA population. These findings have lent support to the continued use of UKA for unicompartmental gonarthrosis.

2 Technical Issues Leading to Success or Failure

Implant thickness of over 6 mm has been recommended as a minimum for prosthetic design. Proper implant position and joint restoration will also dictate long term results. Prior to 1980, instrumentation for performing a UKA was crude or nonexistent and the removal of bone and implant insertion left to the skill of the operating surgeon. For varus knees, the best results have been noted with slight under correction of the deformity [5, 12]. Furthermore, tibial bone resection and seating of the implant on the cortical rim has been more reproducible than burring and insetting the implant into the tibial bone [18].

Fixation of the tibial component has been enhanced with pegs or keels on the undersurface of the component.

Polyethylene wear has been a major concern for arthroplasty engineers and surgeons. In fixed bearing UKA, the best results have been obtained with a relatively flat articular surface manufactured from an all polyethylene component greater than 6 mm thick. The LCS and Oxford designs utilize a conforming polyethylene bearing that moves on a track or plate [7, 10]. These implants have been shown to reduce polyethylene wear and breakage.

On the femoral side, implants have been designed to mimic the sagittal condylar anatomy. The use of 1 or 2 pegs on the bone surface has provided satisfactory stability and allowed long-term fixation when used with polymethylmethacrylate. The coronal articular surface of the femur has varied from flat to curved in geometry. Flat articular implants can cause edge loading if malaligned and have been a cause of failure. For this reason, most contemporary implants incorporate a curved coronal cross section at the articular surface. While this causes fairly high polyethylene stresses by reducing the contact area, it is more tolerant of errors in component position.

In general, perioperative complications with UKA through a parapatellar arthrotomy are less than TKA through a comparable incision. The most common cause for a second surgery is wear of a polyethylene liner on a metal tibial base plate. Range of motion has been excellent (average 122 degrees of flexion) and knee scores have been maintained over 10 years.

3 The LCS UKA Experience

The designers of the original LCS total knee replacement first implanted the unicompartmental LCS in

1977. The design of the femoral component features the same progressively diminishing radius of curvature as is seen in the LCS total knee replacement. The tibial platform contains a dovetail track to allow anteroposterior (A/P) movement of the meniscus bearing but also to inhibit dislocation. This permitted A-P movement again closely follows the kinematics of the normal meniscus. The LCS UKA can be used easily on either the medial or lateral side of the joint (Fig. 1, 2, 3, 4).

These design features of the LCS UKA are different from the only other widely used mobile bearing knee – the Oxford.

In 1990 Buechel, Keblish, Lee and Papas presented their successful LCS UKA results to the AAOS and this was published in 1994 [3].

In the LCS UKA surgical procedure manual written by Briard, Keblish and Buechel the authors emphasize that avoiding lengthy releases and balancing flexion and

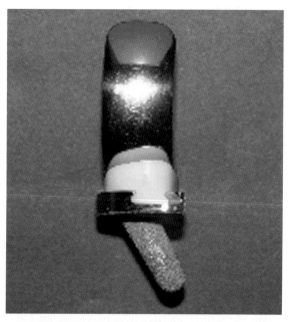

Fig. 1. AP view of LCS UKA

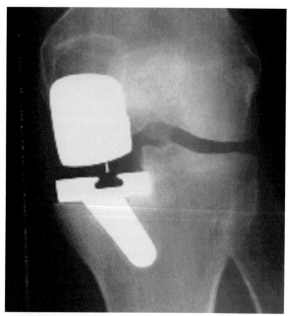

Fig. 3. AP radiograph LCS UKA

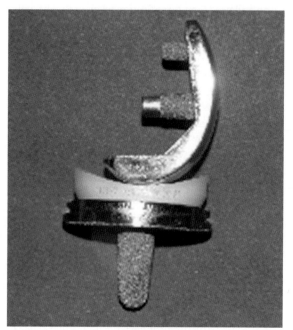

Fig. 2. Lateral view of LCS UKA

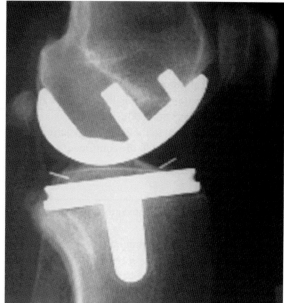

Fig. 4. Lateral radiograph LCS UKA

extension gaps are important principals. They also state that the cruciates should be intact and the MCL normal or minimally contracted. They emphasize correcting alignment to *normal ligament tension* and avoiding over correction and over load of the opposite compartment. They further state that physiological valgus (mechanical axis) is desirable *but should not be forced.*

One of us (GK) has performed 448 open LCS unicompartmental knee replacements between March 1994 and August 2000. A review of 100 of those patients 5 years post surgery (unpublished data) revealed 88% good to excellent results. There was a mean range of motion of 3 to 126 degrees. There were 6 complications (1 tibial loosening, 1 fracture of the medial tibial plateau, 2 with residual varus and pain, 2 deep venous thrombosis with pulmonary embolus). The first 4 were successfully revised to total knee prostheses without any major surgical difficulty confirming other authors reports that revision of a UKA is similar to a primary total knee replacement.

The most striking feature or our LCS experience is the significant improvement in range of motion achieved with many patients achieving a normal or near normal range in marked contrast to TKR patients where this is rarely the case. Buechel et al. who had 122 degrees in the cementless group and 123 degrees in the cemented group also reported this feature. We have also seen a progressive reduction in length of hospital stay through our LCS experience and this has at all times been about half the length of stay of TKA patients.

4   Overview of Minimally Invasive Surgery

Interest in unicompartmental replacement has increased recently with the era of minimally invasive surgical procedures. Compared to the standard parapatellar arthrotomy required for a TKA, the minimally invasive concept works well with UKA. The size of the implants and the limited bone work allow much smaller incisions to perform the procedure. This has further shortened hospital stay and facilitated rehabilitation. In fact, many of these procedures can now be performed in an outpatient surgical setting. While a great deal of public interest has been generated over the concept, little or no data is available yet on the perioperative complications and long term results of these minimally invasive procedures.

Concerns over minimally invasive UKA procedures include limited visibility, bone preparation techniques, accuracy of implant placement, removal of PMMA debris, and soft tissue balancing. Clearly the greatest concerns regard access to adequately perform the procedure. With the limited visibility of a smaller incision, instrumentation to help the surgeon perform the procedure becomes a necessity. Preparation of bone surfaces, implant alignment, and joint line restoration are key determinants of long term success. The ability to achieve these goals with accuracy and consistency must be proven for the minimally invasive UKA to become a common procedure.

5   Preoperative Planning

X-ray templating of the AP and lateral X-rays before surgery provides an estimate of minimal tibial cut thickness (depending on prosthesis choice), femoral component size and A/P slope of the tibial cut which significantly affects the flexion gap.

6   Instruments and Prostheses

We both started performing minimally invasive UKA (MIU) with a fixed bearing UKA implant in 2000. At the same time, we were members of an 8 surgeon international team developing a new MIU called the *Preservation MIU* (DePuy) which includes the unique use of a fixed or mobile bearing tibial component. This implant uses a universal femoral component that is based on the LCS design, and a fixed or mobile tibial implant. Instrumentation for this knee was designed for use with a minimally invasive surgical approach, using principles of flexion and extension gap balancing and minimal bone resection to accommodate the implants.

Instrumentation for this system uses extramedullary alignment guides and reduced profile cutting jigs to prepare the bone surfaces for the implants. A unique set of instruments allows accurate placement of the joint line and flexion/extension gap balancing for optimal kinematics.

7   Surgical Approach

The surgical approach for a minimally invasive UKA includes either a straight longitudinal medial or lateral parapatellar incision. For a medial UKA, this should extend from the superomedial border of the patella to the superomedial border of the tibial tubercle. The medial retinaculum, fat pad, and synovium are opened in line with the skin incision, approximately 1 cm from the medial patellar border. The meniscus is divided and the meniscotibial attachment is released to facilitate exposure. A curved retractor placed between the bone and

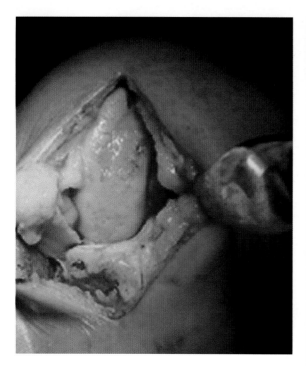

Fig. 5. Minimally invasive knee exposure

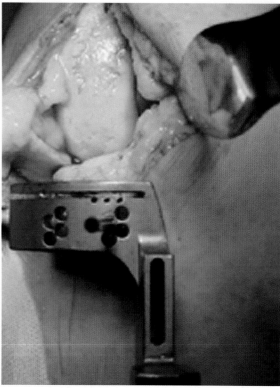

Fig. 6. Tibial cutting guide

the medial collateral ligament protects the ligament during bone preparation. A blunt retractor placed in the intercondylar notch allows leverage on the patella to facilitate medial compartment exposure (Fig. 5). While the patellofemoral joint is readily visible with this approach, the lateral compartment can only be partially visualized. In the event significant damage is present in the patellofemoral or lateral compartments, the incision can be extended proximally and distally to allow a standard parapatellar arthrotomy and perform a TKA.

A minimally invasive lateral UKA requires a lateral arthrotomy. While similar to the medial approach, the retinacular incision may require subcutaneous proximal extension by one or two centimeters to allow medial mobilization of the patella. Again, carefully placed retractors beneath the lateral collateral ligament and in the intercondylar notch allow adequate exposure for the procedure. As the patellofemoral and medial compartments are more difficult to visualize with the lateral approach, the use of an arthroscope can facilitate the evaluation of these compartments prior to performing the arthrotomy. If there is significant disease in the medial or patellofemoral joint mitigating against UKA, then one can proceed to a medial arthrotomy and TKA.

Using the surgical approach previously described, the tibial resection is performed with the aid of an extramedullary cutting guide. This guide allows multidirectional adjustment to create a resection that is perpen-

dicular to the tibial axis in the AP plane, and follows the anatomic posterior slope of the tibia. The depth of resection is controlled by the use of a stylus that contacts the tibial articular surface (Fig. 6).

The next instrument assesses the flexion gap and establishes the joint line. This is a combination spacer and distal femoral cutting guide. With the knee at 90 degrees of flexion, the 7, 9, or 11 mm spacer is placed between the resected tibia and the posterior femoral condyle (Fig. 7). In a knee with medial compartment disease, the damage is usually distal on the condyle with minimal damage to the posterior condyle. Therefore, assessing tibial implant thickness and establishing joint line position is appropriate at this time. For a fixed bearing *Preservation* UKA, tibial implant thickness of 7, 9, 11, or 13 mm are available. Mobile bearing options are 9, 11, and 13 mm.

Once the appropriate thickness of tibial component is chosen, the knee is brought out to full extension. The extension gap is now assessed with the spacer in place. If the knee is loose in extension, shims can be added to the spacer to tighten up the extension gap and lower the distal femoral resection. A modular alignment rod now allows assessment of overall limb alignment and component position in both the AP and ML planes. Once appropriate adjustments have been made, the cutting block is secured and the distal femur can be resected.

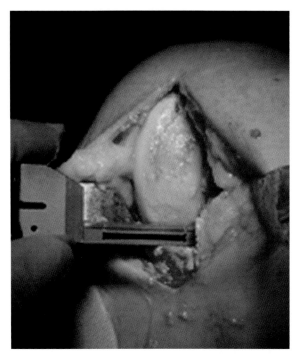

Fig. 7. Combination spacer and distal femoral cutting guide

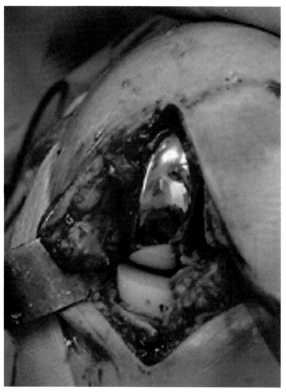

Fig. 8. Implanted UKA

Some surgeons may prefer to assess the extension gap first and 'fit' the flexion gap by shaving the posterior aspect of the femoral condyle to avoid over resecting the tibia if the flexion gap is tight.

Implant sizing is performed with a combination of preoperative templating and intraoperative assessment. Five sizes of universal femoral components are available. The implants are designed to allow up to 10 degrees of internal or external rotation and maintain the same surface contact with the tibial bearing throughout the range of motion. Once the appropriate femoral size is chosen, holes are drilled through the sizing guide, which will establish AP position and rotation. The correctly sized cutting guide is now used to resect the posterior femoral condyle, the posterior chamfer cut, and the anterior inset. The femoral ML position can now be established for a fixed bearing UKA and a drill hole made for the fixation post on the femoral implant. A slot is then cut for the web on the femoral component. The web provides additional strength to the femoral implant and augments fixation. For the mobile bearing UKA, ML position is determined after the tibial preparation and trials have been inserted and the kinematics assessed.

The tibial implant size is now established with overlay templates. Tibial components are available in 5 sizes. Implant fixation is provided by a keel which is seated into the resected tibia. Bone preparation is performed with a gouge and trial punch. Fixed bearing trials are universal and easily slide under the femoral trial. Mobile bearing trials use a metal base with trial bearings that slide on a curved track. As with the real implants, the mobile bearing tibial trials must be inserted before the femoral component. For the mobile UKA, the ML femoral position is now established and the post and slot prepared.

At this time the knee should be balanced in flexion and extension, allowing full range of knee motion. Trials are removed, bone surfaces prepared, and the implants cemented or press fit into place [Figure 8].

8   Wound Closure

Wound closure requires a few retinacular and subcutaneous sutures, followed by subcuticular or interrupted skin closure. While a tourniquet is recommended to improve visibility and enhance PMMA fixation, the use of drains may not be required after this procedure.

9   Rehabilitation

Ambulation with physiotherapy assistance is possible on the day of or day after surgery. Very early discharge from hospital at 1 to 3 days after surgery is possible depending on surgeon, hospital and patient preferences.

We emphasize early achievement of full range of motion and limit heavy or prolonged weight bearing for 6 weeks to facilitate prosthesis bone integration. Some patients will need outpatient physiotherapy to achieve their goals.

10 Differences between Minimally Invasive and Open UKA

Apart from the obvious and major differences of reduced wound length and hospital stay, we have recorded a significant reduction in post operative analgesic requirements and improved early range of motion. Several patients having the minimally invasive Preservation UKA who have had a previous open UKA on their opposite knee have commented that they much prefer the new knee for recovery and function.

11 Early Experience with Preservation UKA

Between us we have performed approximately 150 Preservation UKA's in a 12 month period.

We have found the instrumentation easy to use and provide reliable alignment, joint level, ligament tension and prosthesis component alignment. The fixed and mobile bearing implants have been equally successful in ease of use after the learning curve of several cases.

The Preservation instrument accuracy and choice of bearing insert depending on individual patient needs and surgeon preference, separate the Preservation UKA from all other UKA designs and have enabled us to achieve superior results to other Minimally Invasive UKA implants that we have used.

Postoperative wound healing and early ambulation and return to work and sport easily surpass the result we achieved with open UKA.

12 Summary

In summary, the technology now exists to allow reliable and reproducible minimally invasive unicompartmental knee arthroplasty. Improved implants and instrumentation should provide better long term results. In the future, computer assisted surgery will become more common in orthopedic procedures. One area of application will be arthroplasty surgery. Minimally invasive UKA would seem to be an operation ideally suited to the technology. Computer guidance in bone resection planes, joint line positioning, and implant placement

could significantly improve reproducibility and reliability of these procedures. We look forward to the exploration and development of this technology in the coming years.

References

1. Bernasek T Rand JA, Bryan RS (1988) Unicompartmental porous coated anatomic total knee arthroplasty. Clin Orthop 236: 52–59
2. Bert J (1991) Universal intramedullary instrumentation for unicompartmental total knee arthroplasty. Clin Orthop 271: 79–87
3. Buechel FF et al. (1994) Low contact stress meniscal bearing unicompartmental knee replacement: Long term evaluation of cemented and cementless results. J Orthop Rheumatol 7: 31–41
4. Callahan CM, Drake BG, Heck DA, Dittus RS (1995) Patient outcomes following unicompartmental or bicompartmental knee arthroplasty: A meta-analysis. J Arthroplasty 10(2): 141–150
5. Cartier P Sanouiller JL, Grelsamer RP (1996) Unicompartmental knee arthroplasty surgery: Ten-year minimum follow-up period. J Arthroplasty 11(7): 782–788
6. Christensen NO (1991) Unicompartmental prosthesis for gonarthrosis. A nine-year series of 575 knees from a Swedish hospital. Clin Orthop 273: 165–169
7. Cohen M, Buechel F, Pappas MF (1991) Meniscal-bearing unicompartmental knee arthroplasty. An 11-year clinical study. Orthop Rev 20(5): 443–448
8. Engh G Dwyer KA, Hanes CK (1992) Polyethylene wear of metal-backed tibial components in total and unicompartmental knee prostheses. J Bone Joint Surg 74(1): 9–17
9. Engelbrecht E, Siegel A, Rottger J, Buchholz HW (1976) Statistics of total knee replacement; partial and total knee replacement, design St. Georg: A review of a 4-year observation. Clin Orthop 120: 54–64
10. Goodfellow MS, O'Connor BE (1986) Clinical results of the Oxford knee. Surface arthroplasty of the tibiofemoral joint with a meniscal bearing prosthesis. Clin Orthop 205: 21–42
11. Insall JN, Aglietti P (1980) A five-to-seven year follow-up of unicondylar arthroplasty. J Bone Joint Surg 62 A: 1329–1337
12. Kennedy W, White R (1987) Unicompartmental arthroplasty of the knee. Postoperative alignment and its influence on overall results. Clin Orthop 221: 278–285
13. Kozinn SC, Scott RD (1989) Current concepts review: Unicondylar knee arthroplasty. J Bone Joint Surg 71 A: 145–150
14. MacIntosh DL (1958) Hemiarthroplasty of the knee using a space occupying prosthesis for painful varus and valgus deformities. J Bone Joint Surg 40-A: 1431
15. Marmor L (1988) Unicompartmental knee arthroplasty: Ten-to 13-year follow-up study. Clin Orthop 226: 14–20
16. McKeever DC (1960) Tibial plateau prosthesis. Clin Orthop 18: 86–95
17. Rougraff BT, Heck DA, Gibson AE (1991) A comparison of tricompartmental and unicompartmental arthroplasty for the treatment of gonarthrosis. Clin Orthop 273: 157–164
18. Swank M, Stulberg SD, Jiganti J, Machairas S (1993) The natural history of unicompartmental arthroplasty; An eight-year follow-up study with survivorship analysis. Clin Orthop 286: 130–142

Chapter 23
The Modular LCS Patella Femoral Joint Replacement

A. C. Merchant

1 Introduction

A new modular prosthesis has been designed to treat severely disabled patients who have isolated end-stage arthrosis or failed surgeries of the patellofemoral joint. The younger patients of this group are not good candidates for total knee arthroplasty, and the older patients will benefit from replacement of only those joint surfaces that are damaged. Because this new prosthesis was designed to be modular with the LSC total knee system, it has an important advantage. Some patients who have had successful operations using this modular design will require revision to a total knee arthroplasty in the future due to deterioration of the femorotibial compartments. At that revision surgery, only the trochlear component will need to be removed and replaced by an LCS femoral component. The patellar component can be left intact because it has been designed to articulate exactly with the new femoral component, thus eliminating the high risks and complications associated with patellar component revision.

Eight patients who have had total patellofemoral arthroplasty using this new design have been followed more than two years (24 to 45 months). Seven patients (88%) had excellent or good results, and one was fair. Based on the success of this small initial sample, and the fact that any one surgeon does not perform total patellofemoral arthroplasty frequently, the current author has started a prospective multicenter outcome study. This prospective protocol will use data gathered in a similar manner, the same outcome instrument to measure knee function, and a common database.

2 Design Considerations

During the last two decades various authors [1, 2,4, 6, 9, 11, 16] have reported on three different designs of patellofemoral prostheses. The good or excellent results ranged from a low of 45% [16] to a high of 96% [9]. A careful review of these studies showed that implant design and patient selection are the two most important factors for success.

None of these earlier patellofemoral prostheses have been designed to be modular with a total knee replacement system in order to take advantage of safer and easier revision surgery should it be needed in the future.

Patients disabled by isolated patellofemoral arthritis and failed patellofemoral surgeries tend to be much younger than patients considered to be good candidates for total knee arthroplasty (TKA). Their relative youth demands a prosthetic design that will provide maximum longevity and survivorship. The LCS rotating patella [5] has the best long-term survivorship, greater than 99% at 12-year follow-up, as well as the lowest reported complication rate, 0.9% [8]. The current author modified the polyethylene bearing for use as a patellofemoral implant. Then a trochlear component (Fig. 1) was designed to articulate exactly with that patellar component. This new combination for total patellofemoral arthroplasty (TPFA) takes advantage of the design features that has led to such excellent survivorship and freedom from complications. These design features are:

- An anatomic trochlear groove that is deeper than most other implants, reducing the risk of patellar dislocation.
- Components with broad and congruent area contact loading, as opposed to point or line contact loading, reducing the wear rate.
- The self-aligning feature of the rotating patellar bearing that reduces stress on the bone-implant interface, reducing the risk of loosening.

However, the most important feature of this new prosthesis is the modularity designed into the trochlear component. If a patient with this prosthesis should require revision to a TKA in the future due to deterioration of the femorotibial compartments, then the troch-

Fig. 1. Trochlear components of the modular LCS patello-femoral prosthesis showing the articular surface (left) and the reverse with the three fixation pins (right)

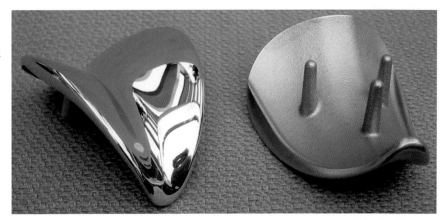

Fig. 2. An LCS femoral component (left) and the modular LCS patellofemoral joint prosthesis (right) demonstrating the modularity of all the components

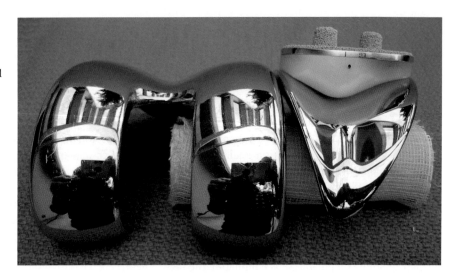

lear component can be removed and the femoral component of the LCS knee system can be implanted, leaving the patellar component intact (Fig. 2). This is not just a theoretical advantage. Berry and Rand [3] have shown that patellar revision has an unacceptably high complication rate of 33%. The new modular knee replacement system avoids this source of complications. Furthermore, the rotating polyethylene bearing can be snapped off from its base plate and exchanged for a new one if wear is found. If a size change is planned, a custom bearing can be ordered.

The trochlear component is inlaid flush with the remaining normal joint surfaces after preparing the osseous bed with small osteotomes and a motorized burr. It is impacted into position secured by its three small fixation pins and bone cement. Because very little bone is removed for implantation, conversion to a total knee femoral component, if necessary at a later date, will be straightforward.

The patella is implanted in the usual manner using a porous coated, press-fit technique or cement at the surgeon's preference. Because the polyethylene patellar bearing slides off the metallic trochlear component to articulate with the remaining normal femoral cartilage during full flexion, the author has redesigned the shape and contour of this bearing. The superior-inferior dimension of the rotating bearing has been increased somewhat so that the bearing will remain in contact with the metal trochlear implant a little longer during acute knee flexion. The sharp, angular superior and inferior edges of the standard LCS rotating bearing have been rounded off or contoured to avoid gouging the femoral articular cartilage during acute flexion (Fig. 3). Because the polyethylene patellar bearing articulates with normal cartilage in full flexion, all patients are warned repeatedly to avoid weight bearing when the knee is flexed more than 90°, that is, avoid full squatting. Half squats are acceptable.

Fig. 3. The modified LCS rotating patella bearing (left) compared to the standard LCS patella (right). Both shown in a side view from the medial aspect

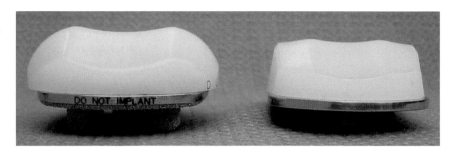

3 Indications

Patellofemoral replacement is a salvage procedure, and patient selection is the single most important factor determining a successful result. There are four major indications for TPFA and all four must be present to qualify a patient for this operation.

- The surgeon must prove that the source of pain is from patellofemoral arthrosis or chondrosis. All other causes for anterior knee pain, such as, tendinitis, neuromata, reflex sympathetic dystrophy, etc., must be ruled out or treated first. The patellar and trochlear damage must be severe, grade III or IV chondromalacia, or true osteoarthrosis. Objective evidence from arthroscopic observation or radiographic joint narrowing, sclerosis, and perhaps osteophytes, must be present.
- The amount of pain must limit the patient's ability to perform the activities of daily living. The goal of TPFA is to return the patient to normal daily activities, not competitive sports.
- The candidate must agree to low demand activities after surgery. Frequently, these patients are relatively young and they tend to over utilize the knee once it is pain free. They must understand the dangers of running, jumping, and squatting. Mild to moderate recreation is allowed, such as, hiking, golf, moderate cycling with the seat adjusted to avoid flexion beyond 90 degrees, and perhaps doubles tennis without tournaments.
- All other alternative treatments must have either been tried and failed or are contraindicated. For instance, a relatively simple lateral release can give significant and long-lasting relief if the patient has a tight lateral retinaculum along with the isolated patellofemoral arthrosis. On the other hand, if the surgeon is considering anterior or anteromedial tibial tubercle transfer, Pidoriano et al. [15] have shown that the presence of proximal patellar articu-

lar lesions is a contraindication to these procedures. In the young patient with patellofemoral plus medial or lateral arthrosis, patellofemoral replacement can be combined with a tibial osteotomy.

4 Contraindications

The usual contraindications for joint replacement also apply to total patellofemoral arthroplasty: infection, reflex sympathetic dystrophy, inflammatory arthritis, and psychogenic pain. Patella infera is a relative contraindication. It must be corrected to normal before the total patellofemoral arthroplasty. If the surgeon has experience with the techniques to correct patella infera and understands the importance of proper extensor mechanism rehabilitatio, these can be performed at the same surgery and the postoperative course modified appropriately.

5 Results

The initial eight patients who met the indications for this new arthroplasty have been followed for an average of 3.8 years (2.5 to 4.25 years). None were lost to follow-up. All were female. The median age at surgery was 47.5 years (range: 26 to 81 years). During hospitalization the patients followed a standard TKA protocol with full weight bearing as tolerated. After discharge, the patients were given a home exercise program to regain knee flexion and quadriceps strength. Understandably, they recovered more rapidly than TKA patients. Because this modular TPFA is a salvage procedure, a simple outcome assessment was used.

- *Excellent:* Able to perform activities of daily living and light recreation using no medication.
- *Good:* Able to perform activities of daily living and light recreation using over-the-counter medications.

- *Fair:* Improved, but still requiring non-narcotic prescription medication for activities of daily living.
- *Poor:* No better, or worse than before surgery.

At the latest follow-up, 7 (88%) patients rated excellent (6) or good (1), and all were very happy with their result. One patient required a prepatellar bursectomy and removal of foreign body suture material under local anesthesia 10 months postoperatively. She continues to have unexplained anterior pain and has a fair result. One patient (Case 1 below) required a patellar tendon lengthening 23 months after her index arthroplasty, changing her good result to excellent. There have been no major complications from the procedure itself, and there have been no implant failures.

6   Illustrative Case Reports

Case 1. A 26-year-old woman had a 6-year history of chronic left anterior knee pain aggravated by an injury 4 years previously. Arthroscopic surgery shortly after that injury revealed a Grade IV lesion of the femoral trochlear cartilage. During the next 4 years she had a total of 5 more unsuccessful surgeries including 2 anteromedializations of the tibial tubercle to treat this severely painful patellofemoral chondrosis. She improved significantly after her modular LCS patellofemoral replacement. Because the severity of a patella infera had not been recognized at the time of her arthroplasty, she required a 1.0 cm Z-plastic patellar tendon lengthening 23 months later, changing her result from good to excellent. At 2.5 years follow-up she is even enjoying mild recreational activities (golf, bicycling, hiking, etc.), without signs of implant loosening or wear.

Case 2. A 41-year-old woman had been involved in sports since childhood and always remembered having had anterior knee pain. She had a solitary dislocation of the right patella at age 14. At age 30 she had a lateral release and patellar exostectomy on the left knee. The diagnosis was bilateral chronic patellar subluxation with secondary patellofemoral arthrosis. A modular LCS patellofemoral replacement on the left produced an excellent result. She has since had the same arthroplasty on the right knee (Fig. 4, 5, 6).

7   Conclusions

The modular LCS patellofemoral arthroplasty offers a more conservative alternative compared to TKA, both for the younger patient for whom TKA is inappropriate and for the older patient who has no disease in the medial or lateral compartments. Laskin and van Steijn [10] and others [13, 14] have advocated TKA for older patients who have only isolated patellofemoral arthritis. It makes no sense to perform a more major operation to remove normal medial and lateral compartments if a less destructive operation, such as TPFA, will provide equally good results.

Based on these encouraging initial results, a prospective multicenter protocol study has been started. Because no one surgeon will perform patellofemoral joint replacement frequently, meaningful numbers of patients cannot be accumulated over a reasonable time without pooled data. All surgeons interested in using this new modular design are being asked to join this prospective study. The data gathering has been simplified to a one-page outcome form. The outcome assessment instrument is a patient-reported Activities of Daily Living (ADL) Scale created by Irrgang et al. [7]. These authors have validated their ADL Scale against the Lysholm Knee Scale and the International Knee Documentation Committee (IKDC) guidelines for global function. Others [12] have confirmed its reliability, validity, and respon-

Fig. 4. The pre-operative axial view radiograph of the right knee of Case No. 2. Diagnosis: chronic subluxation of the patella with secondary patellofemoral osteoarthrosis

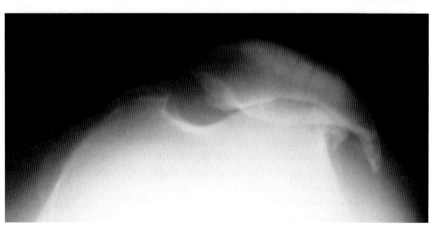

Fig. 5. The post-operative axial view radiograph of the right knee of Case No. 2

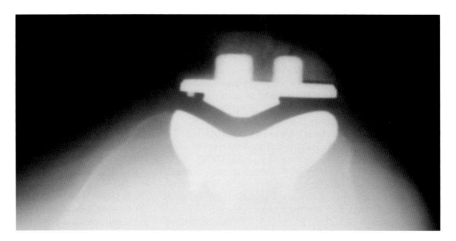

Fig. 6. The post-operative lateral view radiograph of the right knee of Case No. 2

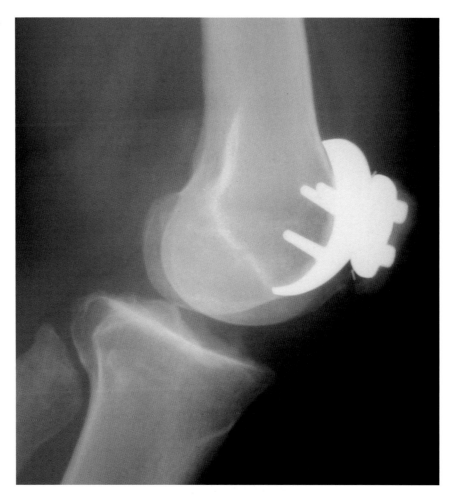

siveness compared to 3 other commonly used knee outcome scales. The ADL Scale expresses the function of the tested knee as a percentage of normal. Pooling this outcome data in a common database will allow a reliable assessment of this new modular LCS patellofemoral joint prosthesis in the future.

References

1. Arciero R, Toomey H (1988) Patellofemoral arthroplasty; a three to nine year follow-up study. Clin Orthop 236: 60–71
2. Argenson J-N A, Guillaume J-M, Aubaniac J-M (1995) Is there a place for patellofemoral arthroplasty? Clin Orthop 321: 162–167

3. Berry DJ, Rand JA (1993) Isolated patellar component revision of total knee arthroplasty. Clin Orthop 286: 110–115
4. Blazina ME, Fox JM, Del Pizzo W, Broukhim B, Ivey FM (1979) Patellofemoral replacement. Clin Orthop 144: 98–102
5. Buechel FF, Rosa RA, Pappas MJ (1989) A metal-backed, rotating-bearing patellar prosthesis to lower contact stress, an 11-year clinical study. Clin Orthop 248: 34–49
6. Cartier P, Sonouiller JL, Grelsamer, R (1990) Patellofemoral arthroplasty. J Arthroplasty 5: 49–55
7. Irrgang JJ, Snyder-Mackler L, Wainner RS, Fu FH, Harner CD (1998) Development of a patient-reported measure of function of the knee. J Bone Joint Surg 80 A: 1132–1145
8. Jordan LR, Olivo JL, Voorhorst PE (2000) Survivorship analysis of a metal-backed rotating anatomic patella in total knee arthroplasty: a 14-year follow-up. Paper No. 183, Am Acad Orth Surg, 67th Annual Meeting, Orlando, FL
9. Krajca-Radcliffe JB, Coker TP (1996) Patellofemoral arthroplasty; a two to eighteen year follow-up study. Clin Orthop 330: 143–151
10. Laskin RS, van Steijn M (1999) Total knee replacement for patients with patellofemoral arthritis. Clin Orthop 367: 89–95
11. Lubinus HH (1979) Patella glide bearing replacement. Orthopedics 2: 119–127
12. Marx RG, Jones EC, Allen AA, Altchek DW, O'Brien SJ, Rodeo SA, Williams RJ, Warren RF, Wickiewicz TL (2001) Reliability, validity, and responsiveness of four knee outcome scales for athletic patients. J Bone Joint Surg 83 A: 1459–1469
13. Mont MA, Haas S, Mullick T, Hungerford DS, Krackow K (2000) Total knee arthroplasty for patellofemoral arthritis. Paper No. 288, Am Acad Orth Surg, 67th Annual Meeting, Orlando, FL
14. Oberlander MA, Baker CL, Morgan BE (1998) Patellofemoral arthrosis: the treatment options. Am J Orthop 27: 263–270
15. Pidoriano AJ, Weinstein RN, Buuck DA, Fulkerson JP (1997) Correlation of patellar articular lesions with results from anteromedial tibial tubercle transfer. Am J Sports Med 25: 533–537
16. Tauro B, Ackroyd CE, Newman JH, Shah NA (2001) The Lubinus patellofemoral arthroplasty, a five- to ten-year prospective study. J Bone Joint Surg 83B: 696–701

Subject Index

- tibia-cut-first flexion space balancing 246, 320
flexion-extension 29
- gap-adjustment 121
- imbalance, extension-flexion 246
fluoroscopy
- dynamic 260
- investigations 231
- video fluoroscopy (in vivo) 59–64, 295, 319
- weight bearing studies (in vivo) 57
Food and Drug Administration, United States
   (FDA) 23–24, 225
forces
- anterior shear force 34
- compressive, loading 32–33
- peak 40
- rotational 33
four-bar linkage 7, 101
fracture 202, 261
future trends with the LCS 309–359

G

gait analysis 57
genu
- valgum
   - supra-condylar varus osteotomy for 84
- varum 84
geomedic / geometric design 42
Gerdy's tubercle 88
Gigli saw 273
graft / grafting, compression-impression bone grafting 227, 283

H

hematoma 163
hemiarthroplasty, unicondylar 311
hinged total knee prostheses
- design 42
- failed hinged prosthesis 281–282
- New Jersey rotating hinge knee 278
- revision of hinge to rotating platform 281–286
- S-ROM Noiles rotating hinge knee system 287
history: "the LCS story" 19–25
hydroxyapatite (see "fixation")

I

International Knee Documentation Committee
   (IKDC) 363
Iliotibial
- band 164
- tract 236

impingement
- anterior 318, 320
- soft tissue impingement, painful replaced
   knee 266–267
- synovial 180
infection 216, 221
- indium111-labeled white cell scan 266
- painful replaced knee 268
Insall, John 25
Insall-method, tibial cut first 136
instability
- flexion instability 129, 175, 236
- ligamentous instability 206, 311
- medial 290
- medial-lateral 244
- painful replaced knee 270
- patellofemoral 260
- posterior cruciate ligament instability 249
instrumentation
- Milestone instrumentation 123
- New Jersey knee instrumentation 122–123

J

joint
- ankle joint 337
- hip joint 380
- knee joint
   - aspiration of the joint 266
   - knee joint simulator 46

K

Kaplan-Meier survivorship 210
kinematics
- of normal knee
   - abduction-adduction 39
   - axial rotation 30, 39
   - flexion-extension 29
   - medial-lateral translation 8, 298
   - polyaxial 14
   - rollback (gliding) 29, 40
- of replaced knee
   - of AP-glide knee prosthesis 313
   - condylar lift-off 37, 64, 303, 317, 319
   - 3D kinematics 59, 62
   - patello-femoral 62
   - rollback (gliding) 57, 97, 101, 108, 306
   - studies
knee (see "joint")

rotating platform 22, 58, 107, 216, 225, 235–240, 273, 281–286, 321
– AP-glide rotating platform 295
– from constraint to rotating platform 281–286
– dislocation / spinout 210, 217, 235–240, 246, 298, 305
– posterior stabilized 64
– wear of rotating platform 67
– S-ROM Noiles rotating hinge knee system 287
rotatory
– axial rotatory laxity 30
– torque 53
Roux's law 304
RSA (see "radiographic assessment")

S
scan
– CT-scan 265–266
– indium111-labeled white cell scan 266
– techneticum diphosphonate bone scan 265
simulators, knee 71
soft tissue
– impingement, painful replaced knee 266
– navigation and soft-tissue balancing 333–342
spacer block 188, 299
stability of the knee 5, 12, 53–55, 304–306
– anterior-posterior 48
– insufficient flexion stability 236
– normal knee 31–32
– patellar-femoral articulations 53–55
stabilizers, extrinsic 34
stem
– intramedullary 37
– modular stem 278, 329–330
sterilization
– gamma in air sterilization 324
– gas plasma sterilization 243, 349
– irradiation 79
stress / stresses
– compressive 4, 44, 303
– contact 17, 35, 42, 51, 53, 74
– tensile 5
– von Mises stress 42
surgical technique
– AP cuts with the CDFF-technique 190
– balancing the ligaments 124
– conservative distal femoral cut first 183–194, 299
– femoral reference points 122
– femoral resection 46, 49, 129–131, 136
– femoral rotation determination 128–129, 171, 175–181
– Insall method of tibial cut first 136

– release
– – iliotibial band release 153
– – medial sleeve release 153–156
– sliding osteotomy of the lateral condyle 153, 159, 236
survivorship 210, 215–216
– analysis 108
– Kaplan-Meier 210
Swedish Knee Arthroplasty Register 202
sympathectomy 269
synovectomy 201
synovial impingement 180
synovitis 244
– hypertrophic 201
– painful 35, 98

T
thrombosis, deep venous 353
tibia
– alignment 209
– axis 175–181
– crest osteotomy 161–166
– high osteotomy 84
– tibial cut first technique 299
– tibial shaft axis method 181
titanium nitrid 349–351

U
UHMWPE (ultra-high molecular weight polyethylene) (see "biomaterials")
unicompartmental knee arthroplasty / replacement
– clinical results of 93–94
– minimally invasive 353
– mobile bearing 83–94
– Oxford unicondylar meniscal bearing device 298
unstable knee 246–252

V
valgus deformity 30, 84, 121, 150, 161, 236
– supra-condylar varus osteotomy for genu valgum 84
varus deformity 141–148, 236
V-Y quadriceps turn down (see "approach")

W
wear
– abrasive 41–42, 75–78
– adhesive 42
– analysis 67–79